Kidney Diseases: A Case-Based Approach

Kidney Diseases:
A Case-Based Approach

Edited by Alice Foster

hayle
medical

New York

Hayle Medical,
750 Third Avenue, 9ᵗʰ Floor,
New York, NY 10017, USA

Visit us on the World Wide Web at:
www.haylemedical.com

ISBN: 978-1-63241-930-9

Cataloging-in-Publication Data

Kidney diseases : a case-based approach / edited by Alice Foster.
   p. cm.
Includes bibliographical references and index.
ISBN 978-1-63241-930-9
1. Kidneys--Diseases. 2. Kidneys--Diseases--Case studies.
3. Nephrology. I. Foster, Alice.
RC902 .K53 2020

616.61--dc23

Table of Contents

Preface

Kidney disease or renal disease refers to a disease of the kidney characterized by a loss of kidney function to varying degrees. It can lead to kidney failure or the complete loss of kidney function, if unresolved. Nephritis, nephrosis, chronic kidney disease and acute kidney disease are common kidney diseases. They may be caused by a deposition of immunoglobulin A antibodies in the glomerulus, xanthine oxidase deficiency, long-term exposure to lead or its salts, and administration of analgesics. A review of medical history, urine test, physical examination and renal ultrasound are required to establish a diagnosis of a kidney disease. Mostly, the management of kidney disease requires dialysis or a kidney transplant. This usually happens when the disease is at its end stage. The objective of this book is to give a general view of the different kinds of kidney diseases, and their diagnosis and treatment. The various studies that are constantly contributing towards advancing technologies and evolution of nephrology are examined in detail. In this book, using case studies and examples, constant effort has been made to make the understanding of the difficult concepts as easy and informative as possible, for the readers.

All of the data presented henceforth, was collaborated in the wake of recent advancements in the field. The aim of this book is to present the diversified developments from across the globe in a comprehensible manner. The opinions expressed in each chapter belong solely to the contributing authors. Their interpretations of the topics are the integral part of this book, which I have carefully compiled for a better understanding of the readers.

At the end, I would like to thank all those who dedicated their time and efforts for the successful completion of this book. I also wish to convey my gratitude towards my friends and family who supported me at every step.

Editor

Genetic Variation at Selected SNPs in the Leptin Gene and Association of Alleles with Markers of Kidney Disease in a Xhosa Population of South Africa

Ikechi G. Okpechi[1]*, Brian L. Rayner[1], Lize van der Merwe[2], Bongani M. Mayosi[1], Adebowale Adeyemo[3], Nicki Tiffin[4], Rajkumar Ramesar[4]

1 Department of Medicine, Groote Schuur Hospital and University of Cape Town, Cape Town, South Africa, 2 Department of Statistics, University of the Western Cape, Cape Town, South Africa, 3 Centre for Research on Genomics and Global Health, National Human Genome Research Institute, Bethesda, Maryland, United States of America, 4 Division of Human Genetics, Institute for Infectious Diseases and Molecular Medicine, University of Cape Town, Cape Town, South Africa

Abstract

Background: Chronic kidney disease (CKD) is a significant public health problem that leads to end-stage renal disease (ESRD) with as many as 2 million people predicted to need therapy worldwide by 2010. Obesity is a risk factor for CKD and leptin, the obesity hormone, correlates with body fat mass and markers of renal function. A number of clinical and experimental studies have suggested a link between serum leptin and kidney disease. We hypothesised that variants in the *leptin* gene (*LEP*) may be associated with markers of CKD in indigenous black Africans.

Methodology/Principal Findings: Black South Africans of Xhosa (distinct cultural Bantu-speaking population) descent were recruited for the study and four common polymorphisms of the *LEP* (rs7799039, rs791620, rs2167270 and STS-U43653 [ENSSNP5824596]) were analysed for genotype and haplotype association with urine albumin-to-creatinine ratio (UACR), estimated glomerular filtration rate (eGFR), Serum creatinine (Scr) and serum leptin level. In one of the four single nucleotide polymorphisms (SNPs) we examined, an association with the renal phenotypes was observed. Hypertensive subjects with the T allele (CT genotype) of the ENSSNP5824596 SNP had a significantly higher eGFR (p = 0.0141), and significantly lower Scr (p = 0.0137). This was confirmed by haplotype analysis. Also, the haplotype GAAC had a modest effect on urine albumin-to-creatinine ratio in normotensive subjects (p = 0.0482).

Conclusions/Significance: These results suggest that genetic variations of the *LEP* may be associated with phenotypes that are markers of CKD in black Africans.

Editor: Zoltán Bochdanovits, VU University Medical Center and Center for Neurogenomics and Cognitive Research, VU University, Netherlands

Funding: This study was supported by the Wyeth Nephrology Funds administered by the University of Cape Town. The funders had no role in study design, data collection and analysis, decision to publish, or preparation of the manuscript.

Competing Interests: The authors have declared that no competing interests exist.

* E-mail: ikokpechi@yahoo.com

Introduction

Chronic kidney disease (CKD) is a significant public health problem. CKD is irreversible and ultimately progresses to end-stage renal disease (ESRD), projected to affect 2 million people worldwide by 2010 worldwide [1,2]. Microalbuminuria, a reversible and early measure of kidney disease marks the initiation of kidney disease and is a significant predictor of cardiovascular events and all-cause mortality in patients with diabetes, hypertension, and in the general population [3,4]. Other measures of renal dysfunctions such as an increase in serum creatinine (Scr) and a reduced estimated glomerular filtration rate (eGFR) have also been shown to predict cardiovascular disease [5]. Estimates of the NHANES III dataset have shown that approximately 3 and 11% of the US population have abnormal Scr levels or microalbuminuria, respectively [6,7].

Recently, obesity has been identified as a major driver for progressive kidney injury [8,9]. A relative risk of 2.3 was reported of incident ESRD or kidney disease-related death in morbidly obese

individuals who participated in the NHANES III survey [8]. Leptin is the obesity hormone synthesized mainly by white adipose tissue in humans [10] and its serum level shows strong correlation with body fat mass [11]. Mutations in the *leptin* gene (*LEP*) have been reported to cause severe obesity [10,12] and may also contribute to the complications associated with obesity. The potential role of serum leptin in the pathogenesis of CKD has become increasingly recognised and a number of studies have demonstrated correlations between serum leptin and markers of renal function [13,14]. Leptin stimulates the proliferation of cultured glomerular endothelial cells and induces mRNA expression and protein secretion of transforming growth factor-β1 (TGF-β1). Long-term infusion with leptin (3 weeks) has led to increased glomerular expression of type IV collagen [15]. Leptin has also been shown to stimulate synthesis of type I collagen in mesangial cells and type IV collagen in glomerular endothelial cells which contributes to extracellular matrix deposition, glomerulosclerosis, and proteinuria [16]. It is therefore possible that genetic variation/s in the *LEP*, possibly related to variation in

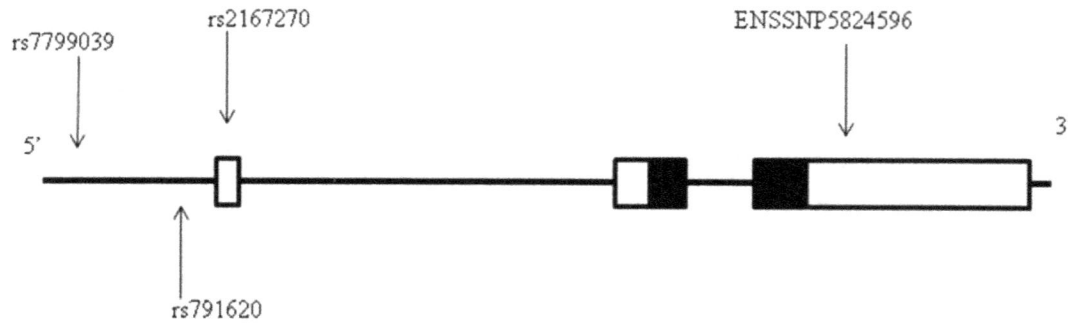

Figure 1. Position of four polymorphisms typed across the leptin (LEP) gene on chromosome 7. Dark shading indicates coding sequence.

serum leptin concentration may be associated with markers of kidney disease such as urine albumin-to-creatinine ratio (UACR), Scr and eGFR. We therefore hypothesized that polymorphisms of the *LEP* may have significant effects on markers of renal function in black Africans.

Methods

The population sampling of this study, which is part of a larger study to determine the effects of obesity through the metabolic syndrome on kidney disease in an indigenous African population, was of a cross-sectional design and was carried out in Cape Town between May 2005 and July 2006. The study was approved by the joint Research Ethics Committee (REC) of the University of Cape Town and Groote Schuur Hospital. Written informed consent (approved by our REC) was obtained from each subject before they could enter the study. The method of recruitment has been previously described [14]. Briefly, two hundred and fifty three (253) ambulatory hypertensive subjects attending the Guguletu hypertension clinic and eighty-three (83) normotensive relatives in the community were recruited for the study. Although 336 subjects were recruited for the entire study, the sample sizes for the different single nucleotide polymorphisms (SNPs) that were examined differed and were fewer than that of the entire study population due to variation in the availability of high quality DNA, and incomplete successfully genotyping. We chose to study these non-coding polymorphisms because they capture the common haplotype variation across the *LEP* (figure 1) and also because they have been the commonly studied of the *LEP* SNPs in other populations, therefore providing a basis for comparison with our population.

The subjects were all of the same indigenous southern African tribal/cultural population group, namely of Xhosa origin, to ensure a homogenous population and to avoid confounding by population admixture which may lead to spurious results in gene

association studies of unrelated individuals [17]. A questionnaire was administered to all participants to obtain relevant demographic information. Height, weight, waist and hip circumference were obtained. Body mass index was calculated from weight (kg) divided by height squared (m²). Blood pressure was measured in all the subjects using the same validated mercury sphygmomanometer. The average of 2 blood pressure measurements taken at least 2 minutes apart in the sitting position after about 5–10 minutes rest was recorded. Blood was drawn in the fasting state for routine chemistry including creatinine, lipids, glucose and for assay of leptin. Spot urine was also taken to measure the urine albumin-to-creatinine ratio (UACR). For all the tests, conventional assays were used in the chemical pathology laboratory on auto-analysers with appropriate quality control. The eGFR was calculated using the Modification of Diet in Renal Disease (MDRD) equation [18]:

$$eGFR = 186 \text{ x } (S_{Cr})^{-1.154} \text{ x } (age)^{-0.203} \text{ x } (0.742 \text{ if } female)$$
$$\text{x } (1.210 \text{ if } black).$$

Serum leptin was measured using a commercially available human leptin radioimmunoassay kit (Linco Research, St. Charles, MO) with sensitivity 0.5 ng/ml, intra-assay precision 3.4–8.3%, and inter-assay precision 3.6–6.2%. All genetic analysis was carried out in the Division of Human Genetics at the University of Cape Town. Genomic DNA was isolated from peripheral blood lymphocytes using the Puregene DNA Isolation Kit (Gentra Systems, USA) according to the manufacturer's protocol. Polymerase Chain Reaction (PCR) was carried out individually for the four SNPs being tested. This was followed by restriction enzyme (RE) digest of the PCR products (table S1, S2, S3, S4). The primers (forward and reverse) used for the SNPs as well as the restriction enzymes used in the digest are shown in Table 1.

Table 1. Primers and the restriction enzymes used for genotyping.

SNP	Forward Primer	Reverse Primer	Restriction Enzyme
rs7799039	5′ TTTCCTGTAATTTTCCCGTGAG 3′	5′ AAAGCAAAGACAGGCATAAAAA 3′	HhaI
rs791620	5′ CAACGAGGGCGCAGCCGTAT 3′	5′ AGTGTGCACCTCGCGGGGCCT 3′	AscI
rs2167270	5′ GCCCCGCGAGGTGCACACTG 3′	5′ GGGCCCTGTGGCCTGCCAAG 3′	MspA1I
ENSSNP5824596	5′ CGACCTGGAGAACCTCCG 3′	5′ GTCCTGGATAAGGGGTGT 3′	HpyCH4IV

Phenotypes of interest had skewed distributions and were quantile normalised for analysis, consequently, only age and gender were adjusted for in the analysis. Untransformed values are summarised, for ease of interpretation. We had to use mixed-effects models for comparing the hypertensive to the normotensive groups, to enable us adjust for the relatedness between the normotensives and the hypertensives.

All genetic association analyses were stratified between hypertensive and normotensives, and adjusted for age and gender. We used linear models on quantile normalised traits. Genotypes were coded as categories (genotype; 2 degrees of freedom) and also as number of minor alleles (allelic; 1 degree of freedom). In cases where no minor allele homozygotes were observed, these analyses were equivalent. Haplotypes were imputed and analysed using an EM algorithm and generalised linear models [19]. We tested haplotype association with hypertension status, as well as for quantile normalised phenotypes stratified by hypertension diagnosis. We tested all possible haplotypes, from two to all four, from adjacent positions. R and R packages were used for statistical modelling; nlme for mixed-effects and haplo.stats for haplotype analyses [19] (R is a free software environment for statistical computing and graphics available from http://www.r-project.org).

Results

The baseline features (demographic, clinical and biochemical) of all the participating subjects are summarised in table 2, stratified by diagnostic group. The median values of kidney disease phenotypes (Scr, eGFR and UACR) were not significantly different between the hypertensive and normotensive individuals. The genotype frequencies of the different polymorphisms are summarised in table 3 and agree closely with the genotype frequencies described at this polymorphism in Yoruba Africans in the Hapmap project [20]. All the typed SNPs were in Hardy-Weinberg equilibrium in the normotensive group (p<0.01), however, the SNP rs2167270 was not in Hardy-Weinberg equilibrium in the hypertensive subjects. No significant association was detected between hypertension status, obesity, the metabolic syndrome, hyperleptinaemia or gender and any of the 4 polymorphisms studied. In the hypertensive group, two phenotypes (Scr and eGFR), were associated with ENNSNP5824596, with the T allele significantly increasing eGFR (p = 0.0137) and decreasing Scr (p = 0.0186) (Table 4).

The haplotypes GCGC and GCAC occurred more frequently than other haplotypes in the hypertensive and normotensive groups, respectively (Table 5). In the hypertensive group, haplotype GCAT yielded significantly higher values of eGFR than GCGC (p = 0.0278). The 3-way haplotype, excluding the first SNP, showed a similar pattern with CAT being associated with significantly higher values of eGFR than both CGC (p = 0.0255). In the last two polymorphisms, AT was also associated with significantly higher eGFR than GC (p = 0.0233) (Table 6).

In the hypertensive group, haplotype GCAT yielded significantly lower values of Scr than GCGC (p = 0.0352). The 3-way haplotype, excluding the first SNP, showed a similar pattern with CAT being associated with significantly lower values of Scr than CGC (p = 0.0318) and in the last two polymorphisms, AT was associated with significantly lower Scr than GC (p = 0.0293) (Table 6).

In the normotensive group, the only significant association was between UACR and the 4-way haplotype. Urine albumin-to-creatinine ratio was significantly higher in GAAC than in GCAC (p = 0.0482) (Table 7). Linkage disequilibrium (LD) plot of the 4 *LEP* SNPs and a comparison with LD of the same region in HapMap YRI population which contains additional markers across the same span, revealed low pairwise r^2 values indicating that LD across the region is weak (figure S1).

Discussion

We show from the results of this study that genetic variation in the *LEP* could have significant effects on renal disease phenotypes (markers of renal disease) in indigenous Africans. On the one hand, a marginal but significant effect was observed on microalbuminuria in normotensive subjects, while on the other hand a moderately significant and what is thought to be a "protective" effect was noticed with Scr and eGFR in hypertensive subjects. The reasons why this gene showed effects only on UACR

Table 2. Characteristics (median and interquartile range) of the study groups.

	Hypertensive				Normotensive				
	n	Median	LQ	UQ	n	Median	LQ	UQ	p-value
Age (yrs)	253	57.0	49.0	63.0	83	32.0	24.0	42.0	<0.0001
BMI (Kg/m²)	252	33.7	28.2	39.9	82	28.2	22.1	33.3	0.0002
SBP (mmHg)	252	151.5	137.0	165.3	83	122.0	114.0	138.0	<0.0001
DBP (mmHg)	252	94.0	87.0	102.0	83	82.0	76.0	89.0	<0.0001
FBG (mmol/L)	249	5.2	4.8	5.5	82	4.7	4.3	5.1	0.0008
TG (mmol/L)	252	1.2	0.8	1.7	83	0.8	0.6	1.1	0.0292
HDL-c (mmol/L)	252	1.4	1.1	1.6	83	1.5	1.3	1.9	0.0027
Leptin (ng/ml)	247	26.9	11.0	45.5	83	20.0	8.6	35.8	0.0986
Scr (µmol/L)	252	75.0	64.8	89.3	83	66.0	58.5	78.0	0.3067
eGFR(ml/min/1.73 m²)	252	99.0	85.8	114.0	78	125.0	109.3	143.8	0.1030
UACR (mg/mmol)	252	0.8	0.3	2.6	83	0.6	0.2	1.4	0.0606

P-values are for test of difference in quantile normalised characteristic between diagnostic groups, adjusted for age and gender and relatedness.
n = Number; Interquartile range is lower quartile (LQ) and upper quartile (UQ). BMI = body mass index; SBP = systolic blood pressure; DBP = diastolic blood pressure; FBG = fasting blood glucose; TG = triglyceride; HDL-c = high density lipoprotein cholesterol Scr = serum creatinine; eGFR = estimated glomerular filtration rate; UACR = urinary albumin-to-creatinine ratio.

Table 3. Genotype counts, allele counts and frequency distributions.

	Hypertensives		Normotensives		p-value
	n	f	n	f	
rs7799039					
Typed	191		59		
G	358	0.94	113	0.96	
A	24	0.06	5	0.04	0.1110
G/G	167	0.87	54	0.92	
G/A	24	0.13	5	0.08	0.1110
rs791620					
Typed	222		71		
C	404	0.91	132	0.93	
A	40	0.09	10	0.07	0.5873
C/C	187	0.84	61	0.86	
C/A	30	0.14	10	0.14	
A/A	5	0.02	0	0	NC
rs2167270					
Typed	219		74		
A	238	0.54	84	0.57	
G	200	0.46	64	0.43	0.8724
A/A	59	0.27	19	0.26	
A/G	120	0.55	46	0.62	
G/G	40	0.18	9	0.12	0.6912
ENSSNP5824596					
Typed	224		77		
C	417	0.93	144	0.94	
T	31	0.07	10	0.06	0.9286
C/C	193	0.86	68	0.88	
C/T	31	0.14	8	0.1	
T/T	0	0	1	0.01	NC

P-values are for test of difference in additive allelic and genotype distributions between diagnostic groups, adjusted for age and gender and relatedness. n = count; f = frequency. NC = could not be calculated, because no minor allele homozygotes observed.

in normotensives and then effects on Scr and eGFR alone in hypertensives are presently unclear. However, other factors associated with the hypertensive state may play a role. Although we consider that the effects of these polymorphisms on the phenotypes may be related to the renal actions of serum leptin, we have not shown that serum leptin has direct effects on the kidneys and can therefore not exclude autocrine and/or paracrine mediated actions of leptin in the kidney. The mechanism of action of serum leptin on the kidney has been previously described [15].

A number of studies have previously assessed the effects of the *LEP* on phenotypes of cardiovascular disease (including obesity) and cancer [21,22,23,24,25]. However, the results from many such studies have been largely inconsistent and difficult to replicate in other populations. For instance, Shintani et al [23] reported a positive association between a polymorphic tetranucleotide repeat (TTTC)$_n$ polymorphism in the 3′ flanking region of the *LEP* and hypertension in a group of Japanese patients with essential hypertension. They found the frequency of the class I allele to be significantly higher in hypertensives compared with normotensive controls. In two other studies in South Americans and Italians

in which the same polymorphism was examined, there was no association between the class I/II genotypes or alleles with hypertension or cardiovascular disease [24,25].

The result of our study may be confirmatory of previous studies that have reported association between the common polymorphisms of the *LEP* and the various phenotypes they have assayed. One such confirmation relates to the "protective" effect of the T allele of the ENSSNP5824596 polymorphism from renal disease. To our knowledge, only one study [26] has reported on this "protective" effect from atherosclerosis in Caucasians. Gaukrodger et al demonstrated a significantly lower carotid intima medial thickness and pulse pressure in subjects with the T allele, compared to subjects without this allele (p = 0.0076 and p = 0.0001 respectively) [26]. Our study may have shown that this so-called "protective" association may exist in a different population using different phenotypes (Tables 4, 6 and 7).

This study was carried out on the assumption that common polymorphisms of the *LEP* may be associated with kidney disease given that serum leptin has been clinically and pathogenetically linked with markers of kidney disease [15,16,27]. As we know it, ESRD is common and more severe in people of African origin,

Table 4. Effect sizes (β) and p-values for genotype and allelic association with quantile normalised traits, adjusted for age and gender.

Hypertensives

	rs7799039 Genotype G/A β	rs7799039 Genotype G/A p-value	rs7799039 Allelic A β	rs7799039 Allelic A p-value	rs791620 Genotype C/A β	rs791620 Genotype A/A β	rs791620 Genotype p-value	rs791620 Allelic A β	rs791620 Allelic A p-value	rs2167270 Genotype A/G β	rs2167270 Genotype G/G β	rs2167270 Genotype p-value	rs2167270 Allelic G β	rs2167270 Allelic G p-value	ENSSNP5824596 Genotype C/T β	ENSSNP5824596 Genotype C/T p-value	ENSSNP5824596 Allelic T β	ENSSNP5824596 Allelic T p-value
Leptin (ng/ml)	-	-	-0.02	0.9159	0.02	-0.16	0.8694	-0.02	0.8500	-0.12	-0.16	0.4814	-0.08	0.2492	-	-	-0.04	0.7923
Scr (µmol/L)	-	-	0.11	0.5206	-0.09	0.24	0.6943	0.00	0.9941	0.10	0.04	0.7038	0.03	0.7182	-	-	-0.37	**0.0186**
GFR(ml/min/1.73 m²)	-	-	-0.14	0.4428	0.02	-0.33	0.6804	-0.06	0.6529	-0.09	-0.04	0.7674	-0.03	0.7275	-	-	0.41	**0.0137**
uACR (mg/mmol)	-	-	-0.01	0.9680	-0.09	-0.70	0.2481	-0.20	0.1682	0.25	0.14	0.2228	0.09	0.3428	-	-	-0.04	0.8240

Normotensives

	rs7799039 Genotype G/A β	rs7799039 Genotype G/A p-value	rs7799039 Allelic A β	rs7799039 Allelic A p-value	rs791620 Genotype C/A β	rs791620 Genotype A/A β	rs791620 Genotype p-value	rs791620 Allelic A β	rs791620 Allelic A p-value	rs2167270 Genotype A/G β	rs2167270 Genotype G/G β	rs2167270 Genotype p-value	rs2167270 Allelic G β	rs2167270 Allelic G p-value	ENSSNP5824596 Genotype C/T β	ENSSNP5824596 Genotype C/T p-value	ENSSNP5824596 Allelic T β	ENSSNP5824596 Allelic T p-value
Leptin (ng/ml)	-	-	-0.28	0.4670	-	-	-	-0.20	0.4603	-0.05	0.21	0.6711	0.07	0.6243	-	-	-0.27	0.2578
Scr (µmol/L)	-	-	-0.11	0.7760	-	-	-	-0.15	0.5833	-0.23	0.16	0.3230	0.02	0.8960	-	-	-0.26	0.2943
GFR(ml/min/1.73 m²)	-	-	0.25	0.5658	-	-	-	0.09	0.7813	0.37	0.02	0.2913	0.10	0.5857	-	-	0.36	0.2252
uACR (mg/mmol)	-	-	-0.10	0.8339	-	-	-	0.56	0.0970	-0.29	0.21	0.2957	0.03	0.8849	-	-	0.08	0.7863

Empty column means genotype result is exactly the same as for allele, because no minor allele homozygotes were observed.

Scr = Serum creatinine, eGFR = Estimated Glomerular filtration rate, UACR = Urine Albumin-to-creatinine ratio.

β (genotype) = effect size (regression coefficient), estimated difference in transformed (quantile normalised) phenotype between individuals with a given genotype and individuals with the major allele homozygote genotype.

β (allelic) = effect size (regression coefficient), estimated difference in transformed (quantile normalised) phenotype for each additional allele.

Table 5. Inferred haplotype frequencies in the study population.

Haplotype *	Frequency	
	Hypertensive	Normotensive
GCAC	0.37	**0.46**
GCGC	**0.42**	0.36
GAAC	0.08	0.07
ACGC	0.04	0.05
GCAT	0.06	0.03
ACAC	0.03	0.00

*- Haplotypes are in their order on chromosome 7 (see Figure 1). Frequencies in bold characters denote the base (common) haplotypes.

although the exact reasons for this remain elusive. Differences in socio-economic status, higher prevalence of hypertension and an increased inherited susceptibility of indigenous Africans to kidney disease are all possible explanations [28,29]. Additionally, as the prevalence of obesity continue to increase, its contribution to kidney disease globally and especially amongst the indigenous Africans cannot be ignored [30]. The overall median BMI of our study population was 32.5 kg/m^2 (33.7 kg/m^2 in the hypertensives and 28.2 kg/m^2 in the normotensive group) (table 2).

This study is important in two ways: firstly, its focus on the relationship between the *LEP* and renal disease phenotypes. However, the value of this is diminished as the only significant effect we observed after multiple testing was the association of the T allele at ENNSNP5824596 among the hypertensives. This may have been due to the smaller sample size in the normotensive group

Table 6. Results of test of association of haplotypes with markers of renal disease, adjusted for age and gender, in the hypertensive subjects.

rs7799039	rs791620	rs2167270	ENNSNP5824596	Scr		eGFR		UACR	
				β	p	β	p	β	p
A	C	A	C	0.29	0.3750	−0.41	0.1760	−0.03	0.9210
A	C	G	C	−0.12	0.7160	0.21	0.5210	−0.16	0.6490
G	A	A	C	0.00	0.9870	−0.06	0.7420	−0.29	0.1480
G	C	A	C	−0.04	0.7230	0.07	0.5340	−0.08	0.4970
G	C	A	T	−0.38	**0.0352**	0.42	**0.0278**	−0.12	0.5960
-	C	A	T	−0.38	**0.0318** †	0.42	**0.0255** †		
-	-	A	T	−0.36	**0.0293** ‡	0.39	**0.0233**‡		
G	C	G	C	**Base haplotype**					

Tests are adjusted for age and sex.
β = estimated difference in transformed phenotype between individuals with a given haplotype and individuals with the base haplotype.
Scr = serum creatinine, eGFR = Estimated Glomerular filtration rate, UACR = Urine Albumin-to-creatinine ratio.
†- 3 –way haplotype analysis between CAT and CGC.
‡- 2 – way haplotype analysis between AT and GC.

Table 7. Results of tests of association of haplotypes with markers of renal disease, adjusted for age and gender, in the normotensive subjects.

rs7799039	rs791620	rs2167270	ENNSNP5824596	Scr		eGFR		UACR	
				β	p	β	p	β	p
A	C	G	C	−0.11	0.7650	0.29	0.4920	0.18	0.6835
G	A	A	C	−0.21	0.4650	0.22	0.4930	0.71	**0.0482**
G	C	A	T	−0.28	0.4790	0.45	0.4820	1.35	0.0743
G	C	G	C	−0.01	0.9480	0.12	0.5380	0.19	0.3194
G	C	G	T	−0.34	0.4540	0.47	0.3000	−0.18	0.6845
G	C	A	C	**Base haplotype**					

β = estimated difference in transformed phenotype between individuals with a given haplotype and individuals with the base haplotype.
Scr = Serum creatinine, eGFR = Estimated Glomerular filtration rate, UACR = Urine Albumin-to-creatinine ratio.

or due to a possible conditional effect in these subjects with hypertension and increased BMI. Secondly, it may be important from the perspective of being carried out in an indigenous African population with no prior similar studies and in whom similar studies are generally under-represented. It therefore provides a prospect to evaluate the relationship between genetic polymorphisms and a specific complex disease (kidney disease) that is common amongst indigenous Africans. The study is however limited by its modest sample size with few SNPs studied and of being a cross-sectional type. A further and probably a more important limitation to it is our inability to show that these polymorphisms have any effect on tissue leptin, especially since we postulated that kidney disease in this population is associated with polymorphisms of the *LEP* through the renal effects of leptin. To demonstrate that these polymorphisms affect tissue (renal) leptin will require the design of further experimental studies. Finally, although modifiable risk factors for kidney disease are well known, a better understanding of obesity-related kidney disease will be necessary to control the progression of chronic renal disease to ESRD in black Africans.

Supporting Information

Table S1   PCR assay of rs7799039

Table S2   PCR assay of rs791620

Table S3   PCR assay of rs2167270

Table S4   PCR assay of ENSSNP5824596

Figure S1   Linkage Disequilibrium (LD) plot visualized as a GOLD heat map

Genetic Variation at Selected SNPs in the Leptin Gene and Association of Alleles with Markers of Kidney...

7

Acknowledgments

We wish to thank Ms Donette Baines, Ms Nicola Baines and Mr. Deane Burton who assisted with collection of the data in Guguletu, Cape Town. We also wish to thank Ms Gabi Solomons, Ms Zeino Latief and Ms Alvera Vorster of the Human Molecular Genetics laboratory of the University of Cape Town who managed and assisted with the analysis of the DNA samples. Finally we wish to thank Drs. Judy King and Helen Vreede of the National Health Laboratory Services (NHLS) at the Groote Schuur Hospital who provided support with chemical and hormone assays.

Author Contributions

Conceived and designed the experiments: IGO BLR BM RR. Performed the experiments: IGO NT. Analyzed the data: IGO BLR LvdM BM AA NT RR. Contributed reagents/materials/analysis tools: IGO BLR LvdM BM AA NT RR. Wrote the paper: IGO BLR LvdM BM AA NT RR.

References

1. Lysaght MJ (2002) Maintenance dialysis population dynamics: Current trends and long-term implications. J Am Soc Nephrol 13: 37–40.
2. Xue J, Ma JZ, Louis TA, Collins AJ (2001) Forecast of the number of patients with end-stage renal disease in United States to the year 2010. J Am Soc Nephrol 12: 2753–2758.
3. Wachtell K, Ibsen H, Olsen MH, Borch-Johnsen K, Lindholm LH, et al. (2003) Albuminuria and cardiovascular risk in hypertensive patients with left ventricular hypertrophy: the LIFE study. Ann Intern Med 139: 901–906.
4. Hillege HL, Fidler V, Diercks GF, van Gilst WH, de Zeeuw D, et al. (2002) Prevention of Renal and Vascular End Stage Disease (PREVEND) Study Group. Urinary albumin excretion predicts cardiovascular and noncardiovascular mortality in general population. Circulation 106: 1777–1782.
5. Santopinto JJ, Fox KA, Goldberg RJ, Budaj A, Piñero G, et al. (2003) on behalf of the GRACE Investigators. Creatinine clearance and adverse hospital outcomes in patients with acute coronary syndromes: findings from the global registry of acute coronary events (GRACE). Heart 89: 1003–1008.
6. Coresh J, Wei GL, McQuillan G, Brancati FL, Levey AS, et al. (2001) Prevalence of high blood pressure and elevated serum creatinine level in the United States: findings from the third National Health and Nutrition Examination Survey (1988–1994). Arch Intern Med 161: 1207–1216.
7. Jones CA, Francis ME, Eberhardt MS, Chavers B, Coresh J, et al. (2002) Microalbuminuria in the US population: third National Health and Nutrition Examination Survey. Am J Kidney Dis 39: 445–459.
8. Stengel B, Tarver-Carr ME, Powe NR, Eberhardt MS, Brancati FL (2003) Lifestyle factors, obesity and the risk of chronic kidney disease. Epidemiology 14: 479–487.
9. Fox CS, Larson MG, Leip EP, Culleton B, Wilson PW, Levy D (2004) Predictors of new-onset kidney disease in a community-based population. JAMA 291: 844–850.
10. Zhang Y, Proenca R, Maffei M, Barone M, Leopold L, Friedman JM (1994) Positional cloning of the mouse obese gene and its human homologue. Nature 372: 425–432.
11. Considine RV, Sinha MK, Heiman ML, Kriauciunas A, Stephens TW, et al. (1996) Serum immunoreactive-leptin concentrations in normal-weight and obese humans. N Engl J Med 334: 292–295.
12. Strobel A, Issad T, Camoin L, Ozata M, Strosberg AD (1998) A leptin missense mutation associated with hypogonadism and morbid obesity. Nat Genet 18: 213–215.
13. Rudberg S, Persson B (1998) Serum leptin levels in young females with insulin-dependent diabetes and the relationship to hyperandrogenicity and microalbuminuria. Horm Res 50: 297–302.
14. Okpechi IG, Pascoe MD, Swanepoel CR, Rayner BL (2007) Microalbuminuria and the metabolic syndrome in non-diabetic black Africans. Diab Vasc Dis Res 4: 365–367.
15. Wolf G, Hamann A, Han DC, Helmchen U, Thaiss F, et al. (1999) Leptin stimulates proliferation and TGF-beta expression in renal glomerular endothelial cells: potential role in glomerulosclerosis. Kidney Int 56: 860–872.
16. Ballerman BJ (1999) A role for leptin in glomerulosclerosis? Kidney Int 56: 1154–1155.
17. Lander ES, Schork NJ (1994) Genetic dissection of complex traits. Science 256: 2037–2048.
18. Levey A, Greene T, Kusek J, Beck G: MDRD Study Group (2001) A simplified equation to predict glomerular filtration rate from serum creatinine [Abstract]. J Am Soc Nephrol 11: 155.
19. Sinnwell JP, Schaid DJ (2008) Haplo Stats (version 1.4.0): Statistical Methods for Haplotypes When Linkage Phase is Ambiguous. Mayo website (2010) http://mayoresearch.mayo.edu/mayo/research/schaid_lab/upload/manualHaploStats.pdf.
20. The International HapMap Project. HapMap website (2010) http://www.hapmap.org.
21. Lucantoni R, Ponti E, Berselli ME, Savia G, Minocci A, et al. (2000) The A19G polymorphism in the 5′ untranslated region of the human obese gene does not affect leptin levels in severely obese patients. J Clin Endocrinol Metab 85: 3589–3591.
22. Skibola CF, Holly EA, Forrest MS, Hubbard A, Bracci PM, et al. (2004) Body Mass Index, Leptin and Leptin Receptor Polymorphisms, and Non-Hodgkin Lymphoma. Cancer Epidemiol Biomarkers Prev 13: 779–786.
23. Shintani M, Ikegami H, Fujisawa T, Kawaguchi Y, Ohishi M, et al. (2002) Leptin gene polymorphism is associated with hypertension independent of obesity. J Clin Endocrinol Metab 87: 2909–2912.
24. Hinuy HM, Hirata MH, Sampaio MF, Armaganijian D, et al. (2006) LEP 3′ HVR is associated with obesity and leptin levels in Brazilian individuals. Molecular Genetics and Metabolism 89: 374–380.
25. Porreca E, Di Febbo C, Pintor S, Baccante G, Gatta V, et al. (2006) Microsatellite polymorphism of the human leptin gene (LEP) and risk of cardiovascular disease. Int J Obes (Lond) 30: 209–213.
26. Gaukrodger N, Mayosi BM, Imrie H, Avery P, Baker M, et al. (2005) A rare variant of the leptin gene has large effects on blood pressure and carotid intima-medial thickness: a study of 1428 individuals in 248 families. J Med Genet 42: 474–478.
27. Briley LP, Szczech LA (2006) Leptin and Renal Disease. Seminars in Dialysis 19: 54–59.
28. Seedat YK (1999) Improvement in treatment of hypertension has not reduced incidence of end-stage renal disease. J Hum Hypertens 13: 747–751.
29. Krop JS, Coresh J, Chambless LE, Shahar E, Watson RL, et al. (1999) A community-based study of explanatory factors for the excess risk for early renal function decline in Blacks vs Whites with diabetes: The Atherosclerosis Risk in Communities Study. Arch Intern Med 159: 1777–1783.
30. Tarver-Carr ME, Powe NR, Eberhardt MS, Laveist TA, Kington RS, et al. (2002) Excess Risk of Chronic Kidney Disease among African-American versus White Subjects in the United States: A Population-Based Study of Potential Explanatory Factors. J Am Soc Nephrol 13: 2363–2370.

2

Regression of Albuminuria and Hypertension and Arrest of Severe Renal Injury by a Losartan-Hydrochlorothiazide Association in a Model of Very Advanced Nephropathy

Simone Costa Alarcon Arias[1], Carla Perez Valente[1], Flavia Gomes Machado[1], Camilla Fanelli[1], Clarice Silvia Taemi Origassa[3], Thales de Brito[2], Niels Olsen Saraiva Camara[3], Denise Maria Avancini Costa Malheiros[1], Roberto Zatz[1]*, Clarice Kazue Fujihara[1]

1 Laboratory of Renal Pathophysiology (LIM-16), Renal Division, Department of Clinical Medicine, Faculty of Medicine, University of São Paulo, São Paulo, Brazil, 2 Department of Pathology, Faculty of Medicine, University of São Paulo, São Paulo, Brazil, 3 Laboratory of Immunology, Nephrology Division, Faculty of Medicine, Federal University of São Paulo, São Paulo, Brazil

Abstract

Treatments that effectively prevent chronic kidney disease (CKD) when initiated early often yield disappointing results when started at more advanced phases. We examined the long-term evolution of renal injury in the 5/6 nephrectomy model (Nx) and the effect of an association between an AT-1 receptor blocker, losartan (L), and hydrochlorothiazide (H), shown previously to be effective when started one month after Nx. Adult male Munich-Wistar rats underwent **Nx**, being divided into four groups: **Nx+V**, no treatment; **Nx+L**, receiving L monotherapy; **Nx+LH**, receiving the L+H association (LH), and **Nx+AHHz**, treated with the calcium channel blocker, amlodipine, the vascular relaxant, hydralazine, and H. This latter group served to assess the effect of lowering blood pressure (BP). Rats undergoing sham nephrectomy (**S**) were also studied. In a first protocol, treatments were initiated 60 days after Nx, when CKD is at a relatively early stage. In a second protocol, treatments were started 120 days after Nx, when glomerulosclerosis and interstitial fibrosis are already advanced. In both protocols, L treatment promoted only partial renoprotection, whereas LH brought BP, albuminuria, tubulointerstitial cell proliferation and plasma aldosterone below pretreatment levels, and completely detained progression of renal injury. Despite normalizing BP, the AHHz association failed to prevent renal damage, indicating that the renoprotective effect of LH was not due to a systemic hemodynamic action. These findings are inconsistent with the contention that thiazides are innocuous in advanced CKD. In Nx, LH promotes effective renoprotection even at advanced stages by mechanisms that may involve anti-inflammatory and intrarenal hemodynamic effects, but seem not to require BP normalization.

Editor: Leighton R. James, University of Florida, United States of America

Funding: This study was supported by grant 2008/55047-3 from the State of São Paulo Foundation for Research Support (FAPESP). RZ is the recipient of a Research Award (No. 304657/2007-7) from the Brazilian Council of Scientific and Technologic Development (CNPq). The funders had no role in study design, data collection and analysis, decision to publish, or preparation of the manuscript.

Competing Interests: The authors have declared that no competing interests exist.

* E-mail: r.zatz@uol.com.br

Introduction

Although several experimental treatments intended to detain the progression of CKD have been proposed in the past few decades, only a small minority could be translated into clinical practice. One possible reason for this is that, in general, treatment is initiated in concomitance with the onset of the disease or a few days thereafter, artificially increasing the effectiveness of therapy, since in this manner the pathogenic factors involved are more easily neutralized. Far less encouraging results are obtained if treatment is initiated at later stages, when the much more complex interaction between these factors would require more vigorous therapy and the association of two or more drugs [1–3].

Five-sixths renal ablation (Nx), a widely employed model of chronic kidney disease (CKD), is characterized by severe glomerular and interstitial injury, accompanied by marked hypertension and renal functional loss. Both hemodynamic and inflammatory phenomena are thought to participate in the pathogenesis of renal injury in the Nx model [4,5]. Accordingly, treatment with inhibitors of the renin-angiotensin system (RAS) provides significant renoprotection in the Nx model, as well as in other CKD models and in clinical CKD [4,6–12]. However, renoprotection afforded by these compounds is far from complete [1,13,14], which has prompted their association with drugs with different mechanisms of action, such as anti-inflammatory or antilymphocytic agents [1,3]. Nevertheless, chronic associations of RAS inhibitors with potentially toxic drugs are unlikely to be translated into clinical practice.

We showed previously [15] that an association between the Angiotensin-II (AII) receptor blocker, losartan (L), and the thiazide diuretic, hydrochlorotiazide (H), started 30 days after Nx, normalized blood pressure and albuminuria, and provided complete renoprotection for at least 7 months. These results did not support the established concept that thiazide diuretics are ineffective when renal function has declined to 1/3 of normal or less [16], as in the Nx model [4,5,17]. However, these findings may not be applicable to the clinical setting. First, although the Nx model is presumed to mimic advanced CKD because the nephron number is so drastically reduced, it may not reflect the real clinical situation, because in patients with advanced CKD severe nephron loss is due to a long process of inflammation and fibrosis, while in the Nx model nephron reduction is an immediate consequence of surgical removal and, even after 30 days, renal inflammation and fibrosis are still relatively limited. Second, the striking renoprotection afforded by the L+H association might merely reflect normalization of blood pressure [15], and in this case could be entirely attributable to amelioration of the hemodynamic strain to the renal microcirculation.

In the present study, we investigated whether the L+H association would still arrest the progression of renal injury at more advanced stages of CKD in the Nx model, when extensive renal fibrosis is already present, thereby mimicking more closely the situation prevailing in advanced human CKD. In addition, we sought to determine whether control of systemic hypertension would play a central role in a possible renoprotective effect of the combined L+H treatment in this setting.

Methods

Two hundred thirty-two adult male Munich-Wistar rats, weighing between 220 and 260 g were utilized in this study. All rats were obtained from a local facility at the Faculty of Medicine, University of São Paulo. All experimental procedures were specifically approved by the local Research Ethics Committee (Comissão de Ética para Análise de Projetos de Pesquisa do Hospital das Clínicas da Faculdade de Medicina da Universidade de São Paulo, CAPPesq, under process n° 0689/08), and developed in strict conformity with our institutional guidelines and with international standards for manipulation and care of laboratory animals. All rats were monitored daily for body weight and general condition. Rats that were in bad condition, presumably due to end-stage renal failure were euthanized by an overdose of anesthetic. Five-sixths renal ablation (Nx) was performed in a single-step procedure after ventral laparotomy under anesthesia with ketamine 50 mg/kg and xylazine 10 mg/kg im. The right kidney was removed and two or three branches of the left renal artery were ligated, resulting in the infarction of two-thirds of the left kidney. Sham-operated rats underwent anesthesia and manipulation of the renal pedicles, without any removal of renal mass. After surgery, all animals received enrofloxacin and, after full recovery, were given free access to tap water, fed regular rodent chow containing 0.5 Na and 22% protein (Nuvital Labs, Curitiba, Brazil), and kept at $23 \pm 1°C$ and $60 \pm 5\%$ relative air humidity, under an artificial 12–12 hour light/dark cycle.

The possibility of regression or prevention of renal injury was analyzed in 2 protocols representing a moderately advanced (Protocol 1) and a very advanced (Protocol 2) stage of chronic nephropathy.

Protocol 1

Sixty days after Nx, tail-cuff pressure (TCP) and daily urinary albumin excretion ($U_{alb}V$) were determined in all Nx rats. Those failing to increase TCP above 170 mmHg or $U_{alb}V$ above 40 mg/day were not included in the study. Fifteen Nx rats were killed at this time and were used as pretreatment control subjects (group Nx_{pre}). The remaining 74 Nx rats were divided into 4 experimental groups: Nx+V (n = 22); Nx+L (n = 15), Nx receiving losartan potassium (L), 50 mg/kg diluted in the drinking water; Nx+LH (n = 17), receiving L 50 mg/kg plus hydrochlorothiazide (H) 6 mg/kg diluted in the drinking water; Nx+AHHz (n = 20),

receiving amlodipine besylate 5 mg/kg plus H 6 mg/kg plus hydralazine chloride (Hz) 12 mg/kg. This last group was included to evaluate the degree of renal protection that would be afforded by decreasing TCP to a similar extent as in group LH, without suppressing the renin-angiotensin system. Nx rats were distributed in such a way that initial body weight (BW), TCP and $U_{alb}V$ were similar among experimental groups. All treatments were maintained for 90 days. A group of 15 Sham-operated rats receiving no treatment was followed for the same time.

Protocol 2

One hundred twenty days after Nx, TCP and $U_{alb}V$ were determined in all Nx rats. Twenty Nx rats were utilized at this time as pretreatment controls (Nx_{pre}). The remaining 85 Nx rats were distributed in the same way as for Protocol 1, among groups: Nx+V (n = 26); Nx+L (n = 19); Nx+LH (n = 20); and Nx+AHHz (n = 20), treatments being maintained for 90 days. A group of 23 untreated sham-operated rats was followed for the same time.

Long-term Studies and Preparation of Renal Tissue for Histological Evaluation

Monthly $U_{alb}V$ was evaluated by radial immunodiffusion and TCP was measured using an optoelectronic automated device (Visitech Systems, Apex, NC) under light restraining and after light warming. To avoid any interference of stress, all rats were preconditioned to the procedure, and were invariably calm at the time of TCP determination. In addition, TCP was taken as the average of at least three consecutive measurements that varied by no more than 2 mmHg, to ensure that BP was stable before readings. At the end of the study, blood glucose (BG) and plasma triglycerides (Tg) were measured in blood taken from a tail vein after 12-hour fasting. On the following day, rats were anesthetized with ketamine, 50 mg/kg and xylazine 10 mg/kg im, and blood was collected from the abdominal aorta for measurement of serum creatinine (S_{Cr}), aldosterone (ALDO) and potassium (K^+) concentration. The kidneys were then retrogradely perfusion-fixed through the abdominal aorta with Dubosq-Brazil solution after a brief washout with saline to remove blood from the renal vessels. After weighing, two midcoronal renal slices were postfixed in buffered 4% formaldehyde and embedded in paraffin using conventional sequential techniques. Histomorphometric and immunohistochemical analyses of the renal tissue were performed in 4-μm-thick sections.

Biochemical Analyses

Tg and BG were measured in blood samples obtained from a tail vein Tg was measured using a commercially available enzymatic kit (Labtest Diagnostica, São Paulo, Brazil). BG concentration was determined using a reflectometric method (Advantage, Roche Diagnostics, USA).

S_{Cr} was determined using a commercially available kit (Labtest Diagnostica, São Paulo, Brazil). A radioimmunoassay kit (Diagnostic Systems Laboratories, Inc., Texas, USA) was used to determine ALDO. Serum K^+ was measured using an electrolyte analyzer (AVL Medical Instruments).

Histomorphometric Analysis

Morphometric evaluations were always performed in a blinded manner by a single observer. The extent of glomerular injury was estimated by determining the frequency of glomeruli with sclerotic lesions, as described previously [9,18] in sections stained by the periodic acid-Schiff reaction. At least 120 glomeruli were examined for each rat. The percentage of the renal cortical area occupied by interstitial tissue, used as a measure of the degree of interstitial expansion (%INT), was estimated in 25 consecutive microscopic fields of Masson-stained sections by a point-counting technique [19], at a final magnification of 100×, under a 144-point grid.

Immunohistochemical Analysis

Immunohistochemistry was performed on 4-µm-thick sections, mounted on glass slides precoated with 2% silane. Sections were deparaffinized and rehydrated by conventional techniques, then heated in citrate buffer for antigen retrieval and incubated overnight with the primary antibody at 4°C. For the negative control experiments, incubation with the primary antibody was not performed. The following primary antibodies were used: monoclonal mouse anti-rat ED-1 antibody for macrophage detection (Serotec, Oxford, United Kingdom); monoclonal mouse anti-rat proliferating cell nuclear antigen (PCNA) (Dako, Glostrup, Denmark); monoclonal mouse anti-alpha-smooth muscle actin (α-SMA) (Sigma, Missouri, USA); polyclonal rabbit anti-human AII (Peninsula Laboratories, San Carlos, USA), polyclonal rabbit Anti-Collagen I (Abcam, Cambridge, United Kingdom) and polyclonal rabbit anti-rat thiazide-sensitive Na-Cl cotransporter, NCC (Chemicon International, Temecula, USA).

For ED-1 detection, sections were preincubated with 5% normal rabbit serum to prevent nonspecific binding, then incubated overnight at 4°C with the primary antibody diluted in bovine serum albumin (BSA) at 1%. After rinsing with Tris-buffered saline (TBS), sections were incubated with an appropriate secondary antibody, then with an alkaline phosphatase anti-alkaline phosphatase (APAAP) complex (Dako, Glostrup, Denmark). Sections were developed with a fast-red dye solution (Sigma-Aldrich, Saint Louis, MO). For AII and α-SMA detection a streptavidin-biotin complex for alkaline phosphatase (DakoCytomation, Glostrup, Denmark) was used. Nonspecific binding was prevented with normal horse serum diluted at 1:20 in nonfat milk at 2% in TBS. Primary antibodies for AII and α-SMA were diluted in BSA at 1:400 and 1:800, respectively. Sections were developed in the same manner as for ED-1 detection. For assessment of PCNA-positive cells and the percentage of the renal area occupied by collagen I, sections were pretreated with 30% hydrogen peroxide in methanol and preincubated with normal horse serum as described. The primary antibodies were diluted at 1:100 (PCNA) and 1:200 (collagen I), in nonfat milk at 2% in TBS. The EnVision Labelled Polymer for peroxydase (Dako, Glostrup, Denmark) was used before development with DAB substrate (Dako, Glostrup, Denmark).

Double immunostaining was used to visualize the proliferation activity of distal convoluted tubules (DCT). Identification of DCT was performed by detection of NCC. Sections were pretreated with 30% hydrogen peroxide in methanol and preincubated with avidin and biotin blocking solutions (Vector, Burlingame, CA). Nonspecific staining was then prevented with normal goat serum diluted at 5% in BSA at 1% in TBS. Sections were incubated overnight with primary antibody against NCC diluted at 1% in BSA at 1% in TBS. Appropriate biotinylated secondary antibody was applied and Streptavidin-AP solution (DakoCytomation, Glostrup, Denmark) was used, followed by development with fast-red dye solution (Sigma-Aldrich, Saint Louis, MO). Sections were then preincubated once again with avidin and biotin blocking solutions, followed by prevention of nonspecific staining with a mixture of normal horse and rabbit sera diluted at 2 and 5%, respectively, in 2% nonfat milk in TBS. Sections were then incubated overnight with the primary antibody against PCNA, 0.01% in a solution containing 1% BSA and 2% nonfat milk

diluted in TBS. Appropriate biotinylated secondary antibodies were applied and the LSAB-HRP kit (DakoCytomation, Glostrup, Denmark) was used for PCNA detection. Sections were developed with DAB substrate (Dako, Glostrup, Denmark). All sections were counterstained with Mayer's hematoxylin, dehydrated and covered with Permount Mounting Media (Thermo Fisher Scientific, New Jersey, USA).

The renal density of macrophages, proliferating cells and AII positive cells was evaluated in a blinded manner at 200× magnification. For each section, 50 microscopic fields (corresponding to a total area of 1.6 mm^2) were examined. The percentage of cortical interstitial area occupied by α-SMA was estimated by the same point-counting technique employed to evaluate %INT, excluding positively stained blood vessels, while interstitial area occupied by collagen I was measured with an image processing software (Image Pro Plus®, version 7.01).

Statistical Analysis

Differences among different groups were analyzed using one-way analysis of variance (ANOVA) with pairwise post-test comparisons by the Neuman-Keuls method [20]. Since $U_{alb}V$, ALDO, AII and PCNA+NCC rates exhibited a strong non-Gaussian distribution, log transformation of these data was performed prior to statistical analysis. Mortalities were analyzed using a Kaplan-Meier approach. p values less than 0.05 were considered significant. Results are presented as Mean±1 SE. Calculations were performed using Prism® 4.0 (GraphPad® Software, USA).

Results

Survival data for Protocol 1 are shown in Figure 1a. In group Nx+V, mortality 150 days after renal ablation was 41%, whereas in the groups treated with L and LH it was reduced to 7% and 6%, respectively (p<0.05 vs. Nx+V). AHHz treatment promoted no improvement in survival, which reached 30% (p>0.05 vs. Nx+V). In Protocol 2 (Fig. 1b), the mortality rate at 210 days after nephrectomy was 70%, while in Groups Nx+L and Nx+LH rates were 40% and 25%, respectively (p<0.05 vs. Nx+V). Treatment with AHHz did not attenuate mortality, which remained at 69% (p>0.05 vs. Nx+V). No deaths occurred in Group S.

Body weights observed in Protocol 1 are shown in Table 1. In all Nx groups, body growth was stunted compared with the S group (p<0.05). There was no significant difference among the treated groups. In Protocol 2 (Table 2), body weight was also reduced compared with S, again without differences among treated groups.

Figure 2a shows the behavior of TCP over time in Protocol 1. Group Nx+V exhibited hypertension along the entire period of observation, reaching 210±4 mmHg at the end of the study (p<0.05 vs. S). Treatment with L had little effect on TCP, which was comparable to that observed in Group Nx+V 150 days after nephrectomy (p>0.05). By contrast, TCP was brought to normal along the whole study in rats receiving the LH treatment, which remained normotensive even at 150 days after renal ablation. TCP in animals treated with AHHz was indistinguishable from that in Group Nx+LH at the end of the study. Results for Protocol 2 are shown in Figure 2b. Nx+V animals remained severely hypertensive along the entire study, TCP reaching 212±4 mmHg 210 days after ablation (p<0.05 vs S). L treatment failed to lower TCP, which was similar to that observed in untreated rats at the end of the observation period. Again, Groups Nx+LH and Nx+AHHz exhibited low values for TCP along the whole study (p<0.05 vs. Nx+V and Nx+L).

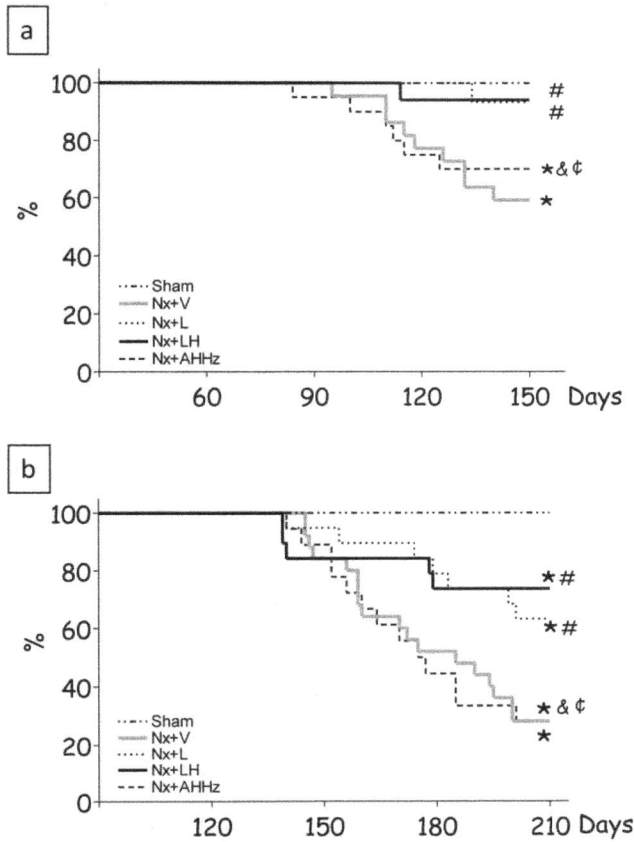

Figure 1. Percent Survival in Protocol 1 (a) and Protocol 2 (b). S, Sham-operated; Nx+V, untreated Nx; Nx+L, losartan-treated Nx; Nx+LH, Nx treated with losartan and hydrochlorothiazide; Nx+AHHz, Nx treated with amlodipine, hydrochlorothiazide, and hydralazine. *, p<0.05 vs. Sham; #, p<0.05 vs. Nx+V; & p<0.05 vs. Nx+L and ¢, p<0.05 vs. Nx+LH.

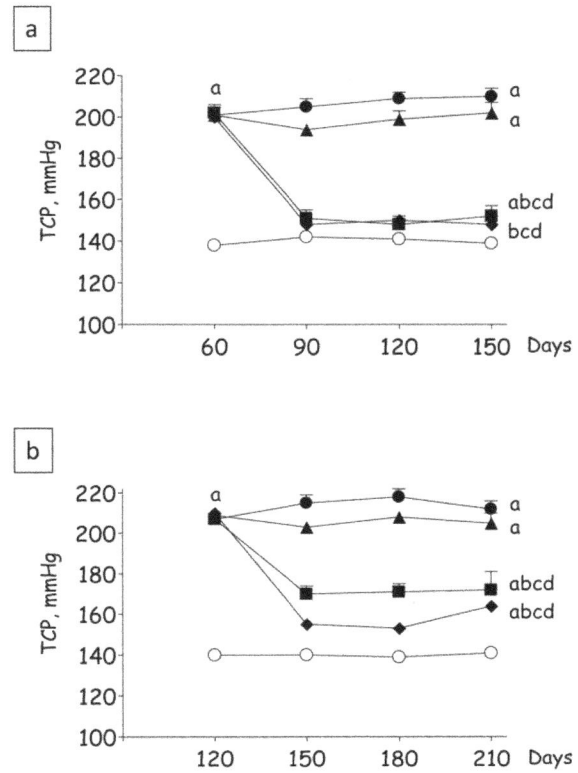

Figure 2. Tail-cuff pressures (TCP, mmHg) in Protocol 1 (a) and Protocol 2 (b). S, Sham-operated (clear circles); Nx$_{pre}$, pretreatment Nx (60 or 120 days after renal ablation); Nx+V (filled circles), untreated Nx; Nx+L (triangles), losartan-treated Nx; Nx+LH (diamonds), Nx treated with losartan+hydrochlorothiazide; Nx+AHHz (squares), Nx treated with amlodipine, hydrochlorothiazide, and hydralazine. Results expressed as Mean ± SE. ^{a}, p<0.05 vs. Sham; ^{b}, p<0.05 vs. Nx$_{pre}$; ^{c}, p<0.05 vs. Nx+V; ^{d}, p<0.05 vs. Nx+L and ^{e}, p<0.05 vs. Nx+LH.

Table 1. Functional and morphologic parameters in Protocol 1 (treatments started 60 days after renal ablation).

	BW	S$_{cr}$	K$^+$	%INT	M	AII+	BG	Tg
Sham	395±7	0.6±0.1	4.9±0.1	0.1±0.1	20±2	0.5±0.1	97±2	64±4
Nx$_{pre}$	284±6^a	1.0±0.1^a	5.8±0.1^a	3.0±0.3^a	128±17^a	6.7±1.2^a	98±3	70±3
Nx+V	297±12^a	1.7±0.1^{ab}	5.8±0.3^a	4.3±0.4^a	191±15^{ab}	16.0±1.8^{ab}	104±3	92±7^{ab}
Nx+L	314±9^a	1.3±0.1^{ac}	6.0±0.1^a	3.8±0.6^a	131±13^{ac}	13.9±1.3^{ab}	108±2^a	75±6
Nx+LH	296±6^a	1.1±0.1^{ac}	5.6±0.1^a	3.0±0.3^a	113±11^{ac}	9.5±1.5^{acd}	105±2	64±4^c
Nx+AHHz	306±10^a	1.5±0.2^{abe}	4.7±0.1^{bcde}	4.1±0.4^a	180±20^{abde}	14.1±1.5^{abe}	108±3^a	79±8

BW, body weight, g; S$_{cr}$, serum creatinine, mg/dL; K$^+$, serum potassium, mmol/L; %INT, fractional cortical interstitial area; MØ, density of tubulointerstitial macrophages, cells/mm^2; AII+, density of tubulointerstitial cells staining positively for AII, cells/mm^2; BG, blood glucose, mg/dL; Tg, triglycerides, mg/dL; S, Sham-operated; Nx$_{pre}$, pretreatment Nx (60 days after renal ablation); Nx+V, untreated Nx; Nx+L, losartan-treated Nx; Nx+LH, Nx treated with losartan+hydrochlorothiazide; Nx+AHHz, Nx treated with amlodipine, hydrochlorothiazide, and hydralazine. Group Nx+V and all Nx treated groups studied 150 days after renal ablation. Results expressed as Mean ±1 SE;
^{a}p<0.05 vs. Sham;
^{b}p<0.05 vs. Nx$_{pre}$;
^{c}p<0.05 vs. Nx+V;
^{d}p<0.05 vs. Nx+L and
^{e}p<0.05 vs. Nx+LH.

The variation of $U_{alb}V$ with time in Protocol 1 is shown in Figure 3a. Nx+V animals showed a progressive increase in $U_{alb}V$, reaching values tenfold higher than in S at 150 days (p<0.05 vs. S). In Group Nx+L, $U_{alb}V$ remained markedly elevated along the study, although final values were nearly 30% lower than in Group Nx+V (p<0.05). By contrast, combined LH treatment promoted $U_{alb}V$ regression, keeping it close to S values until the end of the study (p>0.05), although it should be noted that, since the nephron number had been reduced to 1/6th of normal, albuminuria per nephron was still higher in this group compared to S. Treatment with AHHz was unable to lower $U_{alb}V$, which was always similar to that seen in Group Nx+V. The evolution of $U_{alb}V$ in Protocol 2 is represented in Figure 3b. Again, $U_{alb}V$ was always elevated in Group Nx+V, being lowered by a small but significant amount by L treatment. Triple AHHz therapy had little effect on $U_{alb}V$. Even at this advanced stage, the LH treatment reduced $U_{alb}V$ to levels that approached those observed in S, remaining at these low levels until the end of the observation period (p>0.05 vs. S).

Serum creatinine concentrations (S_{Cr}) for Protocol 1 are shown in Table 1. Sixty days after renal ablation (Group Nx_{pre}) S_{Cr} was

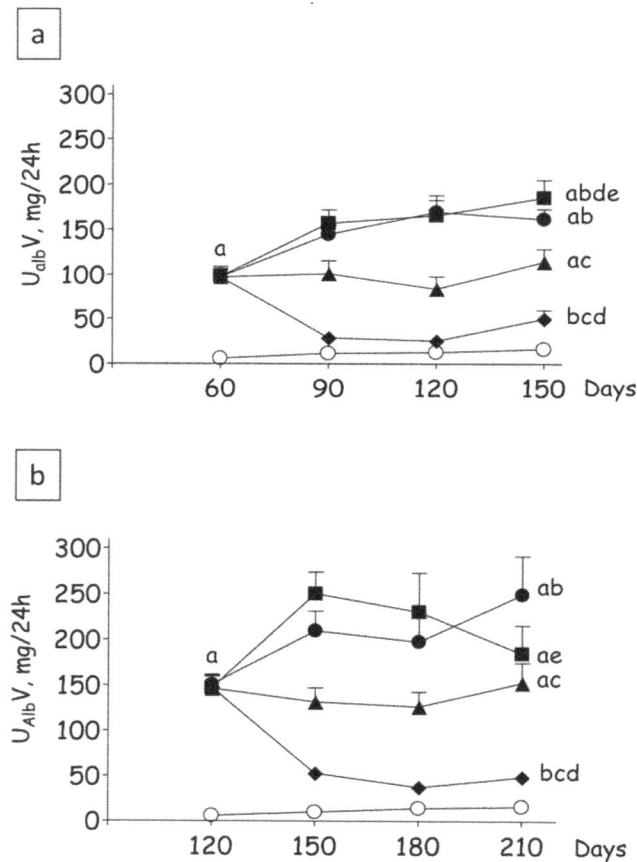

twice as high as in Group S (p<0.05). At the end of Protocol 1, 150 days after renal ablation, S_{cr} was increased further (p<0.05 vs. S and Nx_{pre}), indicating progression of the nephropathy. Treatment with L attenuated the loss of renal function, maintaining S_{cr} at levels comparable to those observed in the pretreatment group (p>0.05 vs Nx_{pre} and p<0.05 vs. Nx+V). Similar functional protection was observed with the LH association (p>0.05 vs Nx+L). The AHHz scheme had no effect on S_{Cr}, which increased over time and was indistinguishable from the Nx+V value at the end of the study. In Protocol 2 (Table 2) S_{cr} was increased in the Nx_{pre} group, which was studied 120 days after nephrectomy (p<0.05 vs S). Animals in Group Nx+V showed severe loss of renal function 210 days after renal ablation, as indicated by a marked increase in S_{cr} (p<0.05 vs. Nx_{pre}). Treatment with L or AHHz had little effect on S_{cr}, which attained levels similar to those seen in Group Nx+V at the end of the study (p>0.05). By contrast, rats treated with the LH combination exhibited final S_{cr} levels that were significantly lower than in the remaining groups, and similar to those verified in Group Nx_{pre} (p>0.05).

Serum K^+ concentrations for Protocol 1 are shown in Table 1. Sixty days after renal ablation (Group Nx_{pre}) serum K^+ was significantly increased compared to S. Animals in group Nx, at both 60 and 150 days after nephrectomy, showed an increase in serum potassium (p<0.05 vs S). Treatments with L or LH had no effect on serum K^+ at the end of the period of observation. The AHHz regimen strongly decreased serum K^+, which was similar to that observed in the S group 150 days after renal ablation. Values for Protocol 2 are shown in Table 2. Again, hyperkalemia was seen in the Nx_{pre} group, 120 days after nephrectomy (p<0.05 vs. S), and in Group Nx+V, examined at the end of the study. Treatment with L aggravated hyperkalemia, serum K^+ reaching values significantly higher than those observed in the Nx_{pre} group (p<0.05). In animals receiving LH therapy, serum K^+ was ameliorated compared to the Nx+L group (p<0.05), being similar to that seen in the Nx_{pre} group (p>0.05). As observed in Protocol 1, treatment with AHHz significantly reduced serum K^+, which was brought to levels similar to those observed in the S group (p>0.05).

The values for aldosterone (ALDO) in both protocols are shown in Figure 4. In Protocol 1, ALDO was numerically higher in Nx animals at 150 days, compared to 60 days, after renal ablation. Treatment with L significantly reduced the final concentration of ALDO (p<0.05 vs. Nx+V). The LH association reduced ALDO to values lower than in Nx_{pre} (p<0.05 vs. Nx_{pre}, Nx+V and p>0.05 vs. S). Triple therapy promoted no change in ALDO concentration, which remained comparable to that in Group Nx+V (p>0.05). In Protocol 2, the pretreatment ALDO concentration (Group Nx_{pre}) was significantly higher than in Group S (p<0.05), a difference that persisted in Group Nx+V. Monotherapy with L promoted a significant reduction compared to Group Nx+V (p<0.05). LH treatment drastically reduced circulating ALDO below pretreatment levels (p<0.05 vs. Nx_{pre}, Nx+V and p>0.05 vs. S). In Group Nx+AHHz serum ALDO was similar to that in Group Nx+V.

Representative glomeruli seen at the end of Protocol 1 (150 days after renal ablation) are shown in Fig. 5 (a, e, i, m, q and u), while analogous microphotographs for Protocol 2 are shown in Fig. 6 (a, e, i, m, q and u). The frequency of sclerotic glomeruli (% GS) in both protocols is given in Figure 7. In Protocol 1, almost 10% of glomeruli exhibited sclerotic lesions 60 days after renal ablation (Group Nx_{pre}). Glomerular injury progressed in untreated animals, %GS exceeding 30% in Group Nx+V 150 days after nephrectomy (p<0.05 vs. Nx_{pre}). Treatment with L alone partially prevented the

Figure 3. Urinary albumin excretion rates ($U_{alb}V$, mg/24 h) in Protocol 1 (a) and Protocol 2 (b). S, Sham-operated (clear circles); Nx_{pre}, pretreatment Nx (60 or 120 days after renal ablation); Nx+V (filled circles), untreated Nx; Nx+L (triangles), losartan-treated Nx; Nx+LH (diamonds), Nx treated with losartan+hydrochlorothiazide; Nx+AHHz (squares), Nx treated with amlodipine, hydrochlorothiazide, and hydralazine. Results expressed as Mean ± SE. [a], p<0.05 vs. Sham; [b], p<0.05 vs. Nx_{pre}; [c], p<0.05 vs. Nx+V; [d], p<0.05 vs. Nx+L and [e], p<0.05 vs. Nx+LH.

Regression of Albuminuria and Hypertension and Arrest of Severe Renal Injury...

13

Table 2. Functional and morphologic parameters in Protocol 2 (treatments started 120 days after renal ablation).

	BW	S_{cr}	K^+	%INT	M	AII+	BG	Tg
Sham	406 ± 7	0.6 ± 0.1	4.9 ± 0.1	0.1 ± 0.1	22 ± 2	0.7 ± 0.1	97 ± 1	54 ± 4
Nx$_{pre}$	305 ± 6^a	1.4 ± 0.1^a	5.5 ± 0.1^a	4.2 ± 0.5^a	188 ± 18^a	12.7 ± 1.8^a	94 ± 2	77 ± 2^a
Nx+V	279 ± 6^a	2.5 ± 0.1^{ab}	5.9 ± 0.2^a	7.2 ± 0.5^{ab}	250 ± 18^{ab}	19.8 ± 2.0^{ab}	123 ± 10^{ab}	95 ± 5^a
Nx+L	293 ± 9^a	2.1 ± 0.2^{ab}	6.2 ± 0.2^{ab}	6.9 ± 0.7^{ab}	189 ± 12^{ac}	17.3 ± 1.4^{ab}	114 ± 5^{ab}	84 ± 10^a
Nx+LH	283 ± 7^a	1.6 ± 0.1^{acd}	5.7 ± 0.1^{ad}	4.0 ± 0.5^{acd}	149 ± 13^{ac}	11.9 ± 1.7^{acd}	116 ± 2^{ab}	64 ± 5^c
Nx+AHHz	291 ± 8^a	2.1 ± 0.2^{abe}	5.1 ± 0.2^{bcde}	6.5 ± 0.6^{abe}	188 ± 14^{ac}	20.6 ± 1.4^{abe}	132 ± 6^{ab}	100 ± 15^{ae}

BW, body weight, g; S_{cr}, serum creatinine, mg/dL; K^+, serum potassium, mmol/L; %INT, fractional cortical interstitial area; MØ, density of tubulointerstitial macrophages, cells/mm^2; AII+, density of tubulointerstitial cells staining positively for AII, cells/mm^2; BG, blood glucose, mg/dL; Tg, triglycerides, mg/dL; S, Sham-operated; Nx$_{pre}$, pretreatment Nx (120 days after renal ablation); Nx+V, untreated Nx; Nx+L, losartan-treated Nx; Nx+LH, Nx treated with losartan+hydrochlorothiazide; Nx+AHHz, Nx treated with amlodipine, hydrochlorothiazide, and hydralazine. Group Nx+V and all Nx treated groups studied 210 days after renal ablation. Results expressed as Mean ±1 SE;
[a] $p<0.05$ vs. Sham;
[b] $p<0.05$ vs. Nx$_{pre}$;
[c] $p<0.05$ vs. Nx+V;
[d] $p<0.05$ vs. Nx+L and
[e] $p<0.05$ vs. Nx+LH.

progression of glomerular lesions, although %GS in Group Nx+L was not significantly different from that seen in untreated rats ($p>0.05$ vs. Nx$_{pre}$ and Nx+V). Glomerular protection was evident in the group receiving the LH association, in which the value for %GS was nearly identical to that observed in Group Nx$_{pre}$. In the group treated with the AHHz association, the frequency of glomerular sclerotic lesions was not limited, progressing in a similar fashion as in the untreated group. In Protocol 2, %GS already reached 27% 120 days after renal ablation (Group Nx$_{pre}$). After 210 days post-ablation, almost 60% of glomeruli exhibited

sclerotic lesions ($p<0.05$ vs. Nx$_{pre}$). Treatment with L failed to prevent the progression of %GS, which reached values that were lower than those found in untreated rats, but significantly higher than pretreatment values. In rats treated with LH, %GS reached final values that were significantly lower than in Group Nx+V or Nx+L, and similar to those seen in Group Nx$_{pre}$. In animals treated with AHHz, %GS behaved in a similar manner as in the untreated group.

Representative microphotographs of cortical interstitial area are shown in Fig. 5 (b, f, j, n, r, and v) for Protocol 1 and Fig. 6 (b, f, j,

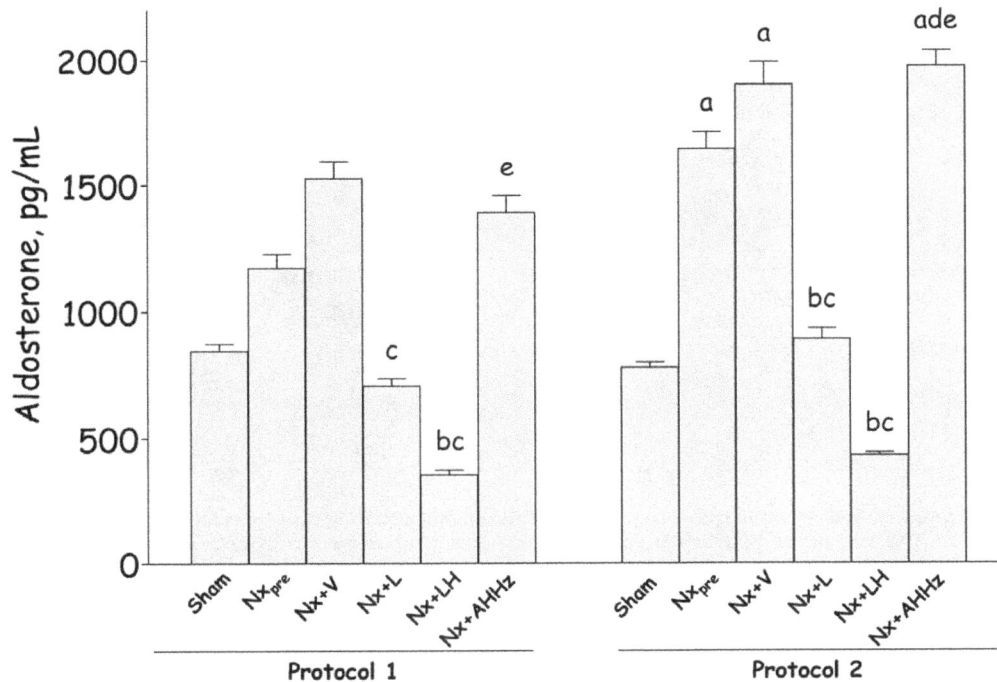

Figure 4. Plasma aldosterone (ALDO, pg/mL) in Protocol 1 and Protocol 2. S, Sham-operated; Nx$_{pre}$, pretreatment Nx (60 or 120 days after renal ablation); Nx+V, untreated Nx; Nx+L, losartan-treated Nx; Nx+LH, Nx treated with losartan+hydrochlorothiazide; Nx+AHHz, Nx treated with amlodipine, hydrochlorothiazide, and hydralazine. Results expressed as Mean $\pm$ SE. [a], $p<0.05$ vs. Sham; [b], $p<0.05$ vs. Nx$_{pre}$; [c], $p<0.05$ vs. Nx+V; [d], $p<0.05$ vs. Nx+L and [e], $p<0.05$ vs. Nx+LH.

Protocol 1

	PAS	% INT	COLLAGEN-I	α-SMA

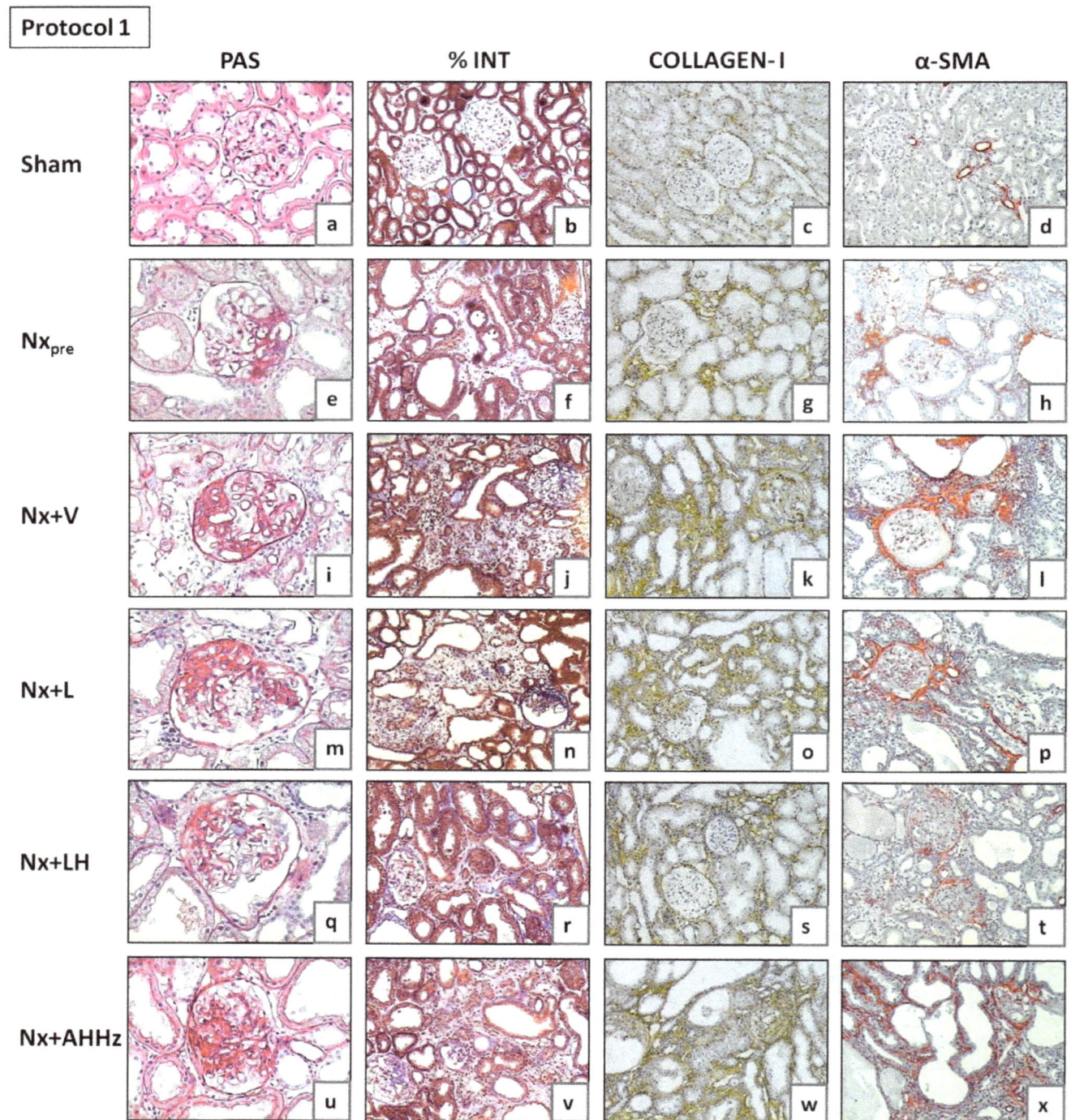

Figure 5. Representative microphotographs of renal tissue from Nx$_{pre}$ (60 days after renal ablation) and from all other groups (150 days after renal ablation) in Protocol 1. PAS, Periodic Acid-Schiff; %INT, percent cortical area occupied by interstitium in sections stained with Masson trichrome; α-SMA, alpha-smooth muscle actin.

n, r, and v) for Protocol 2. Quantitative analysis of the percent cortical interstitium for Protocol 1 (%INT) is shown in Table 1. Group Nx$_{pre}$ exhibited high %INT values compared to S (p<0.05). Little progression was seen in untreated rats 150 days after ablation (p<0.05 vs. Nx$_{pre}$). None of the treatments had a significant effect on %INT at this phase. Table 2 shows the quantitative analysis of %INT for Protocol 2. Values for %INT

were significantly higher in Group Nx$_{pre}$ in comparison with S. At 210 days post-ablation, %INT was significantly increased in Group Nx+V compared with pretreatment values (p<0.05 vs. Nx$_{pre}$). L monotherapy was unable to attenuate the progression of interstitial expansion, %INT reaching similar values as in Group Nx+V. By contrast, the LH association completely prevented the progression of %INT, which remained at similar levels as in

Regression of Albuminuria and Hypertension and Arrest of Severe Renal Injury...

15

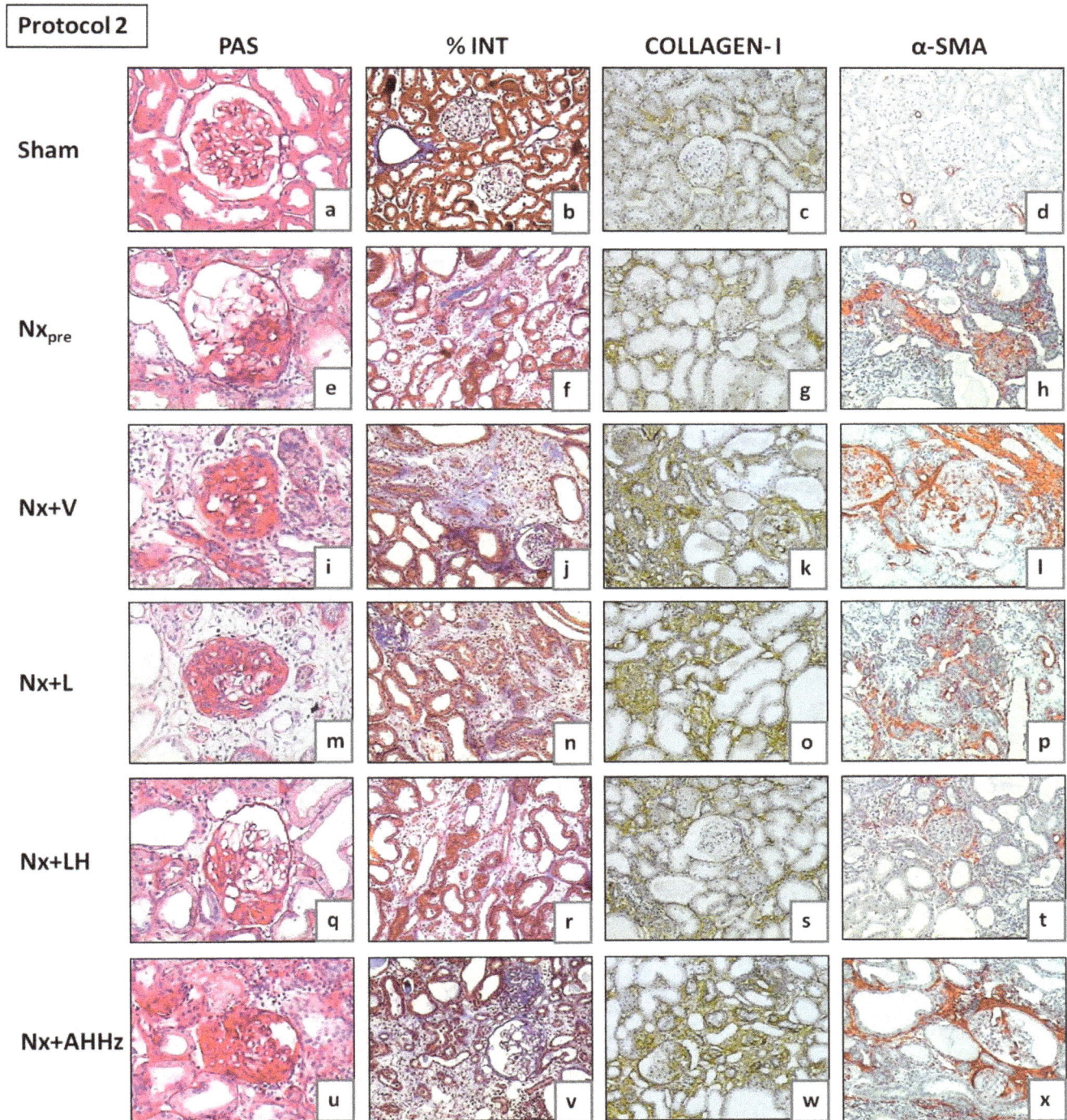

Figure 6. Representative microphotographs of renal tissue from Nx$_{pre}$ (120 days after renal ablation) and from all other groups (210 days after renal ablation) in Protocol 1. PAS, Periodic Acid-Schiff; %INT, percent cortical area occupied by interstitium in sections stained with Masson trichrome; α-SMA, alpha-smooth muscle actin.

Group Nx$_{pre}$. No protection against interstitial expansion was obtained in rats treated with the AHHz association.

The presence of collagen I in the renal tissue, detected by immunohistochemistry, is shown in Fig. 5 (c, g, k, o, s, and w) for Protocol 1, and 6 (c, g, k, o, s, and w) for Protocol 2. The intensity of collagen 1 deposition (Fig. 8) paralleled the fraction of cortical area occupied by interstitial tissue, indicating that at least part of

the interstitial expansion observed in Nx rats was due to fibrosis. No regression of collagen I deposition was seen with any of the treatments. However, renal interstitial fibrosis was arrested at pretreatment levels by the LH treatments in both Protocol 1 and 2.

Representative microphotographs of interstitial α-SMA obtained 150 days (Protocol 1) and 210 days (Protocol 2) after renal ablation are shown in Fig. 5 (d, h, l, p, t and x) and Fig. 6 (d, h, l, p,

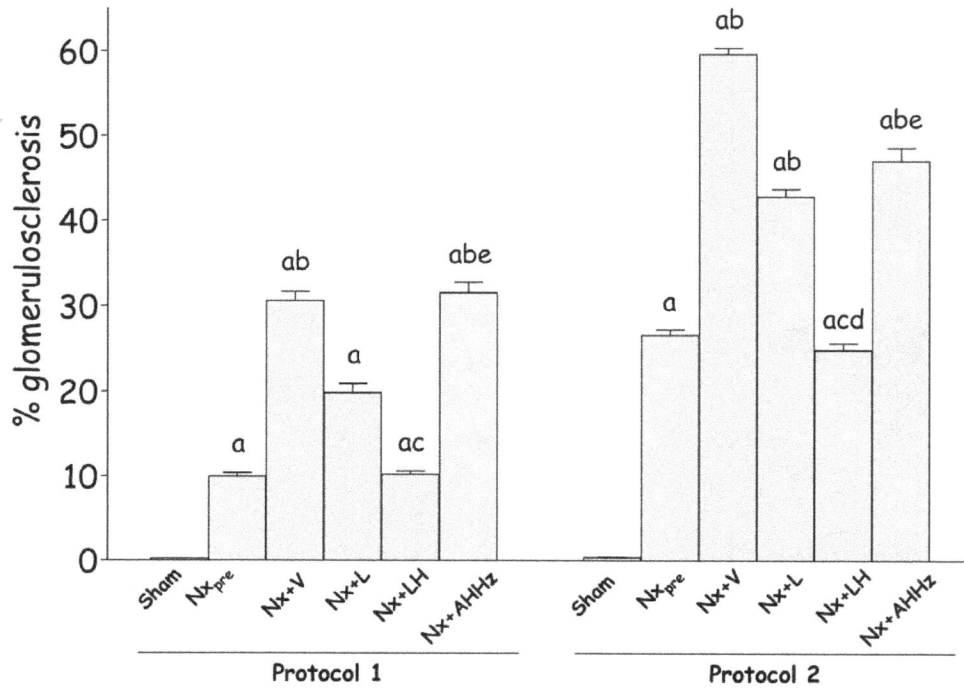

Figure 7. Percent glomerulosclerosis (%GS) in Protocol 1 and Protocol 2. S, Sham-operated; Nx$_{pre}$, pretreatment Nx (60 days or 120 after renal ablation); Nx+V, untreated Nx; Nx+L, losartan-treated Nx; Nx+LH, Nx treated with losartan+hydrochlorothiazide; Nx+AHHz, Nx treated with amlodipine, hydrochlorothiazide, and hydralazine. Results expressed as Mean $\pm$ SE. [a], $p<0.05$ vs. Sham; [b], $p<0.05$ vs. Nx$_{pre}$; [c], $p<0.05$ vs. Nx+V; [d], $p<0.05$ vs. Nx+L and [e], $p<0.05$ vs. Nx+LH.

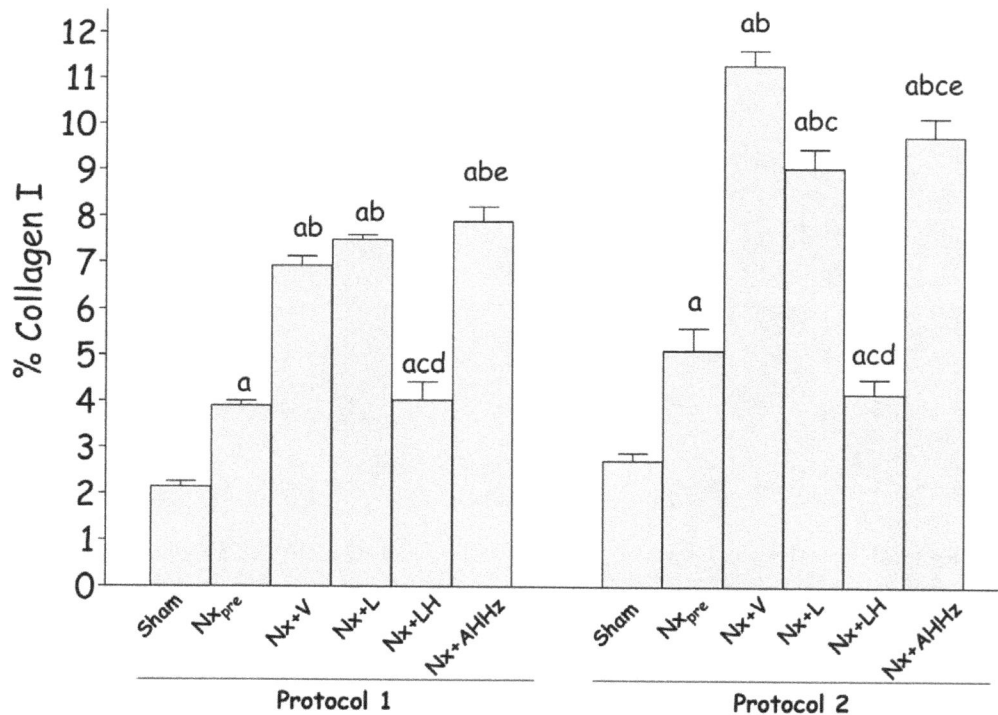

Figure 8. Quantitative analysis of percent renal area occupied by collagen I in Protocol 1 and Protocol 2. S, Sham-operated; Nx$_{pre}$, pretreatment Nx (60 or 120 days after renal ablation); Nx+V, untreated Nx; Nx+L, losartan-treated Nx; Nx+LH, Nx treated with losartan+hydrochlorothiazide; Nx+AHHz, Nx treated with amlodipine, hydrochlorothiazide, and hydralazine. Results expressed as Mean $\pm$ SE. [a], $p<0.05$ vs. Sham; [b], $p<0.05$ vs. Nx$_{pre}$; [c], $p<0.05$ vs. Nx+V; [d], $p<0.05$ vs. Nx+L and [e], $p<0.05$ vs. Nx+LH.

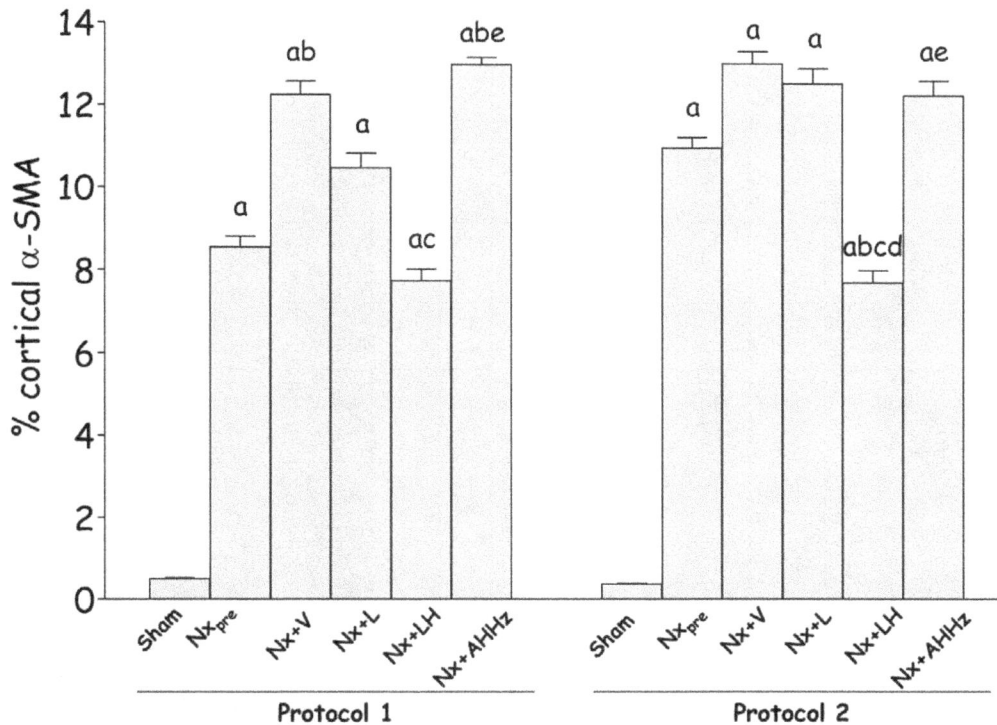

Figure 9. Percent cortical alpha-smooth muscle actin (α-SMA) in Protocol 1 and Protocol 2. S, Sham-operated; Nx$_{pre}$, pretreatment Nx (60 or 120 days after renal ablation); Nx+V, untreated Nx; Nx+L, losartan-treated Nx; Nx+LH, Nx treated with losartan+hydrochlorothiazide; Nx+AHHz, Nx treated with amlodipine, hydrochlorothiazide, and hydralazine. Results expressed as Mean ± SE. [a], $p < 0.05$ vs. Sham; [b], $p < 0.05$ vs. Nx$_{pre}$; [c], $p < 0.05$ vs. Nx+V; [d], $p < 0.05$ vs. Nx+L and [e], $p < 0.05$ vs. Nx+LH.

t and x), respectively. Figure 9 shows the fraction of the interstitial area occupied by α-SMA. In Protocol 1, pretreatment values (60 days after Nx) were significantly higher than in S, and continued to grow until 150 days post-Nx ($p < 0.05$ vs. Nx$_{pre}$). Rats treated with L only or with the AHHz association showed values that were similar to those seen in Group Nx+V ($p > 0.05$), whereas combined LH treatment effectively prevented the increase of interstitial α-SMA with time ($p > 0.05$ vs. Nx$_{pre}$). Parallel results were observed in Protocol 2, with the only difference that the fractional α-SMA area at the end of the study was significantly smaller in Group Nx+LH than in Group Nx$_{pre}$.

Table 1 shows data on macrophage infiltration for Protocol 1. Sixty days after Nx, the density of macrophages at the tubulointerstitial compartment was markedly elevated in Group Nx$_{pre}$ compared to S ($p < 0.05$). This parameter showed a progressive nature, reaching final values (150 days after ablation) that were significantly higher than those observed in Group Nx$_{pre}$. L and LH treatments, but not the AHHz association, prevented the intensification of tubulointerstitial macrophage infiltration ($p > 0.05$ vs. Nx$_{pre}$). Data for Protocol 2 are shown in Table 2. Marked tubulointerstitial macrophage infiltration was observed in the pretreatment group (Nx$_{pre}$) 120 days after renal ablation ($p < 0.05$ vs. S), with progression to final values (210 days after Nx) that were significantly higher than in the Nx$_{pre}$ group. All treatments prevented progression of macrophage infiltration, although this parameter was numerically lower in Group Nx+LH.

Representative microphotographs showing cells staining positively for AII are depicted in Fig. 10 (a, d, g, j, m and p) for Protocol 1, and in Fig. 11 (a, d, g, j, m and p) for Protocol 2. The density of AII-positive cells in Protocol 1 (Table 1) was already significantly higher than in S 60 days post-ablation (Group Nx$_{pre}$),

exhibiting further elevation 150 days after Nx ($p < 0.05$ vs. Nx$_{pre}$). Neither L monotherapy nor the AHHz association were able to prevent the increase in the number of AII-positive cells, while the LH combined therapy reduced this parameter to values that were similar to those found in Group Nx$_{pre}$, and significantly lower than in each of the other Nx groups. Entirely parallel results were obtained in Protocol 2 (Table 2).

Representative microphotographs of renal proliferating cells are shown in Fig. 10 (b, e, h, k, n and q) for Protocol 1, and 11 (b, e, h, k, n and q) for Protocol 2. Figure 12 represents the quantitative data on cell proliferation, obtained by analysis of cells staining positively for PCNA. In Protocol 1, the intensity of cell proliferation in the tubular and interstitial compartments was significantly increased compared to S in the pretreatment group (Nx$_{pre}$). Interstitial, but not tubular proliferation was significantly increased in untreated Nx rats compared to Nx$_{pre}$. Among treatments, only the LH association was able to prevent, and even reverse, cell proliferation in both tubular and interstitial compartments, bringing these parameters to levels that were similar to those found in S. In Protocol 2, pretreatment values for tubular and interstitial proliferation were higher than in S. No progression of these parameters was seen in untreated Nx rats 210 days after renal ablation. At this time, interstitial proliferation was less intense in rats that received L monotherapy or the AHHz combined therapy than in Group Nx+V, but remained at levels similar to those observed prior to treatments. No difference was observed at this time among Groups Nx+V, Nx+L and Nx+AHHz regarding tubular cell proliferation. In rats treated with the LH association, values for PCNA-positive cells in all three compartments were significantly lower than in the Nx+V group, and even

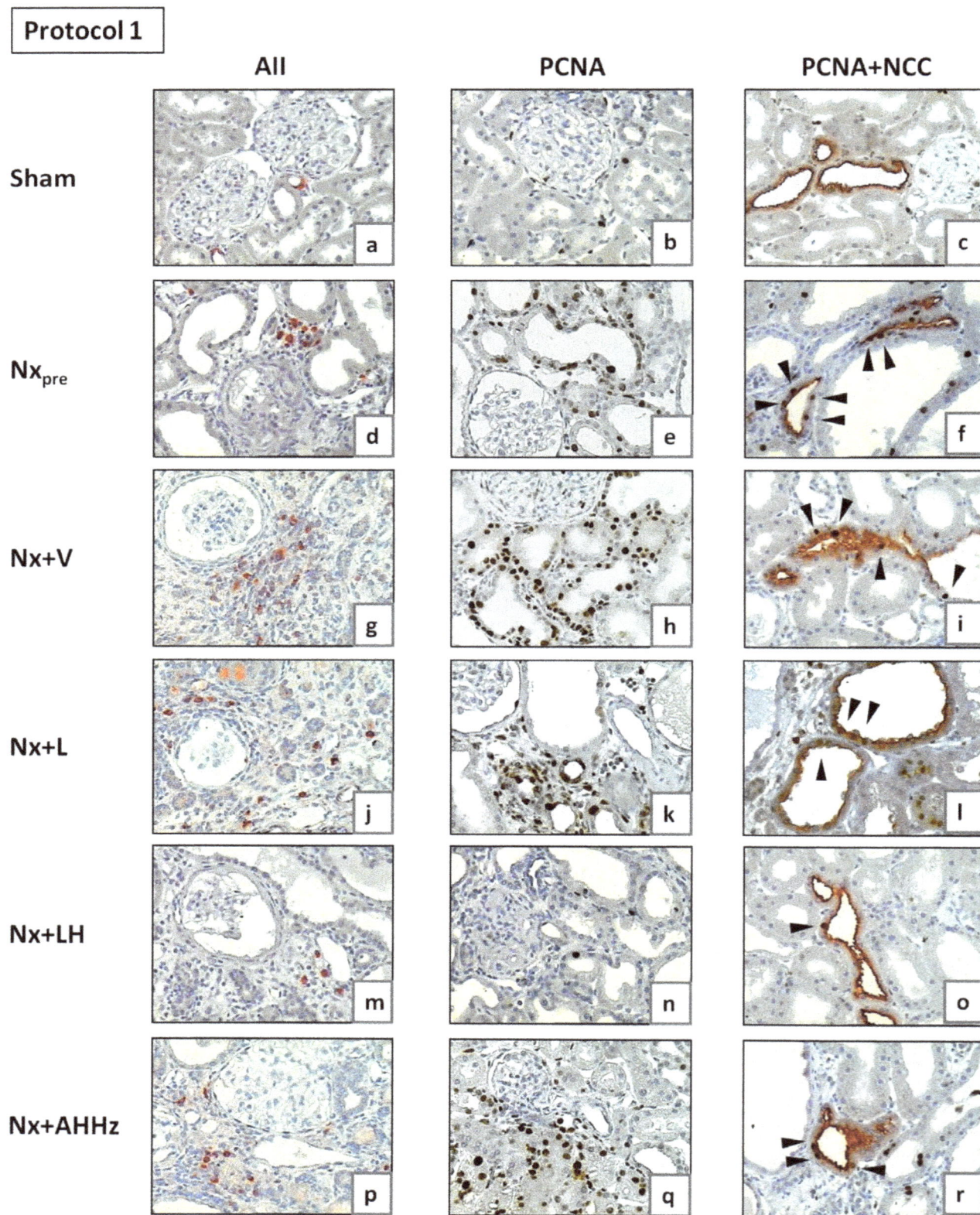

Figure 10. Representative microphotographs of renal tissue obtained for Nx$_{pre}$ (60 days after renal ablation) and for all other groups (150 days after renal ablation) in Protocol 1. All, tubulointerstitial cells staining positively for AII; PCNA, proliferating-cell nuclear antigen; NCC, sodium-chloride cotransporter, specific for distal convoluted tubule (DCT). Arrowheads in Figs. 10c, f, i, l, o and r (double staining for PCNA and NCC) indicate examples of PCNA-positive cells in DCT.

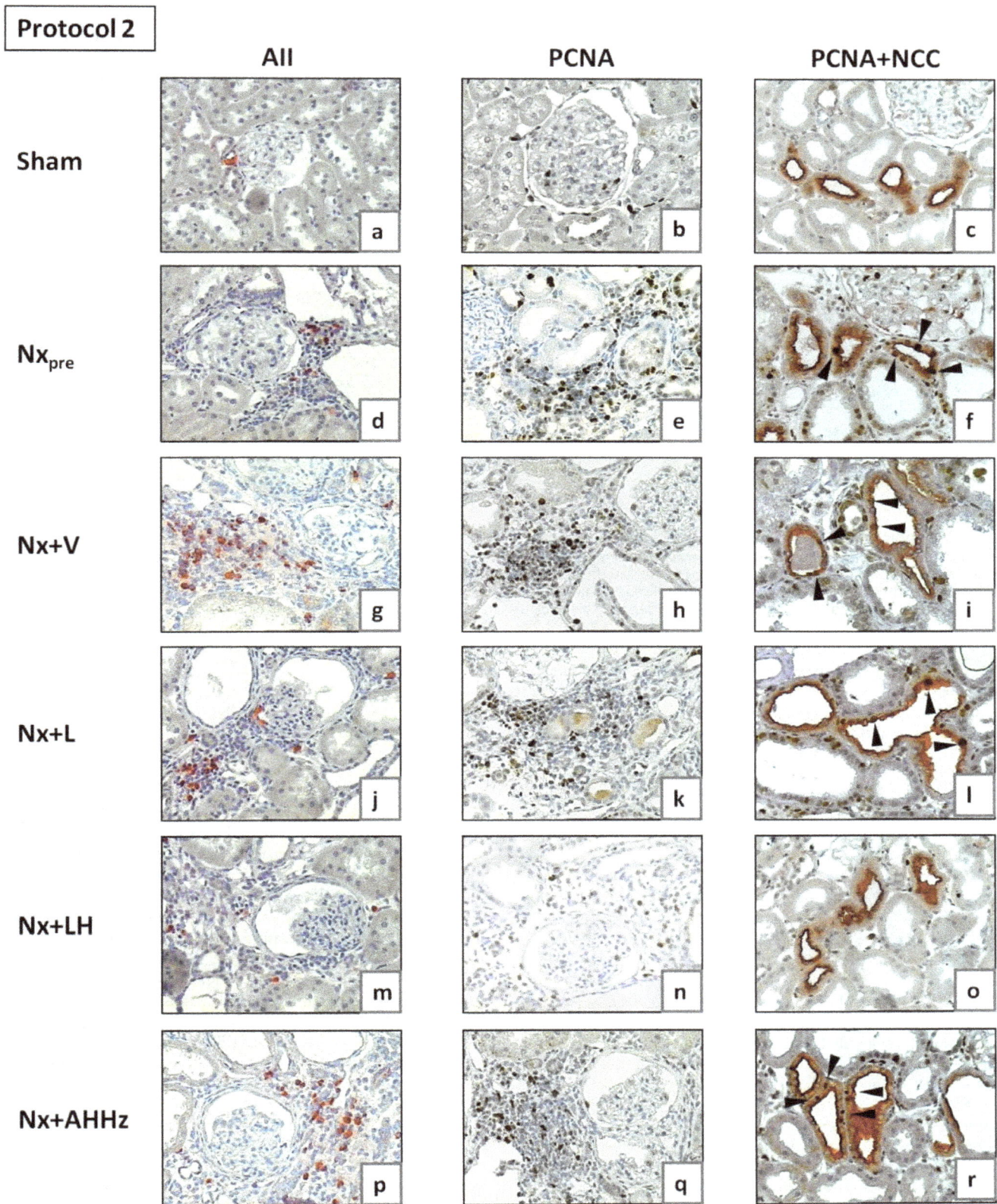

Figure 11. Representative microphotographs of renal tissue obtained for Nx_pre (120 days after renal ablation) and for all other groups (210 days after renal ablation) in Protocol 2. AII, tubulointerstitial cells staining positively for AII; PCNA, proliferating-cell nuclear antigen; NCC, sodium-chloride cotransporter, specific for distal convoluted tubule (DCT). Arrowheads in Figs. 11c, f, i, l, o and r (double staining for PCNA and NCC) indicate examples of PCNA-positive cells in DCT.

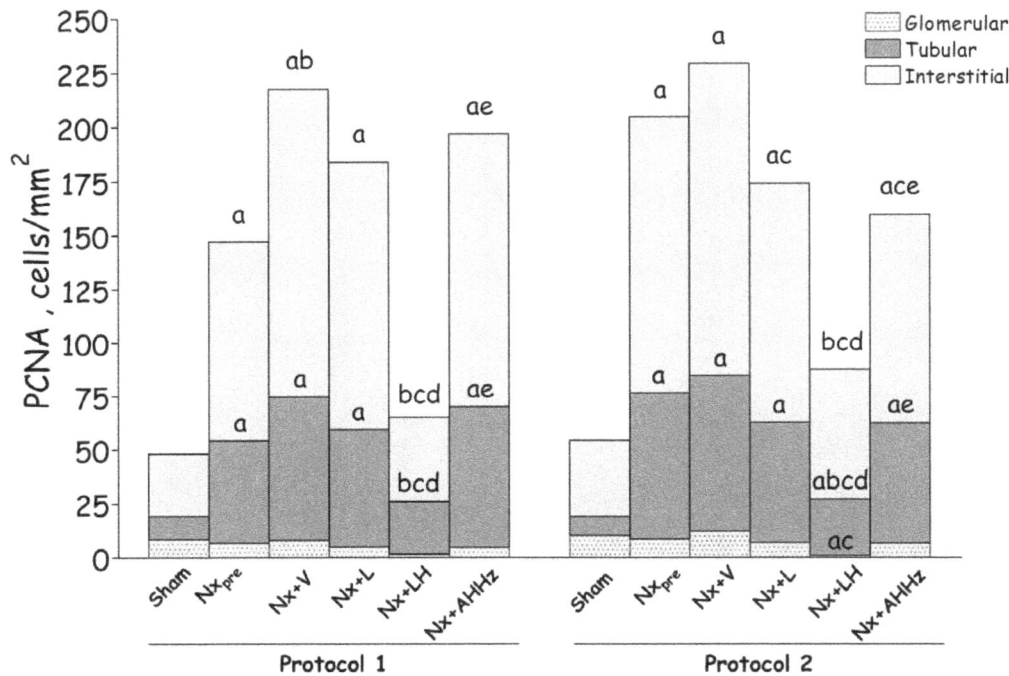

Figure 12. PCNA (Proliferating-cell nuclear antigen)-positive cells in glomerular (dotted areas), tubular (dark grey areas) and interstitial (light grey areas) compartments in Protocol 1 and Protocol 2. S, Sham-operated; Nx_{pre}, pretreatment Nx (60 or 120 days after renal ablation); Nx+V, untreated Nx; Nx+L, losartan-treated Nx; Nx+LH, Nx treated with losartan+hydrochlorothiazide; Nx+AHHz, Nx treated with amlodipine, hydrochlorothiazide, and hydralazine. Results expressed as Mean ± SE. [a], $p<0.05$ vs. Sham; [b], $p<0.05$ vs. Nx_{pre}; [c], $p<0.05$ vs. Nx+V; [d], $p<0.05$ vs. Nx+L and [e], $p<0.05$ vs. Nx+LH. Letters denoting significance are placed immediately above the corresponding bar area.

lower than in the pretreatment group, indicating that treatment promoted regression of cell proliferation in this group.

Representative microphotographs of proliferation in the DCT, obtained through simultaneous staining for PCNA and NCC, are shown in Fig. 10 (c, f, i, l, o and r) for Protocol 1, and Fig. 11 (c, f, i, l, o and r) for Protocol 2. The corresponding quantitative data are shown in Fig. 13. In Protocol 1, pretreatment DCT proliferation (60 days after renal ablation) was significantly increased compared with S. DCT proliferation remained elevated in untreated rats at the end of the study, with no progression compared to Nx_{pre}. L monotherapy and the AHHz regimen promoted no significant change in DCT proliferation. By contrast, the LH association reduced DCT proliferation below pretreatment levels, indicating regression of this parameter. Parallel results were obtained in Protocol 2, with the exception that the differences between Group Nx+LH and either Nx+L and Nx+AHHz were now significant.

In Protocol 1 (Table 1), BG levels were unchanged in Group Nx_{pre} compared with S. At the end of the study (150 days after Nx) BG was slightly elevated in all groups, although only in Groups Nx+L and Nx+AHHz was this value significantly different from that in S. In Protocol 2 (Table 2), BG was again similar in Nx_{pre} and S. At the end of the study (210 days after renal ablation), BG was significantly increased in untreated Nx+V rats ($p<0.05$ vs. S). None of the treatments was able to normalize BG, which remained significantly increased compared to S in all groups of treated rats. Serum triglyceride concentrations (Tg) for Protocol 1 are given in Table 1. Tg was unaltered in the pretreatment group compared to S. Final Tg values were significantly increased in Group Nx+V ($p<0.05$ vs. S). Although L and AHHz treatments tended to normalize Tg, only the LH association was able to bring this parameter to values significantly lower than in the Nx+V group. In Protocol 2 (Table 2) Tg was significantly higher than S in the

pretreatment group (Nx_{pre}), and remained elevated at the end of the study. Only with the LH therapy did Tg fall to values significantly lower than in the Nx+V group, and similar to pretreatment values.

Discussion

As described earlier [2–6,15], reduction of renal mass in 5/6 resulted in systemic hypertension, heavy albuminuria, progressive glomerulosclerosis (GS), interstitial expansion/collagen deposition, marked tubulointerstitial proliferation, as well as interstitial infiltration by macrophages, myofibroblasts, and cells staining positively for AII. Mortality was very high in the untreated group, exceeding 40% at 150 days and 70% 210 days after nephrectomy, thus mimicking the picture observed in clinical practice. Serum aldosterone rose progressively in untreated Nx rats and, in view of its well-known profibrotic actions [21–23] likely made a substantial contribution to the progression of renal injury. Although the main factor stimulating the synthesis of aldosterone are circulating levels of AII, its production by the adrenals was probably influenced by potassium retention as well [24], helping to maintain the balance of this ion at the cost of worsening renal injury.

In most previous studies of the Nx model, treatments intended to prevent or ameliorate CKD were initiated immediately after nephrectomy or at most a few weeks after the procedure. At this initial phase, structural injury in the remaining renal tissue is incipient or only mild, and can be more easily prevented. We showed previously [25] that treatment with losartan and mycophenolate mofetil during the first 30 days after 5/6 nephrectomy strongly attenuated the progression of CKD, and that this protective effect persisted long after treatment was terminated. The same treatment had a much smaller impact when

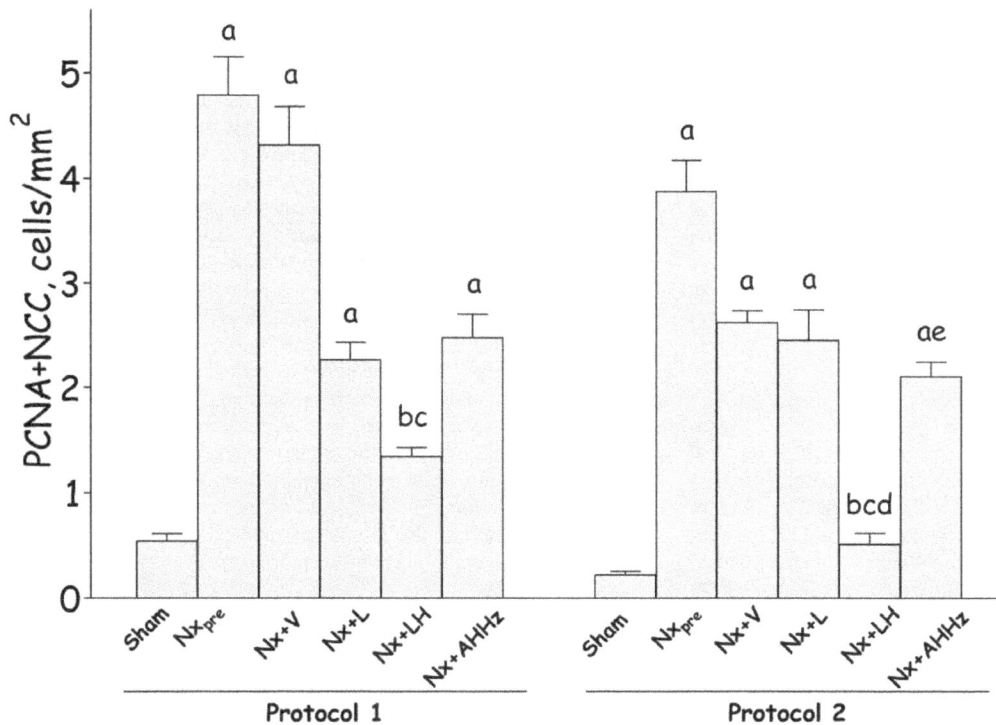

Figure 13. Frequency of proliferating cells in distal convoluted tubule, evaluated by double staining for PCNA (Proliferating-cell nuclear antigen) and NCC (distal convoluted tubule-specific sodium-chloride cotransporter) in Protocol 1 and Protocol 2. S, Sham-operated; Nx_{pre}, pretreatment Nx (60 or 120 days after renal ablation); Nx+V, untreated Nx; Nx+L, losartan-treated Nx; Nx+LH, Nx treated with losartan+hydrochlorothiazide; Nx+AHHz, Nx treated with amlodipine, hydrochlorothiazide, and hydralazine. Results expressed as Mean ± SE. [a], $p < 0.05$ vs. Sham; [b], $p < 0.05$ vs. Nx_{pre}; [c], $p < 0.05$ vs. Nx+V; [d], $p < 0.05$ vs. Nx+L and [e], $p < 0.05$ vs. Nx+LH.

instituted between the 30th and 60th day after nephrectomy, indicating that early events determine the long-term outcome in this model. These findings may help explain the relative failure, in the clinical context, of treatments that appeared promising in experimental models.

In the present study, we compared the response of Nx rats to L monotherapy and the LH association, started at two different times after nephrectomy –60 and 120 days. Whereas the first time point simulated a condition of low nephron number with relatively mild renal inflammation, the second one –120 days after nephrectomy, never used before as a starting point for therapy – represented a situation in which drastic nephron reduction leads to high mortality and coexists with severe ongoing renal injury, with extensive glomerulosclerosis, interstitial inflammation and tubular atrophy, thus mimicking more closely the conditions prevailing in patients with advanced CKD, and their response to therapy.

Monotherapy with L provided only partial protection against mortality and the progression of renal injury/inflammation, especially when started 120 days after ablation. These results are consistent with previous observations [13,26], and contrast sharply with studies in which L treatment, started concomitantly with renal ablation or shortly thereafter, exerted a much clearer renoprotective effect. Taken together, these findings strengthen the concept that, once set in motion, the mechanisms that operate in CKD can no longer be controlled by inhibition of the RAS only, requiring association with other drugs or procedures to be arrested.

In both protocols, the effectiveness of treatment with L was sharply increased when associated with H, promoting regression of $U_{alb}V$ and hypertension to levels below those observed before

treatment, arresting the progression of renal injury and the decline of renal function, and dramatically reducing mortality. The factors that might explain this remarkable synergistic action are unclear. One obvious possibility is the striking BP reduction obtained with LH treatment [27,28]. However, AHHz treatment promoted a similar decrease in BP without corresponding renoprotection (although it limited macrophage infiltration), indicating that the beneficial effects of L+H treatment did not derive from its antihypertensive effect. Intracapillary hypertension is another important pathogenic factor in the Nx model, promoting mechanical stress and associated inflammatory events [29–31]. In the present study, measurement of intraglomerular pressure was impossible due to the severe alteration of the renal surface, made extremely irregular by advanced disease. Since we showed previously that LH treatment started 30 days after Nx, unlike L monotherapy, completely reversed glomerular hypertension [15], it is plausible that a similar effect may have occurred in the present study. Another possible explanation for the renoprotection afforded by the LH combination is its dramatic action on plasma aldosterone, which in both protocols was reduced to levels lower than those observed before treatment and similar to those seen in S. Previous studies showed that blockade of the mineralocorticoid receptor attenuates chronic renal injury in the Nx model [32,33], although inhibition of aldosterone synthesis has not been used in this context. Besides limiting fibrosis, normalization of aldosterone levels may have enhanced the natriuretic effect of H by inhibiting sodium reabsorption at principal cells and by a direct effect on NCC [34], thus exerting a protective effect by two distinct mechanisms. This strong inhibition of aldosterone production may have resulted from a synergistic interaction between L and H: on one hand, blockade of adrenal AT-1 receptors directly neutralized a major stimulus for the synthesis of aldosterone; on the other, H treatment, by facilitating kaliuresis, may have lessened a second important factor for aldosterone production. Finally, the antiproliferative effect of the LH association, bringing rates for glomerular, tubular and interstitial cell proliferation to levels lower than those observed at baseline, should be considered, since multiplication of local cells, including myofibroblasts and their precursors, is an important part of the inflammatory response triggered by renal mass removal [5,35]. This striking effect may also reflect the observed regression of albuminuria, which may have removed the inflammatory stimulus of filtered protein to proximal tubular cells [36,37]. Additionally, the remarkable reduction of DCT proliferation in the LH-treated group may have resulted from a local effect of H [38].

Insulin resistance and dyslipidemia may accompany CKD, aggravating renal injury [39–41]. Corroborating these clinical data, we observed an increase in plasma glucose and triglycerides in untreated Nx rats with advanced CKD (Protocol 2). Although thiazides may worsen these metabolic abnormalities [42], we did not observe such effects in association with LH treatment, which, on the contrary, reversed hypertriglyceridemia. Neither L monotherapy nor the AHHz regimen had any effect on circulating glucose or triglyceride levels, suggesting that the beneficial effect of the LH treatment on triglycerides resulted from the synergistic effect of the two drugs, perhaps reflecting amelioration of renal function.

Although thiazides have been used for decades in the treatment of hypertension, and although their value as antihypertensive agents in CKD has recently been affirmed [43,44], a possible renoprotective effect of these compounds in CKD has not been systematically investigated. We showed previously that H monotherapy initiated 30 days after renal ablation attenuated systemic hypertension and renal injury without preventing their progression, an effect comparable to that obtained with L monotherapy [15]. Likewise, the association of thiazides with inhibitors of the RAS has not been evaluated as a possible resource against

progression of advanced CKD, possibly as a corollary to the widespread notion that thiazides lack any effect at this phase. The present observations are once again at odds with this concept, which had already been challenged by the observations made in our laboratory [15], and by a few clinical studies [43,45]. Thus, further studies focused on the possible effect of the L+H association on CKD progression are warranted.

In summary, the present results suggest that the L+H association arrests the progression of renal injury in the Nx model, even when initiated at advanced stages of the nephropathy, with ongoing GS and interstitial inflammation and fibrosis. Our results do not support the concept that thiazides lose their effect in advanced CKD, nor do they reproduce the metabolic effects attributed to chronic thiazide use. The renoprotective action of the LH association cannot be explained by its antihypertensive effect. Mechanisms possibly involved in this protective action are a fall in intraglomerular pressure, the sharp decrease observed in the filtration of albumin and in the production of aldosterone, as well as an antiproliferative effect. Additional studies are needed to investigate whether these renoprotective effects can also be obtained in human CKD even when treatment is initiated at very advanced stages.

Acknowledgments

Preliminary results of this study were presented at the Annual Meeting of the American Society of Nephrology, November 8–13, 2011, and published in abstract form (J Am Soc Nephrol 22:755A, 2011). We thank Cristiene Okabe, Claudia Ramos Sena, Grasiela Barlette, Vivian Viana, Janice Pião, Walcy Rosolia Teodoro and Ricardo Mazzonetto for expert technical assistance.

Author Contributions

Conceived and designed the experiments: SCAA DMACM RZ CKF. Performed the experiments: SCAA CPV FGM CF NOSC CSTO DMACM. Analyzed the data: SCAA DMACM NOSC RZ CKF. Contributed reagents/materials/analysis tools: TB NOSC. Wrote the paper: SCAA FGM CF RZ CKF.

References

1. Fujihara CK, Noronha IL, Malheiros, Antunes GR, de Oliveira IB, et al. (2000) Combined mycophenolate mofetil and losartan therapy arrests established injury in the remnant kidney. J Am Soc Nephrol 11: 283–290.

2. Fujihara CK, Velho M, Malheiros DM, Zatz R (2005) An extremely high dose of losartan affords superior renoprotection in the remnant model. Kidney Int 67: 1913–1924.

3. Goncalves AR, Fujihara CK, Mattar AL, Malheiros DM, Noronha Ide L, et al. (2004) Renal expression of COX-2, ANG II, and AT1 receptor in remnant kidney: strong renoprotection by therapy with losartan and a nonsteroidal anti-inflammatory. Am J Physiol Renal Physiol 286: F945–954.

4. Anderson S, Meyer TW, Rennke HG, Brenner BM (1985) Control of glomerular hypertension limits glomerular injury in rats with reduced renal mass. J Clin Invest 76: 612–619.

5. Fujihara CK, Malheiros DM, Zatz R, Noronha IL (1998) Mycophenolate mofetil attenuates renal injury in the rat remnant kidney. Kidney Int 54: 1510–1519.

6. Lafayette RA, Mayer G, Park SK, Meyer TW (1992) Angiotensin II receptor blockade limits glomerular injury in rats with reduced renal mass. J Clin Invest 90: 766–771.

7. Wu LL, Cox A, Roe CJ, Dziadek M, Cooper ME, et al. (1997) Transforming growth factor beta 1 and renal injury following subtotal nephrectomy in the rat: role of the renin-angiotensin system. Kidney Int 51: 1553–1567.

8. Fujihara CK, Sena CR, Malheiros DM, Mattar AL, Zatz R (2006) Short-term nitric oxide inhibition induces progressive nephropathy after regression of initial renal injury. Am J Physiol Renal Physiol 290: F632–640.

9. Teles F, Machado FG, Ventura BH, Malheiros DM, Fujihara CK, et al. (2009) Regression of glomerular injury by losartan in experimental diabetic nephropathy. Kidney Int 75: 72–79.

10. Anderson S, Rennke HG, Brenner BM (1986) Therapeutic advantage of converting enzyme inhibitors in arresting progressive renal disease associated with systemic hypertension in the rat. J Clin Invest 77: 1993–2000.

11. Lewis EJ, Hunsicker LG, Bain RP, Rohde RD (1993) The effect of angiotensin-converting-enzyme inhibition on diabetic nephropathy. The Collaborative Study Group. N Engl J Med 329: 1456–1462.

12. Maschio G, Alberti D, Janin G, Locatelli F, Mann JF, et al. (1996) Effect of the angiotensin-converting-enzyme inhibitor benazepril on the progression of chronic renal insufficiency. The Angiotensin-Converting-Enzyme Inhibition in Progressive Renal Insufficiency Study Group. N Engl J Med 334: 939–945.

13. Meyer TW, Anderson S, Rennke HG, Brenner BM (1987) Reversing glomerular hypertension stabilizes established glomerular injury. Kidney Int 31: 752–759.

14. Noda M, Matsuo T, Fukuda R, Ohta M, Nagano H, et al. (1999) Effect of candesartan cilexetil (TCV-116) in rats with chronic renal failure. Kidney Int 56: 898–909.

15. Fujihara CK, Malheiros DM, Zatz R (2007) Losartan-hydrochlorothiazide association promotes lasting blood pressure normalization and completely arrests long-term renal injury in the 5/6 ablation model. Am J Physiol Renal Physiol 292: F1810–1818.

16. Reubi FC, Cottier PT (1961) Effects of reduced glomerular filtration rate on responsiveness to chlorothiazide and mercurial diuretics. Circulation 23: 200–210.

17. Romero F, Rodriguez-Iturbe B, Parra G, Gonzalez L, Herrera-Acosta J, et al. (1999) Mycophenolate mofetil prevents the progressive renal failure induced by 5/6 renal ablation in rats. Kidney Int 55: 945–955.

18. Fujihara CK, Avancini Costa Malheiros DM, de Lourdes Noronha II, De Nucci G, Zatz R (2001) Mycophenolate Mofetil Reduces Renal Injury in the Chronic Nitric Oxide Synthase Inhibition Model. Hypertension 37: 170–175.

19. Jepsen FL, Mortensen PB (1979) Interstitial fibrosis of the renal cortex in minimal change lesion and its correlation with renal function. A quantitative study. Virchows Arch A Pathol Anat Histol 383: 265–270.

20. Wallenstein S, Zucker CL, Fleiss JL (1980) Some statistical methods useful in circulation research. Circ Res 47: 1–9.

21. Brown NJ, Nakamura S, Ma L, Nakamura I, Donnert E, et al. (2000) Aldosterone modulates plasminogen activator inhibitor-1 and glomerulosclerosis in vivo. Kidney Int 58: 1219–1227.

22. Greene EL, Kren S, Hostetter TH (1996) Role of aldosterone in the remnant kidney model in the rat. J Clin Invest 98: 1063–1068.

23. Nagai Y, Miyata K, Sun GP, Rahman M, Kimura S, et al. (2005) Aldosterone stimulates collagen gene expression and synthesis via activation of ERK1/2 in rat renal fibroblasts. Hypertension 46: 1039–1045.

24. Haning R, Tait SA, Tait JF (1970) In vitro effects of ACTH, angiotensins, serotonin and potassium on steroid output and conversion of corticosterone to aldosterone by isolated adrenal cells. Endocrinology 87: 1147–1167.

25. Fujihara CK, Vieira JM, Jr., Sena CR, Ventura BH, Malheiros DM, et al. (2010) Early brief treatment with losartan plus mycophenolate mofetil provides lasting renoprotection in a renal ablation model. Am J Nephrol 32: 95–102.

26. Yamamoto M, Fukui M, Shou I, Wang LN, Sekizuka K, et al. (1997) Effects of treatment with angiotensin-converting enzyme inhibitor (ACEI) or angiotensin II receptor antagonist (AIIRA) on renal function and glomerular injury in subtotal nephrectomized rats. J Clin Lab Anal 11: 53–62.

27. Bidani AK, Griffin KA, Bakris G, Picken MM (2000) Lack of evidence of blood pressure-independent protection by renin-angiotensin system blockade after renal ablation. Kidney Int 57: 1651–1661.

28. Soto K, Gomez-Garre D, Largo R, Gallego-Delgado J, Tejera N, et al. (2004) Tight blood pressure control decreases apoptosis during renal damage. Kidney Int 65: 811–822.

29. Harris RC, Haralson MA, Badr KF (1992) Continuous stretch-relaxation in culture alters rat mesangial cell morphology, growth characteristics, and metabolic activity. Lab Invest 66: 548–554.

30. Riser BL, Cortes P, Heilig C, Grondin J, Ladson-Wofford S, et al. (1996) Cyclic stretching force selectively up-regulates transforming growth factor-beta isoforms in cultured rat mesangial cells. Am J Pathol 148: 1915–1923.

31. Riser BL, Varani J, Cortes P, Yee J, Dame M, et al. (2001) Cyclic stretching of mesangial cells up-regulates intercellular adhesion molecule-1 and leukocyte adherence: a possible new mechanism for glomerulosclerosis. Am J Pathol 158: 11–17.

32. Piecha G, Koleganova N, Gross ML, Geldyyev A, Adamczak M, et al. (2008) Regression of glomerulosclerosis in subtotally nephrectomized rats: effects of monotherapy with losartan, spironolactone, and their combination. Am J Physiol Renal Physiol 295: F137–144.

33. Aldigier JC, Kanjanbuch T, Ma LJ, Brown NJ, Fogo AB (2005) Regression of existing glomerulosclerosis by inhibition of aldosterone. J Am Soc Nephrol 16: 3306–3314.

34. Rozansky DJ, Cornwall T, Subramanya AR, Rogers S, Yang YF, et al. (2009) Aldosterone mediates activation of the thiazide-sensitive Na-Cl cotransporter through an SGK1 and WNK4 signaling pathway. J Clin Invest 119: 2601–2612.

35. Floege J, Burns MW, Alpers CE, Yoshimura A, Pritzl P, et al. (1992) Glomerular cell proliferation and PDGF expression precede glomerulosclerosis in the remnant kidney model. Kidney Int 41: 297–309.

36. Tang S, Leung JC, Abe K, Chan KW, Chan LY, et al. (2003) Albumin stimulates interleukin-8 expression in proximal tubular epithelial cells in vitro and in vivo. J Clin Invest 111: 515–527.

37. Takase O, Marumo T, Imai N, Hirahashi J, Takayanagi A, et al. (2005) NF-kappaB-dependent increase in intrarenal angiotensin II induced by proteinuria. Kidney Int 68: 464–473.

38. Stanton BA, Kaissling B (1988) Adaptation of distal tubule and collecting duct to increased Na delivery. II. Na+ and K+ transport. Am J Physiol 255: F1269–1275.

39. Vaziri ND (2006) Dyslipidemia of chronic renal failure: the nature, mechanisms, and potential consequences. Am J Physiol Renal Physiol 290: F262–272.

40. Wright JT, Jr., Harris-Haywood S, Pressel S, Barzilay J, Baimbridge C, et al. (2008) Clinical outcomes by race in hypertensive patients with and without the metabolic syndrome: Antihypertensive and Lipid-Lowering Treatment to Prevent Heart Attack Trial (ALLHAT). Arch Intern Med 168: 207–217.

41. Syrjanen J, Mustonen J, Pasternack A (2000) Hypertriglyceridaemia and hyperuricaemia are risk factors for progression of IgA nephropathy. Nephrol Dial Transplant 15: 34–42.

42. Reungjui S, Roncal CA, Mu W, Srinivas TR, Sirivongs D, et al. (2007) Thiazide diuretics exacerbate fructose-induced metabolic syndrome. J Am Soc Nephrol 18: 2724–2731.

43. Dussol B, Moussi-Frances J, Morange S, Somma-Delpero C, Mundler O, et al. (2012) A pilot study comparing furosemide and hydrochlorothiazide in patients with hypertension and stage 4 or 5 chronic kidney disease. J Clin Hypertens (Greenwich) 14: 32–37.

44. (2002) Major outcomes in high-risk hypertensive patients randomized to angiotensin-converting enzyme inhibitor or calcium channel blocker vs diuretic: The Antihypertensive and Lipid-Lowering Treatment to Prevent Heart Attack Trial (ALLHAT). JAMA 288: 2981–2997.

45. Dussol B, Moussi-Frances J, Morange S, Somma-Delpero C, Mundler O, et al. (2005) A randomized trial of furosemide vs hydrochlorothiazide in patients with chronic renal failure and hypertension. Nephrol Dial Transplant 20: 349–353.

3

Renal Function at Hospital Admission and Mortality due to Acute Kidney Injury after Myocardial Infarction

Rosana G. Bruetto[1], Fernando B. Rodrigues[2], Ulysses S. Torres[1], Ana P. Otaviano[3], Dirce M. T. Zanetta[4⑨], Emmanuel A. Burdmann[1*⑨¤]

1 Division of Nephrology, Hospital de Base, Sao Jose do Rio Preto Medical School (FAMERP), Sao Jose do Rio Preto, São Paulo, Brazil, 2 Department of Internal Medicine - Division of Emergency and Chest Pain Center, Hospital de Base, Sao Jose do Rio Preto Medical School (FAMERP), Sao Jose do Rio Preto, São Paulo, Brazil, 3 Division of Cardiology, Hospital de Base, Sao Jose do Rio Preto Medical School (FAMERP), Sao Jose do Rio Preto, São Paulo, Brazil, 4 Public Health School, University of São Paulo, São Paulo, Brazil

Abstract

Background: The role of an impaired estimated glomerular filtration rate (eGFR) at hospital admission in the outcome of acute kidney injury (AKI) after acute myocardial infarction (AMI) has been underreported. The aim of this study was to assess the influence of an admission eGFR<60 mL/min/1.73 m^2 on the incidence and early and late mortality of AMI-associated AKI.

Methods: A prospective study of 828 AMI patients was performed. AKI was defined as a serum creatinine increase of $\geq 50\%$ from the time of admission (RIFLE criteria) in the first 7 days of hospitalization. Patients were divided into subgroups according to their eGFR upon hospital admission (MDRD formula, mL/min/1.73 m^2) and the development of AKI: eGFR≥ 60 without AKI, eGFR<60 without AKI, eGFR≥ 60 with AKI and eGFR<60 with AKI.

Results: Overall, 14.6% of the patients in this study developed AKI. The admission eGFR had no impact on the incidence of AKI. However, the admission eGFR was associated with the outcome of AMI-associated AKI. The adjusted hazard ratios (AHR, Cox multivariate analysis) for 30-day mortality were 2.00 (95% CI 1.11–3.61) for eGFR<60 without AKI, 4.76 (95% CI 2.45–9.26) for eGFR≥ 60 with AKI and 6.27 (95% CI 3.20–12.29) for eGFR<60 with AKI. Only an admission eGFR of <60 with AKI was significantly associated with a 30-day to 1-year mortality hazard (AHR 3.05, 95% CI 1.50–6.19).

Conclusions: AKI development was associated with an increased early mortality hazard in AMI patients with either preserved or impaired admission eGFR. Only the association of impaired admission eGFR and AKI was associated with an increased hazard for late mortality among these patients.

Editor: Vineet Gupta, University of Pittsburgh Medical Center, United States of America

Funding: EAB is partially supported by grants from Foundation for the Support of Research in the State of São Paulo (Fundação de Amparo à Pesquisa do Estado de São Paulo, FAPESP), Brazil, and from the National Council for Scientific and Technological Development (Conselho Nacional de Desenvolvimento Científico e Tecnológico, CNPq), Brazil. RGB received a master's degree grant from Coordenação de Aperfeiçoamento de Pessoal de Nível Superior (CAPES), Brazil (process 0076/2007). UST received a young investigator award (process 2008/57115-6) from Foundation for the Support of Research in the State of São Paulo (Fundação de Amparo à Pesquisa do Estado de São Paulo, FAPESP). The funders had no role in study design, data collection and analysis, decision to publish, or preparation of the manuscript.

Competing Interests: The authors have declared that no competing interests exist.

* E-mail: burdmann@usp.br

⑨ These authors contributed equally to this work.

¤ Current address: Division of Nephrology, University of São Paulo Medical School, São Paulo, Brazil

Introduction

Recent North American and European epidemiological studies have shown that the incidence of acute kidney injury (AKI) is increasing at an alarming rate [1,2]. The development and validation of the new AKI diagnostic criteria, namely RIFLE (Risk, Injury, Failure, Loss, and End-Stage Kidney Disease) [3] and AKIN (Acute Kidney Injury Network) [4], were significant advancements in the study of the AKI syndrome and permit accurate comparisons among different studies. The RIFLE criteria [3] classify AKI into increasing levels of severity. The first level, Risk, is defined as an abrupt (within 1–7 days) and sustained

(>24 h) serum creatinine (SCr) increase of at least 1.5 from the reference SCr or a greater than 25% decrease in the glomerular filtration rate (GFR) compared to the reference GFR or a urine output of less than 0.5 mL/kg/h for more than 6 h.

Ischemic heart disease is the leading cause of death among adults in high-income countries and accounts for a substantial fraction of the total disease burden globally. AKI is an important and common complication after acute myocardial infarction (AMI), affecting from 10 to 55% of the patients (this latter number referring to patients suffering from cardiogenic shock) [5–7]. The development of AKI is associated with unfavorable outcomes and higher mortality after an AMI [5–10]. The mechanisms causing AKI in the first few days after an AMI are multifactorial, including systemic and renal hemodynamic changes secondary to an impaired cardiac output and an imbalance of vasodilators and vasoconstrictors, the use of contrast media, and immunological and inflammatory kidney damage resulting from crosstalk between the heart and the kidney [11].

The effect of pre-existing renal dysfunction on AKI mortality remains controversial and conflicting results have been published [12–16]. Similarly, very few studies have assessed the role of impaired estimated glomerular filtration rates (eGFRs) at hospital admission on the mortality of patients with AMI-associated AKI, and no studies have been explicitly designed to assess whether an impaired admission eGFR affects the prognosis of AMI-induced AKI as defined by the RIFLE criteria.

The purpose of this study was to evaluate the association of a decreased admission eGFR with the incidence and early and late mortality of patients developing AKI, as defined by the RIFLE criteria, in the acute phase of a myocardial infarction.

Results

Population characteristics

We evaluated 828 patients with a median age of 65 years (interquartile range: 54 to 74), 65.5% of whom were male. Our study population was composed of 7.7% black patients and 92.3% non-black patients. Overall, at the time of the study, 69% of the patients had a history of hypertension, 36.7% smoked, 25.7% were diabetic, 22.6% were dyslipidemic, 41.7% had previously used angiotensin-converting enzyme inhibitors (ACEIs)/angiotensin II receptor blockers (ARBs), 8.8% had prior percutaneous coronary intervention (PCI), 15.5% had been affected by prior coronary artery disease (CAD) with greater than 50% stenosis, 16.3% had suffered from prior infarction and 8.5% of the patients had previously undergone coronary artery bypass graft (CABG) surgery. The median SCr of patients upon hospital admission was 1.2 mg/dl (interquartile range: 1.0–1.5 mg/dL), and the admission median eGFR was 63.1 mL/min/1.73 m^2 (interquartile range: 47.5–81.3 mL/min/1.73 m^2).

The systolic left ventricular function (LVF) was measured in 709 patients and was classified as normal in 29.7%, mildly dysfunctional in 28.6%, moderately dysfunctional in 22.1% and severely dysfunctional in 19.6% of them. ST elevation myocardial infarction (STEMI) was diagnosed in 50.2% of the patients, 20.9% of whom presented with a Killip class >I and 54.5% of whom presented with an anterior wall infarction. The overall in-hospital mortality was 13.6%.

AKI incidence and mortality

AKI occurred in 121 (14.6%) of the patients, with 76 patients of these patients (9.2%) in the Risk category, 37 patients (4.5%) in the Injury category and 8 patients (1%) in the Failure category. The 30-day mortality rate was 38.8% (8.8% in the group without AKI, p<0.001), and the 30-day to 1-year mortality rate was 25.4% (13% in the group without AKI, p-value = 0.006).

Comparison between patients with impaired and non-impaired admission eGFRs

Patients with an impaired eGFR had a median admission SCr of 1.5 mg/dl (interquartile range: 1.3–1.8 mg/dL) and a median admission eGFR of 46.1 mL/min/1.73 m^2 (interquartile range: 36.7–52.8 mL/min/1.73 m^2). Patients with non-impaired eGFR had a median admission SCr of 1.0 mg/dL (interquartile range: 0.8–1.2 mg/dl) and a median admission eGFR of 79.2 mL/min/1.73 m^2 (interquartile range: 68.5–96.1 mL/min/1.73 m^2).

Among the study population, 46% had an admission eGFR<60 mL/min/1.73 m^2. When compared to the group of patients with an admission eGFR≥60 mL/min/1.73 m^2, this group was composed of a smaller proportion of men; was significantly older; and had a significantly increased prevalence of hypertension, diabetes, prior infarction, prior use of ACEIs/ARBs and previously documented CAD, PCI or CABG. A significantly higher number of patients with an admission eGFR≥60 mL/min/1.73 m^2 had an admission heart rate (HR) >100 beats/min and a systolic blood pressure (SBP) <100 mmHg. These patients were also more likely to have non-ST elevation myocardial infarction (NSTEMI). When presenting with STEMI, these patients exhibited a higher frequency of Killip class >I (Table 1).

Patients with an impaired admission eGFR were significantly less likely to receive β-blockers, ACEIs/ARBs, and clopidogrel and were more likely to receive diuretics. Additionally, they were significantly less likely to undergo coronary angiography, PCI, CABG or any revascularization interventions during their hospitalization than those with an admission eGFR≥60 mL/min/1.73 m^2. STEMI patients with an impaired admission eGFR were significantly less likely to receive thrombolytic treatment or any type of reperfusion therapy than subjects with an admission eGFR≥60 mL/min/1.73 m^2. There was no difference between the two groups in the thrombolysis in myocardial infarction (TIMI) 3 flow rate or in the favorable reperfusion criteria after reperfusion treatment (table 2).

Impaired admission eGFR had no impact on the incidence of AKI, which was similar between the two groups. Patients with an impaired admission eGFR were hospitalized significantly longer and had significantly greater 30-day and 30-day to 1-year mortality rates than those with an admission eGFR≥60 mL/min/1.73 m^2 (Table 2).

Comparison of demographic and clinical characteristics based on admission eGFR and the presence of AKI

Among the patients who had an admission eGFR≥60 mL/min/1.73 m^2, those who had AKI tended to be older (p<0.001), were more likely to have a HR>100 beats/min (p = 0.013) and were more likely to have a history of diabetes (p = 0.009). Among patients with admission eGFRs<60 mL/min/1.73 m^2, there were no significant differences between subgroups with and without AKI (Table 3).

Influence of admission eGFR and AKI on mortality—univariate analysis

Among the patients who did not develop AKI, an impaired admission eGFR was associated with significantly higher 30-day and 30-day to 1-year mortality rates compared to patients with an admission eGFR≥60 mL/min/1.73 m^2 (figures 1 and 2 and Table 4).

Among the patients who developed AKI, the 30-day mortality rate was similar between the groups with preserved or impaired admission eGFR. The 30 day to 1-year mortality rate was significantly higher in patients with an impaired admission eGFR and AKI compared to patients with an admission eGFR≥60 mL/min/1.73 m^2 and AKI (figures 1 and 2 and Table 4).

Influence of admission eGFR and AKI on mortality—Cox multivariate analyses

The association between mortality and impaired admission eGFR and/or AKI development was evaluated among the four groups.

Table 1. Comparison of admission characteristics upon hospitalization between patients with not-impaired or impaired admission eGFR.

Characteristics	Total Cohort (n = 828)	a-eGFR≥60 (n = 447)	a-eGFR<60 (n = 381)	p-value**
Age (y)	65 (54–74)	59 (49–71)	70 (61–75)	<0.001
Male	65.5%	72.0%	57.7%	<0.001
History of hypertension	69%	57.9%	81.9%	<0.001
Current smoker	36.7%	44.5%	27.6%	<0.001
History of diabetes	25.7%	19.2%	33.3%	<0.001
Previous PCI	8.8%	6.7%	11.3%	0.021
Previous CABG	8.5%	5.1%	12.3%	<0.001
Prior CAD (stenosis >50%)	15.5%	10.7%	21.0%	<0.001
Previous AMI	16.3%	12.3%	21.0%	0.001
Prior use of ACEI/ARB*	41.7%	31.1%	54.1%	<0.001
STEMI	50.2%	55.9%	43.6%	<0.001
aSBP<100 mm Hg†	6.3%	3.6%	9.5%	0.001
aHR (beats/min)	80 (70–95)	80 (70–92)	80 (70–100)	0.249
aHR >100 beats/min	16.5%	13.2%	20.5%	0.005
Killip class >1 ‡	20.9%	15.6%	28.9%	0.001

a-eGFR, admission estimated glomerular filtration rate (mL/min/1.73 m^2); PCI, percutaneous coronary intervention; CABG, coronary artery bypass graft; CAD, coronary artery disease; AMI, acute myocardial infarction; ACEI, angiotensin-converting enzyme inhibitors; ARB, angiotensin II receptor blockers; STEMI, ST elevation myocardial infarction; aSBP, admission systolic blood pressure; aHR, admission heart rate. Continuous variables are presented as median values (with interquartile ranges). Categorical variables are presented as percentages.
*n = 821 for the total cohort, n = 444 for a-eGFR≥60 mL/min/1.73 m^2, and n = 377 for a-eGFR<60 mL/min/1.73 m^2.
†n = 827 for the total cohort; n = 380 for a-eGFR<60 mL/min/1.73 m^2.
‡n = 416 (STEMI patients).
**comparison between eGFR≥60 and <60 mL/min/1.73 m^2.

Table 2. Comparison between patients with not impaired and impaired admission eGFR regarding treatment, incidence of AKI, length of hospitalization and mortality.

Variables	Total Cohort (n = 828)	a-eGFR≥60 (n = 447)	a-eGFR<60 (n = 381)	p-value
ß-blockers	93.5%	95.1%	91.6%	0.043
ACEI/ARB	97.2%	98.7%	95.5%	0.006
Diuretics	57.2%	48.5%	67.5%	<0.001
Clopidogrel	82.2%	85.7%	78.2%	0.005
Coronary angiography	82%	89.3%	73.5%	<0.001
PCI	49%	53.7%	43.6%	0.004
CABG	6.4%	8.5%	3.9%	0.007
Any revascularization*	55.2%	61.5%	47.8%	<0.001
Thrombolytic treatment	33.6%	40%	23%	<0.001
Primary PCI for STEMI	48.3%	47.6%	47.6%	0.998
Any reperfusion therapy†	81%	86.4%	69.9%	<0.001
TIMI 3 flow rate after reperfusion treatment	86.5%	83.7%	90.8%	0.131
Favorable reperfusion criteria	73%	76.5%	66.9%	0.064
Incidence of AKI	14.6%	13.4%	16.0%	0.293
Length of hospitalization (d)	7.43 (4.4–13.3)	6.9(4.3–12.2)	8.1(4.4–15.1)	0.014
30-day mortality	13.2%	8.9%	18.1%	<0.001
30-day to 1-year mortality	14.4%	8.5%	22.5%	<0.001

a-eGFR, estimated glomerular filtration rate upon admission (mL/min/1.73 m^2); PCI, percutaneous coronary intervention; CABG, coronary artery bypass graft; ACEI, angiotensin-converting enzyme inhibitors; ARB, angiotensin II receptor blockers. Continuous variables are presented as median values (with interquartile ranges). Categorical variables are presented as percentages.
*With PCI or CABG.
†With primary PCI or a thrombolytic.

Table 3. Comparison of demographic and clinical characteristics based on admission eGFR and AKI development.

Characteristics	admission eGFR≥60		admission eGFR<60		
	without AKI (n=387)	with AKI (n=60)	without AKI (n=320)	with AKI (n=61)	p-value
Age (y)	59 (48–70)	70 (55–78)*	69 (61–75)	72 (61–77)	<0.001
Male	73.1%	65.0%	57.8%	57.4%	<0.001
Hypertension	56.6%	66.7%	81.3%	85.2%	<0.001
Current smoker	45.7%	36.7%	26.9%	31.1%	<0.001
Diabetes	17.3%	31.7%†	32.2%	39.3%	<0.001
Previous PCI	6.2%	10.0%	12.5%	4.9%	0.019
Previous CABG	5.4%	3.3%	12.2%	13.1%	0.003
Prior CAD	10.9%	10.0%	20.9%	21.3%	0.001
Previous AMI	21.0%	13.3%	21.3%	19.7%	<0.009
Prior use of ACEIs/ARBs	29.9%	38.3%	54.7%	50.8%	<0.001
STEMI	55.0%	61.7%	41.3%	55.7%	<0.001
Admission SBP<100 mm Hg	2.8%	8.3%	8.2%	16.4%	<0.001
Admission HR ‡	80 (70–92)	86 (70–100)	80 (70–97)	88 (77–110)	0.047
Admission HR >100 ‡	11.6%	23.3%**	19.4%	26.2	0.002

eGFR, estimated glomerular filtration rate (mL/min/1.73 m²); PCI, percutaneous coronary intervention; CABG, coronary artery bypass graft; CAD, coronary artery disease; AMI, acute myocardial infarction; ACEI, angiotensin-converting enzyme inhibitors; ARB, angiotensin II receptor blockers; STEMI, ST elevation myocardial infarction; aSBP, systolic blood pressure; HR, heart rate. Continuous variables are presented as median values (with interquartile ranges) and were analyzed by the Kruskal-Wallis test followed by Dunn's post-test. Categorical variables are presented as percentages and were analyzed by χ^2 statistics with Bonferroni correction for post-test multiple comparisons.
*p<0.001,
†p=0.009,
**p=0.013, admission eGFR≥60, with AKI versus without AKI,
‡(beats/min).

30-day survival. An admission eGFR<60 mL/min/1.73 m² without AKI was associated with an adjusted hazard ratio (AHR) for death of 2.00 (95% CI 1.11–3.61). Patients with a non-impaired admission eGFR and AKI had a death AHR of 4.76 (95% CI 2.45–9.26). The patients with an impaired admission eGFR and AKI had the worst outcome with a mortality AHR of 6.27 (95% CI 3.20–12.29). The reference group was composed of patients with an admission eGFR≥60 mL/min/1.73 m² without AKI (figures 1 and 3 and table 5).

30-day to 1-year survival. The 30-day to 1-year survival rate was estimated for those patients who survived for 30 days after AMI. Neither an impaired admission eGFR without AKI nor a non-impaired admission eGFR with AKI were associated with late mortality. In contrast, an impaired admission eGFR with AKI was associated with a death AHR of 3.05 (95% CI 1.50–6.19) (figures 2 and 4 and table 6).

Discussion

Influence of admission eGFR on mortality due to AKI

Previous studies have demonstrated that either an impaired renal function at admission or the subsequent development of AKI negatively affects the outcome of patients suffering from an AMI [9,10,17,18]. However, none of the studies prospectively and

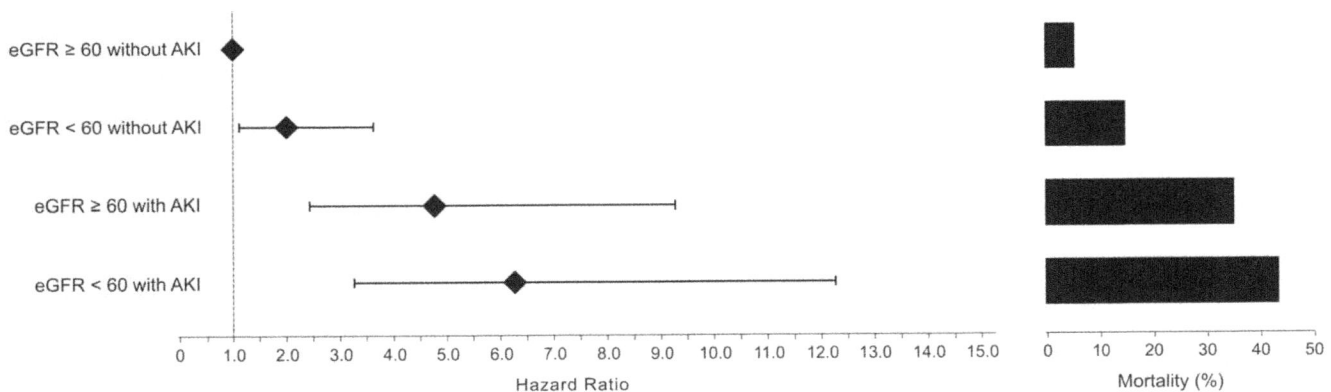

Figure 1. Hospital admission eGFR, AKI development and 30-day mortality rates after acute myocardial infarction. Hazard ratio (Cox multivariate analysis, left) and crude mortality (right).

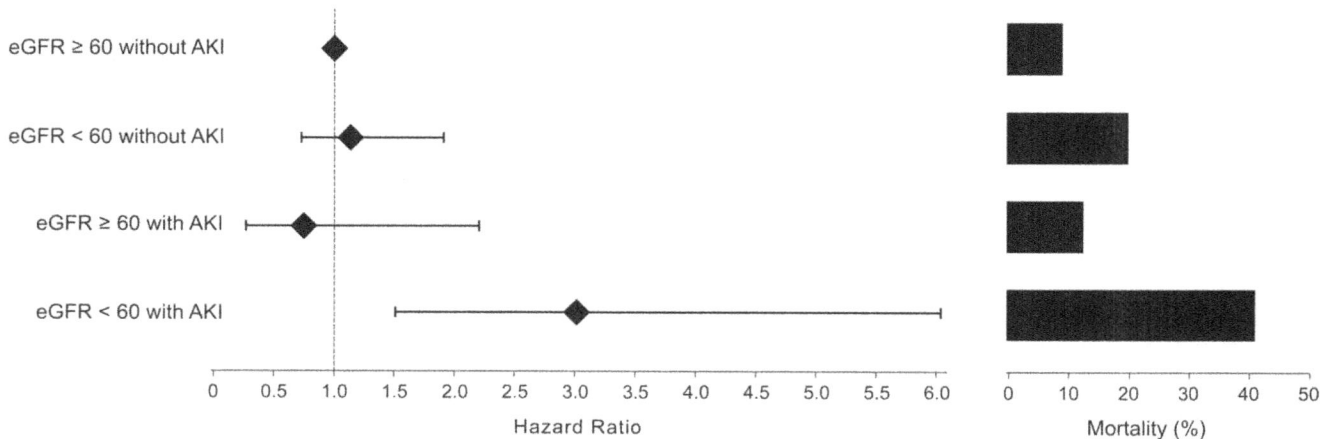

Figure 2. Hospital admission eGFR, AKI development and 30-day to 1-year mortality rates after acute myocardial infarction. Hazard ratio (Cox multivariate analysis, left) and crude mortality (right). Note that only the combination of an admission eGFR<60 mL/min/1.73 m^2 with AKI was associated with a higher late mortality. * 30-day to 1-year mortality rates were estimated for patients who survived for 30 days after AMI.

simultaneously assessed the role of an impaired admission eGFR and AKI development, as defined by RIFLE criteria, on the outcome of AMIs.

In this study, the use of Cox multivariate analysis clearly revealed that the development of AKI was the predominant factor associated with increased 30-day mortality, while an impaired admission eGFR was strikingly associated with an increased long-term mortality in patients with AMI-associated AKI. In fact, during the period from 30 days to one year after hospital admission, only the patients with an impaired admission eGFR and AKI had significantly lower survival rates. These results suggest that early mortality was largely related to the effects of AKI, while long-term outcomes were influenced by AKI development in addition to previously impaired renal function.

The factors leading to the remarkably higher mortality among patients with an impaired admission eGFR and AMI-associated AKI are not evident. One possible explanation for these poorer outcomes may be the combination of a powerful AKI-induced surge of inflammation along with the high prevalence of cardiovascular risk factors, such as older age, diabetes, hypertension and a pro-inflammatory milieu already present in the group of patients with impaired admission eGFR [11,19]. In addition, we observed differences in the AMI treatment received in the two groups; patients in the group with admission eGFRs<60 mL/min/1.73 m^2 were less likely to receive pharmacological therapy

or to undergo interventional procedures. Other authors have also observed that AMI patients with an impaired admission eGFR were offered less AMI treatment [20–23]. More severe cardiac disease was also associated with higher mortality in the current study. However, an association between an impaired admission eGFR and the development of AKI remained independently associated with a higher mortality hazard after controlling for variables possibly related to cardiac function, past history and treatment. Similarly, the overlap between impaired admission eGFR and AKI continued to be independently associated with a higher mortality hazard after correction for the characteristics that distinguish the group with impaired admission eGFRs from the rest of the patient groups.

A limited number of studies have assessed the role of admission eGFR on the outcome of AMI-associated AKI. A study on STEMI patients [5] revealed that AKI, arbitrarily defined as a creatinine elevation >0.5 mg/dL during hospitalization, was associated with increased 30-day and 1-year mortality rates. The study did not find any effect of the admission renal function on mortality due to AKI. It is important to note the differences between this study and our own. We used the RIFLE definition and a time frame of seven days for AKI diagnosis, and we compared the mortality data among the groups by a multivariate Cox proportional hazards regression. On the other hand, Goldberg et al. non-discriminately used an arbitrary absolute SCr

Table 4. Influence of impaired admission eGFR on 30-day and 30-day to 1-year mortality rates with and without AKI development (univariate analysis).

	a-eGFR≥60		a-eGFR<60		p-value
Mortality at day 30	n	% (n)	n	% (n)	
Without AKI	387	4.9% (19)	320	13.4% (43)	<0.001
With AKI	60	35% (21)	61	42.6% (26)	0.39
Mortality at 30-days to 1-year*	n	% (n)	n	% (n)	
Without AKI	308	8.1% (25)	217	19.8% (43)	<0.001
With AKI	35	11.4% (4)	32	40.6% (13)	0.006

a-eGFR, admission estimated glomerular filtration rate (mL/min/1.73 m^2); AKI, acute kidney injury.
*estimated for those surviving at day 30 and who had complete follow-ups for up to one year or death.

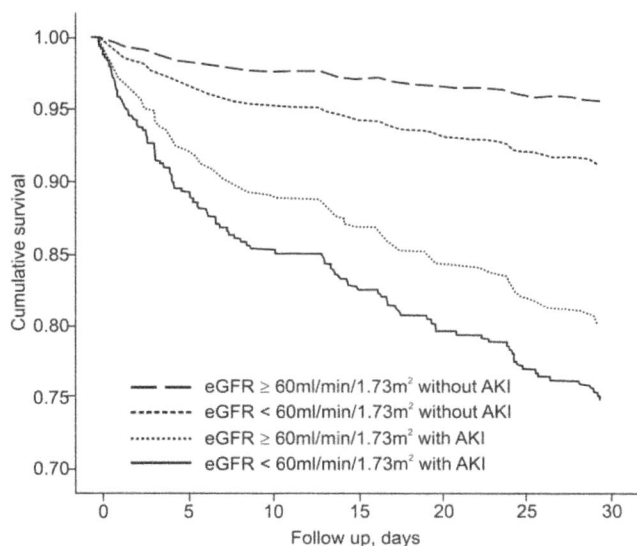

Figure 3. COX curve for 30-day survival among the four groups divided into admission eGFR and AKI development. Admission eGFR, estimated glomerular filtration rate upon admission (mL/min/1.73 m^2); AKI, acute kidney injury. For the comparison between admission eGFR≥60 without AKI and admission eGFR<60 without AKI, p = 0.020; between admission eGFR≥60 without AKI and admission eGFR≥60 with AKI, p<0.001; for admission eGFR≥60 without AKI and admission eGFR<60 with AKI, p<0.001.

Table 5. Cox proportional hazards model for 30-day mortality.

Groups	AHR (95% CI)	p-value
admission eGFR≥60 without AKI (n = 387)	1.0	
admission eGFR<60 without AKI (n = 320)	2.00 (1.11–3.61)	0.020
admission eGFR≥60 with AKI (n = 60)	4.76 (2.45–9.26)	<0.001
admission eGFR<60 with AKI (n = 61)	6.27 (3.20–12.29)	<0.001

eGFR, estimated glomerular filtration rate (mL/min/1.73 m^2); AKI, acute kidney injury; AHR, adjusted hazard ratio; CI, confidence interval.
The model was adjusted for age creatine phosphokinase-MB, and admission glycemia (categorized by quartiles with the first as a reference), gender (females were used as the reference), history of prior coronary artery bypass graft, ST elevation myocardial infarction, history of diabetes, history of hypertension, admission Killip class >I, systolic blood pressure <100 mmHg, admission heart rate >100 beats/min, clopidogrel use during hospitalization, use of diuretics, coronary angiography during hospitalization, reinfarction, severe systolic left ventricular dysfunction and any percutaneous coronary intervention performed during hospitalization.

increase during any time point of hospitalization for AKI diagnosis and compared the mortality by logistic regression. Another study [24] evaluating AMI patients showed that AKI, defined as a ≥25% decrease in eGFR at any point during hospitalization, was associated with a higher 1-year mortality rate. The authors used univariate analysis to assess the relationship between AKI and chronic kidney disease (CKD), diagnosed as an admission eGFR between 15 and 59 mL/min, and they concluded that AKI was a risk factor for 1-year mortality independent of admission eGFR. This conclusion must be taken with reservations because they did not control for any potential confounding variables in their analysis. Parikh et al. [6] examined the long-term mortality rate after post-MI AKI in a large cohort of patients. In a secondary analysis, the authors suggested that AKI in addition to CKD was associated with a lower risk of death compared to AKI without CKD. The inconsistency of these results with those of the present study could be due to the design differences between the two studies and to the limitations of the study by Parikh et al. [25]. We used RIFLE criteria during the first week of hospitalization to diagnose AKI, while Parikh et al. defined AKI by graded absolute changes in the serum creatinine at any point during hospitalization. As the authors acknowledged in their manuscript, "sicker patients are more likely to have longer hospitalizations and thus undergo more blood work and assessment of renal function, increasing the probability of detecting a change in serum creatinine level". Another important difference between ours and Parikh's studies is that we assessed data from 2004 to 2008 in a prospective database, and Parikh et al. used a retrospective database to assess patients hospitalized from 1994 to 1996. As they indicated in their manuscript, the treatment of AMI has substantially improved in the last decade. Further limitations that may affect their secondary analysis are acknowledged by the authors, including the high number of excluded patients (93,784–40% of the total cohort) and the lack of information concerning

the pharmacological treatment of these patients, making it impossible to control for these therapies in the Cox analysis, as was done in the present study. Finally, the left ventricular ejection fraction (a strong predictor of long-term survival after AMI) was unavailable in 39.4% of the non-AKI patients in this previous study.

Overall, studies regarding the prognostic effect of pre-existing renal dysfunction on mortality after AKI have reported conflicting results. Some reported a decrease in early mortality in patients with overlapping AKI and CKD compared to the controls in unselected cohorts of critically ill patients [26–28]. Conversely, a

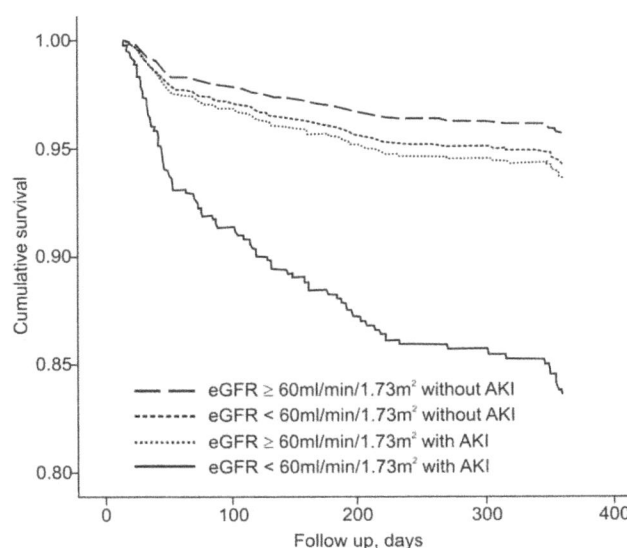

Figure 4. COX curve for 30-day to 1-year survival among the four groups divided into admission eGFR and AKI development. Admission eGFR, estimated glomerular filtration rate upon admission (mL/min/1.73 m^2); AKI, acute kidney injury. P = 0.002 for the comparison between admission eGFR≥60 without AKI and admission eGFR<60 with AKI, while the differences between the others groups with an admission eGFR≥60 without AKI were non-significant. * 30-day to 1-year mortality rates were estimated for patients who survived for 30 days after AMI.

Table 6. Cox proportional hazards model for 30-day to 1-year mortality*.

Groups	AHR (95% CI)	p-value
admission eGFR≥60 without AKI (n = 308)	1.0	
admission eGFR<60 without AKI (n = 217)	1.12 (0.65–1.89)	0.696
admission eGFR≥60 with AKI (n = 35)	0.75 (0.26–2.16)	0.588
admission eGFR<60 with AKI (n = 32)	3.05 (1.50–6.19)	0.002

*Estimated for patients who survived for 30 days after AMI.
eGFR, estimated glomerular filtration rate (mL/min/1.73 m²); AKI, acute kidney injury; AHR, adjusted hazard ratio; CI, confidence interval.
The model was adjusted for age, admission glycemia (categorized by quartiles with the first as a reference), gender (females were used as the reference), ST elevation myocardial infarction, history of diabetes, history of hypertension, prior use of angiotensin-converting enzyme inhibitors or angiotensin II receptor blockers, admission Killip class >I, admission heart rate >100 beats/min, clopidogrel use during hospitalization, diuretics use, coronary angiography during hospitalization, reinfarction, severe systolic left ventricular dysfunction and any percutaneous coronary intervention performed during hospitalization.

study by Kolli et al, assessing 1,359 cardiac surgery patients [13] showed that an impaired admission eGFR (<60 mL/min) was associated with a higher mortality rate in patients who developed AKI. Similarly, a study by Wu et al, which analyzed a very large cohort of patients who developed postoperative AKI showed that those patients with previous CKD had a higher risk of long-term mortality than the patients without CKD [16]. Recently, an interesting and elegant experimental study by Skott et al, showed that even mild CKD led to an increased mortality rate in a rodent model of AKI and multiple organ failure [14].

Influence of admission eGFR on the incidence of AKI

In this study, there was no difference in the incidence of AKI between patients with an admission eGFR<60 mL/min or an eGFR≥60 mL/min. Similarly, Lombardi et al. [29] studied 1,749 patients after cardiac surgery and found no difference in the rates of AKI development (41.9 versus 43.4%, respectively) between patients with an admission eGFR<60 or an eGFR≥60 mL/min. Other studies have reported an association between pre-existing CKD and AKI development [5,30]. It is unclear whether this association exists as a true primary cause-and-effect relationship or if this association is due to confounding secondary comorbidities that are associated with CKD, the increased exposure of this population to nephrotoxic insults or the study bias. In fact, most of the studies correlating increased AKI incidence with previous CKD utilized a retrospective design with methodological short-comings, including improper adjustments for comorbidities in multivariate analyses. Furthermore, these studies often lack a standardized protocol for the diagnosis of CKD and AKI.

Although not assessed in the present study, proteinuria, a marker of renal injury, has been recently identified as an important risk factor for the development of AKI in various situations, such as following cardiac surgery [31–35].

Study limitations

This was a single-center observational prospective cohort study.

Systolic left ventricular function as assessed by echocardiography was not always determined by the same observer.

The present study cannot be used to determine the effect of CKD on the incidence and mortality of AKI because the definition of CKD [36] requires the documentation of kidney damage for three or more months. This time assessment is obviously difficult to obtain in this type of study, as most patients have not undergone a renal function evaluation prior to their admission for an acute illness.

AKI incidence was probable underestimated. The reference SCr used for AKI diagnosis was the one obtained at the hospital admission. It is likely that some patients were hospitalized already with AKI, but because there was no SCr increase from the reference SCr during the hospital stay, they were misdiagnosed as non-AKI.

Finally, SCr measurements were performed on a clinical need basis after discharge from the intensive care unit, which could also lead to an underestimation of the incidence of AKI.

Conclusions

AKI development was negatively associated with the early outcomes of AMI in patients with either non-impaired or impaired admission eGFR. On the other hand, the presence of a low admission eGFR in patients with acute myocardial infarction-associated AKI was clearly associated with a significantly poorer long-term prognosis. Additionally, this study confirmed, using RIFLE criteria that AKI development in AMI patients is frequent and is associated with a high mortality rate.

These results strongly suggest that patients with an impaired admission eGFR should have their renal function monitored closely after an acute myocardial infarction. Clinical measures for the prevention and early diagnosis of AKI must be taken to potentially increase the survival rates of these patients. Moreover, patients with an impaired admission eGFR who develop AKI must have an extremely careful and detailed long-term follow-up to try to avoid the poor long-term outcomes described in this study.

Methods

Ethics statement

The study protocol was approved by the Institutional Ethics Committee on September 21, 2009 ("Comitê de Ética em Pesquisa em Seres Humanos da Faculdade de Medicina de Sao José do Rio Preto", Sao José do Rio Preto, Brazil, process 4988/2009), who agreed that informed consent was unnecessary due to the purely observational and non-interventional nature of this study ("Resolução CNS 196/96").

Patients

A total of 1,012 consecutive patients (October 2004–December 2008) with a STEMI or with a NSTEMI [37] were assessed using a prospective database on thoracic pain from a single center.

Among the 1,012 patients, 184 were not included in the study because they met the following exclusion criteria: admission SCr≥6.0 mg/dL, admission eGFR<15.0 mL/min/1.73 m² or chronic dialysis (21 patients); death within 48 hours of admission (49 patients); lack of at least two SCr measurements in the first seven days of hospitalization (94 patients); obstructive AKI (3 patients); and a hospital stay <48 hours (17 patients).

Only the first hospital admission was considered if a patient had more than one hospitalization for AMI during the study period.

Systolic left ventricular function

Systolic left ventricular function was classified as either normal function or mild, moderate or severe dysfunction and was assessed by echocardiography (based on medical need) in 85.6% of the patients [38].

SCr measurements, eGFR calculation and diagnostic criteria for AKI

The SCr level was obtained at the time of hospital admission and daily during the intensive care unit (ICU) stay. After ICU discharge, the SCr was measured as needed. The SCr was assessed using the Jaffé colorimetric method (ADVIA™ 1650, Bayer, Germany).

The admission eGFR was assessed by the Modification of Diet in Renal Disease (MDRD) formula [39] (mL/min/1.73 m^2): GFR = 186.3×SCr$^{-1.154}$ * age$^{-0.203}$ * 1.212 (if patient is black) * 0.742 (if female). It should be noted that this equation was not specifically validated for this study population.

Patients were divided into 4 subgroups:

admission eGFR≥60 without AKI

admission eGFR<60 without AKI

admission eGFR≥60 with AKI

admission eGFR<60 with AKI

Patients were diagnosed with AKI if they had a SCr increase of ≥1.5-fold over the admission value within the first seven days of hospitalization (RIFLE criteria, stage Risk). The RIFLE criteria definition of AKI using urinary output (<0.5 mL/kg for 6 h for Risk) was not used in this study [40].

Outcomes

The primary endpoints were death from any cause within 30 days and 30-day to 1-year mortality for those patients who survived after 30 days. Patient follow-up after discharge was conducted either by an electronic hospital system records review or by mail or telephone contact of patients.

Statistical Analysis

Patients were categorized based on their admission eGFR (<60 or ≥60 mL/min/1.73 m^2) and on whether they developed AKI during their hospitalization. The demographics and clinical characteristics (presented as median values with interquartile ranges) were compared by the Student's t-test, Mann-Whitney test or Kruskal-Wallis test followed by Dunn's post-test for continuous variables. The categorical variables (presented as numbers and percentages) were compared using either χ^2 statistics or Fisher's exact test. Bonferroni corrections were used for post-test multiple comparisons.

Separate analyses were performed on the 30-day mortality rates after the onset of AMI (n = 828) and on the 30-day to 1-year

mortality rates for those patients (n = 699) who survived past day 30. Patients who had been part of the follow-up period for less than one year were not included (n = 107) in the descriptive and univariate analyses of the mortality rates at that time point.

We performed multivariate Cox proportional hazards regression analyses to evaluate the two mortality periods. The association between mortality and admission eGFR and AKI development in the four subgroups in which patients were divided was evaluated, controlling for clinically important variables and for variables with a p-value<0.15 in the univariate analyses of mortality in each period. The proportional hazards test and the plotted cumulative survival estimate after the ln (-ln) transformation suggested that the hazards of these variables were proportional for the period analyzed.

In the first period of multivariate Cox proportional hazards regression analysis, the follow-up was censored at day-30 and was adjusted for age, creatine phosphokinase MB (CPK-MB) and admission glycemia (categorized by quartiles with the first as a reference), gender (females were used as the reference), history of prior CABG, STEMI, history of diabetes, history of hypertension, admission Killip class >I, SBP<100 mmHg, admission HR >100 beat/min, clopidogrel use during the hospitalization, use of diuretics, coronary angiography during the hospitalization, reinfarction, severe systolic left ventricular dysfunction (LVD) and any PCI performed during the hospitalization.

The multivariate Cox proportional hazards regression analysis of 30-day to 1-year mortality rates included all patients who survived for 30 days after AMI with censoring at 365 days. The controlling variables were the same used for the 30-day analysis with the exception of CPK-MB, history of prior CABG, SBP<100 mmHg and reinfarction. The prior use of ACEIs or ARBs was also controlled in this analysis.

Differences were considered statistically significant by a two-tailed p-value<0.05 and a confidence interval (CI) of 95%.

Analyses were performed with SPSS statistical software (version 15.0, Chicago, IL, USA).

Author Contributions

Conceived and designed the experiments: EAB RGB FBR. Performed the experiments: EAB RGB FBR UST APO DMTZ. Analyzed the data: EAB RGB FBR DMTZ. Contributed reagents/materials/analysis tools: EAB RGB FBR DMTZ. Wrote the paper: EAB RGB FBR UST APO DMTZ.

References

1. Ali T, Khan I, Simpson W, Prescott G, Townend J, et al. (2007) Incidence and outcomes in acute kidney injury: a comprehensive population-based study. J Am Soc Nephrol 18: 1292–1298.
2. Collins AJ, Foley RN, Herzog C, Chavers B, Gilbertson D, et al. (2009) United States Renal Data System 2008 Annual Data Report. Am J Kidney Dis 57: S1–374.
3. Hoste EA, Clermont G, Kersten A, Venkataraman R, Angus DC, et al. (2006) RIFLE criteria for acute kidney injury are associated with hospital mortality in critically ill patients: a cohort analysis. Crit Care 10: R73.
4. Mehta RL, Kellum JA, Shah SV, Molitoris BA, Ronco C, et al. (2007) Acute Kidney Injury Network: report of an initiative to improve outcomes in acute kidney injury. Crit Care 11: R31.
5. Goldberg A, Hammerman H, Petcherski S, Zdorovyak A, Yalonetsky S, et al. (2005) Inhospital and 1-year mortality of patients who develop worsening renal function following acute ST-elevation myocardial infarction. Am Heart J 150: 330–337.
6. Parikh CR, Coca SG, Wang Y, Masoudi FA, Krumholz HM (2008) Long-term prognosis of acute kidney injury after acute myocardial infarction. Arch Intern Med 168: 987–995.
7. Marenzi G, Assanelli E, Campodonico J, De Metrio M, Lauri G, et al. (2010) Acute kidney injury in ST-segment elevation acute myocardial infarction complicated by cardiogenic shock at admission. Crit Care Med 38: 438–444.
8. Newsome BB, Warnock DG, McClellan WM, Herzog CA, Kiefe CI, et al. (2008) Long-term risk of mortality and end-stage renal disease among the elderly after small increases in serum creatinine level during hospitalization for acute myocardial infarction. Arch Intern Med 168: 609–616.
9. Goldberg A, Kogan E, Hammerman H, Markiewicz W, Aronson D (2009) The impact of transient and persistent acute kidney injury on long-term outcomes after acute myocardial infarction. Kidney Int 76: 900–906.
10. Amin AP, Spertus JA, Reid KJ, Lan X, Buchanan DM, et al. (2010) The prognostic importance of worsening renal function during an acute myocardial infarction on long-term mortality. Am Heart J 160: 1065–1071.
11. Ronco C, Haapio M, House AA, Anavekar N, Bellomo R (2008) Cardiorenal syndrome. J Am Coll Cardiol 52: 1527–1539.
12. Khosla N, Soroko SB, Chertow GM, Himmelfarb J, Ikizler TA, et al. (2009) Preexisting chronic kidney disease: a potential for improved outcomes from acute kidney injury. Clin J Am Soc Nephrol 4: 1914–1919.
13. Kolli H, Rajagopalam S, Patel N, Ranjan R, Venuto R, et al. (2010) Mild acute kidney injury is associated with increased mortality after cardiac surgery in patients with eGFR<60 mL/min/1.73 m^2. Ren Fail 32: 1066–1072.
14. Skott M, Norregaard R, Sorensen HB, Kwon TH, Frokiaer J, et al. (2010) Pre-existing renal failure worsens the outcome after intestinal ischaemia and reperfusion in rats. Nephrol Dial Transplant 25: 3509–3517.

15. Ishani A, Xue JL, Himmelfarb J, Eggers PW, Kimmel PL, et al. (2009) Acute kidney injury increases risk of ESRD among elderly. J Am Soc Nephrol 20: 223–228.

16. Wu VC, Huang TM, Lai CF, Shiao CC, Lin YF, et al. (2011) Acute-on-chronic kidney injury at hospital discharge is associated with long-term dialysis and mortality. Kidney Int 80: 1222–1230.

17. Goldenberg I, Subirana I, Boyko V, Vila J, Elosua R, et al. (2010) Relation between renal function and outcomes in patients with non-ST-segment elevation acute coronary syndrome: real-world data from the European Public Health Outcome Research and Indicators Collection Project. Arch Intern Med 170: 888–895.

18. Szummer K, Lundman P, Jacobson S, Schön S, Lindbäck J, et al. (2010) Relation between renal function, presentation, use of therapies and in-hospital complications in acute coronary syndrome: data from the SWEDEHEART register. J Intern Med 268: 40–49.

19. Sarnak MJ, Levey AS, Schoolwerth AC, Coresh J, Culleton B (2003) Kidney disease as a risk factor for development of cardiovascular disease: a statement from the American Heart Association Councils on Kidney in Cardiovascular Disease, High Blood Pressure Research, Clinical Cardiology, and Epidemiology and Prevention. Hypertension 42: 1050–1065.

20. Rodrigues F, Bruetto R, Torres U, Otaviano A, Zanetta D, et al. (2010) Effect of kidney disease on acute coronary syndrome. Clin J Am Soc Nephrol 5: 1530–1536.

21. Shlipak MG, Heidenreich PA, Noguchi H, Chertow GM, Browner WS, et al. (2002) Association of renal insufficiency with treatment and outcomes after myocardial infarction in elderly patients. Ann Intern Med 137: 555–562.

22. Reddan DN, Szczech L, Bhapkar MV, Moliterno DJ, Califf RM, et al. (2005) Renal function, concomitant medication use and outcomes following acute coronary syndromes. Nephrol Dial Transplant 20: 2105–2112.

23. Inrig JK, Patel UD, Briley LP, She L, Gillespie BS, et al. (2008) Mortality, kidney disease and cardiac procedures following acute coronary syndrome. Nephrol Dial Transplant 23: 934–940.

24. Lazaros G, Tsiachris D, Tousoulis D, Patialiakas A, Dimitriadis K, et al. (2012) In-hospital worsening renal function is an independent predictor of one-year mortality in patients with acute myocardial infarction. Int J Cardiol 155: 97–101.

25. Bouzas-Mosquera A, Vazquez-Rodriguez JM, Peteiro J, Alvarez-Garcia N (2009) Acute kidney injury and long-term prognosis after acute myocardial infarction. Arch Intern Med 169: 87.

26. Waikar SS, Curhan GC, Wald R, McCarthy EP, Chertow GM (2006) Declining mortality in patients with acute renal failure, 1988 to 2002. J Am Soc Nephrol 17: 1143–1150.

27. Chertow GM, Christiansen CL, Cleary PD, Munro C, Lazarus JM (1995) Prognostic stratification in critically ill patients with acute renal failure requiring dialysis. Arch Intern Med 155: 1505–1511.

28. Waikar SS, Liu KD, Chertow GM (2008) Diagnosis, epidemiology and outcomes of acute kidney injury. Clin J Am Soc Nephrol 3: 844–861.

29. Lombardi R, Ferreiro A (2008) Risk factors profile for acute kidney injury after cardiac surgery is different according to the level of baseline renal function. Ren Fail 30: 155–160.

30. Singh P, Rifkin DE, Blantz RC (2010) Chronic kidney disease: an inherent risk factor for acute kidney injury? Clin J Am Soc Nephrol 5: 1690–1695.

31. Grams ME, Astor BC, Bash LD, Matsushita K, Wang Y, et al. (2010) Albuminuria and estimated glomerular filtration rate independently associate with acute kidney injury. J Am Soc Nephrol 21: 1757–1764.

32. James MT, Hemmelgarn BR, Wiebe N, Pannu N, Manns BJ, et al. (2010) Glomerular filtration rate, proteinuria, and the incidence and consequences of acute kidney injury: a cohort study. Lancet 376: 2096–2103.

33. Doi K, Negishi K, Ishizu T, Katagiri D, Fujita T, et al. (2011) Evaluation of new acute kidney injury biomarkers in a mixed intensive care unit. Crit Care Med 39: 2464–2469.

34. Huang TM, Wu VC, Young GH, Lin YF, Shiao CC, et al. (2011) Preoperative proteinuria predicts adverse renal outcomes after coronary artery bypass grafting. J Am Soc Nephrol 22: 156–163.

35. Coca SG, Jammalamadaka D, Sint K, Thiessen Philbrook H, Shlipak MG, et al. (2012) Preoperative proteinuria predicts acute kidney injury in patients undergoing cardiac surgery. J Thorac Cardiovasc Surg 143: 495–502.

36. Levey AS, Eckardt KU, Tsukamoto Y, Levin A, Coresh J, et al. (2005) Definition and classification of chronic kidney disease: a position statement from Kidney Disease: Improving Global Outcomes (KDIGO). Kidney Int 67: 2089–2100.

37. Thygesen K, Alpert JS, White HD (2007) Universal definition of myocardial infarction. J Am Coll Cardiol 50: 2173–2195.

38. Cheitlin MD, Alpert JS, Armstrong WF, Aurigemma GP, Beller GA, et al. (1997) ACC/AHA guidelines for the clinical application of echocardiography: executive summary. A report of the American College of Cardiology/American Heart Association Task Force on practice guidelines (Committee on Clinical Application of Echocardiography). Developed in collaboration with the American Society of Echocardiography. J Am Coll Cardiol 29: 862–879.

39. Levey A, Bosch J, Lewis J, Greene T, Rogers N, et al. (1999) A more accurate method to estimate glomerular filtration rate from serum creatinine: a new prediction equation. Modification of Diet in Renal Disease Study Group. Ann Intern Med 130: 461–470.

40. Bellomo R, Ronco C, Kellum JA, Mehta RL, Palevsky P (2004) Acute renal failure - definition, outcome measures, animal models, fluid therapy and information technology needs: the Second International Consensus Conference of the Acute Dialysis Quality Initiative (ADQI) Group. Crit Care 8: R204–212.

4

Immunosuppressive Treatment for Nephrotic Idiopathic Membranous Nephropathy

Guoqiang Xie⁹, Jing Xu⁹, Chaoyang Ye⁹, Dongping Chen, Chenggang Xu, Li Yang, Yiyi Ma, Xiaohong Hu, Lin Li, Lijun Sun, Xuezhi Zhao, Zhiguo Mao*, Changlin Mei*

Kidney Institute of CPLA, Division of Nephrology, Changzheng Hospital, Second Military Medical University, Shanghai, China

Abstract

Background: Idiopathic membranous nephropathy (IMN) is the most common pathological type for nephrotic syndrome in adults in western countries and China. The benefits and harms of immunosuppressive treatment in IMN remain controversial.

Objectives: To assess the efficacy and safety of different immunosuppressive agents in the treatment of nephrotic syndrome caused by IMN.

Methods: PubMed, EMBASE, Cochrane Library and *wanfang, weipu, qinghuatongfang,* were searched for relevant studies published before December 2011. Reference lists of nephrology textbooks, review articles were checked. A meta-analysis of randomized controlled trials (RCTs) meeting the criteria was performed using Review Manager.

Main Results: 17 studies were included, involving 696 patients. Calcineurin inhibitors had a better effect when compared to alkylating agents, on complete remission (RR 1.61, 95% CI 1.13, to 2.30 P = 0.008), partial or complete remission (effective) (CR/PR, RR 1.29, 95% CI 1.09 to 1.52 P = 0.003), and fewer side effects. Among calcineurin inhibitors, tacrolimus (TAC) was shown statistical significance in inducing more remissions. When compared to cyclophosphamide (CTX), leflunomide (LET) showed no beneficial effect, mycophenolate mofetil (MMF) showed significant beneficial on effectiveness (CR/PR, RR: 1.41, 95% CI 1.16 to 1.72 P = 0.0006) but not significant on complete remission (CR, RR: 1.38, 95% CI 0.89 to 2.13 P = 0.15).

Conclusions: This analysis based on Chinese adults and short duration RCTs suggested calcineurin inhibitors, especially TAC, were more effective in proteinuria reduction in IMN with acceptable side effects. Long duration RCTs were needed to confirm the long-term effects of those agents in nephrotic IMN.

Editor: Krisztian Stadler, Pennington Biomedical Research Center, United States of America

Funding: This work was supported by Shanghai Higher Education Outstanding Young Teacher Scientific Research Special Fund, Shanghai Municipal Education Commission; Outstanding Young Scholars project, Second Military Medical University; Medical Educational Reforming and Research Grant of Changzheng Hospital. This work was funded in part by the National Nature Science Fund of China (81000281). The funders had no role in study design, data collection and analysis, decision to publish, or preparation of the manuscript.

Competing Interests: The authors have declared that no competing interests exist.

* E-mail: chlmei1954@126.com (CM); maozhiguo93@gmail.com (ZM)

⁹ These authors contributed equally to this work.

Introduction

Idiopathic membranous nephropathy (IMN) is the most common cause of nephrotic syndrome for adults in western counties, as well as in China. Although 30% patients showed spontaneous complete or partial remission of nephrotic syndrome [1], 30–40% of patients progress toward end-stage renal disease (ESRD) within 5–15 years [2].

A meta-analysis [3] included 18 worldwide RCTS have been made to assess the effects and safety of immunosuppressive treatment of nephrotic idiopathic membranous nephropathy (IMN) in 2004, glucocorticoids improved proteinuria but did not induce remission. Combined corticosteroids with cytotoxic agents showed effectiveness to nephrotic IMN patients in many trials [4–7] and was considered a standard treatment.

Immunosuppressive treatment has been widely used in the treatment of IMN worldwide. However, there are still big controversies over the efficacy and safety of different immunosuppressive agents treatments in IMN, especially for those relatively new agents like, tacrolimus (TAC) and leflunomide (LET). So a meta-analysis comparing the efficacy and safety of different immunosuppressive agents in the treatment of Chinese adults with nephrotic IMN makes sense. China is the country with largest population of the world. To exclude the interferences caused by the ethnic variety, this meta-analysis was made on Chinese adults base.

Methods

Information Sources and Search Strategy

We tried to include all the RCTs that assess the efficacy and tolerability associated with the comparison of different immunosuppressive agents for the treatment of Chinese adults with nephrotic IMN. PubMed (up to December 2011), EMBASE (1980 to December 2011), and Cochrane Library (Issue12, 2011) and the databases in Chinese including *wanfang, weipu, qinghuatongfang* (up to December 2011) were searched, and reference lists of nephrology textbooks, review articles were checked.

Inclusion Criteria

1. Prospective RCTs compared different immunosuppressive agents.
2. The selected patients were Chinese adults suffering from IMN, aged 16 years or older, with nephrotic syndrome.
3. The diagnosis of IMN was made by renal needle biopsy.

Exclusion Criteria

1. Study design without randomization, own control or compared with different usage of the same agent.
2. Secondary types of membranous nephropathy or not Chinese patients.
3. Trials including the use of traditional Chinese medicine were excluded,for its unknown additional effects on immunosuppressive agents and uncertain dose of active components. We also excluded studies where it was impossible to identify how many patients had nephrotic syndrome, after checking the baseline evaluations and contacting with the authors.

Study Selection

Two reviewers(G. Xie and J. Xu) independently assessed the eligibility of each article to be included in this meta-analysis, and this work was checked by another author (Z. Mao).

Data Collection Process and Data Items

Data were extracted from each identified trial by two researchers (G. Xie and J. Xu) with a predesigned review form (Microsoft Office Excel 2007) independently, and any disagreement was resolved by discussion. Authors of the original studies were consulted through emails for suggestions if any problem occurred.

The following data were included: the authors of each study, the year of publication, the design of the trial, the duration of the study, the sample size, the age and gender of the patients, the interventions (mainly immunosuppressive agents, dose and usage), the baseline proteinuria/serum creatinine/serum albumin values, the final proteinuria/serum creatinine/serum albumin values, and the therapeutic remission of participants (complete remission, partial remission). In addition, we retrieval the side effects including elevated liver enzymes, renal toxicity, infections, digestive symptoms, leukocytopenia, and other recorded.

Risk of Bias

The quality of included studies were evaluated by two authors (C Ye and D Chen) independently based on the standard criteria (randomization, blinding, and loss to follow-up)using the scoring system developed by Jadad [8]. The quality scoring system was as follows: (1) Was the study described as randomized? (2 = Properly with detailed description of randomization, 1 = randomized but detail not reported); (2) Was the blind method used? (2 = Double-blind, 1 = single-blind, 0 = open-label); (3) Were dropout and follow-up reported? (1 = Numbers and reasons reported, 0 = not reported). The publication bias was assessed by examining the funnel plot. A sensitivity analysis was performed by omitting low quality studies and investigating the influence on the overall meta-analysis estimate.

Data Analysis and Statistical Methods

Statistical analyses were performed with Review Managerver 5.0.20 (Cochrane Collaboration, Oxford, UK). We assessed the heterogeneity of the trial results by calculating a chi-square test of heterogeneity and the I^2 measure of inconsistency. Dichotomous data were summarized as risk ratio (RR) and 95% confidence intervals (CIs), continuous ones (final proteinuria) as weighted mean difference (WMD) and 95% CIs as well.

The Flowchart of this meta-analysis was shown in Figure 1.

Results

Study Characteristics

All included trials were prospective RCTs, 3 [9–11] were published in English and 14 were published in Chinese. The included studies involved 696 patients. Only one study [11] used blindness and it is the only one published as conference abstract without full text. In 15 of 17 studies, cyclophosphamide(CTX) was involved in the comparison. 6 studies compared MMF with alkylating agents, 5 of them with CTX, the other one with chlorambucil. 7 studies compared calcineurin inhibitors with alkylating agents (only CTX). 3 studies compared leflunomide (LET) with CTX. 1 study compared LET with TAC. Characteristics of the included trials are shown in Table 1.

Effects of Interventions

Calcineurin inhibitors versus alkylating agents. Seven trials [10–16] involving 282patients compared calcineurin inhibitors with alkylating agents, 5 [10–13,15] for comparing TAC with CTX, 2 [14,16] for comparing CyA with CTX. Calcineurin inhibitors showed statistically significant higher rate on inducing remission, on complete remission (CR, RR: 1.61, 95% CI 1.13 to 2.30, P = 0.008) figure 2.1, on complete/partial remission (CR/PR, RR: 1.29, 95% CI 1.09 to 1.52, P = 0.003) figure 2.2.

Comparison of Two Agents

MMF versus CTX. 5 studies [17–21] involving 224 patients compared MMF with CTX. MMF was given at 1.0–2.0 g/d orally for the first period (3 to 6 months), and then gradually tapered. Immunosuppressive treatment lasted for 12 months. MMF showed significant benefit on effectiveness (CR/PR, RR: 1.41, 95% CI 1.16 to 1.72, P = 0.0006) figure 3.2 but no significant on complete remission (CR, RR: 1.38, 95% CI 0.89 to 2.13, P = 0.15) [figure 3.1].

TAC versus CTX. 5 studies [10–13,15] involving 166 patients compared TAC with CTX. TAC was given at 0.1 mg/kg/d initially and adjusted to a blood trough concentration level at 5 to 10 ng/mL for the first period (mostly 6 months), then reduced. TAC induced more remission than CTX (CR, RR 1.75, 95% CI 1.12 to 2.72, P = 0.01; CR/PR, RR 1.22, 95% CI 1.00 to 1.48, P = 0.01) (figure 2), with lower final proteinuria (WMD 1.12, 95% CI 0.53 to 1.71).

LET versus CTX. 3 studies [22–24] involving 150 patients compared LET with CTX. LET was given orally 50 mg/d for 3 days, followed by 20–30 mg/d for 3 months, and then tapered. LET showed no benefit in inducing remissions compared to

PRISMA 2009 Flow Diagram

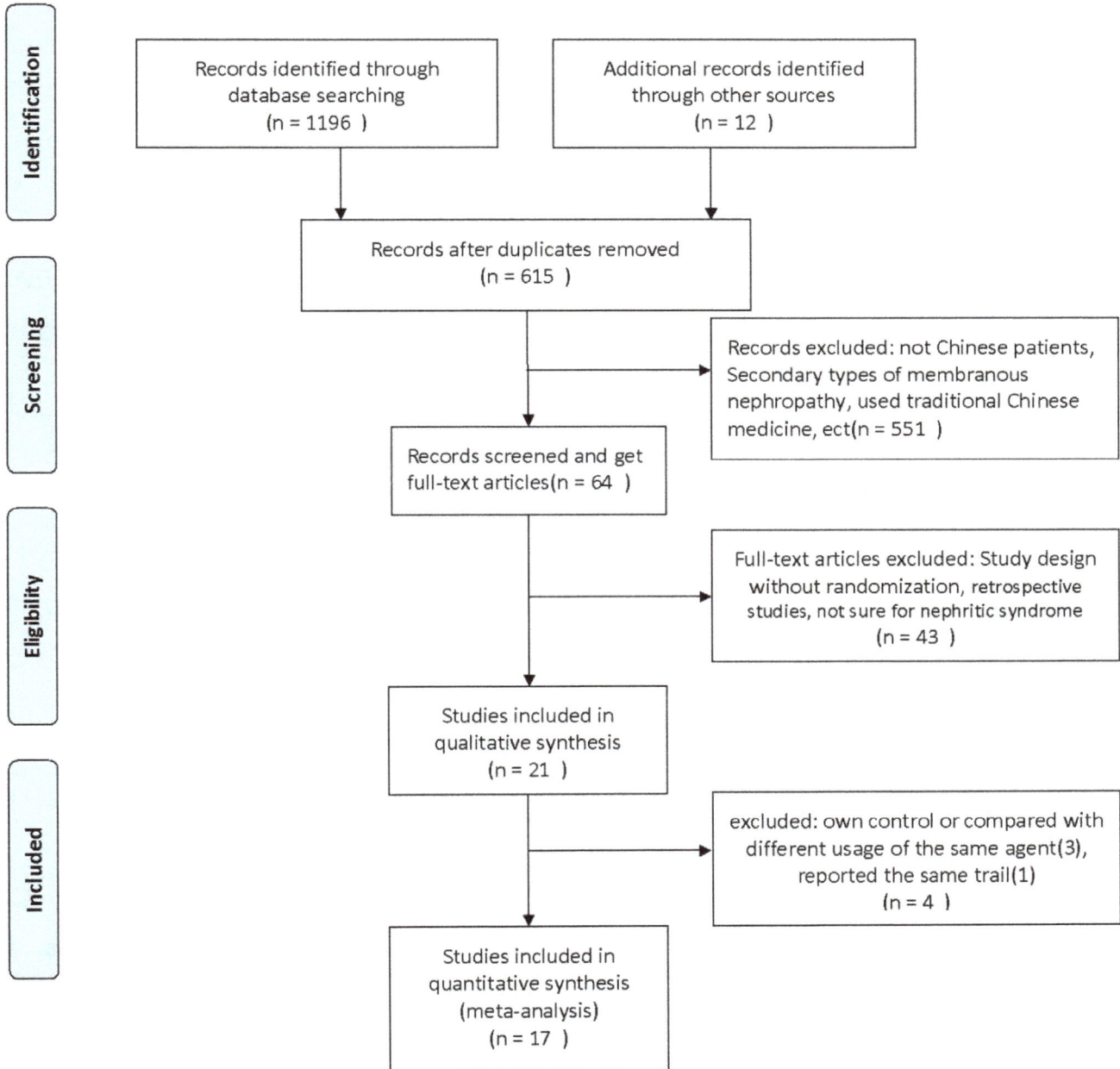

Figure 1. PRISMA Flowchart.

cyclophosphamide. (CR, RR 0.92, 95% CI 0.59 to 1.44, P = 0.71; CR/PR, RR 1.13,95% CI 0.94 to 1.37, P = 0.19) figure 4.

CyA versus CTX. Only 2 studies [14,16] involving 116 patients compared CyA with CTX. CyA was given at 3–5 mg/kg/ d initially and adjusted to a blood trough concentration level at 100 to 200 µg/L during the induction period (all 3 months),then tapered the doses. CyA showed better responsiveness (CR/PR,

RR: 1.41, 95% CI 1.05 to 1.90, P = 0.002) figure 2.2 but no significant on complete remission (CR, RR: 1.42, 95% CI 0.79 to 2.55, P = 0.25) figure 2.1.

TAC versus LET. Only 1 study [25] involving 20 patients compared TAC with LET. TAC was given at 0.1 mg/kg/ d initially and adjusted to a blood trough concentration level at 5 to 10 ng/mL for 6 months; LET was given orally at 50 mg/

Table 1. Characteristics of the included trials.

Trials	Number	Length	Mean age(year)	Gender male/ female	Baseline proreinuria (g/day)	Initial steroids dose	Quality grade
CyA versus CTX							
Li GF 2011 [14]	76	12 months	45.2/44.8	49/27	5.4±2.3/5.0±2.1	PDN0.5 mg/kg/d	2
Wu QX 2011 [16]	40	12 months	36.2	29/11	6.2±3.5/5.9±4.1	aPDN0.8 mg/kg/d	2
LET versus CTX							
Li GF 2011 [24]	80	6 months	48.3/47.6	63/17	3.59±1.18/3.72±1.23	PDN0.5 mg/kg/d	2
Zhou W 2009 [22]	30	12 months	42.8/41.6	15/15	7.84±3.73/7.78±3.67	Prednisolone 0.8–1.0 mg/kg/d	3
Zhu KY 2009 [23] MMF versus CTX	40	>6 months	51	24/16	6.15±2.36/6.17±2.53	aPDN30 mg/d	2
Zhang W 2011 [20]	60	12 months	43.6/43.6	38/22	7.55±3.66/7.48±3.63	PDN0.5/1.0 mg/kg/d	3
Zhou W 2009 [21]	40	12 months	43.8/42.6	17/23	7.93±3.82/7.62±3.55	Prednisolone 0.8–1.0 mg/kg/d	3
Li MX 2004 [18]	40	12 months	45.5	29/11	5.01±1.78/5.15±1.87	PDN1.0 mg/kg/d	2
An WW 2009 [17]	32	12 months	53.6	20/12	8.4±2.2/NC	Prednisolone60 mg/d	2
Ren Y 2011 [19]	52	12 months	46.6/41.1	36/16	NC	PDN0.8–1.0 mg/kg/d	1
TAC versus CTX							
Bai GZ 2011 [12]	32	9 months	48.2	21/11	NC	PDN15–60 mg/d	1
Xu J 2010 [11]	24	24 months	55.0/54.6	15/9	NC	NC	>3
Chen M 2010 [10]	73	12 months	47.2/48.6	41/32	7.11±3.93/7.28±3.91	PDN1 mg/kg/d	3
Chen WZ 2009 [13]	17	9 months	NC	NC	4.0±0.7/3.9±1.6	PDN15–60 mg/d	2
Liu JP 2009 [15]	20	6 months	51.3	13/7	NC	PDN1 mg/kg/d	2
MMF versus chlorambucil							
Chan TM 2007 [9]	20	15 months	49.5	13/7	4.9(3.4–6.9)/5.8(4.1–8.1) median (range)/median (range)	Prednisolone 0.8/ mPDN1g×3 days then Prednisolone 0.4 mg/kg/d	3
TAC versus LET							
Sun GD 2008 [25]	20	6 months	49.5	14/6	9.87±2.45/8.96±1.79	PDN30 mg/d	2

Abbreviations: PDN, prednisone; aPDN, prednisone acetate; NC, not clear.

d for 3 days, then 50 mg/d for 6 months, 1 hour before breakfast. TAC showed borderline advantage on complete remission (CR, RR: 2.50, 95% CI 0.63 to 10.00, P = 0.20), and on complete/partial remission (CR/PR, RR: 1.80, 95% CI 0.94 to 3.46, P = 0.08).

Side Effects

As side effects in a single comparison was not easy to make a statistical analysis, the major side effects of each agents were showed as following. 325 patients were given cyclophosphamide in total, and adverse events in 309 patients were reported: 42(13.6%) with dysfunction of liver, 37(12.0%) with leukocytopenia, 28(9.1%) with digestive symptoms. Hypertrichosis was the most frequent side effect of CyA (9/60, 15%). Elevated blood glucose happened in 18/78(23.1%) patients treated with TAC, 3 of which developed diabetes mellitus. 8/78(10.3%) patients treated with TAC got elevated blood pressure, and were treated with increased anti-hypertension drugs.

Eight among 112 (7.1%) patients given MMF got digestive symptoms. 6/75(8.0%) patients given LET got elevated liver enzymes, anther 8% got digestive symptoms.

There was no obvious nephrotoxicity directly related to immunosuppressive agents. 3 patients reported transient elevation of Scr in the comparison of "TAC versus CTX", 2 for CTX, 1 for TAC, and none of them progressed to renal failure. Sun GD et al

[25] reported increased serum creatinine concentration in 5 patients, 2 for TAC and 3 for LET. The very high proteinuria in this study (mean 9.87 g/24 h in TAC group, 8.96 g/24 h in LET group) should be taken into account.

Sensitivity Analysis

The funnel plots (Figure 5) did not show significant visual asymmetry.

We conducted a sensitivity analysis focus on the quality and patients of trials to assess the robustness of this meta-analytical results.

An analysis was performed by excluding low quality trials. As shown in Table 1, the quality score of all included trials is not high, only in one study [11] blindness was used. So we excluded the trials scoring less than 2 points. 2 studies [12,19] were excluded. The inferior position of cyclophosphamide have not changed in the analyses of "calcineurin inhibitors versus alkylating agents", on complete remission (CR, RR 1.53, 95% CI 1.06 to 2.20), on complete/partial remission (CR/PR, RR 1.25, 95% CI 1.05 to 1.48). In the analyses of "TAC versus CTX", the comparison on CR maintained (RR 1.61, 95% CI 1.01 to 2.56), on CR/PR became not statistical significant (RR 1.16, 95% CI 0.95 to 1.41). This sensitivity analysis did not substantially change the results of other comparisons.

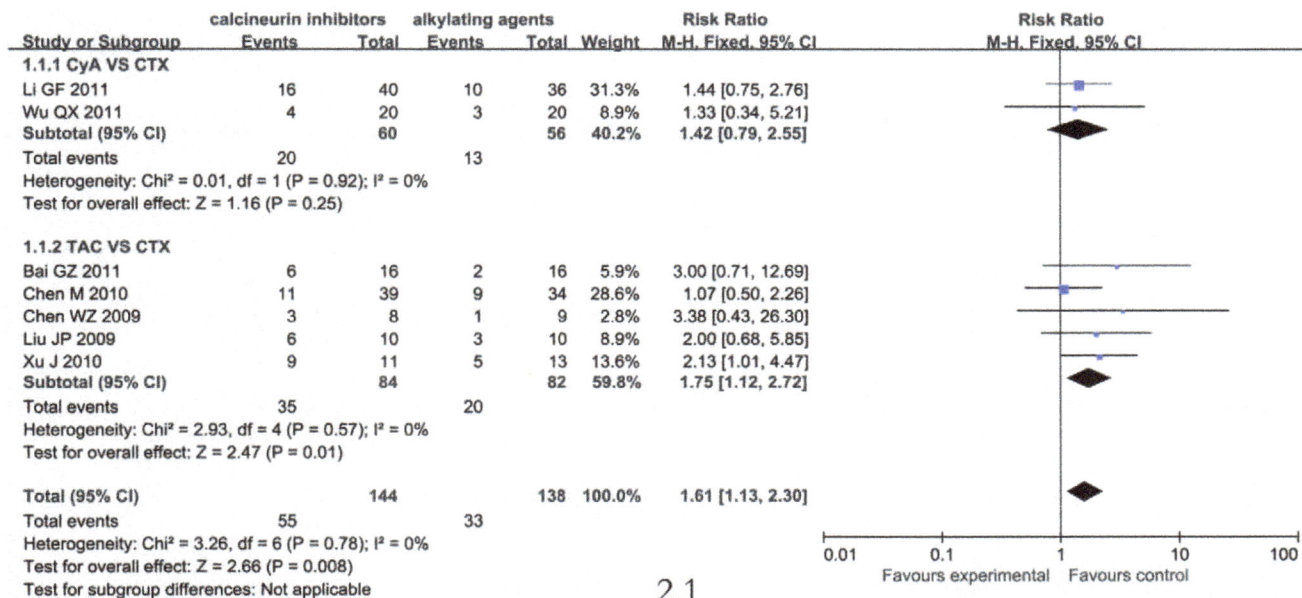

Figure 2.1:

Study or Subgroup	calcineurin inhibitors Events	Total	alkylating agents Events	Total	Weight	Risk Ratio M-H, Fixed, 95% CI
1.1.1 CyA VS CTX						
Li GF 2011	16	40	10	36	31.3%	1.44 [0.75, 2.76]
Wu QX 2011	4	20	3	20	8.9%	1.33 [0.34, 5.21]
Subtotal (95% CI)		60		56	40.2%	1.42 [0.79, 2.55]
Total events	20		13			

Heterogeneity: Chi² = 0.01, df = 1 (P = 0.92); I² = 0%
Test for overall effect: Z = 1.16 (P = 0.25)

Study or Subgroup	Events	Total	Events	Total	Weight	Risk Ratio M-H, Fixed, 95% CI
1.1.2 TAC VS CTX						
Bai GZ 2011	6	16	2	16	5.9%	3.00 [0.71, 12.69]
Chen M 2010	11	39	9	34	28.6%	1.07 [0.50, 2.26]
Chen WZ 2009	3	8	1	9	2.8%	3.38 [0.43, 26.30]
Liu JP 2009	6	10	3	10	8.9%	2.00 [0.68, 5.85]
Xu J 2010	9	11	5	13	13.6%	2.13 [1.01, 4.47]
Subtotal (95% CI)		84		82	59.8%	1.75 [1.12, 2.72]
Total events	35		20			

Heterogeneity: Chi² = 2.93, df = 4 (P = 0.57); I² = 0%
Test for overall effect: Z = 2.47 (P = 0.01)

Total (95% CI)		144		138	100.0%	1.61 [1.13, 2.30]
Total events	55		33			

Heterogeneity: Chi² = 3.26, df = 6 (P = 0.78); I² = 0%
Test for overall effect: Z = 2.66 (P = 0.008)
Test for subgroup differences: Not applicable

2.1

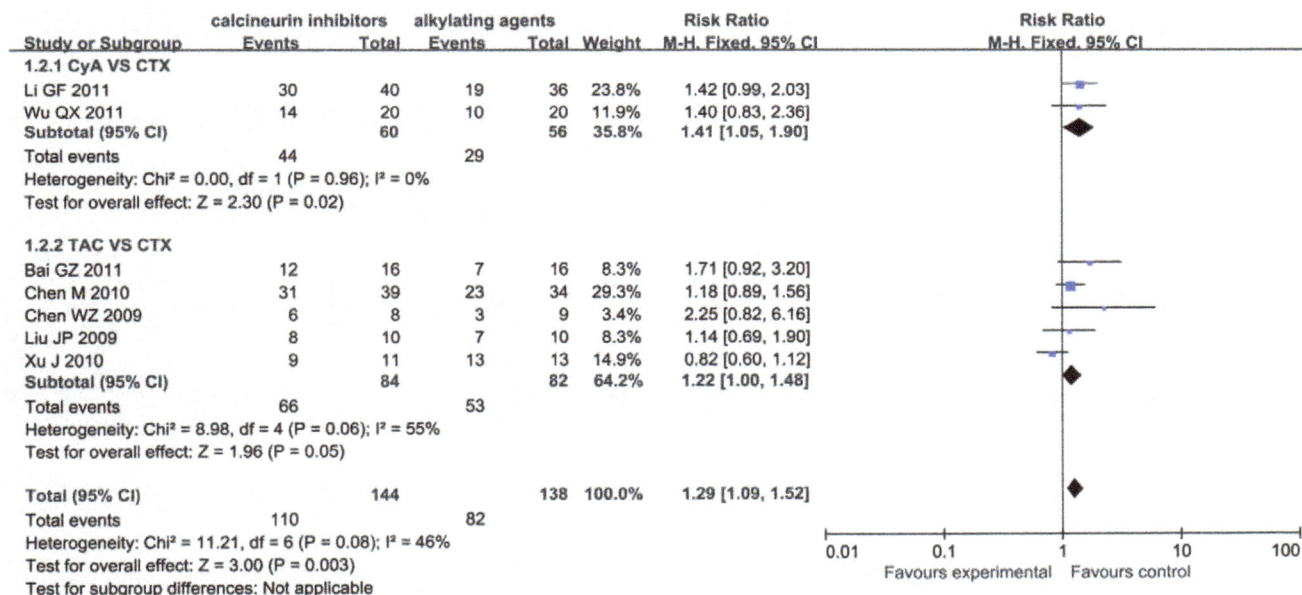

Figure 2.2:

Study or Subgroup	calcineurin inhibitors Events	Total	alkylating agents Events	Total	Weight	Risk Ratio M-H, Fixed, 95% CI
1.2.1 CyA VS CTX						
Li GF 2011	30	40	19	36	23.8%	1.42 [0.99, 2.03]
Wu QX 2011	14	20	10	20	11.9%	1.40 [0.83, 2.36]
Subtotal (95% CI)		60		56	35.8%	1.41 [1.05, 1.90]
Total events	44		29			

Heterogeneity: Chi² = 0.00, df = 1 (P = 0.96); I² = 0%
Test for overall effect: Z = 2.30 (P = 0.02)

Study or Subgroup	Events	Total	Events	Total	Weight	Risk Ratio M-H, Fixed, 95% CI
1.2.2 TAC VS CTX						
Bai GZ 2011	12	16	7	16	8.3%	1.71 [0.92, 3.20]
Chen M 2010	31	39	23	34	29.3%	1.18 [0.89, 1.56]
Chen WZ 2009	6	8	3	9	3.4%	2.25 [0.82, 6.16]
Liu JP 2009	8	10	7	10	8.3%	1.14 [0.69, 1.90]
Xu J 2010	9	11	13	13	14.9%	0.82 [0.60, 1.12]
Subtotal (95% CI)		84		82	64.2%	1.22 [1.00, 1.48]
Total events	66		53			

Heterogeneity: Chi² = 8.98, df = 4 (P = 0.06); I² = 55%
Test for overall effect: Z = 1.96 (P = 0.05)

Total (95% CI)		144		138	100.0%	1.29 [1.09, 1.52]
Total events	110		82			

Heterogeneity: Chi² = 11.21, df = 6 (P = 0.08); I² = 46%
Test for overall effect: Z = 3.00 (P = 0.003)
Test for subgroup differences: Not applicable

2.2

Figure 2. The complete remission rate (CR; figure 2.1) and the complete/partial remission rate (CR/PR; figure 2.2) comparison between calcineurin inhibitors and alkylating agents.

Discussion

Idiopathic membranous nephropathy (IMN) is the most common form of nephrotic syndrome in adults. Immunosuppressive agents acts predominate in its treatment for its benign or indolent course. As single-use glucocorticoids showed no benefit on IMN [3], several immunosuppressive agents in combination with glucocorticoids widely be used in China, namely CTX, CyA, LET, MMF and TAC. There was no good evidence for the choices of immunosuppressive agents in treating nephrotic IMN.

The object of this meta-analysis was to compare the efficacy and safety of different immunosuppressive in the treatment of Chinese adults with nephrotic IMN, providing some updated references to nephrologists for making optimal therapy. By limiting trials conducted in Chinese adults, we aimed to exclude the interference of ethnic differences on the response to immunosuppressive treatment, as some studies [26–28] showed that Asian might have better prognosis in IMN compared to Caucasian.

None of the studies involved reported the long-term outcome, like mortality or ESRD requiring initiation of dialysis or kidney transplantation. This analysis only viewed the short-term parameters to evaluate efficacy, including the final proteinuria/serum creatinine/serum albumin values and the therapeutic remission of participants (complete remission, partial remission). Serum creat-

Study or Subgroup	MMF Events	Total	CTX Events	Total	Weight	Risk Ratio M-H, Fixed, 95% CI
An WW 2009	8	16	7	16	29.2%	1.14 [0.54, 2.40]
Li MX 2004	2	20	1	20	4.2%	2.00 [0.20, 20.33]
Ren Y 2011	11	26	7	26	29.2%	1.57 [0.72, 3.42]
Zhang W 2011	8	30	5	30	20.8%	1.60 [0.59, 4.33]
Zhou W 2009	4	20	4	20	16.7%	1.00 [0.29, 3.45]
Total (95% CI)		112		112	100.0%	1.38 [0.89, 2.13]
Total events	33		24			

Heterogeneity: Chi² = 0.80, df = 4 (P = 0.94); I² = 0%
Test for overall effect: Z = 1.42 (P = 0.15)

3.1

Study or Subgroup	MMF Events	Total	CTX Events	Total	Weight	Risk Ratio M-H, Fixed, 95% CI
An WW 2009	12	16	11	16	18.0%	1.09 [0.71, 1.69]
Li MX 2004	18	20	11	20	18.0%	1.64 [1.07, 2.50]
Ren Y 2011	23	26	15	26	24.6%	1.53 [1.07, 2.19]
Zhang W 2011	21	30	13	30	21.3%	1.62 [1.01, 2.59]
Zhou W 2009	12	20	11	20	18.0%	1.09 [0.64, 1.86]
Total (95% CI)		112		112	100.0%	1.41 [1.16, 1.72]
Total events	86		61			

Heterogeneity: Chi² = 3.23, df = 4 (P = 0.52); I² = 0%
Test for overall effect: Z = 3.42 (P = 0.0006)

3.2

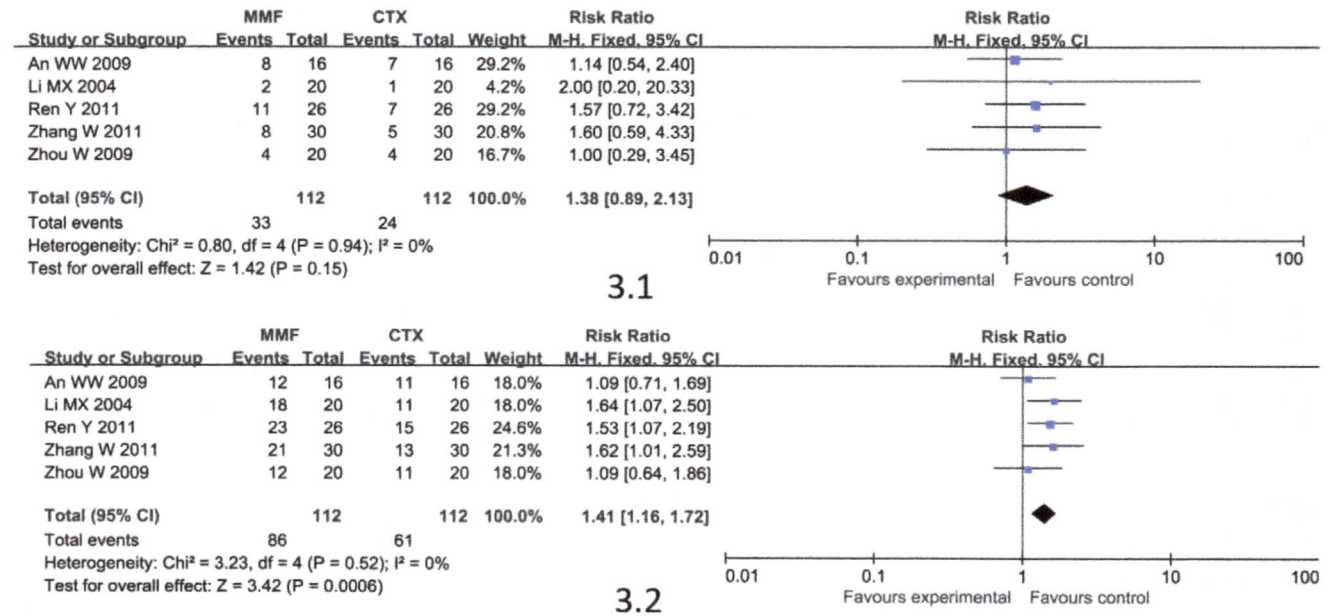

Figure 3. The complete remission rate (CR; figure 3.1) and complete/partial remission rate (CR/PR; figure 3.2) comparison between MMF and CTX.

inine is a value determined by multifactor, and has not showed obvious change during short-term follow up. Final proteinuria and serum albumin has correlation with the therapeutic remission, so the authors mainly analysed the latter. The most frequent definition usually adopted for "partial remission" was proteinuria between 0.3–2.0 g/24 h or decreased to lower by half. For "complete remission" the usual definition was proteinuria of less than 0.3 g/24 h and serum albumin more than 35 g/L and a normal renal function. However these definitions can be heterogeneous.

Cyclophosphamide as a classical immunosuppressive agent used in Chinese nephrotic IMN patients, was compared with other relatively new immunosuppressive agents, including LET, MMF, TAC and CyA. There were heterogeneous in the usage of cyclophosphamide: in 3 trials [10,18,19] received daily oral CTX 100 mg/d for 6 months then reduced half for another 6 months; in the other 12 trials, CTX was given intravenously (1g/month, for single dose or divided into two times). Through the comparison "calcineurin inhibitors versus alkylating agents", IMN patients showed a better treatment response to calcineurin inhibitors. In the analysis of two different agents, tacrolimus was in optimistic position, showing better response than CTX, statistically significant higher rate on inducing remission than CTX, and with tolerable side effects. When compared to CTX, MMF and CyA

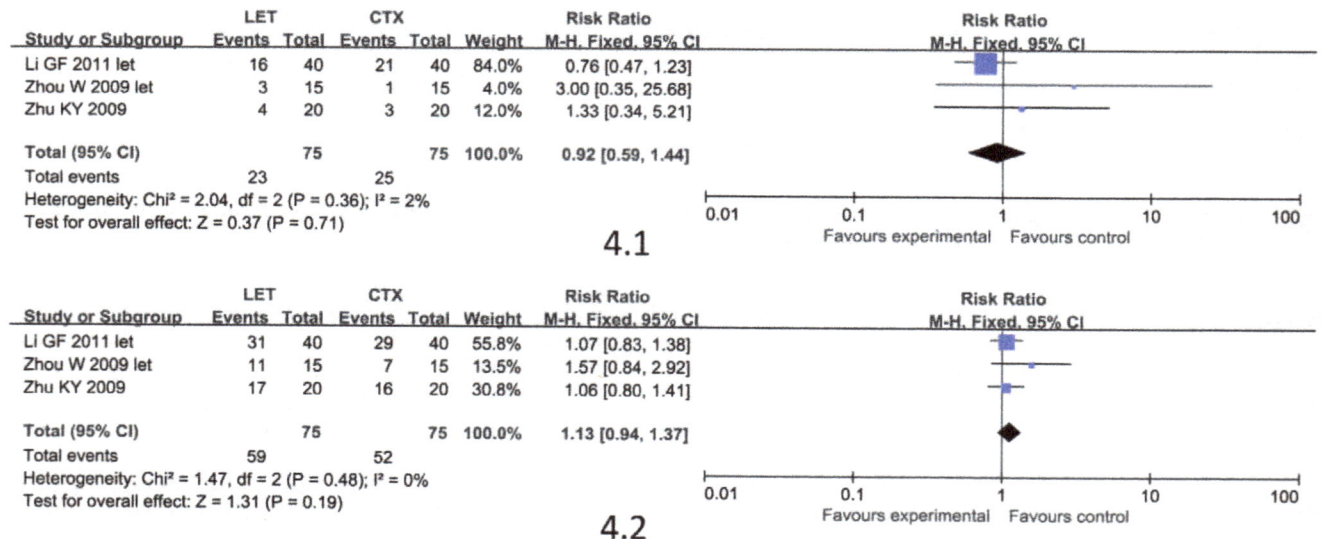

Study or Subgroup	LET Events	Total	CTX Events	Total	Weight	Risk Ratio M-H, Fixed, 95% CI
Li GF 2011 let	16	40	21	40	84.0%	0.76 [0.47, 1.23]
Zhou W 2009 let	3	15	1	15	4.0%	3.00 [0.35, 25.68]
Zhu KY 2009	4	20	3	20	12.0%	1.33 [0.34, 5.21]
Total (95% CI)		75		75	100.0%	0.92 [0.59, 1.44]
Total events	23		25			

Heterogeneity: Chi² = 2.04, df = 2 (P = 0.36); I² = 2%
Test for overall effect: Z = 0.37 (P = 0.71)

4.1

Study or Subgroup	LET Events	Total	CTX Events	Total	Weight	Risk Ratio M-H, Fixed, 95% CI
Li GF 2011 let	31	40	29	40	55.8%	1.07 [0.83, 1.38]
Zhou W 2009 let	11	15	7	15	13.5%	1.57 [0.84, 2.92]
Zhu KY 2009	17	20	16	20	30.8%	1.06 [0.80, 1.41]
Total (95% CI)		75		75	100.0%	1.13 [0.94, 1.37]
Total events	59		52			

Heterogeneity: Chi² = 1.47, df = 2 (P = 0.48); I² = 0%
Test for overall effect: Z = 1.31 (P = 0.19)

4.2

Figure 4. The complete remission rate (CR; figure 4.1) and the complete/partial remission rate (CR/PR; figure 4.2) comparison between LET and CTX.

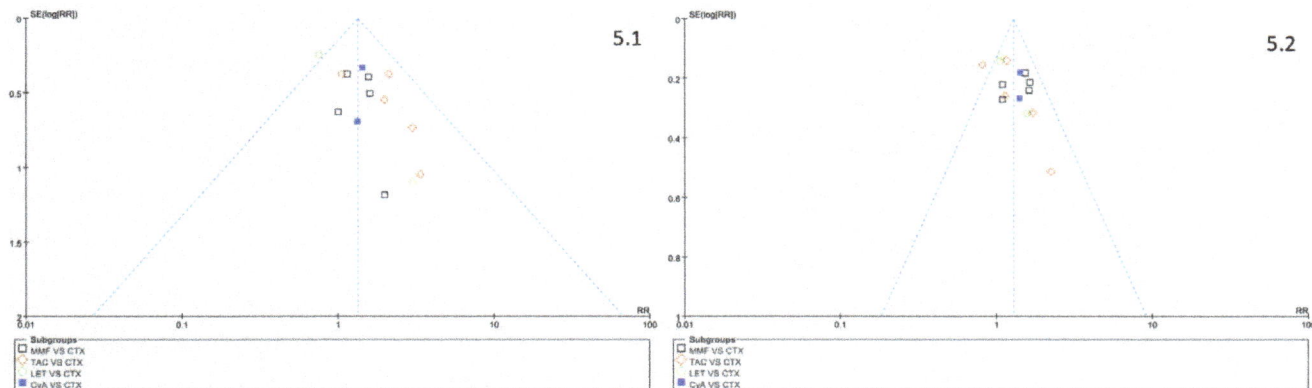

Figure 5. Funnel plot of complete remission (CR; figure 5.1) and complete/partial remission (CR/PR; figure 5.2) in four comparisons.

induced more response but not significant in inducing complete remission, LET shown no significant difference both on complete remission and complete/partial remission. But only 2 studies involving 116 patients compared CyA with CTX, more high quality RCTs were needed to determine their effects. Only one study was included in the analysis on "TAC versus LET" and "MMF versus modified Ponticelli regimen", both shown no significant difference.

Sensitivity analysis was performed by excluding low quality trials, did not substantially change the main results. This meta's result "calcineurin inhibitors inducing more remission than alkylating agents" coincided with the earlier meta [3]. "TAC's favor position" was supported by data from previous TAC monotherapy effect [29]. The funnel plots did not show obvious publishing bias of mainly comparisons.

Short-term duration (6–24 mouths), only one trial [11] used blindness, not large-sample participants (696 in total), absence comparison between some agents(mostly compared to CTX), no

advanced subgroup analyses of different level proteinuria (only definition was "nephrotic") led to limitations of this meta. The probable explain for non-blindness was those agents have a relative high adverse rate and blood drug concentration level need to be checked. CTX have been compared in most studies, possibly for its classical position.

In conclusion, based on Chinese adults and short duration RCTs, calcineurin inhibitors, especially TAC, showed superior potency to induce remission in nephrotic IMN with tolerable adverse effects, compared to alkylating agent (CTX).

Author Contributions

Conceived and designed the experiments: GX JX CY ZM CM. Analyzed the data: GX JX CY ZM CM DC XH LL LS XZ. Contributed reagents/materials/analysis tools: CX YM LY. Wrote the paper: GX JX ZM CY LY.

References

1. Schieppati A, Mosconi L, Perna A, Mecca G, Bertani T, et al. (1993) Prognosis of untreated patients with idiopathic membranous nephropathy. N Engl J Med 329: 85–89.
2. Honkanen E, Tornroth T, Gronhagen-Riska C (1992) Natural history, clinical course and morphological evolution of membranous nephropathy. Nephrol Dial Transplant 7 Suppl 1: 35–41.
3. Schieppati A, Perna A, Zamora J, Giuliano GA, Braun N, et al. (2004) Immunosuppressive treatment for idiopathic membranous nephropathy in adults with nephrotic syndrome. Cochrane Database Syst Rev: CD004293.
4. Jha V, Ganguli A, Saha TK, Kohli HS, Sud K, et al. (2007) A randomized, controlled trial of steroids and cyclophosphamide in adults with nephrotic syndrome caused by idiopathic membranous nephropathy. J Am Soc Nephrol 18: 1899–1904.
5. Ponticelli C, Altieri P, Scolari F, Passerini P, Roccatello D, et al. (1998) A randomized study comparing methylprednisolone plus chlorambucil versus methylprednisolone plus cyclophosphamide in idiopathic membranous nephropathy. J Am Soc Nephrol 9: 444–450.
6. Ponticelli C, Zucchelli P, Passerini P, Cagnoli L, Cesana B, et al. (1989) A randomized trial of methylprednisolone and chlorambucil in idiopathic membranous nephropathy. N Engl J Med 320: 8–13.
7. Ponticelli C, Zucchelli P, Passerini P, Cesana B, Locatelli F, et al. (1995) A 10-year follow-up of a randomized study with methylprednisolone and chlorambucil in membranous nephropathy. Kidney Int 48: 1600–1604.
8. Jadad AR, Moore RA, Carroll D, Jenkinson C, Reynolds DJ, et al. (1996) Assessing the quality of reports of randomized clinical trials: is blinding necessary? Control Clin Trials 17: 1–12.
9. Chan TM, Lin AW, Tang SCW, Qian JQ, Lam MF, et al. (2007) Prospective controlled study on mycophenolate mofetil and prednisolone in the treatment of membranous nephropathy with nephrotic syndrome. Nephrology 12: 576–581.
10. Chen M, Li H, Li XY, Lu FM, Ni ZH, et al. (2010) Tacrolimus combined with corticosteroids in treatment of nephrotic idiopathic membranous nephropathy:

A multicenter randomized controlled trial. American Journal of the Medical Sciences 339: 233–238.
11. Xu J, Zhang W, Xu Y, Chen N (2010) A double-blinded prospective randomised study on the efficacy of corticosteroid plus cyclophosphamide or FK506 in idiopathic membranous nephropathy patients with nephrotic syndrome. Nephrology 15: 43.
12. Bai GZ, Fan W, Yuan YJ, Wang JH, Zhang SH (2011) An observation of tacrolimus in combination with low dose steriod in idiopathic membranous nephropathy. Journal of Guiyang College of Traditional Chinese Medicine 33: 52–53.
13. Chen WZ, Chen DJ, Xu GB (2009) An observation of tacrolimus in idiopathic membranous nephropathy treatment The Journal of Practical Medicine 25: 1674–1675.
14. Li GF, Liu T, Bao BY (2011) Comparison on the therapeutic effect of cyclosporin A and cyclophosphamide in the creatment of idiopathic membranous nephropathy. Chinese Journal of Integrated Traditional and Western Nephrology 12: 522–525.
15. Liu J, Li D (2009) The study on the treatment of idiopathic membranous nephropathy with tacrolimus. graduation dissertation.
16. Wu QX, Gong ZF (2011) Middle or small dose tacrolimus in the treatment of 20 membranous nephropathy patients. China Pharmacist 14: 115–117.
17. An WW, Tu YK, Wang T (2009) Clinical research of mycophenolate mofetil and glucocorticoid in treatment of membranous nephropathy. Occupation and Health 25: 2009–2010.
18. Li MX, Song JW, Yu YW, Shi XY (2004) Effects of mycophenolate mofetil in combination of prednesone on the early stage of membranous nephropathy. journal of Clinical nephrology 4: 160–162.
19. Ren Y, Hu ZX, Luo YH, Shan W (2011) Clinical observation of mycophenolate mofetil combined with low-dose prednisone on idiopathic membranous nephropathy. Journal of modern Chinese doctor 49: 73–74.

20. Zhang W, Zhang XT, Ma JW, Liu HF (2011) Mycophenolate mofetil plus small dose steroid in the treatment of membranous nephropathy. Chinese Journal of Integrated Traditional and Western Nephrology 12: 59–60.

21. Zhou W, Zhang WX, Zhang ZM, Zhang ZQ, Shi XY (2009) Mycophenolate mofetil in the treatment of 20 membranous nephropathy patients. Journal of Clinical Internal Medicine 26: 479–481.

22. Zhou W, Zhang WX, Zhang ZM, Zhang ZQ, Shi XY (2009) Clinical trial on the effect of leflunomide in treating primary membranous nephropathy. Sichuan Medical Journal 30: 1889–1891.

23. Zhu KY, Bi CY (2009) The clinical efficacy observation of leflunomide in the treatment of membranous nephropathy. China Practical Medicine 4: 99–100.

24. Li GF, Liu T, Bao BY (2011) Efficacy comparison of lefluomide and cyclophosphamine treatment on idiopathic nephropathy. Chinese Journal of Integrated Traditional and Western Nephrology 12: 872–874.

25. Sun GD, Xu ZG, Luo P, Miao LN (2008) The clinical efficacy of tacrolimus in the treatment of idiopathic membranous nephropathy. Chinese Journal of Gerontology 28: 469–471.

26. Shiiki H, Saito T, Nishitani Y, Mitarai T, Yorioka N, et al. (2004) Prognosis and risk factors for idiopathic membranous nephropathy with nephrotic syndrome in Japan. Kidney Int 65: 1400–1407.

27. Donadio JV Jr, Torres VE, Velosa JA, Wagoner RD, Holley KE, et al. (1988) Idiopathic membranous nephropathy: the natural history of untreated patients. Kidney Int 33: 708–715.

28. Reichert LJ, Koene RA, Wetzels JF (1998) Prognostic factors in idiopathic membranous nephropathy. Am J Kidney Dis 31: 1–11.

29. Praga M, Barrio V, Juarez GF, Luno J (2007) Tacrolimus monotherapy in membranous nephropathy: a randomized controlled trial. Kidney Int 71: 924–930.

5

Conformational Changes of Blood ACE in Chronic Uremia

Maxim N. Petrov[1], **Valery Y. Shilo**[2], **Alexandr V. Tarasov**[1], **David E. Schwartz**[3], **Joe G. N. Garcia**[4], **Olga A. Kost**[1], **Sergei M. Danilov**[3,4,5]*

1 Department of Chemistry, Lomonosov Moscow State University, Moscow, Russia, 2 Department of Nephrology, Moscow University for Medicine and Dentistry, Moscow, Russia, 3 Department of Anesthesiology, University of Illinois at Chicago, Chicago, Illinois, United States of America, 4 Institute for Personalized Respiratory Medicine, University of Illinois at Chicago, Chicago, Illinois, United States of America, 5 National Cardiology Research Center, Moscow, Russia

Abstract

Background: The pattern of binding of monoclonal antibodies (mAbs) to 16 epitopes on human angiotensin I-converting enzyme (ACE) comprise a conformational ACE fingerprint and is a sensitive marker of subtle protein conformational changes.

Hypothesis: Toxic substances in the blood of patients with uremia due to End Stage Renal Disease (ESRD) can induce local conformational changes in the ACE protein globule and alter the efficacy of ACE inhibitors.

Methodology/Principal Findings: The recognition of ACE by 16 mAbs to the epitopes on the N and C domains of ACE was estimated using an immune-capture enzymatic plate precipitation assay. The precipitation pattern of blood ACE by a set of mAbs was substantially influenced by the presence of ACE inhibitors with the most dramatic local conformational change noted in the N-domain region recognized by mAb 1G12. The "short" ACE inhibitor enalaprilat (tripeptide analog) and "long" inhibitor teprotide (nonapeptide) produced strikingly different mAb 1G12 binding with enalaprilat strongly increasing mAb 1G12 binding and teprotide decreasing binding. Reduction in S-S bonds via glutathione and dithiothreitol treatment increased 1G12 binding to blood ACE in a manner comparable to enalaprilat. Some patients with uremia due to ESRD exhibited significantly increased mAb 1G12 binding to blood ACE and increased ACE activity towards angiotensin I accompanied by reduced ACE inhibition by inhibitory mAbs and ACE inhibitors.

Conclusions/Significance: The estimation of relative mAb 1G12 binding to blood ACE detects a subpopulation of ESRD patients with conformationally changed ACE, which activity is less suppressible by ACE inhibitors. This parameter may potentially serve as a biomarker for those patients who may need higher concentrations of ACE inhibitors upon anti-hypertensive therapy.

Editor: Dulce Elena Casarini, Federal University of São Paulo (UNIFESP), Escola Paulista de Medicina, Brazil

Funding: This work was partly financially supported by the Russian Fund for Basic Research (grant number 11-04-01923-a). The funders had no role in study design, data collection and analysis, decision to publish, or preparation of the manuscript. No additional external funding received for this study.

Competing Interests: The authors have declared that no competing interests exist.

* E-mail: danilov@uic.edu

Introduction

Angiotensin I-converting enzyme (ACE, CD143, EC 3.4.15.1), a zinc-metallopeptidase, is a key regulator of blood pressure participating in the development of vascular pathology and remodeling [1–3]. The somatic isoform of ACE (sACE) is highly expressed as a type-I transmembrane glycoprotein in endothelia [4–7], epithelia and neuroepithelia [8–10], as well as immune cells – macrophages and dendritic cells [11–12]. ACE has been designated as a CD marker – CD143 [13–14]. Somatic ACE also presents as a soluble form, for example, in plasma, cerebrospinal and seminal fluids, that lacks the transmembrane domain responsible for membrane attachment [15].

In healthy individuals, the level of ACE in the blood is very stable [16], whereas significant increase (2-4-fold) in blood ACE activity was observed in granulomatous diseases such as sarcoidosis and Gaucher's disease [15,17–20]. Less dramatic, but still significant increase in blood ACE activity was reported in patients with renal diseases and at uremia [21–23].

Under normal conditions, serum ACE likely originates from ACE released from endothelial cells [24], perhaps, mainly lung capillaries [7] by proteolytic cleavage by still unidentified membrane-bound secretase [25].

Two homologous domains (N and C domains) within a single polypeptide chain comprise the majority of the structure of sACE, each containing a functional active center [26]. The three-dimensional crystal structure of sACE is still unknown. However, the models of the two-domain ACE has been recently suggested [27–29], based on the solved crystal structures of the C and N domains [30–31], epitope mapping of monoclonal antibodies (mAbs) to ACE [27], and on the electron microscopy picture of sACE [28].

To provide structure-function information on ACE molecule, we previously developed a set of ~40 mAbs directed to sequential and conformational epitopes to human, rat and mouse ACE [27,32–36], which proved useful for ACE quantification in solution by ELISA [37] and by flow cytometry [12,38]. These mAbs have facilitated the investigation of the structure and function of ACE [27,32,39–45] and were successfully used for the detection of carriers of novel ACE gene mutations such as Pro1199Leu [46], Trp1197Stop [47], Gln1069Arg [48], and Tyr465Asp [29].

Recent ACE studies with mAbs recognizing different conformational epitopes on the surface of the catalytically active N domain (eight mAbs) and the C domain (eight mAbs) of human ACE molecule revealed that the pattern of mAb binding to ACE is potentially a very sensitive marker of the local conformation of ACE globule. The changes of this pattern could be definitely attributed to the changes of the epitopes for the distinct mAbs due to denaturation of ACE globule, chemical modification, inhibitor binding, mutations, and different glycosylation/deglycosylation [49].

Based on these systematic studies of ACE epitopes [27,32,42–45,49–50], we hypothesized that the pattern of precipitation of ACE activity by this set of mAbs, i.e. the "conformational fingerprinting of ACE", may detect conformationally changed ACE in the blood as a result of a disease. Uremia is characterized by an elevated level of toxic compounds [51] and therefore served as a disorder of interest for assessing blood ACE conformation.

Here we report the findings which support this hypothesis and suggest that ACE "conformational fingerprinting" provides a potential tool for the future selection of a subgroup of ESRD patients, whose ACE inhibitor therapy, if needed, should be more aggressive in order to be effective.

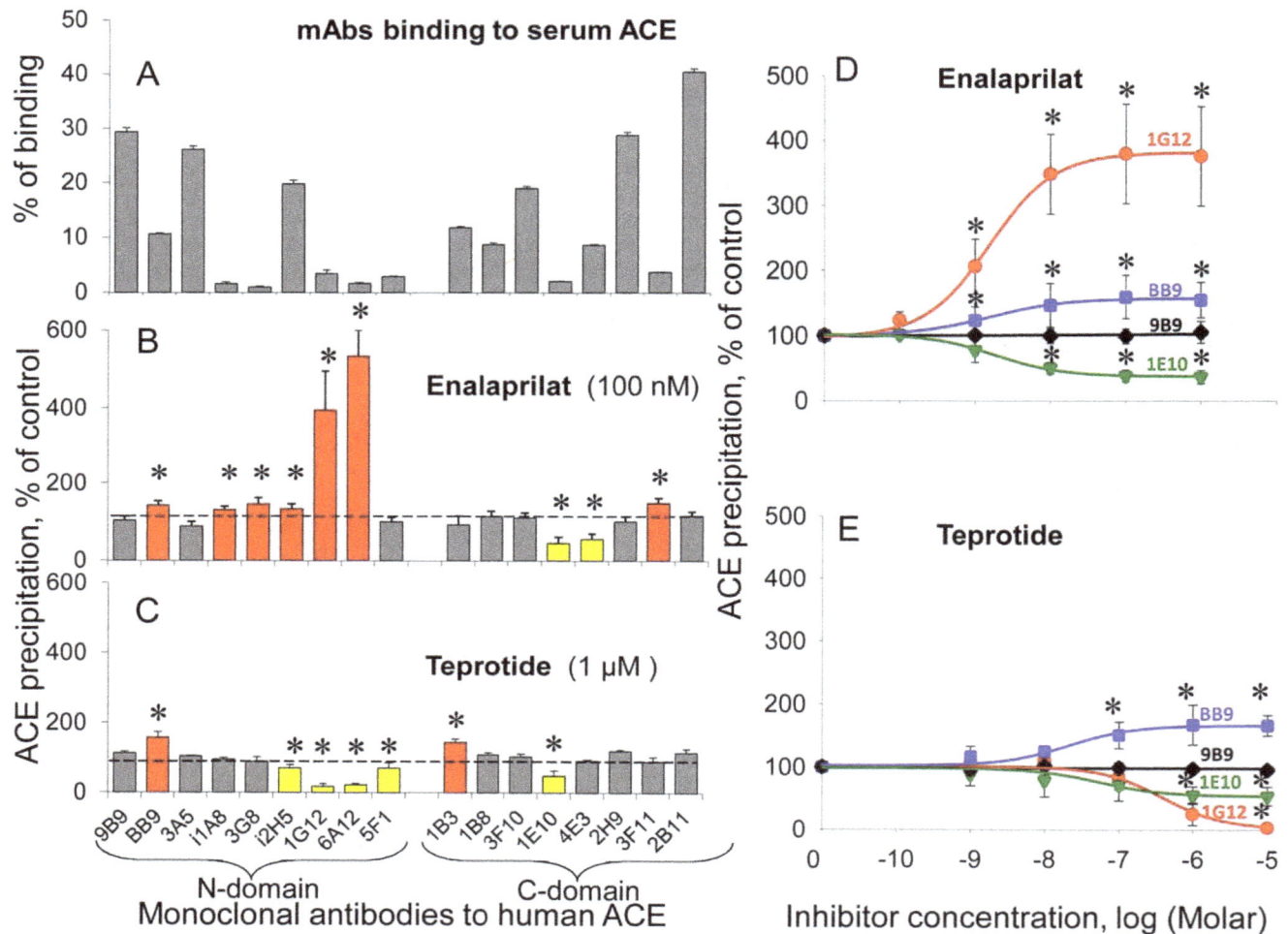

Figure 1. Effect of ACE inhibitors on the binding of a set of anti-ACE mAbs to blood ACE. The binding of a set of 17 mAbs to the N and C domains of human sACE to the human serum ACE was determined using plate precipitation assay [32,49] with ZPHL as a substrate. Serum pooled from 30 healthy donors and diluted 1/5 in PBS (50 µl) was incubated with or without ACE inhibitors for 1 hour at 37oC and then was incubated overnight with microtiter plate coated with different anti-ACE mAbs (3 µg/ml) via goat-anti-mouse bridge. Serum components, inhibitors, as well as unbound ACE, were then eliminated by washing. ACE activity precipitated by each of tested mAbs was determined by adding ZPHL solution (in 100 mM potassium phosphate buffer, containing 300 mM KCl, 1 µM ZnSO4, pH 8.3) directly into the wells. After 1–4 hours at 37°C the product of the enzymatic reaction, His-Leu, was quantified by reaction with o-phthaldialdehyde spectrofluorometrically directly in the wells. **A.** Comparative binding of the mAbs set to serum ACE. **B–C.** Data are expressed as a percentage of precipitated ACE activity from serum pre-incubated with enalaprilat (100 nM - **B**) or teprotide (1 µM - **C**) by a given mAb from that w/o inhibitor. The colored columns show antibodies which binding to blood ACE in the presence of ACE inhibitor differed (more than 20%) from that to without the inhibitor: mAbs increasing or decreasing their binding to ACE in the presence of inhibitor are marked by red or yellow, respectively. **D–E.** Effect of different concentrations of enalaprilat (**D**) or teprotide (**E**) on mAbs binding to serum ACE. Data are mean ± SD of 3–8 independent experiments (each in duplicates). *, p<0.05 in comparison with mean values for samples without ACE inhibitors.

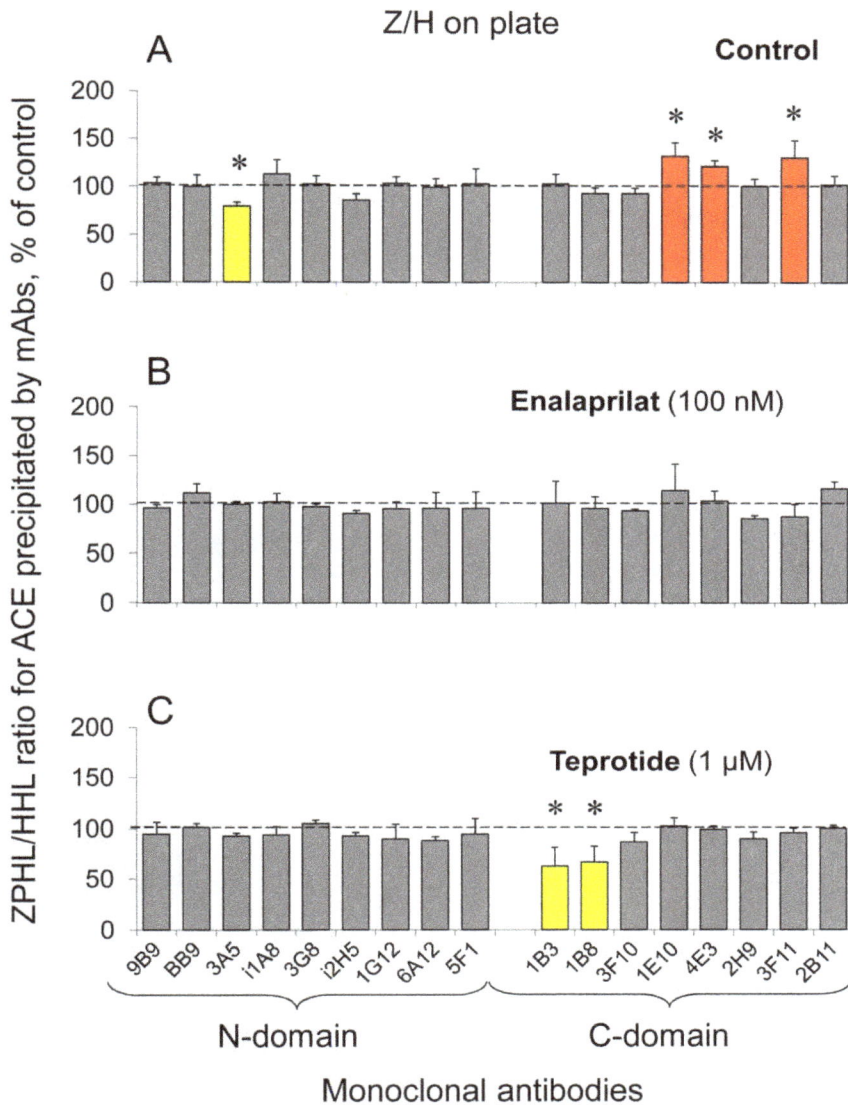

Figure 2. Effect of ACE inhibitors on the comparative rates of ZPHL and HHL hydrolysis by blood ACE bound by mAbs on the plate.
A. ACE activity precipitated from citrated pooled plasma by each given mAb was determined spectrofluorometrically directly in the wells (as in Fig. 1) with two substrates for ACE, HHL and ZPHL. Data are expressed as the ratio of the rates of the hydrolysis of two substrates (ZPHL/HHL ratio) by ACE bound by mAbs in comparison with the mean value obtained for all 17 mAbs. * - $p < 0.05$ in comparison with mean value for the whole set of mAbs.
B–C. Effect of enalaprilat (100 nM – **B**) and teprotide (1 μM – **C**) on ZPHL/HHL ratio determined for ACE bound with each mAb. * - $p < 0.05$ in comparison with mean values for samples without ACE inhibitors. All other terms and conditions are as in Fig. 1. Red colored columns show those mAbs which binding with ACE increased (and yellow – decreased) ZPHL/HHL ratio. Data are mean ± SD from 3–8 independent experiments (each in duplicates). $p < 0.05$ in comparison with mean values for samples without ACE inhibitors.

Experimental Section

ACE Activity Assay

ACE activity in citrate plasma, serum, cell lysates or culture medium was measured by fluorimetric assay [52–53]. Briefly, 20–40 μl aliquots of ACE source, diluted correspondingly in PBS-BSA (0.1 mg/ml), were added to 200 μl of ACE substrate (5 mM Hip-His-Leu or 2 mM Z-Phe-His-Leu) in phosphate buffer, pH 8.3 (with 300 mM NaCl) and incubated for the appropriate time at 37°C. His-Leu product was quantified with o-phthaldialdehyde spectrofluorometrically (365 nm excitation and 500 nm emission wavelengths). Determination of the ratio of the rates of the hydrolysis of two substrates (ZPHL/HHL) was performed as

described [54]. ACE activity in serum/plasma was also determined with 0.3 mM angiotensin I as a substrate as described above.

Isolation and Cultivation of ACE-expressing Cells

Plasmids carrying the coding sequence for wild-type (WT) ACE (based on pcDNA3.1, Invitrogen Corp., Carlsbad, CA) containing the full-length somatic ACE cDNA controlled by CMV early promoter [55] or mutant ACEs – i) WTΔ –without transmembrane anchor [56], kindly provided by Dr. F. Alhenc-Gelas (then INSERM Unit 352, Paris, France); ii) truncated N domain - D629 [57]; iii) testicular ACE –tACE [58], kindly provided by Dr. E.

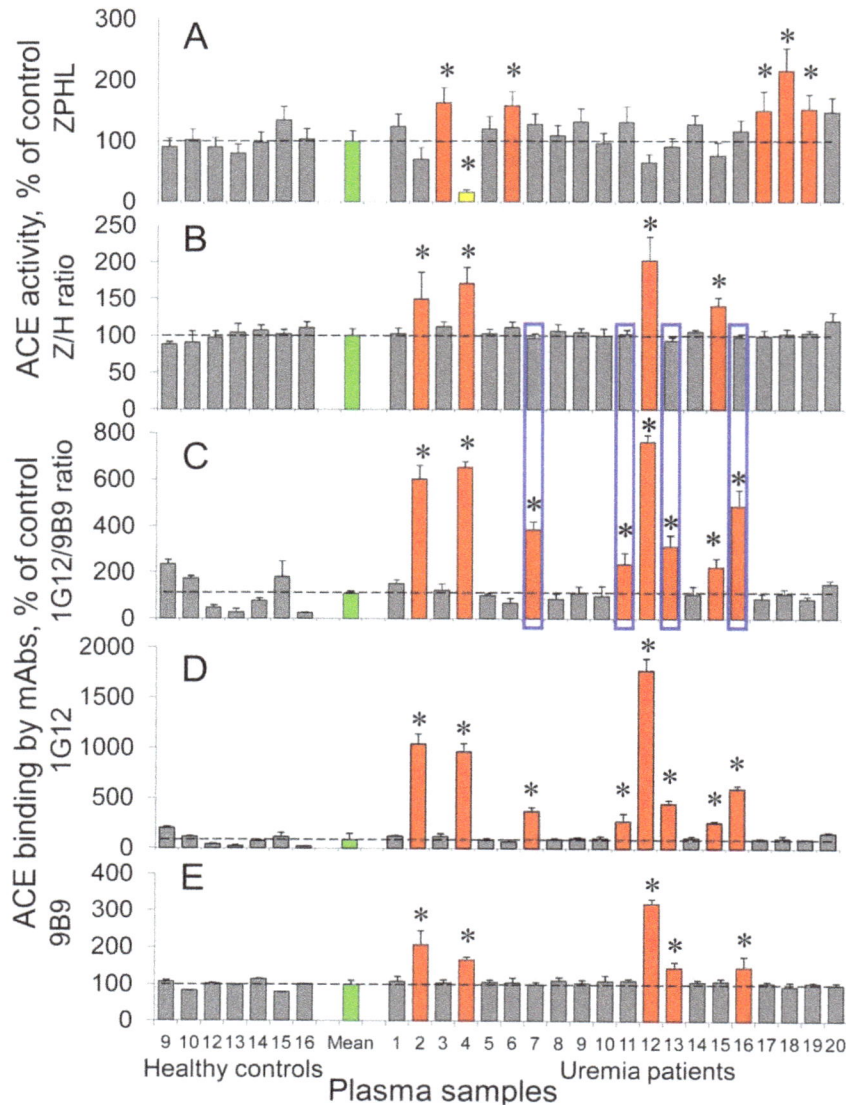

Figure 3. Blood ACE phenotyping in uremia. A. ACE activity in the citrated plasma (diluted 5-fold) of patients with uremia (versus that of healthy volunteers) was determined spectrofluorometrically using 20 μl of diluted plasma with 100 μl of ACE substrate ZPHL at 1 hour of incubation with substrate. B. **The ratio of the rates of the hydrolysis of two substrates (ZPHL/HHL ratio) for ACE from the blood of patients with uremia and from the blood of healthy persons. C-E**. ACE activity precipitated by different mAbs from citrated plasma of uremic patients (versus that from plasma of healthy donors: **E** - by mAb 9B9; **D** - by mAb 1G12 and **C** – their ratio for each plasma sample. Results are shown as mean ± SD from 3 to 10 independent experiments, each in duplicates or triplicates. The red color of the columns shows plasma of those patients whose blood parameter (ACE activity, Z/H ratio, 1G12/9B9 ratio/mAb 9B9 or 1G12 binding) was significantly higher (and yellow bar-significantly lower) than mean value for healthy donors. The green bars shows mean values for healthy controls. Boxes show those patients which have increased 1G12/9B9 ratio while normal ZPHL/HHL ratio. All other terms and conditions are as in Fig. 1. * - p<0.05 in comparison with mean value for healthy controls.

Sturrock (University of Cape Town, South Africa) were stably expressed in CHO cells (ATCC, Manassas, VA) using Plus Reagent (Invitrogen Corp., Carlsbad, CA) as described [55]. Stable transfected cells expressing ACE at confluence were washed gently with PBS and incubated 24–48 hours with "complete culture medium" (Mediatech, Inc, Herndon, VA) or Ultra-CHO medium (Cambrex Bio-Science Walkersville, Inc, Walkersville, MD) without fetal bovine serum (FBS). Culture medium was collected as a source of soluble ACE. Cell lysates were used as a source of a membrane form of wild-type and mutant ACEs for biochemical and immunological characterization. After 24 hours of the culturing the culture medium was aspirated and centrifuged

(to precipitate possible detached cells) and the cells, after washing by PBS, were lysed with 50 mM Tris-HCl buffer, pH 7.5, containing 150 mM NaCl and 0.5% Triton X-100. ACE activity in the lysates and culture medium was determined with two ACE substrates as described above.

Immunological Characterization of ACE from Different Sources (Plate Immunoprecipitation Assay)

Plastic 96-well plates (Corning, Corning, NY) were coated with 50 μl of 10 μg/ml affinity-purified goat anti-mouse IgG (Pierce, Rockford, IL) and stored overnight at 4°C. After washing with PBS/0.05% Tween 20, the wells were incubated with different

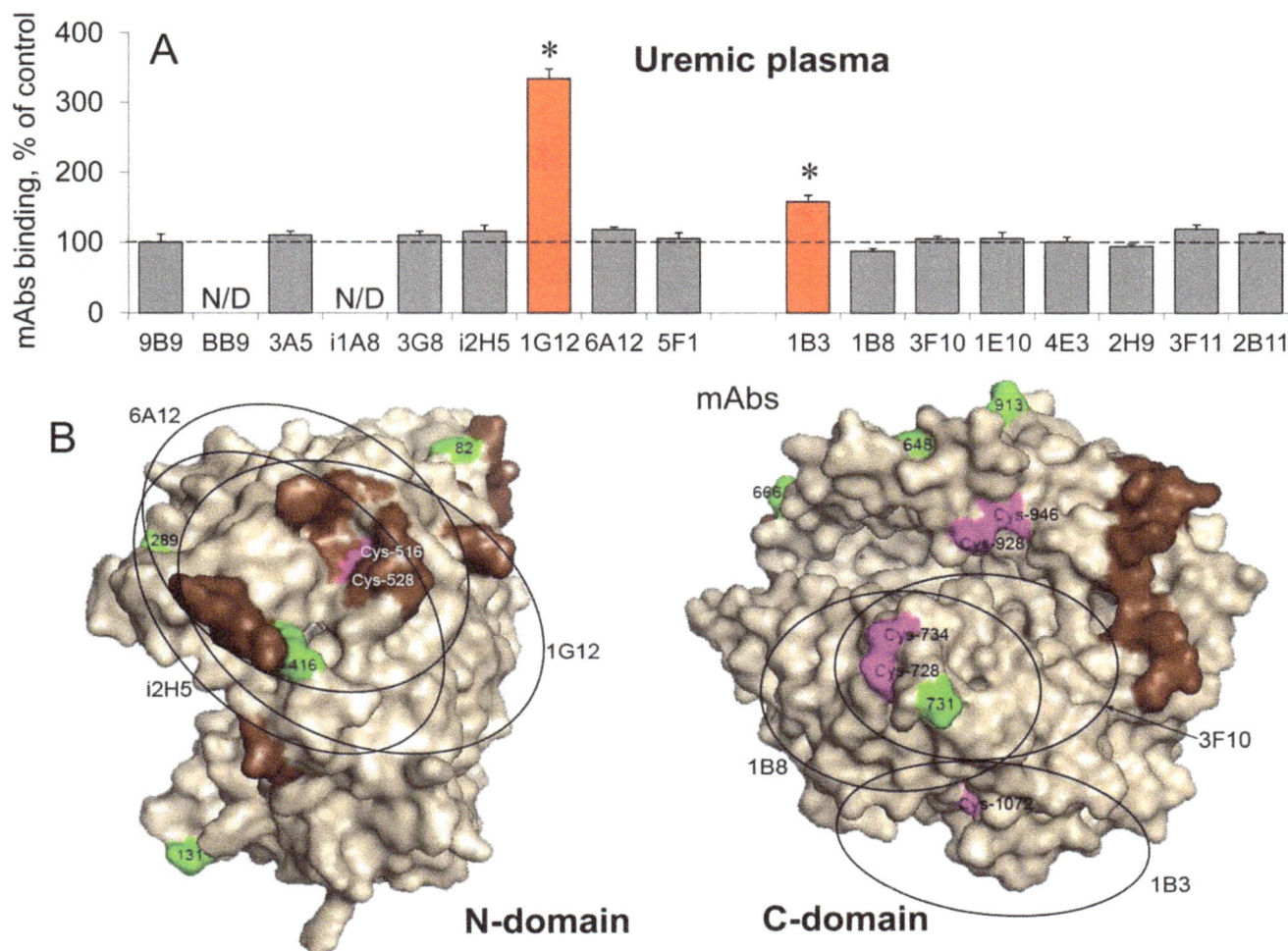

Figure 4. Conformational fingerprinting of uremic plasma with highly elevated 1G12/9B9 ratio and normal Z/H ratio. A. ACE activity precipitated by different mAbs from plasma of uremic patients with highly elevated 1G12/9B9 ratio and normal Z/H ratio (mean data for uremic samples #7 and #16 from Fig. 3) as a percentage from that for plasma from uremic persons with normal 1G12/9B9 and ZPHL/HHL ratios (mean data of two uremic samples #5 and #18 from Fig. 3) taken as control. Data presented are mean ± SD of duplicates from 2 experiments. The red-colored columns show those antibodies which binding to blood ACE in uremic patients with high 1G12/9B9 ratio differ more than 20% from that for patients with normal 1G12/9B9 ratio. * – parameter from the test sample was statistically different ($p < 0.05$) from the healthy control. **B**. Localization of disulfide bridges and free cysteine residues in the epitopes for mAbs 1G12 together with overlapping epitopes for mAbs 6A12 and i2H5 on the N domain of ACE (left) and mAb 1B3 together with adjacent epitopes for mAbs 1B8 and 3F10 (on the C domain of ACE). The regions of the epitopes for different mAbs were marked by circles with diameter of approximately 30Å, which corresponds to the square of 600–900 Å². Cysteine residues are marked magenta; potential glycosylation sites are marked green; amino acid residues participating in hinge-bending movement of domains are marked brown.

anti-ACE mAbs (2 μg/ml) in PBS/BSA (0.1 mg/ml) for 2 hrs at RT and washed. mAb BB9 to the N domain of ACE [59] which has an epitope overlapping with epitopes of 9B9 and 3A5 (Danilov et al., unpublished observation) was kindly provided by Dr. P. Simmons (Brown Foundation Institute of Molecular Medicine (IMM), University of Texas Health Science Center, Houston, TX). Wells were then incubated with 50 μl of ACE from any source (plasma/serum from volunteers or patients, soluble ACE secreted from cells transfected with wild type or mutant ACEs, lysate from these cells, or ACE purified from serum or seminal fluid by affinity chromatography on lisinopril-Sepharose as in [10]). Some samples (e.g., soluble ACE versus membrane-bound

ACE) were preliminarily equilibrated by ACE activity with Z-Phe-His-Leu as a substrate. After washing of unbound ACE, plate-bound ACE activity was measured by adding a substrate (Hip-His-Leu or Z-Phe-His-Leu) directly into the wells [49].

In some experiments, the source of ACE (pure ACE from serum or seminal fluid, plasma/serum, seminal fluid, soluble or membrane form of recombinant ACE) was preliminarily incubated with the effectors (ACE inhibitors, glutathione, dithiotreitol, etc.) and then added to the 96-well plate covered by different anti-ACE mAbs. Hemolysis of erythrocytes was performed as follows: several drops of distilled water were added to the whole blood (9 ml), the blood was vigorously shaken for 10 minutes, incubated at 4° for 14 hours and then centrifuged to obtain hemolysed serum.

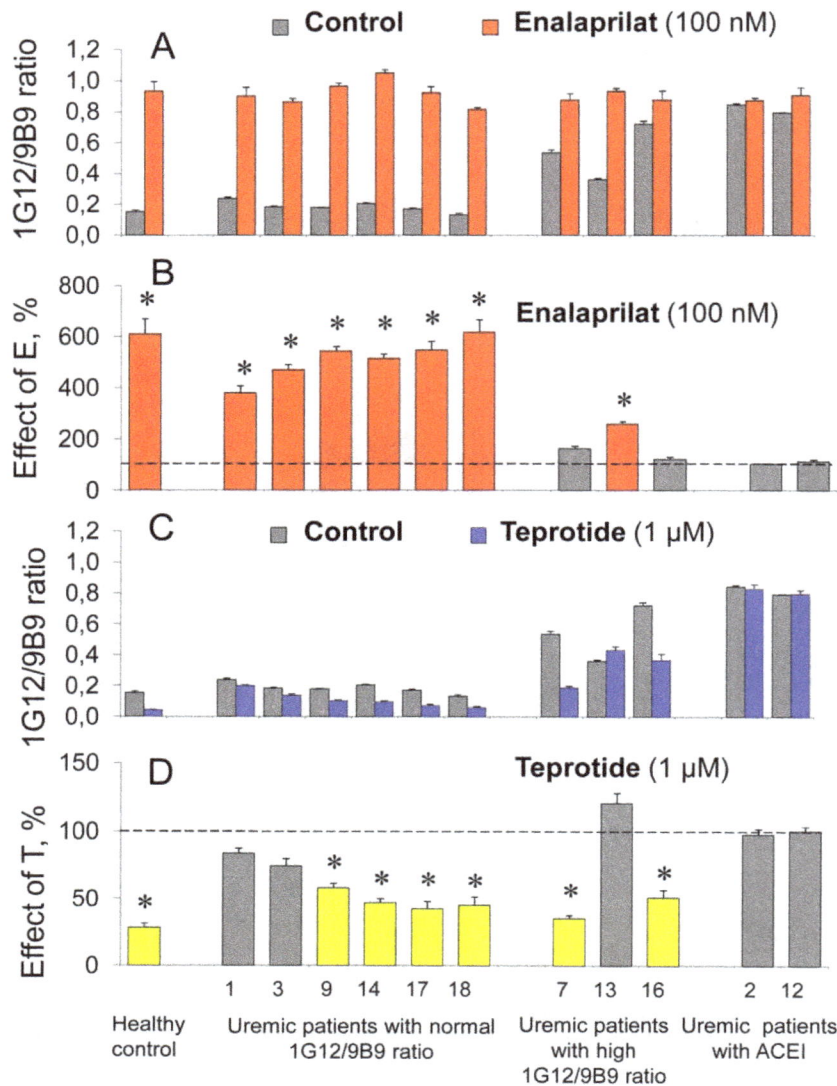

Figure 5. Effect of ACE inhibitors on the local conformation of blood ACE in uremia. A. The ratio of ACE activities precipitated from the citrated plasma of uremic patients by mAbs 1G12 and 9B9 (1G12/9B9 ratio) and from pooled plasma from healthy volunteers in the presence of enalaprilat (100 nM) – red bars and without the inhibitor – grey bars. **B.** The data presented on Fig. 5A were also expressed as a percentage of the effect of enalaprilat on the values of 1G12/9B9 ratio for different patients. The red columns show those mAbs for which enalaprilat effect (increase of mAb binding) exceeded 20%. **C.** The ratio of ACE activities precipitated from the citrated plasma of uremic patients by mAbs 1G12 and 9B9 (1G12/9B9 ratio) and from pooled plasma from healthy volunteers in the presence of teprotide (1 μM) – blue bars and without the inhibitor – grey bars. **D.** The data presented on Fig. 5C were also expressed as a percentage of the effect of teprotide on the values of 1G12/9B9 ratio for different patients. The yellow columns show those mAbs for which teprotide effect (decrease of mAb binding) exceeded 20%. All other terms and conditions – as in Figure 1. Data are mean ± SD of 3 independent experiments (each in duplicates). *, p<0.05 in comparison with mean value obtained without inhibitor.

Analysis of ACE Activity in Blood from Healthy Volunteers and Uremic Patients

This non-interventional pilot study was approved by the Institutional Review Boards of Moscow State University, clinical base of Moscow University for Medicine and Dentistry - Euromedic International Dialysis Centers, and University of Illinois at Chicago, and the procedures followed were in accordance with institutional guidelines. After providing informed consent regarding blood samples and data processing, citrated plasma or serum was obtained from healthy donors, from 20 patients with End Stage Renal Disease (ERSD) on maintenance hemodialysis (HD) or from age-match control patients without kidney diseases. Samples were kept at $-18°$ not longer than 3 months until further determination of ACE activity and immuno-chemical characterization of ACE. All ESRD patients were on maintenance HD with standard dialysis prescription (4 h × 3 times per week schedule), mean age of patients (mean±SD) was $58.3±8.5$ years, mean dialysis vintage was $151±32$ months. Hemodialysis procedures were performed on Fresenius 4008S dialysis machines with low flux polysulfone dialyzers F-series. All

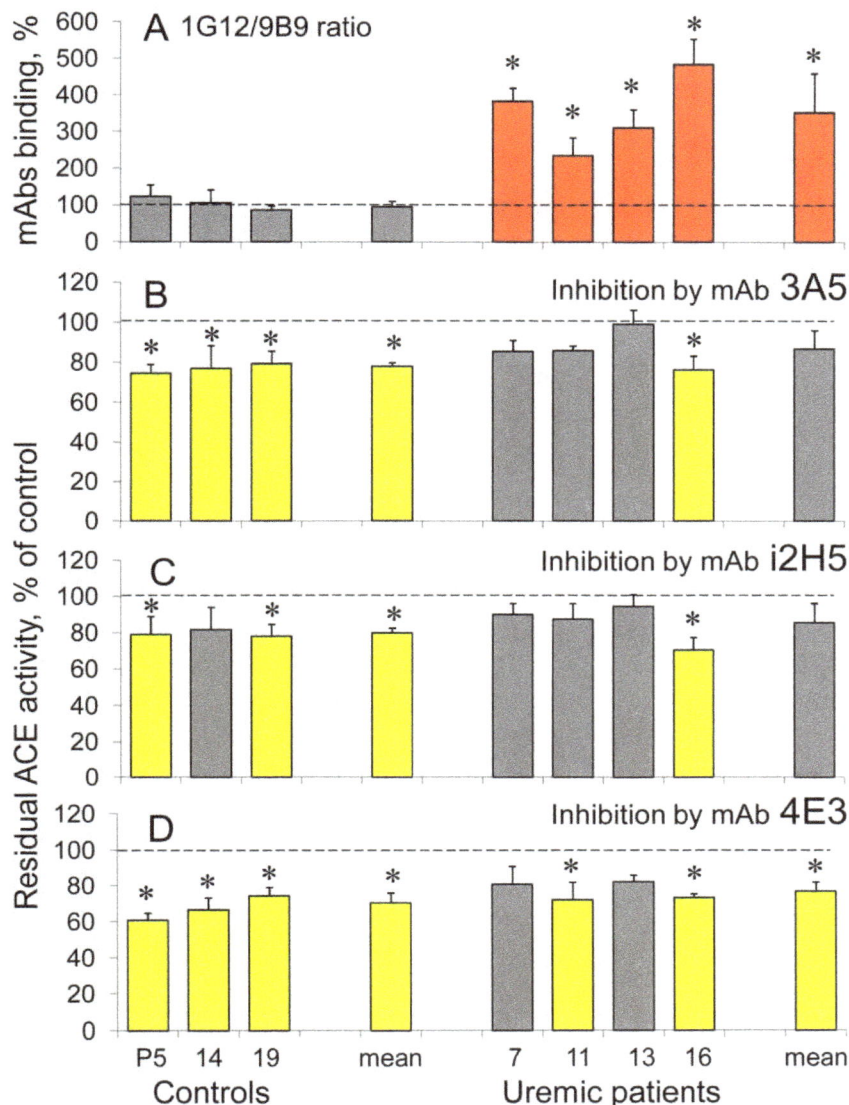

Figure 6. Effect of anti-catalytic mAbs on plasma ACE in uremia. A. The ratio of ACE activities precipitated from the citrated plasma of uremic patients with high 1G12/9B9 ratio and normal ZPHL/HHL ratio and from healthy controls (P5– pooled citrated plasma, #14 and #19– individual plasmas) by mAbs 1G12 and 9B9 (1G12/9B9 ratio. Grey bars – healthy controls; red bars – uremic patients with high 1G12/9B9 ratio with p<0.05 in comparison with mean value. **B-D**. Effect of anti-catalytic mAbs on ACE activity. The effects of anti-N domain mAbs 3A5 and i2H5 [42] were determined with ZPHL as a substrate. The effect of anti-C domain mAb 4E3 [27] was determined with HHL as a substrate. Data are presented as a residual ACE activity after incubation of tested mAbs (10 µg/ml) with citrated plasma (diluted 5-fold). Grey bars – ACE inhibition less than 20%, yellow bars – more than 20% of ACE inhibition. Data are mean ± SD of 3 independent experiments (each in duplicates), with p<0.05 in comparison with mean value obtained without anti-catalytic mAb.

patients match major dialysis adequacy criteria - Urea Reduction Rate (URR)>65%, Gotch dialysis index (KT/V)>1.4 and maintain stable Hb level from 10 to 12 g/dl on low dose epoetin beta and i.v. iron (iron sucrose) preparations. Concomitant therapy included calcium salt as a phosphate binder, active vitamin D and/or cinacalcet in some patients with secondary hyperparathyreosis. Though all patients had a past history of severe hypertension, some patients continued to intake antihypertensive medications at the time of the study - ACE inhibitors, AT2 receptor blockers (ARBs), calcium channel blockers (CCBs) or beta blockers.

Results and Discussion

Effect of ACE Inhibitors on ACE Conformational Fingerprinting

The presence of toxic compounds in the blood could influence the pattern of mAbs binding to blood ACE. Thus, in the course of mAbs 1G12 and 6A12 (to the N domain of ACE) epitope mapping we determined that the binding of these mAbs to blood ACE increased dramatically in the presence of common ACE inhibitors (captopril, lisinopril, enalaprilat), even facilitating the development of a sensitive assay for detection/quantification of ACE inhibitors in blood [43].

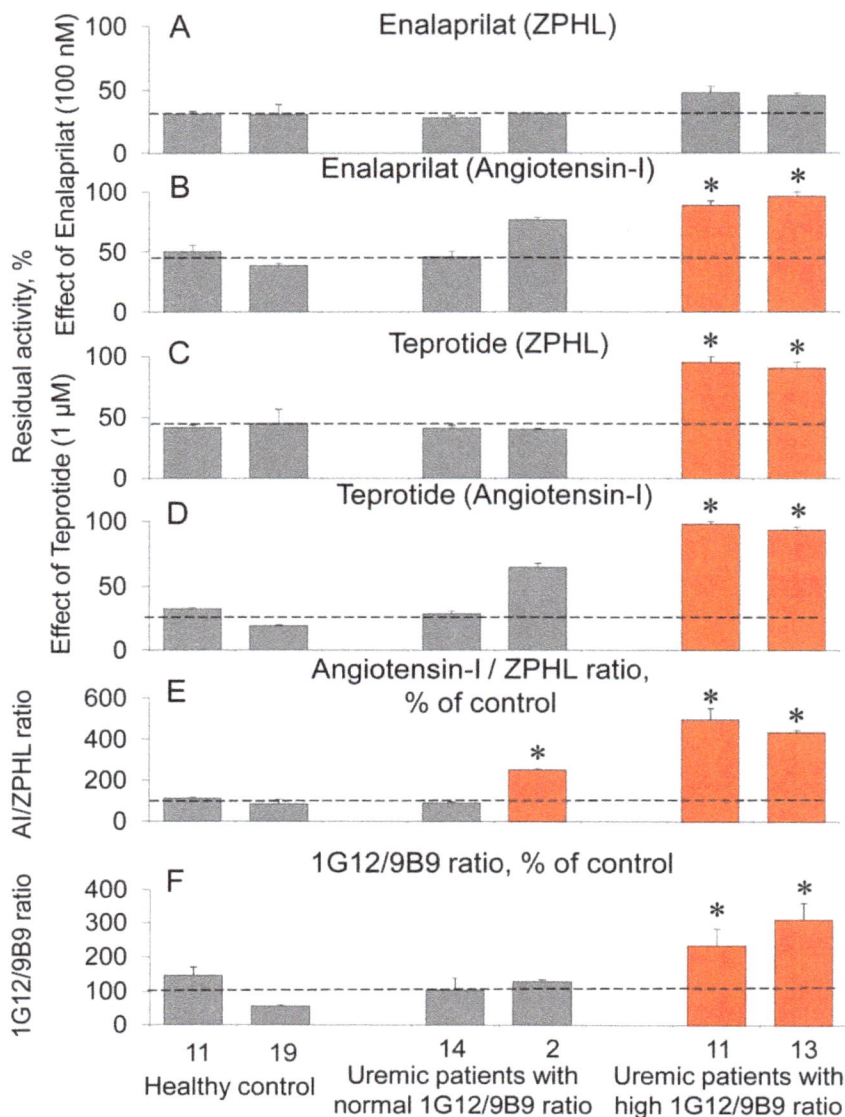

Figure 7. Effect of ACE inhibitors on the activity of plasma ACE in uremia. A–D Citrated plasma samples of uremic patients with normal (patients #14 and #2) and high (patients #11 and #13) 1G12/9B9 ratio (versus healthy controls, #11 and #19) were incubated with "short" ACE inhibitor enalaprilat (100 nM, **A** and **B**) and "long" ACE inhibitor teprotide (1 µM, **C** and **D**) for 1 hour. Data are presented as a residual ACE activity determined with "short" substrate ZPHL (0.5 mM, **A** and **C**) and "long" substrate angiotensin I (0.3 mM, **B** and **D**). Data are presented as a residual ACE activity. **E**. The ratio of the rates of the hydrolysis of angiotensin I and ZPHL (angiotensin I/ZPHL ratio) for corresponding samples. **F**. mAb1G12/9B9 binding ratio for corresponding samples expressed as % from the mean value for healthy persons. Grey bars – inhibition of ACE activity (A–D) or parameters measured in E–F in uremic samples was not differed from that for healthy patients with low 1G12/9B9 ratio. Red bars –measured parameters were statistically higher than that in healthy patients with low (normal) 1G12/9B9 ratio *, $p < 0.05$ in comparison with mean value for healthy patients. Data are mean ± SD from 3 independent experiments (each in duplicates).

We performed a study of ACE inhibitor effects on the binding of a panel of 17 mAbs to blood ACE ("conformational fingerprinting" approach) revealed by ACE activity precipitated by each mAb. The relative binding of strong mAbs (2B11, 9B9, 3A5, 2H9) dramatically differed compared to weak mAbs (i1A8, 3G8, 1E10, 3F11), likely reflecting difference in affinity constants for these mAbs (Fig. 1A). Figure 1B demonstrates that in addition to dramatic effect of enalaprilat on the binding of mAbs 1G12 and 6A12 [43] this commercially available and commonly used "short" (tripeptide analog) ACE inhibitor weakly (but significantly) increased precipitation of ACE activity with 5 other mAbs - 4 to the N domain (BB9, i1A8, 3G8, i2H5) and 1 to the C domain

(3F11) but decreased measured precipitated ACE activity with two mAbs - 1E10 and 4E3 to the C domain. The colored columns show those antibodies which binding to serum ACE in the presence of enalaprilat differ from that without ACE inhibitor.

Interestingly, the effect of the "long" (nonapeptide) ACE inhibitor teprotide (BPP9a, Glp-Trp-Pro-Arg-Pro-Gln-Ile-Pro-Pro) on the precipitation of serum ACE activity was different - teprotide increased mAb BB9 and decreased mAb 1E10 binding to ACE similar to enalaprilat but dramatically decreased the binding of mAbs 1G12 and 6A12 (with partially overlapping epitopes) as opposite to enalaprilat (Figure 1C). The effects of both inhibitors on mAbs binding to ACE were confirmed at a wide

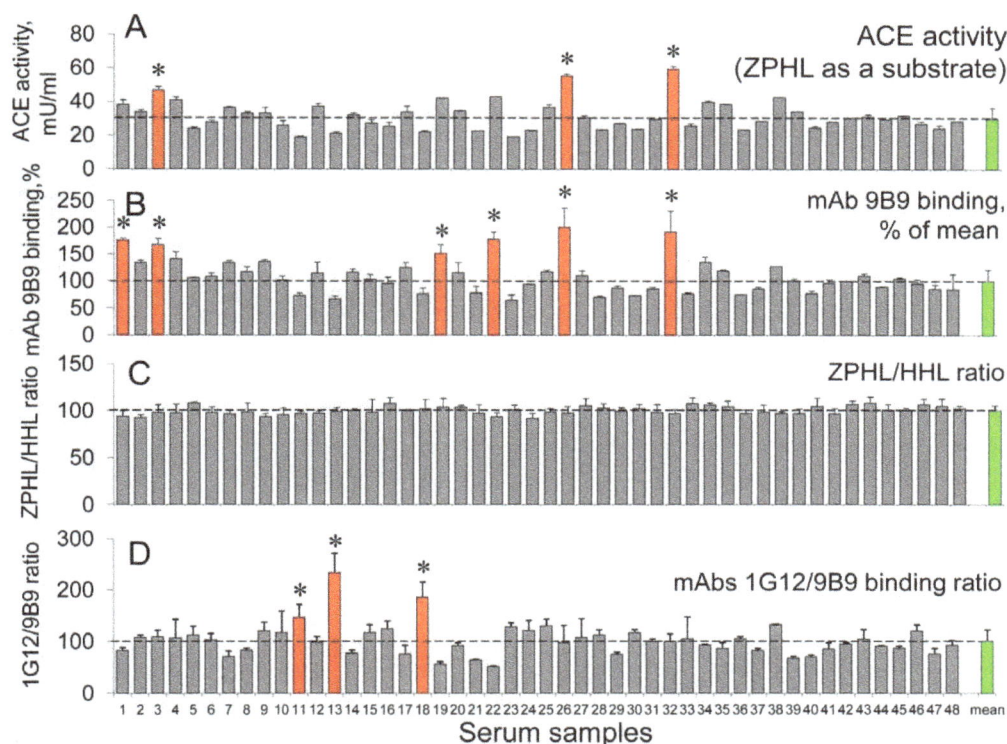

Figure 8. Blood ACE phenotyping in healthy donors. A. ACE activity in serum of healthy young donors was determined as in Figure 3. B. **ACE activity precipitated from serum of healthy donors by mAb 9B9 (estimation of relative ACE protein content). C. The ratio of the rates of the hydrolysis of two substrates (ZPHL/HHL ratio) for tested serum samples was determined as in Figure 3. D**. ACE activity precipitated from serum of healthy donors by mAbs 9B9 and 1G12 and expressed as their ratio for each serum sample. The red color of the bar shows serum of those patients whose tested parameters were significantly higher (and yellow bar – significantly lower) than mean value for all samples (green bars). Results are shown as mean ±SD of 4 independent experiments, each in duplicates or triplicates. *, statistically significant difference (p<0.05) from the mean value.

range of their concentrations (Figures 1D and 1E), thus demonstrating that the binding of the inhibitors with different structures within ACE active centers causes strikingly different conformational changes of the surface of ACE globule.

The increase in precipitated ACE activity in the presence of ACE inhibitor (most visibly seen in the case of mAbs 1G12/6A12 and enalaprilat, Figures 1B and 1D) could be only due to the increase in ACE binding by a particular mAb. However, when ACE activity precipitated by any mAb decreased in the presence of inhibitor the situation was not so simple. The decrease in ACE activity precipitated by any particular mAb and measured directly in the well could be attributed either to a decrease of the efficiency of ACE binding with this mAb or just to some retention of ACE inhibitor within ACE active centers induced by mAb binding.

In order to clarify this point we used previously described approach that the relative rate of the hydrolysis of two ACE substrates Z-Phe-His-Leu (ZPHL) and Hip-His-Leu (HHL) can indicate the presence of ACE inhibitors in the reaction media as the ratio ZPHL/HHL dramatically increased in the presence of inhibitors [54]. Fig. 2A shows that ZPHL/HHL ratio for blood ACE (without any additional inhibitor) precipitated by most mAbs did not differ from the corresponding value obtained for blood ACE in solution. This ratio was lower for ACE precipitated by anti-catalytic mAbs for the N domain, 3A5 and i2H5, due to selective inhibition by these mAbs of the N domain [32,42] and was higher in the case of anti-catalytic mAbs for the C domain, 1E10 and 4E3, due to selective inhibition of the C domain [27],

similarly to the effect of these mAbs on ZPHL/HHL ratio for ACE in solution [54] (and Fig. S1). In addition, we noticed that this ratio significantly increased in the case of mAb 3F11 to the C domain (Fig. 2A) - an effect that was not noticed for blood ACE in solution (not shown). Interestingly, in contrast to blood ACE, ZPHL/HHL ratio for recombinant ACE precipitated by mAb 1B8 decreased – for both soluble or membrane ACEs (Figure S1B and S1C), whereas an increase in ZPHL/HHL ratio precipitated by mAb 3F11 was not seen in the case of soluble recombinant ACE (Figure S1B). We consider these findings as an indication that two mAbs, 1B8 and 3F11, to the C domain are capable to induce conformational changes in ACE globule accompanying by the change of ZPHL/HHL ratio, however, the local conformation of the epitope for the particular mAb on the ACE surface, as well as capability for conformational changes induced by mAbs binding, are ACE-type specific.

Figure 2, B and C, demonstrates that in the presence of high concentration (100 nM) of "short" ACE inhibitor enalaprilat the ZPHL/HHL ratio (after standard washing, 5×200 μl/well) slightly increased only in the case of mAb 1E10, which could be considered as an indication of some retention of enalaprilat inside ACE induced by this particular mAb. After extensive washing (10×200 μl/well) with Cl⁻ free buffer, however, the ZPHL/HHL ratio in case of mAb 1E10 appeared to be equal to that for other mAbs and ACE in solution (data not shown), that is, enalaprilat bound to blood ACE was completely washed out before adding of ACE substrates.

Table 1. Clinical Data.

1st Group Conformationally naïve ACE					2nd Group Conformationally changed ACE					3rd Group Presence of ACE inhibitors				
Patient ##	Age, Years	DV[1] months	SBP[2] mm,Hg	DBP[3] mm,Hg	Patient ##	Age, Years	DV[1] months	SBP[2] mm,Hg	DBP[3] mm,Hg	Patient ##	Age, Years	DV[1] months	SBP[2] mm,Hg	DBP[3] mm,Hg
1	47	147	137	80	7	58	119	156	72	2	43	216	140	90
3	75	161	72	42	11	61	216	158	90	4	65	160	130	80
5	48	190	130	75	13	61	126	130	70	12	57	184	138	77
6	48	98	140	78	16	47	115	137	80	15	63	125	80	45
8	53	228	123	70										
9	39	137	97	56										
10	72	177	162	80										
14	62	120	129	74										
17	58	109	110	60										
18	72	141	140	66										
19	63	128	87	53										
20	73	123	160	60										
Mean	**59.2**	**146.6**	**123.9**	**66.2**		56.8	144.0	145.3	78.0		57.0	171.3	122.0	73.0
SD	12.2	37.1	27.8	12.1		6.7	48.2	13.9	9.1		9.9	38.4	28.3	19.5
p value	For difference with 1st group					0.629	0.926	0.069	0.078		0.217	0.06	0.974	0.547
p value	For difference with 2nd group										0.968	0.411	0.191	0.659

[1]DV- Dialysis Vintage; [2]SBP- Systolic Blood Pressure; [3]DBP- Diastolic Blood Pressure.
Blood pressure was measured before dialysis and before blood sampling.

Moreover, the fact that ZPHL/HHL ratio did not increased for ACE precipitated by mAbs 1G12/6A12 and by 1E10 in the presence of teprotide both after standard and intensive washings could be unequivocally considered as the evidence that there was no any retention of the inhibitor by these mAbs. So, the decrease of the precipitation of blood ACE activity by mAbs 1G12/6A12 and 1E10 in the presence of this inhibitor (Fig. 1) was due to a real decrease of these mAbs binding to blood ACE induced by teprotide binding within ACE active centers.

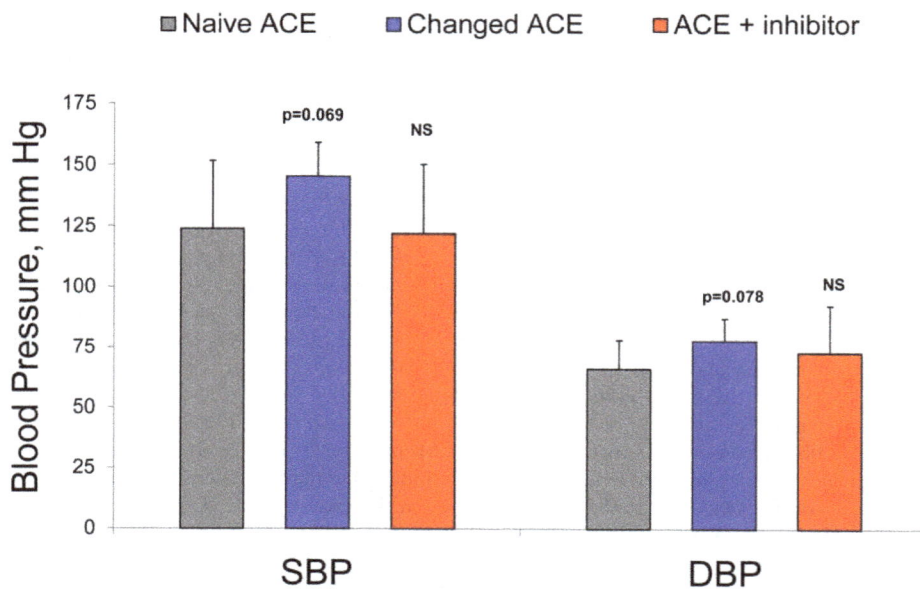

Figure 9. Blood pressure in patients with uremia due to ESRD. Blood pressure was measured in patients with ESRD before dialysis and before blood sampling. According to T test p values for the differences in Systolic Blood Pressure (SBP) and Diastolic Blood Pressure (DBP) between patients with conformationally naïve and conformationally changed ACE were close to the level of significance (p<0.05).

It is necessary to note that the effect of ACE inhibitors on mAbs binding to ACE depends both on the type of ACE inhibitor and the source of ACE. Thus, "long" ACE inhibitor teprotide similarly changed the pattern of mAbs binding to ACE from serum, seminal fluid or soluble recombinant human sACE, as well as truncated N or C domain expressed in CHO cells: the binding of mAbs 1G12 and 6A12 to the N domain dramatically decreased, 2–3 folds, in all cases, whereas the binding of mAb 1B3, directed to the C terminal part of the C domain, significantly increased (Figure S2 and S3). "Short" inhibitor enalaprilat showed more difference. This inhibitor similarly decreased the binding of mAbs 1E10 and 4E3 (directed to the C domain) to blood ACE, ACE from seminal fluid or soluble recombinant ACE. However, while the binding of mAbs 1G12 and 6A12 to blood ACE sharply increased in the presence of enalaprilat, the binding of mAb 1G2 to ACE from seminal fluid or soluble recombinant human ACE practically did not change and the amplitude of the effect of enalaprilat on mAb 6A12 binding was much less pronounced (Figures S2 and S3).

Therefore, data presented on Figures 2, S1–S3 demonstrated clearly, that the effects of ACE inhibitors on the mAbs binding, while ACE-type specific, confirmed one more time that the pattern of mAbs binding to ACE is the most sensitive marker for even subtle local conformational changes in ACE molecule.

The main goal of this study was to find putative conformational changes in ACE at disease/pathology by use of a conformational fingerprinting of blood ACE with a set of mAbs. Therefore processing of blood ACE for the future analysis could be a very important technological and methodological issue. By classical biochemical approach, an isolation of pure ACE from plasma/serum of patients with a disease seemed an ideal. However, when we performed purification of ACE from plasma or seminal fluid by lisinopril affinity chromatography we found that the pattern of mAbs binding (conformational fingerprint, i.e. local conformation of ACE) was rather different for purified ACE and the corresponding ACE in the content of biological fluid (Figure S4). Therefore we decided to use unprocessed serum/plasma as the source of naive blood ACE conformation from a given patient. It is important that ACE from serum, citrate plasma or heparinized plasma (but not EDTA-plasma) exhibited similar "conformational fingerprint" (data not shown), that is this particular blood processing did not influence ACE local conformation.

Effect of Different Compounds on mAbs Binding to Blood ACE

Sensitivity of the pattern of binding of a set of mAbs to local conformational changes induced by glycan moiety [49] or by binding of ACE inhibitors ([43] and this study) inspired us to hypothesize that the disease(s) characterized by high concentration of toxic compounds can be accompanied by the conformational changes in ACE in the blood. Therefore we performed screening of several compounds for their effect on mAbs binding to ACE.

Somatic ACE molecule contains 6 paired cysteine residues (Cys) forming S-S bridges [60]- Cys128-Cys136, Cys330-Cys348 and Cys526-Cys528 in the N domain, as well as Cys728-Cys734, Cys928-Cys946 and Cys1114-Cys1126 in the C domain, and two unpaired cysteines, Cys 474 and Cys 1072, which theoretically can participate in the creation of homo- or hetero- ACE dimers via disulfide bridges. Therefore, at first we tested compounds that can affect the disulfide bridge formation, dithiothreitol (DTT) and reduced glutathione (GSH).

Figure S5 demonstrates the effects of DTT and GSH on blood ACE conformational fingerprint. The reduction of S-S bridges by both reagents (Fig. S5, A and B) resulted in rather similar changes in mAbs binding pattern: the most significant effect was observed with mAbs 1G12 and i2H5 to the N domain and mAb 1B3 to the C domain which binding to ACE significantly increased as a result of the treatment. Epitopes for mAbs 1G12 and i2H5 contain the disulfide bridge Cys516-Cys528, therefore we can conclude that the reduction of this bridge resulted in the effect observed. The epitope for mAb 1B3 does not contain any S-S bridge, but the bridge Cys728-Cys734 is located nearby. The binding of mAb 3F11 to the C domain also increased after GSH (not DTT) treatment, its epitope containing Cys1114-1126; mAb BB9 slightly increased and mAb 1E10 decreased the binding to ACE due to GSH treatment, however, epitopes for these mAb do not contain any S-S bridge. Other mAbs, 3G8 (no S-S bridges in the epitope) and 5F1 (Cys330-Cys348 in the epitope) to the N domain, 1B8 and 3F10 (Cys728-Cys734 in epitopes) and 2H9 (no S-S bridges in the epitope) to the C domain decreased the binding with blood ACE due to DTT treatment. Similar but less pronounced effects of DTT and GSH on mAbs binding to ACE we obtained with purified ACE from seminal fluid (data not shown).

Another compound, 5,5'-dithiobis(2-dinitrobenzoic acid), capable to interact with free Cys residues, induced the only change in mAbs binding pattern – the 40%-decrease of the binding of mAb 1B3 (data not shown), epitope of which is localized on the C-terminal end of the C domain and contains free Cys 1072 [27].

Thus, these experiments demonstrated that the state of Cys residues and S-S bridges can play a remarkable role in the conformational fingerprint of ACE. It is known that the hemolysis of erythrocytes causes liberation of intracellular GSH to plasma thus increasing both GSH and GSSH (oxidized glutathione, due to auto-oxidation of GSH in the extracellular medium) plasma concentrations [61–62]. So, we tested the effect of hemolysis on mAbs binding to blood ACE and showed that the binding of three mAbs to the N domain, 1G12, 6A12 and i2H5 (epitopes of all three contain Cys516-Cys528 bridge), remarkably increased (Fig. S5, C). So, we unequivocally demonstrated that the compounds present in blood can directly influence the conformation of ACE globule as seen by ACE conformational fingerprint. It is worth noting, as a methodological remark, that plasma/serum should not be hemolysed prior this fingerprinting.

Conformational Fingerprinting of Blood ACE in Uremic Patients

Uremia is a pathology characterized by a high content of different toxic compounds [51] due to retention of these compounds and a deficient renal clearance caused by kidneys disease. Patients suffering from chronic renal failure are exposed to increased oxidative stress generated by uremic toxins, further exacerbated by HD, chronic inflammatory state, etc. [63–65]. Specifically, GSH was reported to be significantly elevated in the ESRD and HD patients [66–67]. Therefore, we chose uremic state in HD ESRD patients to be checked for the effect both on the activity and on the conformation of blood ACE.

Figures 3 demonstrates an example of this approach (ACE phenotyping) when patient plasma/serum was tested for 1) ACE activity with two substrates, ZPHL and HHL; 2) the presence of ACE inhibitors in patient's blood using enzymatic assay – ZPHL/HHL ratio [54] and more sensitive antibody-based assay –1G12/9B9 ratio [43]; 3) concentration of ACE protein (using immuno-capture assay with mAb 9B9 [37]); 4) conformational control of the most labile region of ACE – the region of the epitope for mAb 1G12 overlapping with epitopes for mAbs 6A12 and i2H5 [43].

Figure 3A shows ACE activity in 20 ESRD HD patients, whose blood was taken before HD and in 7 healthy volunteers. Five ESRD patients (out of 20) demonstrated an increased ACE activity in their blood which corroborate with several publications that reported increased ACE activity in uremic patients [21–23]. Figure 3B demonstrates the ratio of the rates of hydrolysis of two substrates (ZPHL/HHL ratio) for all these patients. This parameter [54] is very stable in a normal population, $100 \pm 3.0\%$, while ACE activity itself measured with any substrate deviates very significantly, $100 \pm 30\%$, [16,37]. It is clearly seen that ZPHL/HHL ratio was significantly increased in 4 (out of 20, numbers 2, 4, 12 and 15) ESRD patients. This result indicates the presence of ACE inhibitor in the blood of these patients at the time of blood sampling [54] and confirms the necessity of the objective testing of presence of ACE inhibitors in the patient's blood in all clinical trials which can include treatment with ACE inhibitors.

We performed also antibody-based assay and estimated the precipitation of blood ACE from these patients by two mAbs to ACE – mAb 9B9 (Figure 3E) which binding to blood ACE is not affected by the presence of ACE inhibitors and corresponds to the ACE protein in the blood [37], and mAb 1G12 (Figure 3D), which binding to blood ACE remarkably increased (3-5-fold) in the presence of common ACE inhibitors [43]. We confirmed that both the binding of mAb 1G12 (Figure 3D) and, more important, 1G12/9B9 ratio (Figure 3C) increased dramatically in those 4 patients (numbers 2, 4, 12 and 15) that were detected as having ACE inhibitors in their blood with the help of ZPHL/HHL ratio (Figure 3B).

This approach, however, allowed us to discover another four ESRD patients (out of 20, numbers 7, 11, 13 and 16 - boxed in Figures 3B and C), whose 1G12/9B9 ratio increased while ZPHL/HHL ratio was absolutely normal. So, we could consider blood ACE (at least) in these patients as having local conformational changes in 1G12 epitope. It is important that these changes could not be attributed to the presence of ACE inhibitors (as common drugs at hypertension) in the blood of these patients but should be considered as conformational changes of ACE surface caused by some toxic compounds due to uremia.

We tested the binding of the set of mAbs to ACE from plasma of those ESRD patients (numbers 7, 11, 13 and 16) compared to that for healthy persons and found that besides the increase of binding of mAb 1G12 (Figure 3, C and D) only mAb 1B3 to the C domain (2 mAbs out of 15) bound better to ACE from the blood of ESRD patients (Figure 4A). One of the reasons for such an increase could be an effect of putative toxic compounds on the disulfide bridge Cys516-Cys528 in the epitope for mAb 1G12 and on the disulfide bridge Cys728-Cys734 close to epitope for mAb 1B3 and/or on unpaired Cys1072 directly in the epitope for mAb 1B3 (Figure 4B) similar to the effects obtained after hemolysis or after ACE treatment with DTT, GSH and DTNB (Fig. S5). It should be pointed out, however, that the principal difference between the abovementioned effects and uremia effect exists: the binding of mAbs 6A12 and i2H5 (having overlapping epitopes with epitope for mAb 1G12) with ACE from the blood of ESRD patients changed only very slightly (Fig. 4A) compared with the significant increase of the binding of mAb i2H5 after GSH and DTT treatments and increase of the binding of all three mAbs, 1G12, 6A12 and i2H5, due to hemolysis (Fig. S5).

The next logical step was an analysis of the effect of the presence of "short" (enalaprilat) and "long" (teprotide) inhibitors on the local conformation of blood ACE (expressed as 1G12/9B9 ratio) from ESRD patients versus that of healthy volunteers. Figure 5 clearly demonstrates that both healthy donors (mean value for 33 persons) and ESRD patients (numbers 1, 3, 9, 14, 17 and 18) having low 1G12/9B9 ratio responded to enalaprilat in a common way, i.e. by a significant increase of 1G12/9B9 ratio. However, the response of ESRD patients with high 1G12/9B9 ratio (patients 2, 7, 13, 16, 2 and 12, the last two having ACE inhibitors in the

blood as shown above) did not show significant response (if any) to the presence of enalaprilat (Fig. 5, A and B). It seems that in the blood of these ESRD patients ACE possesses the local conformation with most accessible epitope for mAb 1G12, otherwise partially buried/hidden in ACE from healthy persons. The action of enalaprilat on ACE, besides activity inhibition, is the increase of accessibility of this epitope to the mAb which appeared to be impossible for these ESRD patients (including persons having ACE inhibitors in the blood) as 1G12 epitope on ACE from their blood is already fully accessible.

A rather different situation was observed with teprotide: the effect of the inhibitor on mAbs binding with ACE from uremic patients in both groups, with low and high 1G12/9B9 ratios, was less pronounced than that for healthy persons (Fig. 5, C and D). However, the response to teprotide appeared to be individual, as in both groups there were patients with very weak (numbers 1, 3, and 13) and almost normal (number 7) decrease of mAb 1G12 binding to ACE in the presence of teprotide. The binding of mAb 1G12 to ACE from the blood of patients (numbers 2 and 12) having ACE inhibitors did not decrease at all in the presence of teprotide, indicating that teprotide could not reverse the effect of ACE inhibitors in the blood.

The fact that ACE inhibitors became unable to induce conformational changes on the surface of ACE from blood from some ESRD patients (Figures 3,4,5) put the question about ACE response to these inhibitors regarding inhibition of the enzyme activity. At first we tested an effect of anti-catalytic mAbs to ACE on the rate of the hydrolysis of substrates ZPHL (with mAbs 3A5 and 12H5 to the N domain) and HHL (with mAb 4E3 to the C domain) by ACE from uremic plasma and several samples of plasma from healthy donors. Figure 6 demonstrates that at least three (out of 4) ESRD patients with elevated 1G12/9B9 ratio exhibited significantly diminished efficacy of anti-catalytic action of mAbs 3A5 and i2H5 to the N domain and two ESRD patients exhibited diminished efficacy of mAb 4E3 as anti-catalytic mAbs to the C domain (Fig. 6).

The most important results were obtained in the experiments with inhibition of ACE from the blood of ESRD patients compared with that from healthy donors with both ZPHL and angiotensin I as substrates (Fig. 7). First of all, the activity of ACE in the blood of some ESRD patients, especially with high 1G12/9B9 ratio, in the reaction of the hydrolysis of angiotensin I appeared to be much higher (up to 5-fold) than the activity of ACE in the blood of healthy donors (Fig. 7E). This result couldn't be explained by higher level of ACE in uremic plasma, as we did not find any increase in ACE binding with mAb 9B9 (Fig. 3E). Besides, the activity of these patients with ZPHL as a substrate was similar to that of healthy donors (Fig. 3A).

Figure 7A and B shows that patients with high 1G12/9B9 ratio are slightly less susceptible to inhibition of the hydrolysis of ZPHL by "short" ACE inhibitor enalaprilat (Fig. 7 A) and even less susceptible to the inhibition of the hydrolysis of angiotensin I by this inhibitor (Fig. 7B). "Long" ACE inhibitor teprotide distinguished patients with low and high 1G12/9B9 ratios even more effectively and less dependently on the structure of the substrate: blood ACE from patients with high 1G12/9B9 ratio was inhibited by 1 µM teprotide only slightly with both ZPHL and angiotensin I as substrates (Fig. 7, C and D). Moreover, in the latter case inhibition could be considered as negligible. To prove it true, we diluted plasma from ESRD patients 5-fold to make it equal to normal plasma by ACE activity with angiotensin I as a substrate. However, even at this case ACE from blood of ESRD patients with high 1G12/9B9 ratio failed to be inhibited with the same effectiveness as ACE in normal blood (data not shown). It is worth noting that we did not find any dependence of these effects on the age or gender of patients.

It is known, that cardiovascular events are the leading cause of death in adult ESRD patients on maintenance HD with annual mortality rate about 20% [68–69]. The current recommendation is to employ a renin-angiotensin system (RAS)-blocking agents, ACE inhibitors in particular [70–71]. However, the majority of cardiovascular primary and secondary prevention clinical trials have excluded patients with advanced renal insufficiency [72–73]. Therefore, it is less known whether the results of clinical trials could be also applied to those patients, who are on maintenance HD with a mixture of uremic toxic compounds in their serum. In a retrospective study, patients with renal failure on HD treated with ACE inhibitors had a lower mortality rate as compared to those who were not treated [74–75]. However, observational analyses alone are not sufficient to assess the efficacy and safety of ACE inhibitor use in this setting [72]. In randomized controlled Fosinopril Study in Dialysis (FOSIDIAL) no significant benefit for Fosinopril was observed in the intent-to-treat analysis after adjusting for independent predictors of cardiovascular events [72]. Similar conclusion, but with different ACE inhibitors, was made in HEMO study representing randomized clinical trial of HD patients regarding flux and dose of dialysis [72]. This study fail to show an association of ACE inhibitors use with less cardiovascular morbidity and mortality of HD patients, while beneficial effect of ACE inhibitors on CVE risk reduction in general populations was repeatedly and clearly demonstrated [76]. In another study, in children with chronic renal failure, the use of ACE inhibitors in ESRD patients failed to decrease plasma angiotensin II level at all [77].

Different mechanisms underlying therapy resistance to ACE inhibitors have been suggesting so far: ACE gene polymorphism [78–79], the extent of renal damage prior to ACE inhibition [80], different drug clearance in responders and non-responders [81]. We can hypothesize, however, on the base of obtained results, that in uremic state the response to ACE inhibitors could be markedly attenuated by uremic toxicity and possible reason might be conformational changes in ACE molecule, induced by elevated levels of toxic substances in the uremic serum.

Therefore, we can consider that simple and technological control of ACE conformation - determination of 1G12/9B9 ratio for blood ACE in the conjunction with the simultaneous determination of ZPHL/HHL ratio, altogether with determination of ACE activity with angiotensin I as a substrate, can identify subpopulation of patients (at least ESRD patients) less sensitive to ACE inhibitor therapy and who, therefore, either should be treated with these drugs more aggressively or use alternative approach to RAS blockade.

In order to estimate the frequency of conformationally changed blood ACE in a wide population we performed ACE phenotyping and determined these parameters, 1G12/9B9 and ZPHL/HHL ratios, in 63 unrelated patients and in 48 healthy young blood donors. The result of the 1st round of such ACE phenotyping (in 48 healthy young donors) is presented in Figure 8. ACE activity in this population (within 95%) differed 2.3-fold (Fig. 8A), and ACE protein in the blood in this population (according to mAb 9B9 binding) differed 2.2-fold (Fig. 8B), which showed high accuracy of the determination of ACE activity and protein and confirmed high diversity of ACE level in population [16,37]. ZPHL/HHL ratio was a very stable parameter (Fig. 8C, 100±4.4%). In this population of 48 patients we found 3 patients (Fig. 8D, numbers 11, 13 and 18) with significantly elevated 1G12/9B9 ratio (with normal ZPHL/HHL ratio).

As a whole, we found 4 patients with elevated 1G12/9B9 ratio, while normal ZPHL/HHL ratio, from 20 ESRD patients (that is 20%); 5 patients of such characteristics from 63 patients without chronic kidney diseases (7.9%), while only 3 healthy donors out of 48 (6.3%) exhibited elevated 1G12/9B9 ratio. Thus, in a normal population the percentage of blood ACE with changed conformation is remarkably lower than that in chronic uremia in ESRD.

The level of 1G12/9B9 ratio reached 240–490% in the blood of ESRD patients from that for healthy controls, while for patients with unrelated diseases and for healthy persons this level did not exceed 230–240% for two persons and was only about 145–185% for other 6 persons with elevated 1G12/9B9 ratio (Fig. S6, F). It is important that those persons exhibiting higher 1G12/9B9 ratio (more than 200% from control) exhibited higher ACE activity towards angiotensin I as well (Fig. S6, E). The inhibition of ACE from the blood of healthy/unrelated patients with lower 1G12/9B9 ratio (145–185%) didn't differ from that for control persons both by enalaprilat and teprotide with ZPHL and angiotensin I as substrates (Fig. S6, A–D). However, the inhibition of blood ACE activity for the patients with higher 1G12/9B9 ratio (230–240% from control) by both enalaprilat (Fig. S6, B) and teprotide (Fig. S6, D) appeared to be less effective than for normal ones with angiotensin I as a substrate, similar to that for ACE from the blood of ESRD patients.

Thus, elevated 1G12/9B9 ratio for blood ACE could be considered as marker for conformationally altered ACE, which inhibition by ACE inhibitors could be impaired in uremic state and, thus, could mark non-responders to ACE inhibitors.

What could be the reason for this particular region on the blood ACE molecule (epitopes for mAb 1G12/6A12) to be so sensitive to conformational changes induced by ACE inhibitors (Fig. 1), SH-reagents (Fig. S5), ACE purification (Fig. S4), uremia (Fig. 3,4,5, 7), whereas binding of these mAbs to recombinant human somatic ACE or individual domains was less influenced by these reagents? Figure S7 shows comparative effects of ACE inhibitor enalaprilat and fetal bovine and human sera on mAbs binding to soluble human recombinant sACE. Effect of enalaprilat on mAbs binding to recombinant ACE (Fig. S7B) was similar to human serum ACE (Fig. S7A) for all mAbs, except mAbs 1G12 and 6A12, which binding to recombinant ACE increased to less extent. Fetal bovine serum (10%) slightly increased the binding of these mAbs to recombinant ACE (Fig. S7C) which can indicate on the presence of endogenous ACE inhibitors in bovine serum that were previously found in plasma from different animals, including human [54, 82–84, and own unpublished data]. However, adding of 10% of human serum to recombinant ACE dramatically decreased the binding of 3 mAbs, 1G12, 6A12 and i2H5, directed to overlapping epitopes on the N domain of ACE (Fig. S7D). We can consider this fact as an indication that some component of human plasma (ACE-binding protein?) binds to the region of the overlapping epitopes for these mAbs on the N domain of recombinant ACE and decrease, therefore, the binding of mAbs. In this case, dramatic increase of mAbs 1G12 and 6A12 binding to blood ACE in the presence of commercial "short" ACE inhibitor, as a result of treatment with GSH or DTT or after action of toxic compounds in the blood of ESRD patients could be partially explained by a possible dissociation of this putative ACE-binding protein from its complex with the enzyme with simultaneous unmasking the epitopes for these mAbs. Several ACE-binding proteins (some of them with ACE-inhibiting properties) were suggested so far: 100 kD protein [85–86], 14 kD protein [87], but the nature of these proteins was not yet identified.

Finally we tried to link our findings with surrogate clinical end-point, such is blood pressure (BP) - Table 1. There was a clear (however, not statistically significant) trend towards differences in pre-dialysis BP in those patients, who demonstrate conformational changes of ACE, and other patients (Fig. 9). Systolic BP for the patients with conformationally changed ACE was 145.3 ± 13.9 mm Hg versus 122.0 ± 28.3 (p = 0,069) for other patients, while diastolic BP was 78.0 ± 9.1 mm Hg versus 66.2 ± 12.1, respectively (p = 0.078).

Conclusions

We demonstrated that the pattern of precipitation of ACE activity by mAbs to ACE (conformational fingerprinting of ACE) is a sensitive parameter characterizing changes in the local ACE conformation. We have shown that this pattern of ACE binding by a set of mAbs was influenced significantly by the presence of ACE inhibitor, common inhibitor (tripeptide analog) and teprotide (nonapeptide) causing different effects. Conformational characteristics of ACE can be also changed by the action of compounds capable to interact with S-S bridges within protein globule or with free Cys residues. The conformational fingerprinting of ACE together with technological enzymatic test – the determination of relative rates of the hydrolysis of two substrates, ZPHL and HHL, appeared to have a potential for the selection of a group of patients among ESRD patients which are not sensitive enough for a common treatment by ACE inhibitors. ACE in the blood of these patients is characterized by elevated 1G12/9B9 ratio (relative binding of two mAbs to different epitopes on the surface of ACE N domain) and elevated activity with angiotensin I as a substrate, while normal activity with ZPHL and normal ZPHL/HHL ratio. ACE activity in the blood of these patients is worse inhibited both by common ACE inhibitor and teprotide.

These findings indicate that conformational fingerprinting of ACE can help to indicate the occurrence of the changes of the protein due to disease and may be considered as an approach for the finding of risk factors at pathology.

Despite obvious limitation of our study that was not designed to evaluate BP in this high risk group of patients, our results in the group of long-term survivals on maintenance HD with long time exposure to chronic uremia reveal that conformational changes of ACE might participate in the mechanism of adverse clinical outcomes in ESRD patients.

Supporting Information

Figure S1   ZPHL/HHL ratio for different ACEs precipitated by mAbs to ACE. Pooled citrated plasma diluted 1/5 with PBS was equilibrated by ACE activity with soluble or membrane form of human recombinant ACE (5 mU/ml with HHL as a substrate) and incubated with microtiter plate coated with 16 different anti-ACE mAbs via goat-anti-mouse IgG bridge as in Figure 1. Precipitation of ACE activity by these mAbs from different ACE sources was expressed as a ratio of precipitated ACE activity with substrate ZPHL to that with substrate HHL (Danilov et al. 2008). Pooled citrated plasma from 30 healthy individuals Culture medium from CHO cells transfected with human recombinant ACE (clone 2C2 -Balyasnikova et al. 1999) – soluble WT ACE. Lysate from CHO cells transfected with human recombinant ACE (clone 2C2 -Balyasnikova et al. 1999) – membrane form of WT ACE. The red color of the bars shows higher ZPHL/HHL ratio – more than 20% (and yellow – lower) obtained for ACE precipitated by corresponding mAb compared to that in solution. * – p<0.05 in comparison with ZPHL/HHL ratio of a given ACE in solution.

Figure S2   Effect of ACE inhibitors on mAbs binding to plasma and seminal fluid ACE. A–B, D–E. The effect of enalaprilat (100 nM, **A** and **B**) or teprotide (1 µM, **D** and **E**) on mAbs binding to seminal fluid ACE (**B** and **E**) in comparison with plasma ACE (**A** and **D**) was determined using plate precipitation assay with ZPHL as a substrate as in Figure 1. The red color of the bars shows higher mAbs binding – more than 20% (and yellow – lower) obtained in the presence of inhibitors. *, p<0.05 in comparison with corresponding values obtained without inhibitor. **C–F.** The ratio of the effects of the inhibitor (enalaprilat, C, and teprotide, F) on mAbs binding with seminal fluid ACE to that for plasma ACE. The red color of the bars shows higher effects ratio – more than 20% (and yellow – lower) in comparison with the mean value for the whole mAbs set. All other terms and conditions are as in Fig. 1. Data are mean ± SD of 3–8 independent experiments (each in duplicates). * - p<0.05 in comparison with mean value for plasma ACE.

Figure S3   Effect of ACE inhibitors on mAbs binding to soluble recombinant two-domain ACE (WTΔ) and individual truncated domains. The effect of enalaprilat (100 nM, **A–C**) or teprotide (1 µM, **D–F**) on mAbs binding to soluble recombinant ACEs expressed in CHO cells was determined using plate precipitation assay with Z-Phe-His-Leu (ZPHL) as a substrate as in Figure 1. **A, D.** Soluble truncated human recombinant two-domain s ACE: 1–1230 WTΔ (Wei et al. 1991). **B, E.** Truncated recombinant N domain: 1–629 (Balyasnikova et al. 2003). **C, F.** Truncated recombinant C domain: 1–4, 613–1203 (Balyasnikova et al. 2005). All other terms and conditions-as in Figure 1. Data are mean ± SD of 3–4 independent experiments (each in duplicates). * - p<0.05 in comparison with values for samples without ACE inhibitors.

Figure S4   Effect of ACE purification on the local conformation of ACE. The effect of the purification of ACE from plasma and from seminal fluid by affinity chromatography on the lisinopril-Sepharose on the conformational fingerprint of ACE was assessed using 16 mAbs to different epitopes on the N and C domains of ACE. Pooled citrated plasma diluted 1/5 with PBS and seminal fluid (diluted 1/150) were equilibrated by activity with corresponding purified ACEs (approximately to 5 mU/ml). Precipitation of ACE activity by the set of mAbs was performed as in Figure 1 and expressed as a ratio of precipitated ACE activity from pure ACE to that from the corresponding source (plasma or seminal fluid). Plasma ACE. Seminal fluid ACE. All other terms and conditions are as in Figure 1. Red columns shows bigger (yellow – lower) precipitation of pure ACE activity (more than 20%) that that of ACE from biological fluid. Data are mean ± SD of 3 independent experiments (each in duplicates). * - p<0.05 in comparison with values for ACE from biological fluids.

Figure S5   Effect of different compounds on mAbs binding to blood ACE. A, B. Reduced glutathione and dithiotreitol at the indicated concentrations were incubated with pooled citrated plasma from 33 healthy volunteers (diluted 5-fold in PBS) for half an hour at 25°C before plate precipitation assay. **C.** Plasma sample was hemolysed by adding water and vigorous stirring and incubated for three days before the assay. Data were expressed as a ratio of precipitated ACE activity from plasma sample with tested compound/hemolysis to that without treatment. Red columns shows bigger (yellow – lower) precipitation of treated ACE activity (more than 20%) that that of ACE without treatment. Mean (+/− SD) from three independent experiments (each in duplicates). * - p<0.05 in comparison with mean values for samples without treatment.

Figure S6 Effect of ACE inhibitors on the blood ACE activity of healthy donors/unrelated patients with normal *versus* high 1G12/9B9 ratio.

A–D Citrated plasma samples of unrelated patients and healthy donors with normal (patients #2 healthy and #19 unrelated), elevated (patients ##11 and 18 healthy; ##20, 32, 46, and 54 - unrelated) and high (patients #13 healthy and #21 unrelated) 1G12/9B9 ratio were incubated with "short" ACE inhibitor enalaprilat (100 nM, **A** and **B**) and "long" ACE inhibitor teprotide (1 µM, **C** and **D**) for 1 hour as in Fig. 7. Data are presented as a residual ACE activity determined with "short" substrate ZPHL (0.5 mM, **A** and **C**) and "long" substrate angiotensin I (0.3 mM, **B** and **D**). **E.** The ratio of the rates of the hydrolysis of angiotensin I and ZPHL (angiotensin I/ZPHL ratio) for corresponding samples. **F.** mAb 1G12/9B9 binding ratio for corresponding samples expressed as % from the mean value for controls. Grey bars – inhibition of ACE activity (A–D) or parameters measured in E–F in tested samples was not differed from that for healthy patients with low 1G12/9B9 ratio (controls). Red bars –measured parameters were statistically higher that in healthy patients with low (normal) 1G12/9B9 ratio *, p<0.05 in comparison with mean value for healthy patients. Data are mean ± SD from 3 independent experiments (each in duplicates).

Figure S7 Effect of ACE inhibitor and bovine/human sera on mAbs binding to ACEs

The effect of enalaprilat (100 nM) on mAbs binding to plasma ACE (**A**) or enalaprilat (100 nM)- **B** or Fetal Bovine Serum - FBS, 10% (**C**) or Human Serum −10% (**D**) on mAbs binding to soluble recombinant sACE was determined using plate precipitation assay with ZPHL as a substrate as in Figure 1. Human serum after incubation with enalaprilat **B–D**. Soluble truncated human recombinant two-domain sACE: 1–1230 WTΔ (Wei et al. 1991), after incubation with enalaprilat (**B**), FBS (**C**) and Human Serum (**D**) for 1 hour. All other terms and conditions-as in Figure 1. Data are mean ± SD of 3–4 independent experiments (each in duplicates). * - p<0.05 in comparison with values for samples without ACE inhibitors.

Acknowledgments

The authors thank Dr. Francois Alhenc-Gelas (then INSERM U367, Paris, France) who kindly provide us with plasmid coding for truncated soluble recombinant human ACE – WTΔ, and Dr. Edward Sturrock (University of Cape Town, South Africa) who kindly provided us with recombinant testicular ACE (tACE). We acknowledge technical assistance of Zhu-Li Sun and Jude Vivin (University of Illinois at Chicago, USA).

Author Contributions

Conceived and designed the experiments: SMD OAK. Performed the experiments: MNP SMD. Analyzed the data: SMD OAK JGNG VYS. Contributed reagents/materials/analysis tools: VYS AVT DES JGNG SMD. Wrote the paper: SMD OAK VYS JGNG.

References

1. Ehlers MWR, Riordan JF (1989) Angiotensin-converting enzyme: new concepts concerning its biological role. Biochemistry 8: 5311–5318.
2. Bernstein KE, Xiao HD, Frenzel K, Li P, Shen XZ, et al. (2005) Six truisms concerning ACE and the renin-angiotensin system educed from the genetic analysis of mice. Circ Res 96: 1135–1144.
3. Sturrock ED, Anthony CS, Danilov SM (2012) Peptidyl-dipeptidase A/ Angiotensin I-converting enzyme. In: Editors-in-Chief: Neil D. Rawlings, Guy Salvesen, *Handbook of Proteolytic Enzymes*, 3rd Edition, Academic Press, Oxford (in press).
4. Caldwell PR, Seegal BC, Hsu KC, Das H, Soffer RL (1976) Angiotensin-converting enzyme: vascular endothelial localization. Science 191: 1050–1051.
5. Ryan US, Ryan JW, Whitaker C, Chiu A (1976) Localization of angiotensin converting enzyme (kininase II). II. Immunocytochemistry and immunofluorescence. Tissue Cell 8: 124–145.
6. Balyasnikova IV, Danilov SM, Muzykantov VR, Fisher AB (1998) Modulation of angiotensin-converting enzyme in cultured human vascular endothelial cells. In Vitro Dev Biol Anim 34: 545–554.
7. Metzger R, Franke FF, Bohle RM, Alhenc-Gelas F, Danilov SM (2011) Heterogeneous distribution of Angiotensin I-converting enzyme (CD143) in the human and rat vascular systems: vessels, organs and species specificity. Microvasc Res 82: 206–215.
8. Defendini R, Zimmerman EA, Weare JA, Alhenc-Gelas F, Erdos EG (1983) Angiotensin-converting enzyme in epithelial and neuroepithelial cells. Neuro-endocrinology 37: 32–40.
9. Bruneval P, Hinglais N, Alhenc-Gelas F, Tricottet V, Corvol P, et al. (1986) Angiotensin I converting enzyme in human intestine and kidney. Ultrastructural immunohistochemical localization. Histochemistry 85: 73–80.
10. Hooper NM, Turner AJ (1987) Isolation of two differentially glycosylated forms of peptidyl-dipeptidase A (angiotensin-converting enzyme) from pig brain: a re-evaluation of their role in neuropeptide metabolism. Biochem J 241: 625–633.
11. Silverstein E, Friedland J, Setton C (1978) Angiotensin-converting enzyme in macrophages and Freund's adjuvant granuloma. Isr J Med Sci 14: 314–318.
12. Danilov SM, Sadovnikova E, Scharenbourg N, Balysnikova IV, Svinareva DA, et al. (2003) Angiotensin-converting enzyme (CD143) is abundantly expressed by dendritic cells and discriminates human monocytes-derived dendritic cells from acute myeloid leukemia-derived dendritic cells. Exp Hem 31: 1301–1309.
13. Danilov SM, Franke FE, Erdos EG (1997) Angiotensin-Converting Enzyme (CD143). In: Leucocyte Typing VI: White Cell differentiation Antigens. (Kishimoto T., et al., Eds.) Garland Publishing Inc.New York. 746–749.
14. Franke FE, Metzger R, Bohle RM, Kerkman L, Alhenc-Gelas F, et al. (1997) Angiotensin I-Converting Enzyme (CD 143) on endothelial cells in normal and in pathological conditions. In: Leucocyte Typing VI: White Cell Differentiation Antigens. (Kishimoto T., et al., Eds.) Garland Publishing Inc. New York. 749–751.
15. Beneteau-Burnat B, Baudin B (1991) Angiotensin-converting enzyme: clinical applications and laboratory investigation in serum and other biological fluids. Crit Rev Clin Lab Sci 28: 337–356.
16. Alhenc-Gelas F, Richard J, Courbon D, Warnet JM, Corvol P (1991) Distribution of plasma angiotensin I-converting enzyme levels in healthy men: Relationship to environmental and hormonal parameters. J Lab Clin Med 117: 33–39.
17. Lieberman J (1975) Elevation of serum angiotensin-converting enzyme level in sarcoidosis. Am J Med 59: 365–372.
18. Lieberman J, Beutler E (1976) Elevation of angiotensin-converting enzyme in Gaucher's disease. N Engl J Med 294: 1442–1444.
19. Silverstein E, Friedland J, Lyons HA, Gourin A (1976) Elevation of angiotensin-converting enzyme in granulomatous lymph nodes and serum in sarcoidosis: clinical and possible pathological significance. Ann NY Acad Sci 278: 498–513.
20. Romer FK (1984) Clinical and biochemical aspects of sarcoidosis. With special reference to angiotensin-converting enzyme (ACE). Acta Med Scand Suppl 690: 3–96.
21. Patel R, Ansari A (1979) Serum angiotensin converting enzyme activity in patients with chronic renal failure on long term hemodialysis. Clin Chem Acta 92: 491–495.
22. Silverstein E, Brunswick J, Rao TK, Friedland J (1984) Increased serum angiotensin-converting enzyme in chronic renal disease. Nephron 37: 206–210.
23. Dux S, Aron N, Boner G, Carmel A, Yaron A, et al. (1984) Serum angiotensin converting enzyme activity in normal adults and patients with different types of hypertension. Isr J Med Sci 20: 1138–1142.
24. Ching SF, Hayes LW, Slakey LL (1983) Angiotensin-converting enzyme in cultured endothelial cells. Synthesis, degradation and transfer to culture medium. Arteriosclerosis 3: 581–588.
25. Parkin ET, Turner AJ, Hooper NM (2004) Secretase-mediated cell surface shedding of the angiotensin-converting enzyme. Protein Pept Lett 11: 423–432.
26. Soubrier F, Alhenc-Gelas F, Hubert C, Allegrini J, John M, et al. (1988) Two putative active centers in human angiotensin I-converting enzyme revealed by molecular cloning. Proc Natl Acad Sci USA 85: 9386–9390.
27. Naperova IA, Balyasnikova IV, Schwartz DE, Watermeyer J, Sturrock DE, et al. (2008) Mapping of conformational mAb epitopes to the C domain of human angiotensin I-converting enzyme (ACE). J Proteome Res 7: 3396–3411.
28. Chen HL, Lunsdorf H, Hecht HJ, Tsai H (2010). Porcine pulmonary angiotensin I-converting enzyme - Biochemical characterization and spatial

arrangement of the N- and C-domains by three-dimensional electron-microscopic reconstruction. Micron 41: 674–685.

29. Danilov SM, Gordon K, Nesterovitch AB, Chen Z, Castellon M, et al. (2011) An angiotensin I-converting enzyme mutation (Y465D) causes a dramatic increase in blood ACE via accelerated ACE shedding. PLoS One 6: e25952.

30. Natesh R, Schwager SL, Sturrock ED, Acharya KR (2003) Crystal structure of the human angiotensin-converting enzyme-lisinopril complex. Nature 421: 551–554.

31. Corradi HR, Schwager SL, Nchinda AT, Sturrock ED, Acharya KR (2006) Crystal structure of the N domain of human somatic angiotensin I-converting enzyme provides a structural basis for domain-specific inhibitor design. J Mol Biol 357: 964–974.

32. Danilov S, Jaspard E, Churakova T, Towbin H, Savoie F, et al. (1994) Structure-function analysis of angiotensin I-converting enzyme using monoclonal antibodies. J Biol Chem 269: 26806–26814.

33. Balyasnikova IV, Metzger R, Visintine DJ, Dimasius V, Sun ZL, et al. (2005) A new set of monoclonal antibodies to rat angiotensin I-converting enzyme (ACE) for the lung endothelial targeting. Pulm Pharm Ther 18: 251–267.

34. Balyasnikova IV, Metzger R, Sun ZL, Berestetskaya YV, Albrecht RFII, et al. (2005) Development and characterization of rat monoclonal antibodies to denatured mouse angiotensin-converting enzyme. Tissue Antigens 65: 240–251.

35. Balyasnikova IV, Sun ZL, Metzger R, Taylor PR, Vicini E, et al. (2006) Monoclonal antibodies to native mouse angiotensin-converting enzyme (CD143): ACE expression; quantification; lung endothelial cell targeting and gene delivery. Tissue Antigens 67: 10–29.

36. Balyasnikova IV, Metzger R, Franke FE, Towbin H, Gordon K, et al. (2008) Epitope mapping of mAbs to denatured human testicular ACE. Tissue Antigens 72: 354–368.

37. Danilov S, Savoie F, Lenoir B, Jeunemaitre X, Azizi M, et al. (1996) Development of enzyme-linked immunoassays for human angiotensin I converting enzyme suitable for large-scale studies. J Hypertens 14: 719–727.

38. Nikolaeva MA, Balyasnikova IV, Alexinskaya MA, Metzger R, Franke FE, et al. (2006) Testicular isoform of angiotensin I-converting enzyme (ACE; CD143) on the surface of human spermatozoa: revelation and quantification using monoclonal antibodies. Am J Reprod Immunol 55: 54–68.

39. Balyasnikova IV, Karran EH, Albrecht RF, Danilov SM (2002) Epitope-specific antibody-induced cleavage of angiotensin-converting enzyme from the cell surface. Biochem J 362: 585–595.

40. Kost OA, Balyasnikova IV, Chemodanova EE, Nikolskaya II, Albrecht RF, et al. (2003) Epitope-dependent blocking of the angiotensin-converting enzyme dimerization by monoclonal antibodies to the N-terminal domain of ACE: possible link of ACE dimerization and shedding from the cell surface. Biochemistry 42: 6965–6976.

41. Balyasnikova IV, Woodman ZL, Albrecht RFII, Natesh R, Acharya KR, et al. (2005) Localization of an N domain region of angiotensin-converting enzyme involved in the regulation of ectodomain shedding using monoclonal antibodies. J Proteome Res 4: 258–267.

42. Skirgello OE, Balyasnikova IV, Binevski PV, Sun ZL, Baskin II, et al. (2006) Inhibitory antibodies to human angiotensin-converting enzyme: fine epitope mapping and mechanism of action. Biochemistry 45: 4831–4847.

43. Balyasnikova IV, Skirgello OE, Binevski PV, Nesterovitch AB, Albrecht RFII, et al. (2007) Monoclonal antibodies 1G12 and 6A12 to the N-domain of human angiotensin-converting enzyme: fine epitope mapping and antibody-based method for revelation and quantification of ACE inhibitors in the human blood. J Proteome Res 6: 1580–1594.

44. Danilov SM, Watermeyer JM, Balyasnikova IB, Gordon K, Kugaevskaya EV, et al. (2007) Fine epitope mapping of mAb 5F1 reveals anticatalytic activity toward the N domain of human angiotensin-converting enzyme. Biochemistry 46: 9019–9031.

45. Gordon K, Balyasnikova IV, Nesterovitch AB, Schwartz DE, Sturrock ED, et al. (2010) Fine epitope mapping of monoclonal antibodies 9B9 and 3G8, to the N domain of human angiotensin I-converting enzyme (ACE) defines a region involved in regulating ACE dimerization and shedding. Tissue Antigens 75: 136–150.

46. Danilov SM, Deinum J, Balyasnikova IV, Sun ZL, Kramers C, et al. (2005) Detection of mutated angiotensin I-converting enzyme by serum/plasma analysis using a pair of monoclonal antibodies. Clin Chem 51: 1040–1043.

47. Nesterovitch AB, Hogarth K, Adarichev VA, Vinokour EI, Schwartz D, et al. (2009) Angiotensin I-converting enzyme mutation (Trp1197Stop) causes a dramatic increase in blood ACE. PLoS One 4: (12) e8282.

48. Danilov SM, Kalinin S, Chen Z, Vinokour EI, Nesterovitch AB, et al. (2010) Angiotensin I-converting enzyme Gln1069Arg mutation impairs trafficking to the cell surface resulting in selective denaturation of the C domain. PLoS One 5: e10438.

49. Danilov SM, Balyasnikova IB, Danilova AS, Naperova IA, Arablinskaya E, et al. (2010) Conformational fingerprinting of the angiotensin-converting enzyme (ACE): Application in sarcoidosis. J. Proteome Res 9: 5782–5793.

50. Balyasnikova IV, Sun ZL, Berestetskaya YV, Albrecht RAII, Sturrock ED, et al. (2005) Monoclonal antibodies 1B3 and 5C8 as probes for monitoring the nativity of C-terminal end of soluble angiotensin-converting enzyme (ACE). Hybridoma 24: 14–26.

51. Vanholder R, De Smet R, Glorieux G, Argilés A, Baurmeister U, et al. (2003) Review on uremic toxins: classification; concentration; and interindividual variability. Kidney Int. 63: 1934–1943.

52. Piquilloud Y, Reinharz A, Roth M (1970) Studies on the angiotensin-converting enzyme with different substrates. Biochim Biophys Acta 206: 136–142.

53. Friedland J, Silverstein E (1976) A sensitive fluorometric assay for serum angiotensin-converting enzyme. Am J Pathol 66: 416–424.

54. Danilov SM, Balyasnikova IV, Albrecht RFI, Kost OA (2008) Simultaneous determination of ACE activity with two substrates provides information on the status of somatic ACE and allows detection of inhibitors in human blood. J Cardiovasc Pharmacol 52: 90–103.

55. Balyasnikova IV, Gavriljuk VD, McDonald TD, Berkowitz R, Miletich DJ, et al. (1999) Antibody-mediated lung endothelium targeting: In vitro model using a cell line expressing angiotensin-converting enzyme. Tumor Targeting 4: 70–83.

56. Wei L, Alhenc-Gelas F, Soubrier F, Michaud A, Corvol P, et al. (1991) Expression and characterization of recombinant human angiotensin I-converting enzyme. Evidence for a C-terminal transmembrane anchor and for a proteolytic processing of the secreted recombinant and plasma enzymes. J Biol Chem 266: 5540–5546.

57. Balyasnikova IV, Metzger R, Franke FE, Danilov SM (2003) Monoclonal antibodies to denatured human ACE (CD 143), broad species specificity, reactivity on paraffin sections, and detection of subtle conformational changes in the C-terminal domain of ACE. Tissue Antigens 61: 49–62.

58. Ehlers MRW, Chen YN, Riordan JF (1991) Spontaneous solubilization of membrane-bound human testis angiotensin-converting enzyme expressed in Chinese hamster ovary cells. Proc Natl Acad Sci USA 88: 1009–1013.

59. Jokubaitis VJ, Sinka L, Driessen R, Whitty G, Haylock DN, et al. (2008) Angiotensin-converting enzyme (CD143) marks hematopoietic stem cells in human embryonic; fetal and adult hematopoietic tissues. Blood 111: 4055–4063.

60. Sturrock ED, Yu XC, Wu Z, Biemann K, Riordan J (1996) Assignment of free- and disulfide-bonded cysteine residues in testis angiotensin-converting enzyme: functional implications. Biochemistry 35: 9560–9566.

61. Jones DP, Carlson JL, Samiec PS, Sternberg P, Mody VC, et al. (1998) Glutathione measurement in human plasma. Evaluation of sample collection; storage and derivatization conditions for analysis of dansyl derivatives by HPLC. Clin Chim Acta 275: 175–184.

62. Giustarini D, Dalle-Donne I, Colombo R, Milzani A, Rossi R (2004) Interference of plasmatic reduced glutathione and hemolysis on glutathione disulfide levels in human blood. Free Rad Res 10: 1101–1106.

63. Himmelfarb J, Stenvinkel P, Ikizler TA, Hakim RM (2002) The elephant in uremia: oxidant stress as a unifying concept of cardiovascular disease in uremia. Kidney Int 62: 1524–1538.

64. Ward RA, McLeish KR (2003) Oxidant stress in hemodialysis patients: what are the determining factors? Artif Organs 27: 230–236.

65. Morena M, Delbosc S, Dupuy AM, Canaud B, Cristol JP (2005) Overproduction of reactive oxygen species in end-stage renal disease patients: a potential component of hemodialysis- associated inflammation. Hemodial Int 9: 37–46.

66. Lucchi L, Bargamini S, Iannone A, Perrone S, Stipo L, et al. (2005) Erythrocyte susceptibility to oxidative stress in chronic renal failure patients under different substitutive treatments. Artif Organs 29: 67–72.

67. Stepniewska J, Dolegowska B, Ciechanowski K, Kwiatkowska E, Millo B, et al. (2006) Erythrocyte antioxidant defense system in patients with chronic renal failure according to the hemodialysis conditions. Arch Med Res 37: 353–359.

68. Herzog CE, Ma JZ, Collins AJ (2002) Long-term survival of dialysis patients in the United States with prosthetic heart valves: should ACC/AHA practice guidelines on valve selection be modified? Circulation 105: 1336–1341.

69. Gendlin GE, Shilo VYu, Tomilina NA, Storogakov GI, Borisovskaya SV, et al. (2009) Left ventricular myocardial hypertrophy and its prognostic role at chronic kidney disease. Clinical Nephrology (Russian) 1: 22–28.

70. Suzuki H (2009) Therapeutic efficacy of renin-angiotensin blockade in patients receiving dialysis. Ther Adv Cardiovasc Dis 3: 397–405.

71. Inrig JK (2010) Antihypertensive agents in hemodialisys patients. Semin Dial 23: 290–297.

72. Zannad F, Kessler M, Lehert P, Grünfeld JP, Thuilliez C, et al. (2006) Prevention of cardiovascular events in end-stage renal disease: results of a randomized trial of fosinopril and implications for future studies. Kidney Int. 70: 1318–1324.

73. Chang TI, Shilane D, Brunelli SM, Cheung AK, Chertow GM, et al. (2011) Angiotensin-converting enzyme inhibitors and cardiovascular outcomes in patients on maintenance hemodialysis. Am Heart J 162: 324–330.

74. Efrati S, Zaidenstein R, Dishy V, Beberashvili I, Sharist M (2002) ACE inhibitors and survival of hemodialysis patients. Am J Kidney Dis 40: 1023–1029.

75. McCullough PA, Sandberg KR, Yee J, Hudson MP (2002) Mortality benefit of angiotensin-converting enzyme inhibitor after cardiac events in patients with end-stage renal disease. J Renin Angiotensin Aldosterone Syst 3: 188–191.

76. Menard J, Patchett AA (2001). Angiotensin-converting enzyme inhibitors. Adv Protein Chem 56: 13–75.

77. Silva ACS, Diniz JSS, Pereira RM, Pinheiro SVB, Santos RAS (2006) Circulating renin angiotensin system in childhood chronic renal failure: marked increase of angiotensin-(1–7) in end-stage renal disease. Ped Res 60: 734–739.

78. Scharplatz M, Puhan MA, Steurer J, Perna A, Bachmann LM (2005) Does the angiotensin-converting enzyme (ACE) gene insertion/deletion polymorphism modify the response to ACE inhibitor therapy? – a systematic review. Curr Control Trials Cardiovasc Med 6: 16.

79. Danser AHJ, Batenburg WW, van den Meiracker AH, Danilov SM (2007) ACE pheno-typing as a first step toward personalized medicine for ACE inhibitors.

Why does ACE geno-typing not predict the therapeutic efficacy of ACE inhibition? Pharm Ther 113: 607–618.

80. Kramer AB, Laverman GD, van Goor H, Navis G (2003) Inter-individual differences in anti-proteinuric response to ACEi in established adriamycin nephritic rats are predicted by pretreatment renal damage. J Pathol 201: 160–167.

81. Windt WA, van Dokkum RPE, Kluppel CA, Jeronimus-Stratingh CM, Hut F, et al. (2008) Therapeutic resistance to angiotensin converting enzyme (ACE) inhibition is related to phar-macodynamic and kinetic factors in 5/6 nephrectomized rats. Eur J Pharmacol 580: 231–240.

82. Ryan JW, Martin LC, Chung A, Pena GA (1979) Mammalian inhibitors of angiotensin-converting enzyme (kininase II). In Advances in Experimental Medicine and Biology. KininsII; 120B; (Fuji S., Moriya M., Suzuki T., Eds.). Plenum: New York, 599–606.

83. Hazato T, Kase R (1986) Isolation of angiotensin-converting enzyme inhibitor from porcine plasma. Biochem Biophys Res Communs 139: 52–55.

84. Lieberman J, Sastre A (1986) An angiotensin-converting enzyme (ACE) inhibitor in human serum. Increased sensitivity of the serum ACE assay for detecting active sarcoidosis. Chest 90: 869–875.

85. Ikemoto F, Song GB, Tominaga M, Yamamoto K (1989) Endogenous inhibitor of angio-tensin-converting enzyme in the rat heart. Biochem Biophys Res Communs 159: 1093–1099.

86. Brecher AS, Thevananter S, Wilson S (1996) Observation of high and low MW inhibitors of angiotensin converting enzyme in rat lung. Arch Int Pharmacodyn Ther 331: 301–312.

87. Thevananter S, Brecher AS (1999) Isolation of angiotensin converting enzyme (ACE) binding protein from human serum with an ACE affinity column. Can J Physiol Pharmacol 77: 216–223.

6

Circulating FGF21 Levels are Progressively Increased from the Early to End Stages of Chronic Kidney Diseases and are Associated with Renal Function in Chinese

Zhuofeng Lin[1,2⁹], **Zhihong Zhou**[3⁹], **Yanlong Liu**[1⁹], **Qi Gong**[1], **Xinxin Yan**[1], **Jian Xiao**[1], **Xiaojie Wang**[1], **Shaoqiang Lin**[1], **Wenke Feng**[1,5], **Xiaokun Li**[1,4]*

1 School of Pharmacy, Wenzhou Medical College, Zhejiang, China, **2** School of Pharmacy, Jinan University, Guanghzou, China, **3** Division of Kidney, the 2nd Affiliated Hospital, Wenzhou Medical College, Zhejiang, China, **4** The Key Lab of Pathobiology, National Ministry of Education, Jilin University, Changchun, China, **5** School of Medicine, University of Louisville, Louisville, Kentucky, United States of America

Abstract

Background: Fibroblast growth factor 21 (FGF21) is a hepatic hormone involved in the regulation of lipid and carbohydrate metabolism. This study aims to test the hypothesis that elevated FGF21 concentrations are associated with the change of renal function and the presence of left ventricular hypertrophy (LVH) in the different stages of chronic kidney disease (CKD) progression.

Methodology/Principal Findings: 240 subjects including 200 CKD patients (146 outpatients and 54 long-term hemodialytic patients) and 40 healthy control subjects were recruited. All CKD subjects underwent echocardiograms to assess left ventricular mass index. Plasma FGF21 levels and other clinical and biochemical parameters in all subjects were obtained based on standard clinical examination methods. Plasma FGF21 levels were significantly increased with the development of CKD from early- and end-stage ($P<0.001$ for trend), and significantly higher in CKD subjects than those in healthy subjects ($P<0.001$). Plasma FGF21 levels in CKD patients with LVH were higher than those in patients without LVH ($P=0.001$). Furthermore, plasma FGF21 level correlated positively with creatinine, blood urea nitrogen (BUN), β2 microglobulin, systolic pressure, adiponectin, phosphate, proteinuria, CRP and triglyceride, but negatively with creatinine clearance rate (CCR), estimated glomerular filtrate rate (eGFR), HDL-c, LDL-c, albumin and LVH after adjusting for BMI, gender, age and the presence of diabetes mellitus. Multiple stepwise regression analyses indicated that FGF21 was independently associated with BUN, Phosphate, LVMI and β2 microglobulin (all $P<0.05$).

Conclusion: Plasma FGF21 levels are significantly increased with the development of early- to end-stage CKD and are independently associated with renal function and adverse lipid profiles in Chinese population. Understanding whether increased FGF21 is associated with myocardial hypertrophy in CKD requires further study.

Editor: Aimin Xu, University of Hong Kong, China

Funding: This work was supported by grants from Changjiang Scholars and Innovative Research Team (to XL), Zhejiang Provincial Natural Science Foundation of China (R2090550, Y2100048), and Natural Science Grant of Zhejiang Province, China (2009J1-C451). No additional external funding was received for this study. The funders had no role in study design, data collection and analysis, decision to publish, or preparation of the manuscript.

Competing Interests: The authors have declared that no competing interests exist.

* E-mail: xiaokunli@163.com

⁹ These authors contributed equally to this work.

Introduction

Chronic kidney disease (CKD) is a growing public health concern that is associated with a markedly increased risk of cardiovascular disease and mortality[1,2]. Although many traditional risk factors for atherosclerosis such as hypertension and diabetes mellitus promote the progression of CKD from early- to end-stage, these classic risk factors do not fully account for the burden of cardiovascular disease in patients with CKD[3,4]. Left ventricular hypertrophy (LVH) is one of several common manifestations of cardiovascular disease that is a major independent risk factor for mortality in patients with CKD[3,4]. Exploring the early mechanism of LVH is necessary to develop therapies that

block the progression of CKD and attenuate cardiovascular disease associated with CKD.

The fibroblast growth factor family is composed of 22 members with a wide range of biological functions, including cell growth, development, angiogenesis, and wound healing[5–9]. FGF21 is a member of the endocrine FGF subfamily, which also includes FGF23, human FGF19, and its mouse homolog FGF15[10–14]. In mice, FGF21 is expressed predominantly in the liver and stimulates glucose uptake through the induction of GLUT1 in adipocytes[13]. In vivo treatment with FGF21 results in amelioration of glucose and regulates lipid metabolism in both murine and nonhuman primate models of diabetes and obesity[15–17]. Taken together, these findings demonstrate an important role of FGF21 as a hepatic hormone in the regulation of lipid metabolism and also suggest that FGF21exhibits the therapeutic characteristic necessary for an effective treatment of obesity and fatty liver disease.

Human studies indicate that circulating levels of FGF21 increased in obese individuals [18], subjects with metabolic syndrome, type 2 diabetes mellitus[19–21] and coronary heart disease[22]. Furthermore, FGF21 was found to closely associated with renal dysfunction in end-stage renal disease subjects[23,24]. On the other hand, previous studies indicated that FGF receptors, particularly FGFR1, are expressed in adult myocardial cells, and their activation by locally secreted growth factors can stimulate myocardial hypertrophy and interstitial fibrosis[25,26]. For example, mice lacking FGF-2 exhibit dilated cardiomyopathy and impaired hypertrophic responses to angiotensin II[27], and adenoviral Gene Transfer of FGF-5 to Hibernating myocardium improves function and stimulates myocytes to hypertrophy and reenter the cell cycle[26]. Recently, FGF-23, one member of FGF-19 subfamilies, was reported to associate with the onset and development of CKD[28–30] as well as LVH in patients with CKD[31]. Take together, all these reports suggested that FGF family members play an important role in the physiopathology of LVH. Whether FGF21, however, is closely associated with the pathological relevance of CKD and LVH in CKD patients remain unclear. To explore the physiological and pathological relevance of FGF21 in patients with CKD, we measured the plasma concentrations of FGF21 in 240 Chinese subjects and analyzed its association with renal function and a cluster of metabolic parameters that related to the change of renal functions.

Materials and Methods

Study Population

The study population consisted of 146 outpatients with CKD and 54 CKD patients with long-term hemodialysis. 146 patients with CKD were recruited from outpatient nephrology clinics at the Second Affiliated Hospital of Wenzhou Medical College, Wenzhou. Patients recruited into this study were ≥25 years of age and had a sustained reduction (≥3 months) in estimated glomerular filtration rate (eGFR) ≤60 ml · min^{-1} · 1.73 m^{-2} based on the simplified Modification of Diet in Renal Disease formula. Patients with preserved eGFR (≥60 ml/min per 1.73 m^2) were also considered as early stage CKD patients if they presented with one or more of the following related symptoms: persistent hematuria and/or proteinuria with biopsy-proven minimal-change disease, membranoproliferative glomerulonephritis, or other relevant nephropathies. 54 CKD patients with long-term hemodialysis (eGFR<15 ml · min^{-1} · 1.73 m^{-2}) were also recruited into the present study. These subjects with long-term hemodialysis were recruited from inpatient services at the Hemodialytic Center of the 2nd Affiliated Hospital of Wenzhou Medical College and were scheduled for an echocardiogram for diagnostic purposes by the primary admitting team. Patients were at least 25 years of age and clinically stable and did not have acute myocardial infarction, known cardiomyopathy or ejection fraction < 40%, or known mitral or aortic valve disease. Exclusion criteria included kidney transplant, history of coronary artery bypass grafting, or an incidence of myocardial infarction within 90 days of enrollment. In addition, to focus on patients with early cardiac disease, patients surpassing criteria for New York Heart Association class 1 heart failure or Canadian Cardiovascular Society class 1 angina were excluded. The comorbidities including diabetes and hypertension were defined on basis of the clinical diagnosis criteria of WHO and American Diabetes Association or

American Society of Hypertension respectively. We also included healthy controls (n = 40) who underwent a routine health examination at 2nd Affiliated Hospital of Wenzhou Medical College, had no history of medical disease, and were not taking regular medication, all control subjects were selected based on the results of physician's questionnaire and clinical biochemical examination. All studies were approved by the Ethics Committee of Wenzhou Medical College, and all patients provided written informed consent.

Clinical Data and Laboratory test

Data on demographic characteristics, medical history, current medications, and blood samples were collected from all subjects at the time of enrollment. Blood was collected from subjects after overnight fasting for at least 10 h. Blood samples were immediately centrifuged, separated into aliquots, and stored at −80°C for future batched assays. Serum creatinine, calcium, phosphate, and albumin were measured with standard commercial assays. Intact parathyroid hormone concentrations were measured with the Roche Elecsys parathyroid hormone assay (Roche, Indianapolis, Ind). Plasma FGF21 (Biovendor, Modrice, Czech Republic) and C-reactive protein (CRP, R&D, USA)concentrations and were measured in duplicate with commercially available enzyme-linked immunosorbent assays according to the manufacturers' instructions in the Core Laboratory of School of Pharmacy, Wenzhou Medical College. All other blood tests in CKD subjects were processed in Clinical Examination Laboratory of the 2nd Affiliated Hospital of Wenzhou Medial College after a single thaw.

Echocardiography

All subjects underwent 2-dimensional transthoracic echocardiograms. The studies were interpreted by a single reviewer at the 2nd Affiliated Hospital of Wenzhou Medial College who was blinded to subjects' clinical and laboratory data. For the primary analysis, left ventricular mass index (LVMI) was calculated with the Devereux formulation[32,33]: Left ventricular hypertension (LVH) was defined as LVMI >135 g/m^2 for men and >110 g/m^2 for women in Chinese population[34]. Left ventricular ejection fraction (LVEF) was determined using biplane-modified Simpson's measurements.

Statistical analysis

All analyses were performed with Statistical Package for Social Sciences version 13.0 (SPSS,Chicago, IL), and the statistical analysis was done similarly as described by Zhang X et al[18]. In brief, normally distributed data were expressed as mean±SD. Data that were not normally distributed, as determined using Kolmogorox-Smirnov test, were logarithmically transformed before analysis and expressed as median with interquartile range. Student's unpaired t test was used for comparison between two groups. Pearson's correlations were used as appropriate for comparisons between groups, and multiple testing was corrected using Bonferroni correction. Linear regression was used to examine the association between LVMI, LVH, CRP and other clinical, and laboratory variables. We used multivariable models to examine the relationship between LVMI and FGF21 concentrations, adjusting for age, gender, body mass index (BMI), diabetes mellitus, hypertension that were significantly ($P<0.05$) associated with LVMI in univariate analyses. The variables that correlated significantly with serum FGF21 (after Bonferroni correction for multiple testing) were selected to enter into multiple linear regression. In all statistical tests, P values <0.05 were considered significant.

Results

Patient Characteristics

Table 1 depicts demographic information, laboratory data and echocardiogram results of the 200 CKD subjects according to level of kidney function and 40 normal control subjects. CKD patients were divided into three groups according to the eGFR, namely early-stage group (preserved renal function, eGFR 60 to 90 ml/min per 1.73 m^2), middle-stage group (eGFR 30 to 60 ml/min per 1.73 m^2) and end-stage group (hemodialytic group, eGFR <30 ml/min per 1.73 m^2). 55 patients with preserved eGFR (>90 ml/min per 1.73 m^2) were also considered as CKD patients (early stage) based on the recruitment standards shown in the Materials and Methods section. Furthermore, relevant biochem-ical and anthropometric parameters in 40 healthy subjects were shown in Table 1. The results of echocardiography and its relevant parameters in normal subjects were not examined in this study, because all these subjects recruited into the present study were underwent a routine health examination, and had no history of disease, and were not taking regular medication based on the results of physician's questionnaire and clinical biochemical examination.

Plasma FGF21 levels are increased in CKD patients

Plasma FGF21 levels ranged from 67.4 to 7232.6 pg/ml amongst subjects in this study, and the median FGF21 concentration in overall subjects was 616.1 pg/ml (interquartile range, 264.4 to 1137.8 pg/ml). No gender differences in plasma FGF21 levels were

Table 1. Description of Subjects by Level of Kidney Function.

Variables	Normal subjects	Early-stage eGFR >60 ml/min per 1.73 m^2	Middle-stage eGFR(30–60) ml/min per 1.73 m^2	End-stage eGFR <30 ml/min per 1.73 m^2	P for trend
N	40	76	36	88	-
Age(years)	49.5±12.3	50.7±15.0	50.7±17.3	50.6±10.0	NS
Women(%)	14(32.5)	25(32.8)	12(33.3)	28(31.8)	NS
BMI(kg/m^2)	21±2.5	23±3.3	23.8±3.6	21±2.9	<0.001
Hypertension					
Systolic blood press	104±18	136±24	149±28	150±31	<0.001
Diastolic blood press	69±11	84±17	88±14	85±19	<0.001
The presence of hypertension	-	36.8	55.6	50.0	NS
Glucose					
fasting glucose	5.08±0.56	4.99±1.37	4.59±1.02	7.59±4.52	<0.001
fasting insulin	4.16(3.01–6.17)	7.62(4.96–11.37)	13.82(8.06–30.95)	12.99(5.08–23.16)	<0.001
HOMA-ir	0.92(0.63–1.44)	1.31(0.77–2.27)	4.63(2.47–5.34)	3.58(1.04–7.26)	<0.001
The presence of diabetes	-	19.7	33.3	46.6*	<0.001
Lipid profiles					
TG	0.92±0.38	2.05±1.20	1.97±1.37	1.93±1.49	0.004
LDL	2.57±0.46	3.30±1.60	3.30±1.23	2.26±0.46	<0.001
HDL	1.39±0.25	1.15±0.50	1.09±0.40	0.94±0.31	<0.001
Laboratory values					
CCR	81.2±13.5	66.2±27.5	28.2±10.7	7.5±3.5	<0.001
Albumin(g/l)	48.7±6.7	30.4±8.8	28.8±7. 4	30.9±4.6	<0.001
Creatinine(μmol/l)	65.8±11.0	103.9±39.3	243.6±47.5	811.3±293.3	<0.001
Calcium (mmol/l)	2.28±0.32	2.13±0.17	2.16±0.12	2.19±0.21	NS
phosphate(mmol/l)	1.24±0.26	1.26±0.22	1.36±0.16	1.78±0.61	<0.001
PTH(pg/ml)	42.3±17.0	76.7±26.0	97.6±64.7	469.0±470.0	<0.001
BUN(mmol/l)	4.1±1.04	6.35±2.67	12.28±4.58	21.44±7.51	<0.001
Uric Acid(μmol/l)	286±51	388±98	431±118	443±120	<0.001
CRP(μg/ml)	0.18±0.16	0.71±0.53	1.17±1.29	2.02±1.68	<0.001
β2 microglobulin(μg/ml)	1.51±0.32	2.62±1.09	5.90±1.24	15.50±9.87	<0.001
Adiponectin(μg/ml)	2.10±0.78	2.26±0.65	2.58±0.59	3.26±1.17	<0.001
FGF21(pg/ml)	127.6(85.7 to 218.4)	317.1(209.9 to 732.8)	517.1(220.3 to 912.0)	1098.8(523.1 to 2467.8)	<0.001
Echocardiography					
LVMI(g/m^2)	-#	100.6±21.7	112.3±14.7	136.6±39.7	<0.001
LVH,%	-#	12.0	28.6	53.7	<0.001
EF,%	-#	66.7±3.5	64.4±6.5	62.8±5.9	<0.001

NS: not significant. Results are expressed as frequencies, mean±SD, or median (interquartile range) as appropriate.
*Percentage of type 2 diabetes mellitus in end-stage CKD patients is significantly higher than those CKD patients in early-and middle-stage.

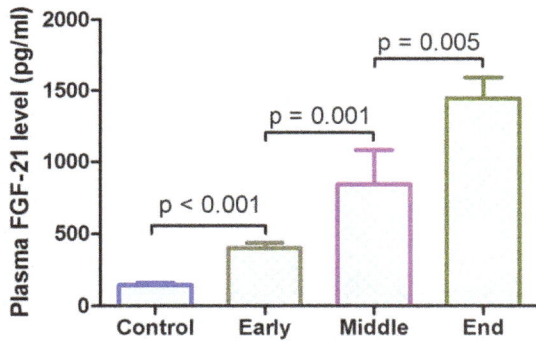

Figure 1. Plasma FGF21concentration in different stage of CKD subjects and normal subjects.

found between men (826.3±100.4 pg/ml, n = 155) and women (789.6±86.5 pg/ml, n = 85; p = 0.470). After adjusting for age, gender, and body mass index (BMI), median circulating FGF21 level in end-stage CKD patients (1447.9±146.5 pg/ml) was 10-fold higher compared with normal subjects (147.3±12.25 pg/ml; $P<0.0001$); and about 3.5-fold higher compared with the early-stage CKD patients (402.9±35.0 pg/ml; $P<0.0001$), and about 1.5-fold higher compared with the middle-stage CKD patients (845.8±238.7 pg/ml; $P<0.0001$; Figure 1). Interestingly, CKD patients recruited into this study with diabetes mellitus (DM) (1253±170.1 pg/ml, n = 68) had significantly higher plasma FGF21 levels ($P = 0.0016$) than those without DM (714± 82.1 pg/ml, n = 132). On the other hand, no significant difference in plasma FGF21 levels was observed between all CKD patients with and without hypertension ($P = 0.7730$), as well with and without CHD ($P = 0.6563$). Furthermore, all CKD

subjects with other comorbidities including DM, hypertension and CHD in this study had significantly higher plasma FGF21 levels (1422±302.9 pg/ml, n = 9) than those without corresponding comorbidities (611.2±111.5 pg/ml, n = 55, p = 0.0091).

FGF21 and left ventricular structure

LVMI values in all CKD subjects of this study ranged from 49.02 to 247.99 g/m^2 with mean LVMI at 118.5 g/m^2 and 31.7% of patients experiencing left ventricular hypertrophy. Compared with early- and middle-stage CKD patients, however, patients with end-stage CKD had significantly higher mean LVMI(110.3 ± 28.7 vs. 132.8 ± 36.1 g/m^2) and lower mean ejection fraction(67.97±3.40 vs. 63.33±4.97%). Mean LVMI and the prevalence of LVH (31.7%) among CKD subjects in this study were lower than in previous studies[35,36] confirming that the majority of patients recruited for this study were free of significant cardiac disease, consistent with the study design. Furthermore, CKD patients with hypertension showed a higher LVMI value than those without hypertension (124.9±34.8 vs.110.9±32.8, $P = 0.006$).

To explore the relationship between FGF21 and ventricular structure, we compared the levels of FGF21 in the CKD patients with and without LVH. Plasma FGF21 levels in CKD patients with LVH (median 923.9 pg/ml, interquartile 363.7 to 1478.7 pg/ml) were significantly higher than those without LVH (median 446.5 pg/ml, interquartile 245.6 to 953.1 pg/ml; $P = 0.001$; Figure 2A).

In univariable analyses, increased log FGF21 concentrations were significantly associated with increased LVMI ($P = 0.007$; Figure 2B). When adjusted for age, gender, BMI, diabetes mellitus, no significant association was found between log FGF21and log LVMI ($P = 0.091$). In the multivariable model, BMI, systolic pressure and LVH were the only three parameters that remained

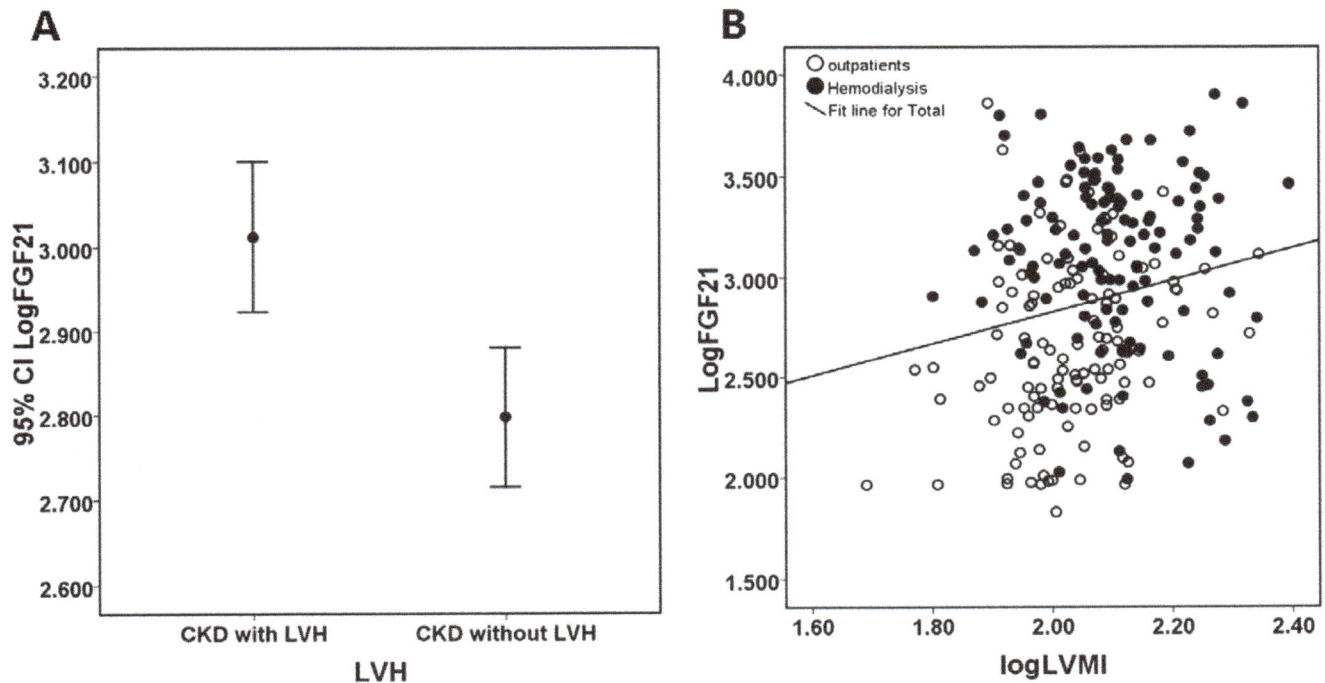

Figure 2. The relationship between FGF21 and LVH. A, circulating levels of FGF21 in CKD patients with LVH were significantly higher than that of CKD subjects without LVH; B, correlation between log-transformed FGF21 and LVMI. ○ indicates outpatients (early-and middle-stage CKD patients); ● hemodialytic patients (end-stage CKD patients).

Table 2. Echocardiographic characteristics and relevant interesting factors by tertile of log FGF21.

variable	Log FGF21(< 2.5) Tertile 1	Log FGF21 (2.5 to 3.0) Tertile 2	Log FGF21 (>3.0) Tertile 3	P for trend
N	52	51	82	-
LVMI,(g/m²)	109±32	119±31	127±35	0.004
LVH, %	21	34	46	0.006
Phosphate(mmol/l)	1.40±0.42	1.46±0.45	1.65±0.63	0.007
CRP(μg/ml)	0.62(0.22–1.28)	0.89(0.82–1.82)	1.47(0.71–3.45)	< 0.001

Results are expressed as mean±SD, frequencies (%) and median (interquartile) as appropriate.

significantly associated with LVMI ($P \leq 0.003$ respectively). Furthermore, when examined in tertiles, mean LVMI increased with increasing tertiles of log FGF21($P = 0.005$ for trend; Table 2).

On the other hand, in univariable analyses, increasing log FGF21 concentration was also significantly associated with the presence of LVH (odd ratio[OR] per 1-SD increase in log FGF21, 0.381; 95% confidence interval [CI], 0.214 to 0.68; $P = 0.001$). When adjusted for age, gender, BMI, hypertension, diabetes mellitus, log FGF21 was still significantly associated with the presence of LVH (OR per 1-SD increase in log FGF21, 0.422; 95% CI, 0.218 to 0.817; $P = 0.010$). Furthermore, the prevalence of LVH increased significantly with ascending tertiles of log FGF21 in univariable analyses (Table 2), but this relationship was attenuated after multivariable adjustment.

FGF21 and Phosphate Concentrations

Hyperphosphatemia with serious inflammatory reaction is a common manifestation of CKD. As shown in Table 3, circulating levels of FGF21 were found to strongly correlate with serum phosphate, creatine and CRP levels in CKD subjects after adjustment for BMI, gender, age and diabetes mellitus. Furthermore, mean FGF21, phosphate and creatinine concentrations were significantly increased with decreasing levels of eGFR(P for trend <0.001 for both). However, the absolute difference in mean serum phosphate concentration between normal subjects and early-stage CKD patients was about 0.01 mmol/l (relative difference, increasing 0.8%, $P = 0.727$; Figure 3A); Furthermore, the absolute difference in mean serum creatinine levels between normal subjects and early-stage CKD patients was about 38.1 μmol/l (relative difference, increasing 57.8%, $P<0.001$; Figure 3B). In contrast, the absolute difference in mean FGF21 concentration between normal subjects and early-stage CKD group was 245 pg/ml (relative difference, increasing 1.5-fold, $P<0.001$). Additionally, a significant difference in FGF21 concentration was found between early-and middle-stage CKD patients (402.4±49.6 *vs.* 904.6±262.0 pg/ml; $P = 0.0014$; Figure 1A).

Plasma FGF21 levels strongly associated with renal function, adverse lipid profiles and other factors in all CKD subjects

As shown in Table 3 and Figure 4, plasma FGF21 levels were strongly correlated with eGFR, endogenous creatinine clearance rate (CCR), creatinine and BUN, suggesting that elevated FGF21 concentrations were closely associated with the renal function in these CKD subjects. On the other hand, plasma FGF21 levels were associated with adverse lipid profiles including HDL-c, LDL-c and triglyceride (all P<0.05) after adjustment for age, gender, BMI and diabetes mellitus in all CKD subjects. Furthermore,

systolic pressure, adiponectin, proteinuria, β2 microglobulin, phosphate, albumin and LVH were significantly correlated with circulating FGF21 levels after adjustment for BMI, gender age and diabetes mellitus in all CKD subjects.

Table 3. Correlations of serum FGF21 levels with anthropometric parameters, biochemical indexes as well as other relevant factors.

Variables	Plasma FGF21 #		Plasma FGF21 # *	
	r	p	r	p
Gender	-0.201	0.004	-	-
BMI	-0.158	0.026	-	-
Age	0.186	0.035		
Diabetes	-0.310	<0.001	-	-
Systolic pressure	0.255	<0.001	0.243	0.001
CCR#	-0.503	<0.001	-0.349	<0.001
eGFR#	-0.469	<0.001	-0.341	<0.001
BUN#	0.413	<0.001	0.306	<0.001
Creatinine#	0.513	<0.001	0.412	<0.001
CRP	0.271	<0.001	0.178	0.013
Adiponectin	0.221	0.008	0.220	0.009
CXCL16	0.24	0.001	0.134	NS
TG	0.147	0.013	0.153	0.015
Cholesterol	-0.151	0.011	-0.095	NS
HDL-c	-0.250	<0.001	-0.189	0.003
LDL-c	-0.250	<0.001	-0.158	0.012
Proteinuria	0.318	0.001	0.302	0.001
Fasting glucose	0.263	<0.001	0.165	0.009
Albumin	-0.165	0.019	-0.145	0.047
β2 microglobulin	0.850	<0.001	0.930	<0.001
Phosphate	0.288	<0.001	0.261	<0.001
LVDd	0.194	0.024	0.171	NS
LVMI	0.221	0.008	0.113	NS
LVH	-0.217	0.001	-0.174	0.009

#Log transformed before analysis;
*adjusted by age, gender, BMI and diabetes; NS, not significant; CCR: endogenous creatinine clearance rate; IVSTd, left ventricular end-systolic dimension; LVDd: left ventricular diastolic dimension; LVMI: left ventricular mass index; LVH: left ventricular hypertrophy.

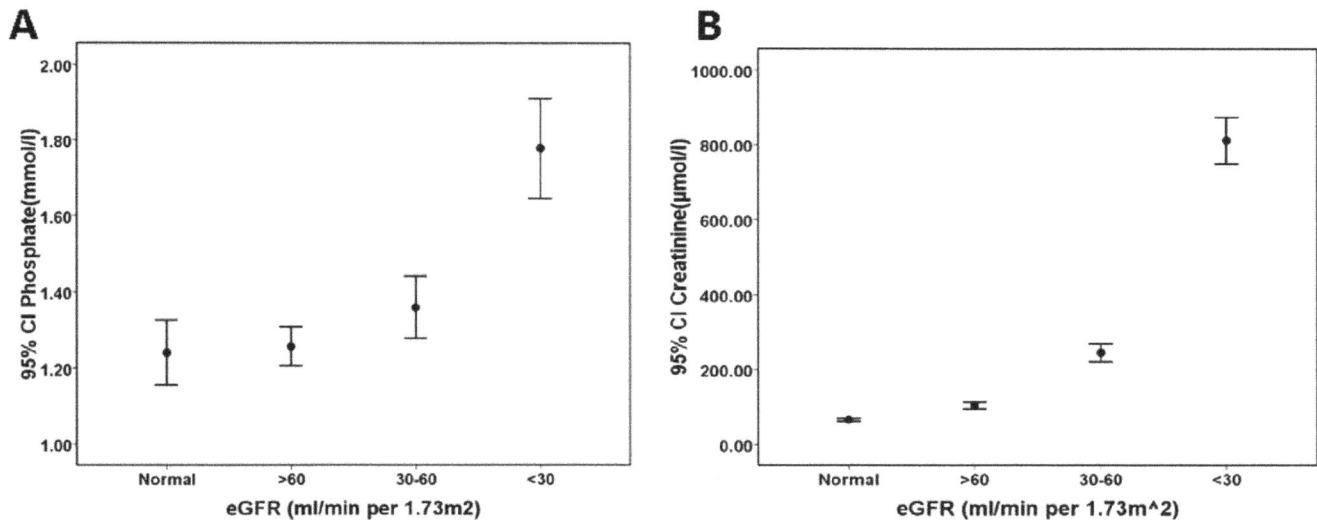

Figure 3. The change tendency of serum phosphate and creatinine according to the level of eGFR in 240 Chinese subjects. Bars represent SDs.

Independent Association of Plasma FGF21 levels with β2 microglobulin, LVMI, and Diabetes Mellitus

To determine whether plasma FGF21 was independently associated with anthropometric parameters and other relevant factors, multiple stepwise regression analysis involving all the parameters with significant correlations with plasma FGF21 was performed. Multiple stepwise regression analysis revealed that plasma FGF21 was independently associated with BUN, Phosphate, LVMI and β2 microglobulin adjustment for age, gender and BMI in all CKD subjects ($P \leq 0.043$, respectively, Table 4), thus all other parameters including gender, BMI, diabetes, systolic pressure, CCR, eGFR, creatinine, BUN, CRP, adiponectin, CXCL16, triglyceride, total cholesterol, LDL, HDL, proteinuria, fasting glucose, albumin, LVDd and LVH were excluded during regression analysis.

Discussion

Although several clinical studies focusing on FGF21 and its relevant human diseases have been reported in recent years[18–24], the definitive mechanism of FGF21 is not fully understood. In the present study, we investigated (1) the clinical correlation of circulating FGF21 in conjunction with physiological and pathological aspects in CKD patients, (2) the relationship between the change of circulation FGF21 levels and the development of CKD from early- to end-stage of disease, and (3) the effect of comorbidities of CKD to plasma FGF21 concentration. Our results suggest that FGF21 is involved in the development of CKD as supported by two novel findings. First, plasma FGF21 concentration is increased with the development of CKD from early- to end-stage following the loss of renal function. Second, relevant comorbidities including DM, hypertension and CHD in CKD patients affected plasma FGF21 concentration. Furthermore, plasma FGF21 levels in CKD patients are significantly correlated with adverse lipid profiles and LVH, but not with LVMI after adjustment for age, gender, BMI and diabetes.

Previous studies indicated that serum FGF21 concentration was 15-fold higher in chronic hemodialytic patients (CKD end-stage) than normal subjects and was associated significantly with the loss of renal function[24]. More recently, a cross-sectional study also indicated that serum FGF21 concentration was associated with residual renal function and insulin resistance in end-stage CKD patients with long-term hemodialysis[23]. These results suggested that FGF21 may be related to renal excretion functions in humans. Consistent with these reports, we show that plasma FGF21 concentration is increased with the development of early- to end-stage CKD following the loss of renal functions in CKD patients. Our data indicated that plasma FGF21 levels in end-stage CKD patients are about 10-fold higher compared with normal subjects (Figure 1). Furthermore, plasma FGF21 levels in end-stage CKD patients are about 4.5-fold higher compared with the early-stage CKD patients; and about 1.5-fold higher compared with the middle-stage CKD patients (Figure 1). These results suggest that circulating FGF21 concentration is associated with the CKD progression.

Diabetes contributes to increased morbidity and mortality in patients with chronic kidney disease[37]. Diabetes is the single leading cause of kidney failure in the U.S., accounting for about 45% of people who start treatment for kidney failure each year[38]. In the present study, we found that diabetes has additional effects on FGF21 levels in CKD patients, which are supported by the fact that plasma FGF21 levels in CKD individuals with DM were significantly higher than those CKD patients without this complication (Figure 1B). Furthermore, stepwise logistic regression analysis revealed that plasma FGF21 was independently associated with diabetes. Take together, these results suggest that plasma FGF21 levels in CKD subjects are affected by relevant comorbidities s and as on.

Hyperphosphatemia with serious inflammatory reaction is a common manifestation of CKD, and has been shown to be significantly associated with FGF-23, one of members of FGF family[28,39]. In the present study, we found that elevated FGF21 levels were associated with increasing serum phosphate and CRP levels. The relative difference in mean serum phosphate concentration between normal subjects and early-stage CKD patients was significantly lower than that of plasma FGF21 levels (relative difference, 0.8% vs.150%). These results suggest that FGF21 is a better biomarker than blood phosphate to reflect the progression of CKD from the early-to middle stage.

Left ventricular hypertrophy (LVH) is one of several common manifestations of cardiovascular disease and is an independent risk

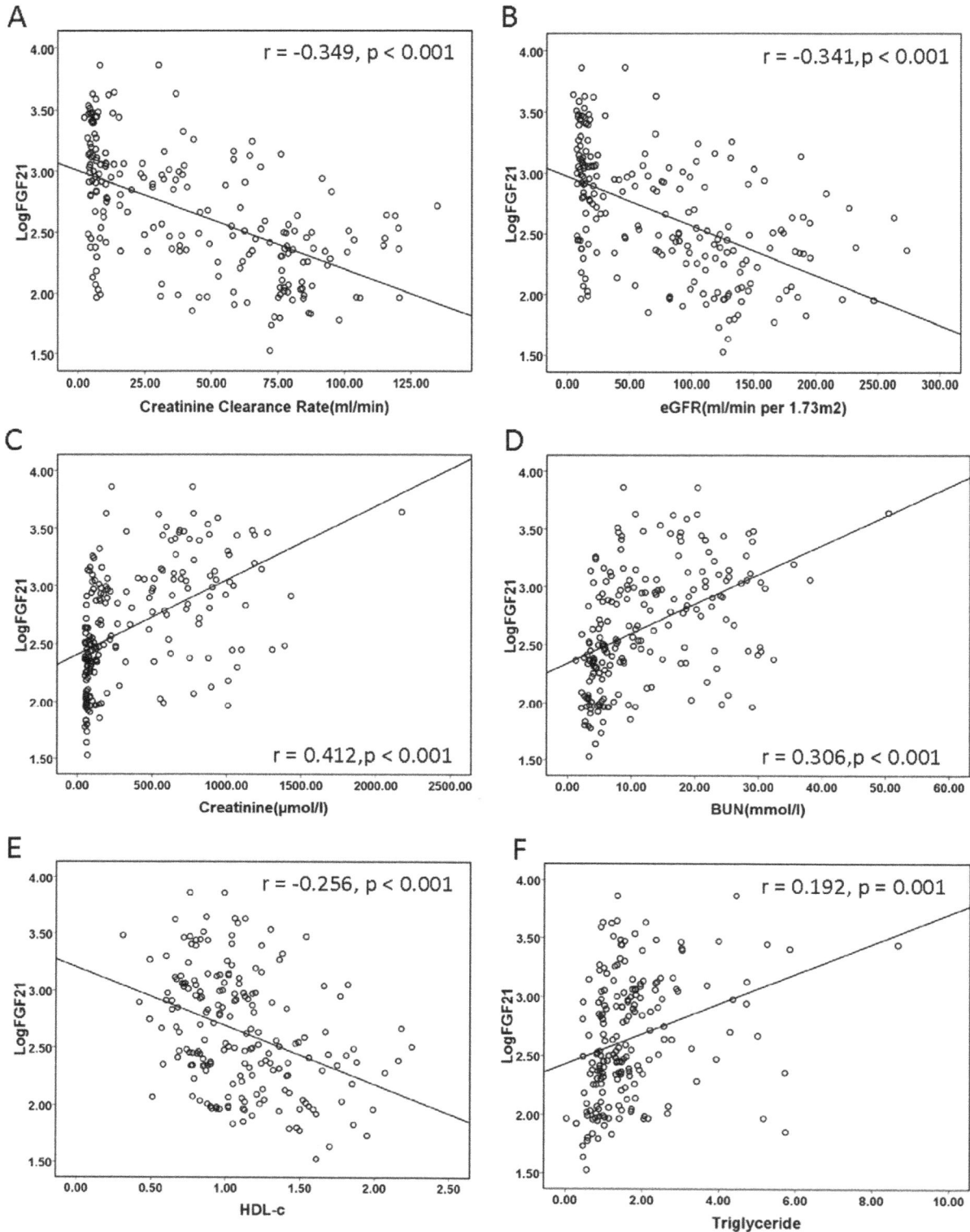

Figure 4. Correlation of plasma level of FGF21(log transformed) with CCR(A), eGFR(B), Creatinine(C), BUN(D), HDL-c(E) and Triglyceride(F) after adjustment for age, gender, BMI and diabetes in 240 Chinese subjects.

factor for mortality in patients with CKD[3,4]. Previous studies showed that approximately 40% of patients with pre-dialysis CKD and up to 80% of patients initiating hemodialysis manifest

LVH[4,36]. Furthermore, FGF-23, one member of the FGF-19 subfamilies, was shown to associated with LVH in patients with CKD[31]. In the present study, the prevalence of LVH (39.7%)

Table 4. Multiple stepwise regression analysis showing variables independently associated with the plasma level of FGF21.

Independent variables	Standardized Coefficients (Beta)	t	Sig.	B (95% CI)
BUN	1.066	3.406	0.004	0.046(0.017 to 0.075)
LVMI	-0.426	-2.676	0.017	-0.007(-0.012 to -0.001)
Phosphates	-0.992	-3.229	0.006	-0.747(-1.240 to -0.254)
β2 microglobulin	0.631	2.209	0.043	4.194E-5(0.000 to 0.000)

The analysis also included gender, BMI, diabetes, systolic pressure, CCR, eGFR, creatinine, BUN, CRP, adiponectin, CXCL16, triglyceride, total cholesterol, LDL, HDL, proteinuria, fasting glucose, albumin, LVDd and LVH, which were excluded during regression analysis.

among all CKD subjects was lower than in previous studies, because the majority of patients recruited for this study were free of significant cardiac disease. Furthermore, our data indicated that CKD patients with hypertension have a higher LVMI level than those of patients without hypertension, suggesting hypertension lead to an increase in the percentage of LVH. However, no significant difference in plasma FGF21 level was found between CKD patients with and without hypertension. These results indicated that hypertension can lead to increase LVMI levels but do not affect circulating levels of FGF21 in CKD patients.

Previous clinical studies indicated that the plasma lipid profile frequently evolves during the course of progression of CKD, and dyslipidemia is a strong predictor of myocardial infarction in sujects with CKD[40,41]. Patients with mild to moderate CKD, especially those with significant proteinuria, commonly exhibit hypercholesterolemia and elevated LDL levels[42]. Serum triglycerides and very low-density lipoprotein (VLDL) levels are elevated, and clearance of VLDL and chylomicrons and their atherogenic remnants is impaired in patients with advanced CKD or end stage renal disease (ESRD)[42,43]. In present study, our data showed that elevation of FGF21 are significantly correlated with adverse lipid profiles including elevating LDL and triglyceride, as well as decreasing HDL after adjustment for age, gender, BMI and diabetes suggesting that the elevation of circulating FGF21 levels may be directly or indirectly linked to the progression of pathophysiology of CKD.

eGFR, CCR, creatinine and BUN are conventional biomarkers reflecting the change of renal function[2,30]. Recent studies indicated that serum levels of cystatin C and β2 microglobulin (β2 MG) as well as urinary β2 MG and N-acetyl-β-Dglucosaminidase (NAG) increase in patients with early and mild renal impairment[44–47]. In the present study, our data indicated that plasma FGF21 levels are independently associated with β2 microglobulin, and were significantly associated with eGFR, CCR, creatinine and

BUN in CKD subjects(Figure 4), suggesting that elevated FGF21 levels are closely related to the injury of glamorous and the change of renal function in CKD patients. However, the mechanisms responsible for the elevation of FGF21 concentration with the progression of CKD are not fully understood. FGF21 is expressed predominantly in liver and adipose tissue[13], and plays an important role in regulating lipid and energy metabolism[15,48]. We speculated that the paradoxical increase in CKD patients is a compensatory mechanism to counteract metabolic stress. Because FGF21 resistance might be found in obesity and in renal failure, leading to compensatory upregulation of this hepatokine[18,24]. Based on these findings, we propose that the mechanism of increased FGF21 levels in kidney disease is similar to those observed in obesity-associated resistance to insulin. Further studies are needed to elucidate the precise mechanism by which CKD subjects elevate circulating FGF21 levels and to reveal the role of increased FGF21 levels in the onset and development of CKD.

In summary, this study provides clinical evidence revealing that plasma concentrations of FGF21 are increased with CKD progression and are independently associated with the loss of renal function. There are several limitations in this study. The sample size of this study cohort is relatively small. Furthermore, the cross-sectional natures of this study do not allow us to address the causal relationship between FGF21 and the development of CKD in patients. Further prospective studies with larger sample sizes are needed to determine whether FGF21 is related to myocardial hypertrophy in patients with CKD.

Author Contributions

Conceived and designed the experiments: XL ZL. Performed the experiments: ZL ZZ YL QG JX XY XW. Analyzed the data: QG YL SL WF. Wrote the paper: ZL XL.

References

1. Hostetter TH (2004) Chronic kidney disease predicts cardiovascular disease. N Engl J Med 351: 1344–1346.
2. Coresh J, Selvin E, Stevens LA, Manzi J, Kusek JW, et al. (2007) Prevalence of chronic kidney disease in the United States. JAMA 298: 2038–2047.
3. Sarnak MJ, Levey AS, Schoolwerth AC, Coresh J, Culleton B, et al. (2003) Kidney disease as a risk factor for development of cardiovascular disease: a statement from the American Heart Association Councils on Kidney in Cardiovascular Disease, High Blood Pressure Research, Clinical Cardiology, and Epidemiology and Prevention. Circulation 108: 2154–2169.
4. Middleton RJ, Parfrey PS, Foley RN (2001) Left ventricular hypertrophy in the renal patient. J Am Soc Nephrol 12: 1079–1084.
5. Smallwood PM, Munoz-Sanjuan I, Tong P, Macke JP, Hendry SH, et al. (1996) Fibroblast growth factor (FGF) homologous factors: new members of the FGF family implicated in nervous system development. Proc Natl Acad Sci U S A 93: 9850–9857.
6. Asplin IR, Wu SM, Mathew S, Bhattacharjee G, Pizzo SV (2001) Differential regulation of the fibroblast growth factor (FGF) family by alpha(2)-macroglobulin:

7. evidence for selective modulation of FGF-2-induced angiogenesis. Blood 97: 3450–3457.
8. Fu X, Cuevas P, Gimenez-Gallego G, Tian H, Sheng Z (1996) Acidic fibroblast growth factor reduces renal morphologic and functional indicators of injury caused by ischemia and reperfusion. Wound Repair Regen 4: 297–303.
9. Fu X, Cuevas P, Gimenez-Gallego G, Sheng Z, Tian H (1995) Acidic fibroblast growth factor reduces rat skeletal muscle damage caused by ischemia and reperfusion. Chin Med J (Engl) 108: 209–214.
10. Beenken A, Mohammadi M (2009) The FGF family: biology, pathophysiology and therapy. Nat Rev Drug Discov 8: 235–253.
11. Fukumoto S (2008) Actions and mode of actions of FGF19 subfamily members. Endocr J 55: 23–31.
12. Jones S (2008) Mini-review: endocrine actions of fibroblast growth factor 19. Mol Pharm 5: 42–48.
13. Nishimura T, Nakatake Y, Konishi M, Itoh N (2000) Identification of a novel FGF, FGF-21, preferentially expressed in the liver. Biochim Biophys Acta 1492: 203–206.

13. Kharitonenkov A, Shiyanova TL, Koester A, Ford AM, Micanovic R, et al. (2005) FGF-21 as a novel metabolic regulator. J Clin Invest 115: 1627–1635.

14. Kharitonenkov A, Shanafelt AB (2009) FGF21: a novel prospect for the treatment of metabolic diseases. Curr Opin Investig Drugs 10: 359–364.

15. Coskun T, Bina HA, Schneider MA, Dunbar JD, Hu CC, et al. (2008) Fibroblast growth factor 21 corrects obesity in mice. Endocrinology 149: 6018–6027.

16. Kharitonenkov A, Wroblewski VJ, Koester A, Chen YF, Clutinger CK, et al. (2007) The metabolic state of diabetic monkeys is regulated by fibroblast growth factor-21. Endocrinology 148: 774–781.

17. Badman MK, Pissios P, Kennedy AR, Koukos G, Flier JS, et al. (2007) Hepatic fibroblast growth factor 21 is regulated by PPARalpha and is a key mediator of hepatic lipid metabolism in ketotic states. Cell Metab 5: 426–437.

18. Zhang X, Yeung DC, Karpisek M, Stejskal D, Zhou ZG, et al. (2008) Serum FGF21 levels are increased in obesity and are independently associated with the metabolic syndrome in humans. Diabetes 57: 1246–1253.

19. Mraz M, Bartlova M, Lacinova Z, Michalsky D, Kasalicky M, et al. (2009) Serum concentrations and tissue expression of a novel endocrine regulator fibroblast growth factor-21 in patients with type 2 diabetes and obesity. Clin Endocrinol (Oxf) 71: 369–375.

20. Li H, Bao Y, Xu A, Pan X, Lu J, et al. (2009) Serum fibroblast growth factor 21 is associated with adverse lipid profiles and gamma-glutamyltransferase but not insulin sensitivity in Chinese subjects. J Clin Endocrinol Metab 94: 2151–2156.

21. Stein S, Stepan H, Kratzsch J, Verlohren M, Verlohren HJ, et al. (2010) Serum fibroblast growth factor 21 levels in gestational diabetes mellitus in relation to insulin resistance and dyslipidemia. Metabolism 59: 33–37.

22. Lin Z, Wu Z, Yin X, Liu Y, Yan X, et al. (2010) Serum Levels of FGF-21 Are Increased in Coronary Heart Disease Patients and Are Independently Associated with Adverse Lipid Profile. PLoS One 5: e15534.

23. Han SH, Choi SH, Cho BJ, Lee Y, Lim S, et al. (2010) Serum fibroblast growth factor-21 concentration is associated with residual renal function and insulin resistance in end-stage renal disease patients receiving long-term peritoneal dialysis. Metabolism.

24. Stein S, Bachmann A, Lossner U, Kratzsch J, Bluher M, et al. (2009) Serum levels of the adipokine FGF21 depend on renal function. Diabetes Care 32: 126–128.

25. Corda S, Mebazaa A, Gandolfini MP, Fitting C, Marotte F, et al. (1997) Trophic effect of human pericardial fluid on adult cardiac myocytes. Differential role of fibroblast growth factor-2 and factors related to ventricular hypertrophy. Circ Res 81: 679–687.

26. Suzuki G, Lee TC, Fallavollita JA, Canty JM, Jr. (2005) Adenoviral gene transfer of FGF-5 to hibernating myocardium improves function and stimulates myocytes to hypertrophy and reenter the cell cycle. Circ Res 96: 767–775.

27. Scheinowitz M, Kotlyar AA, Zimand S, Leibovitz I, Varda-Bloom N, et al. (2002) Effect of basic fibroblast growth factor on left ventricular geometry in rats subjected to coronary occlusion and reperfusion. Isr Med Assoc J 4: 109–113.

28. Gutierrez OM, Mannstadt M, Isakova T, Rauh-Hain JA, Tamez H, et al. (2008) Fibroblast growth factor 23 and mortality among patients undergoing hemodialysis. N Engl J Med 359: 584–592.

29. Imel EA, Econs MJ (2005) Fibroblast growth factor 23: roles in health and disease. J Am Soc Nephrol 16: 2565–2575.

30. Fliser D, Kollerits B, Neyer U, Ankerst DP, Lhotta K, et al. (2007) Fibroblast growth factor 23 (FGF23) predicts progression of chronic kidney disease: the Mild to Moderate Kidney Disease (MMKD) Study. J Am Soc Nephrol 18: 2600–2608.

31. Gutierrez OM, Januzzi JL, Isakova T, Laliberte K, Smith K, et al. (2009) Fibroblast growth factor 23 and left ventricular hypertrophy in chronic kidney disease. Circulation 119: 2545–2552.

32. Devereux RB, Casale PN, Kligfield P, Eisenberg RR, Miller D, et al. (1986) Performance of primary and derived M-mode echocardiographic measurements for detection of left ventricular hypertrophy in necropsied subjects and in patients with systemic hypertension, mitral regurgitation and dilated cardiomyopathy. Am J Cardiol 57: 1388–1393.

33. Devereux RB, Alonso DR, Lutas EM, Gottlieb GJ, Campo E, et al. (1986) Echocardiographic assessment of left ventricular hypertrophy: comparison to necropsy findings. Am J Cardiol 57: 450–458.

34. Yu Yang, Ming Song (2000) Hypertension and left ventricular hypertrophy. In: Zhengqiu Yu SMLZ, ed. Hypertension Beijing Scientific Publishing Company. pp 1428–1441.

35. Khan IA, Fink J, Nass C, Chen H, Christenson R, et al. (2006) N-terminal pro-B-type natriuretic peptide and B-type natriuretic peptide for identifying coronary artery disease and left ventricular hypertrophy in ambulatory chronic kidney disease patients. Am J Cardiol 97: 1530–1534.

36. Verma A, Anavekar NS, Meris A, Thune JJ, Arnold JM, et al. (2007) The relationship between renal function and cardiac structure, function, and prognosis after myocardial infarction: the VALIANT Echo Study. J Am Coll Cardiol 50: 1238–1245.

37. Whaley-Connell A, Sowers JR, McCullough PA, Roberts T, McFarlane SI, et al. (2009) Diabetes mellitus and CKD awareness: the Kidney Early Evaluation Program (KEEP) and National Health and Nutrition Examination Survey (NHANES). Am J Kidney Dis 53: S11–S21.

38. National Kidney Foundation (2010) Diabetes and kidney disease. http://www.kidney.org/kidneydisease/diabetesckd/index.cfm.

39. Kida Y (2003) Fibroblast growth factor 23 in oncogenic osteomalacia and X-linked hypophosphatemia. N Engl J Med 349: 505–506.

40. Liu YB, Wu CC, Lee CM, Chen WJ, Wang TD, et al. (2006) Dyslipidemia is associated with ventricular tachyarrhythmia in patients with acute ST-segment elevation myocardial infarction. J Formos Med Assoc 105: 17–24.

41. Holzmann MJ, Jungner I, Walldius G, Ivert T, Nordqvist T, et al. (2010) Dyslipidemia is a strong predictor of myocardial infarction in subjects with chronic kidney disease. Ann Med.

42. Vaziri ND (2006) Dyslipidemia of chronic renal failure: the nature, mechanisms, and potential consequences. Am J Physiol Renal Physiol 290: F262–F272.

43. Vaziri ND (2010) Lipotoxicity and impaired high density lipoprotein-mediated reverse cholesterol transport in chronic kidney disease. J Ren Nutr 20: S35–S43.

44. Wibell L (1978) The serum level and urinary excretion of beta2-microglobulin in health and renal disease. Pathol Biol (Paris) 26: 295–301.

45. Michelis R, Sela S, Ben-Zvi I, Nagler RM (2007) Salivary beta2-microglobulin analysis in chronic kidney disease and hemodialyzed patients. Blood Purif 25: 505–509.

46. Jovanovic D, Krstivojevic P, Obradovic I, Durdevic V, Dukanovic L (2003) Serum cystatin C and beta2-microglobulin as markers of glomerular filtration rate. Ren Fail 25: 123–133.

47. Hei ZQ, Li XY, Shen N, Pang HY, Zhou SL, et al. (2008) Prognostic values of serum cystatin C and beta2 microglobulin, urinary beta2 microglobulin and N-acetyl-beta-D-glucosaminidase in early acute renal failure after liver transplantation. Chin Med J (Engl) 121: 1251–1256.

48. Xu J, Lloyd DJ, Hale C, Stanislaus S, Chen M, et al. (2009) Fibroblast growth factor 21 reverses hepatic steatosis, increases energy expenditure, and improves insulin sensitivity in diet-induced obese mice. Diabetes 58: 250–259.

7

A Decreased Level of Serum Soluble Klotho is an Independent Biomarker Associated with Arterial Stiffness in Patients with Chronic Kidney Disease

Masashi Kitagawa[1], Hitoshi Sugiyama[1,2]*, Hiroshi Morinaga[1,2], Tatsuyuki Inoue[1¤], Keiichi Takiue[1], Ayu Ogawa[1], Toshio Yamanari[1], Yoko Kikumoto[1], Haruhito Adam Uchida[1], Shinji Kitamura[1], Yohei Maeshima[1], Kazufumi Nakamura[3], Hiroshi Ito[3], Hirofumi Makino[1]

1 Department of Medicine and Clinical Science, Okayama University Graduate School of Medicine, Dentistry and Pharmaceutical Sciences, Okayama, Japan, 2 Department of Chronic Kidney Disease and Peritoneal Dialysis, Okayama University Graduate School of Medicine, Dentistry and Pharmaceutical Sciences, Okayama, Japan, 3 Department of Cardiovascular Medicine, Okayama University Graduate School of Medicine, Dentistry and Pharmaceutical Sciences, Okayama, Japan

Abstract

Background: Klotho was originally identified in a mutant mouse strain unable to express the gene that consequently showed shortened life spans. In humans, low serum Klotho levels are related to the prevalence of cardiovascular diseases in community-dwelling adults. However, it is unclear whether the serum Klotho levels are associated with signs of vascular dysfunction such as arterial stiffness, a major determinant of prognosis, in human subjects with chronic kidney disease (CKD).

Methods: We determined the levels of serum soluble Klotho in 114 patients with CKD using ELISA and investigated the relationship between the level of Klotho and markers of CKD-mineral and bone disorder (CKD-MBD) and various types of vascular dysfunction, including flow-mediated dilatation, a marker of endothelial dysfunction, ankle-brachial pulse wave velocity (baPWV), a marker of arterial stiffness, intima-media thickness (IMT), a marker of atherosclerosis, and the aortic calcification index (ACI), a marker of vascular calcification.

Results: The serum Klotho level significantly correlated with the 1,25-dihydroxyvitamin D level and inversely correlated with the parathyroid hormone level and the fractional excretion of phosphate. There were significant decreases in serum Klotho in patients with arterial stiffness defined as baPWV≥1400 cm/sec, atherosclerosis defined as maximum IMT≥1.1 mm and vascular calcification scores of ACI>0%. The serum Klotho level was a significant determinant of arterial stiffness, but not endothelial dysfunction, atherosclerosis or vascular calcification, in the multivariate analysis in either metabolic model, the CKD model or the CKD-MBD model. The adjusted odds ratio of serum Klotho for the baPWV was 0.60 (p = 0.0075).

Conclusions: Decreases in the serum soluble Klotho levels are independently associated with signs of vascular dysfunction such as arterial stiffness in patients with CKD. Further research exploring whether therapeutic approaches to maintain or elevate the Klotho level could improve arterial stiffness in CKD patients is warranted.

Editor: Karin Jandeleit-Dahm, Baker IDI Heart and Diabetes Institute, Australia

Funding: A portion of this study was supported by a Research Grant from the Kidney Foundation Japan (JKFB10-20 and JKFB12-44) and a 2011 Chronic Kidney Disease Award to M.K., a Research Grant from the Japan Vascular Disease Research Foundation to H.S. and a Grant-in-Aid for Progressive Renal Diseases Research, Research on Intractable Disease, from the Ministry of Health, Labor and Welfare of Japan. The funders had no role in study design, data collection and analysis, decision to publish or preparation of the manuscript.

Competing Interests: The authors have declared that no competing interests exist.

* E-mail: hitoshis@md.okayama-u.ac.jp

¤ Current address: Center for iPS Cell Research and Application, Kyoto University, Kyoto, Japan

Introduction

Chronic kidney disease (CKD) may fundamentally underlie the development of cardiovascular disease (CVD) and appears to be a risk factor for CVD [1]. Patients with CKD are more likely to die of CVD than to develop end-stage renal failure [2]. CKD leads to increased levels of parathyroid hormone (PTH) and fibroblast growth factor 23 (FGF23) and decreased levels of circulating 1,25-dihydroxyvitamin D (1,25D) along with hypocalcemia, hyper-

phosphatemia, bone disease, vascular calcification and cardiovascular morbidities collectively referred to as chronic kidney disease-mineral and bone disorder (CKD-MBD) [3,4,5]. Recent reports suggest that increased levels of FGF23 are a common manifestation of CKD that develop earlier than increased levels of phosphate or PTH [6]. Additionally, the circulating FGF23 level is independently correlated with endothelial dysfunction, possibly due to asymmetrical dimethyl arginine, an endogenous inhibitor of nitric oxide synthase [7].

The Klotho gene, identified as an 'aging suppressor' gene in mice, encodes a single-pass transmembrane protein that is predominantly expressed in the distal tubular epithelial cells of the kidneys, parathyroid glands and choroid plexus of the brain [8,9,10,11]. Klotho was originally identified in a mutant mouse strain that could not express the gene, which developed multiple disorders resembling human aging and had a shortened life span [10]. The aging phenotypes include atherosclerosis, endothelial dysfunction, low bone mineral density, sarcopenia, skin atrophy and impaired cognition. In an atherosclerotic mouse model, the *in vivo* gene delivery of Klotho protects against endothelial dysfunction [12]. HMG-CoA reductase inhibition enhances the Klotho protein expression in the kidneys and inhibits atherosclerosis in rats with chronic blockade of nitric oxide synthase [13]. Emerging evidence suggests that a deficiency of Klotho is an early biomarker for CKD [14,15,16,17] and acute kidney injury [18]. There are two forms of Klotho, a membrane form and a secreted form, and each has distinct functions. Membrane Klotho acts as an obligate co-receptor for FGF23, a bone-derived hormone that induces phosphate excretion into the urine [19]. Secreted Klotho is involved in the regulation of nitric oxide production in the endothelium [20,21], maintenance of endothelial integrity and permeability [22], calcium homeostasis in the kidneys [23] and inhibition of intracellular insulin and insulin-like growth factor-1 signaling [24]. Secreted Klotho proteins are present in human sera and cerebrospinal fluid, suggesting that post-translational cleavage results in the release of Klotho proteins from the cell membrane [25]. The extracellular domain of Klotho is clipped by the membrane-anchored proteases ADAM10 and ADAM17 in order to generate the secreted form [26].

Recently, a sensitive and specific assay was developed for the measurement of soluble Klotho in humans [27]. Low serum Klotho levels have been reported to be associated with poor skeletal muscle strength [28] and the prevalence of CVD [29] and all-cause mortality [30] in community-dwelling adults. The expression of local vascular Klotho has been observed to decrease in human arteries in patients with CKD compared to healthy individuals [31]. Low serum Klotho levels have been reported in patients with diabetes mellitus [32]. However, whether the serum Klotho levels are closely related to signs of vascular dysfunction such as arterial stiffness in patients with CKD is largely unknown. We hypothesized that low serum Klotho levels are associated with signs of vascular dysfunction such as arterial stiffness in patients with CKD. To address this hypothesis, we measured the serum Klotho levels and extensively investigated the relationship between the serum Klotho level and signs of vascular dysfunction, including endothelial dysfunction, arterial stiffness, atherosclerosis and vascular calcification, in CKD patients. The data presented here suggest that a decrease in the serum soluble Klotho level is an independent biomarker of pronounced arterial stiffness in patients with CKD.

Results

Patient characteristics

The baseline characteristics of the study population are shown in **Table 1**. A total of 114 CKD patients with a median age of 58 (47–66) years were included in the study. The background causes of CKD included 54 cases of glomerulonephritis (47%), 27 cases of nephrosclerosis (24%), 13 cases of diabetic nephropathy (11%) and 20 cases of "other" (18%). A total of 83 patients were on antihypertensive therapy (71 patients were being treated with angiotensin receptor blockers (ARBs) or angiotensin converting enzyme inhibitors (ACEIs), 58 with calcium channel antagonists

and 14 with other agents). Antihyperlipidemic agents were administered to 35 patients and antidiabetic agents were administered to 16 patients. The median serum Klotho level was 616.3 pg/mL, with an interquartile range of 460.0 to 755.5 pg/mL, the value of which was comparable to that reported in a previous study of CKD patients [17] and was higher than that in hemodialysis patients [33,34].

Table 1. Baseline characteristics of the study subjects.

	CKD patients (n = 114)
Age (year)	58 (47–66)
Male sex, n (%)	72 (59%)
Cause of CKD, n	
Glomerulonephritis	54 (47%)
Nephrosclerosis	27 (24%)
Diabetic nephropathy	13 (11%)
Others	20 (18%)
Current medication, n	
ARBs/ACEIs	71 (62%)
CCBs	58 (51%)
MBP (mmHg)	94 ± 13
Serum calcium (mg/dL)	9.3 (9.0–9.5)
Serum phosphate (mg/dL)	3.6 ± 0.7
FECa (%)	0.42 (0.26–0.70)
FEPi (%)	16.0 (11.2–29.6)
Intact PTH (pg/mL)	50 (38–84)
25D (ng/mL)	15 (12–23)
1,25D (pg/mL)	35 (24–50)
FGF23 (pg/mL)	44.4 (31.6–90.0)
Serum Klotho (pg/mL)	616.3 (459.9–755.5)
LDL-cholesterol (mg/dL)	119 ± 34
HDL-cholesterol (mg/dL)	51 (41–64)
Triglycerides (mg/dL)	133 (89–183)
HbA1c (NGSP) (%)	5.7 (5.5–6.0)
CRP (mg/dL)	0.05 (0.02–0.15)
eGFR (ml/min/1.73 m^2)	48 ± 29
Albuminuria (mg/day)	439 (128–1381)
Serum albumin (g/dL)	3.9 (3.6–4.2)
Hemoglobin (g/dL)	12.6 ± 2.2
Uric acid (mg/dL)	6.9 ± 1.6
FMD (%)	4.7 (3.1–7.6)
baPWV (cm/sec)	1560 (1331–1796)
Max IMT (mm)	0.85 (0.68–1.10)
ACI (%)	4.2 (0–16.4)

ACEI, angiotensin converting enzyme inhibitor; ACI, abdominal aortic calcification index; ARB, angiotensin receptor blocker; baPWV, brachial-ankle pulse wave velocity; CRP, C-reactive protein; 1,25D, 1,25-dihydroxyvitamin D; 25D, 25-hydroxyvitamin D; eGFR, estimated glomerular filtration rate; FECa, fractional excretion of calcium; FEPi, fractional excretion of phosphate; FGF23, fibroblast growth factor 23; FMD, flow-mediated dilatation; HDL, high density lipoprotein; IMT, intima-media thickness; LDL, low density lipoprotein; MBP, mean blood pressure; NGSP, national glycohemoglobin standardization program.

Relationship between the serum Klotho level and age, renal function, CKD-related mineral metabolism and markers of vascular dysfunction

Age-dependent changes were recognized in the serum Klotho levels in patients with CKD (**Figure 1A**), as has been reported in healthy subjects [27]. The serum Klotho level was significantly correlated with the eGFR (**Figure 1B**) and decreased along with CKD stages (**Figure S1A**). With regard to markers of CKD-MBD, the serum Klotho level was positively correlated with the 1,25-dihydroxyvitamin D (1,25D) level (**Figure 1C**) and negatively correlated with the log intact parathyroid hormone (PTH) and fractional excretion of phosphate (FEPi) (**Figure 1D, 1E**). The FEPi significantly increased along with declines in the eGFR (univariate regression, r = −0.7228, p<0.0001). There were no correlations between the level of serum Klotho and the fractional excretion of calcium (FECa) (**Figure 1F**) or the 25-hydroxyvitamin D (25D) level (**Figure S2C**). However, correlations were observed between the level of serum Klotho and the level of serum calcium (r = 0.1618; p = 0.0855), the level of serum phosphate (r = −0.1454; p = 0.1426) and log intact FGF23 (r = −0.1751; p = 0.0624) (**Figure S2A, Figure S2B** and **Figure S2D**, respectively).

We next investigated the association between the serum Klotho level and various markers of vascular dysfunction, including flow-mediated dilatation (FMD), a marker of nitric oxide-dependent endothelial function, brachial-ankle pulse wave velocity (baPWV), a marker of arterial stiffness, maximum intima-media thickness (max IMT), a marker of atherosclerosis, and the abdominal aortic calcification index (ACI), a marker of vascular calcification (**Figure 2**). The serum Klotho levels tended to be lower in patients with FMD<6.0% compared to those with FMD≥6.0% (p = 0.0863) (**Figure 2A**). The serum Klotho levels were significantly lower in patients with PWV≥1400 cm/s, max IMT≥1.1 mm and ACI>0% compared to those with PWV<1400 cm/s, max IMT<1.1 mm and ACI = 0%, respectively (**Figure 2B–D**).

A multivariate analysis of the determinants of signs of vascular dysfunction, including arterial stiffness, in CKD patients

Separate multiple logistic regression models for markers of various signs of vascular dysfunction were analyzed (**Table 2 and Table S1, S2, S3**). After adjusting for age, gender, mean blood pressure, use of antihypertensive drugs, drinking and current smoking, the serum Klotho level was found to be a significantly independent predictor of baPWV≥1400 cm/sec in a metabolic model that included non-HDL cholesterol, use of antihyperlipidemic agents, hemoglobin A1c and use of antidiabetic agents as other parameters (**Table 2, upper panel**). The serum Klotho level was also found to be a significantly independent predictor of baPWV≥1400 cm/sec in a CKD model that included eGFR, albuminuria and hemoglobin as other parameters (**Table 2, middle panel**) and a CKD-MBD model that included serum calcium, phosphate, intact PTH, 1,25D and FGF23 as other parameters (**Table 2, lower panel**). We performed the same analysis using multiple logistic regression models of the serum Klotho level as a predictor of FMD≥6.0%, max IMT≥1.1 mm and ACI>0%; however, the serum Klotho level was not found to be a significant predictor of any of these parameters (**Table S1, S2, S3**, respectively). Next, a multivariable logistic regression analysis was performed to evaluate the impact of serum Klotho on arterial stiffness assessed by baPWV in CKD patients. This model includes candidate predictors that were selected based on Table 2.

The factors significantly associated with baPWV were age, MBP, albuminuria and serum Klotho. The adjusted odds ratios (ORs) for serum Klotho (per 100 pg/mL increase) and albuminuria (per 500 mg/day increase) were 0.60 (95% CI: 0.39 to 0.98; p = 0.0075) and 1.97 (95% CI: 1.16 to 3.73; p = 0.0219), respectively (**Figure 3**).

Discussion

In this study, we measured the serum Klotho levels and determined the relationships between the serum Klotho level and markers of CKD-MBD and vascular dysfunction, including FMD, baPWV, max IMT and ACI in patients with CKD. We herein provide the first evidence in CKD patients that: 1) the serum soluble Klotho level is significantly correlated with markers of CKD-MBD, including the levels of PTH, 1,25D and FEPi; 2) decreased levels of serum Klotho are significantly associated with signs of vascular dysfunction such as pronounced arterial stiffness evaluated by baPWV; and 3) in a multivariate analysis, the serum Klotho level was found to be an independent determinant of marked arterial stiffness, which has been reported to be associated with increased cardiovascular mortality and morbidity.

In this study, the group with lower levels of serum Klotho exhibited significantly lower eGFR levels, as previously reported in CKD patients [17] and patients on hemodialysis [34]. It has been reported that the mRNA and protein expression levels of Klotho are severely reduced in the kidneys of patients with chronic renal failure compared to control subjects [35]. However, it seems that the serum Klotho levels are not completely depleted, even in patients with stage 5 CKD on hemodialysis [34]. This finding suggests that a basal level of Klotho production from other organs than the kidneys, such as the brain and parathyroid glands, might exist in humans, as has been previously reported in mice [8,9,10]. A recent study indicated that the transcriptional suppression of Klotho by a protein-bound uremic toxin, indoxyl sulfate, results from CpG hypermethylation of the Klotho gene [36]. Since indoxyl sulfate may play a significant role in the vascular disease and higher mortality observed in CKD patients [37], epigenetic modification of the Klotho gene by a uremic toxin such as indoxyl sulfate might be a mechanism underlying the association between the decline of serum Klotho levels and arterial stiffness in CKD patients observed in the current study.

With regard to markers of CKD-MBD, the serum Klotho level was inversely correlated with the FEPi and log intact PTH and positively correlated with the 1,25D level. The FEPi significantly increased along with declines in the eGFR in the CKD patients evaluated in this study and also in the Chronic Renal Insufficiency Cohort (CRIC) study [6]. The serum Klotho is unable to function as a decoy receptor for FGF23, because Klotho alone does not bind to FGF23 with high affinity. Unlike membrane Klotho, serum Klotho cannot efficiently support FGF23-induced activation of FGF signaling [38]. Instead, serum Klotho may inhibit Type 2a Na-phosphate co-transporter (Npt2a) by decreasing the number of cell-surface Npt2a, thereby reducing cellular phosphate uptake in renal proximal tubular cells [39]. The level of serum Klotho might therefore reflect increased phosphate excretion from the kidneys, which is one of the characteristics of disordered mineral metabolism observed in CKD patients.

To date, several markers have been utilized to assess cardiovascular dysfunction in CKD patients, including FMD, baPWV, IMT and ACI [40,41,42,43,44]. In the current study, we demonstrated that the level of serum Klotho is an independent determinant of arterial stiffness only defined as baPWV≥1400 cm/s, even after adjusting for age, gender, mean

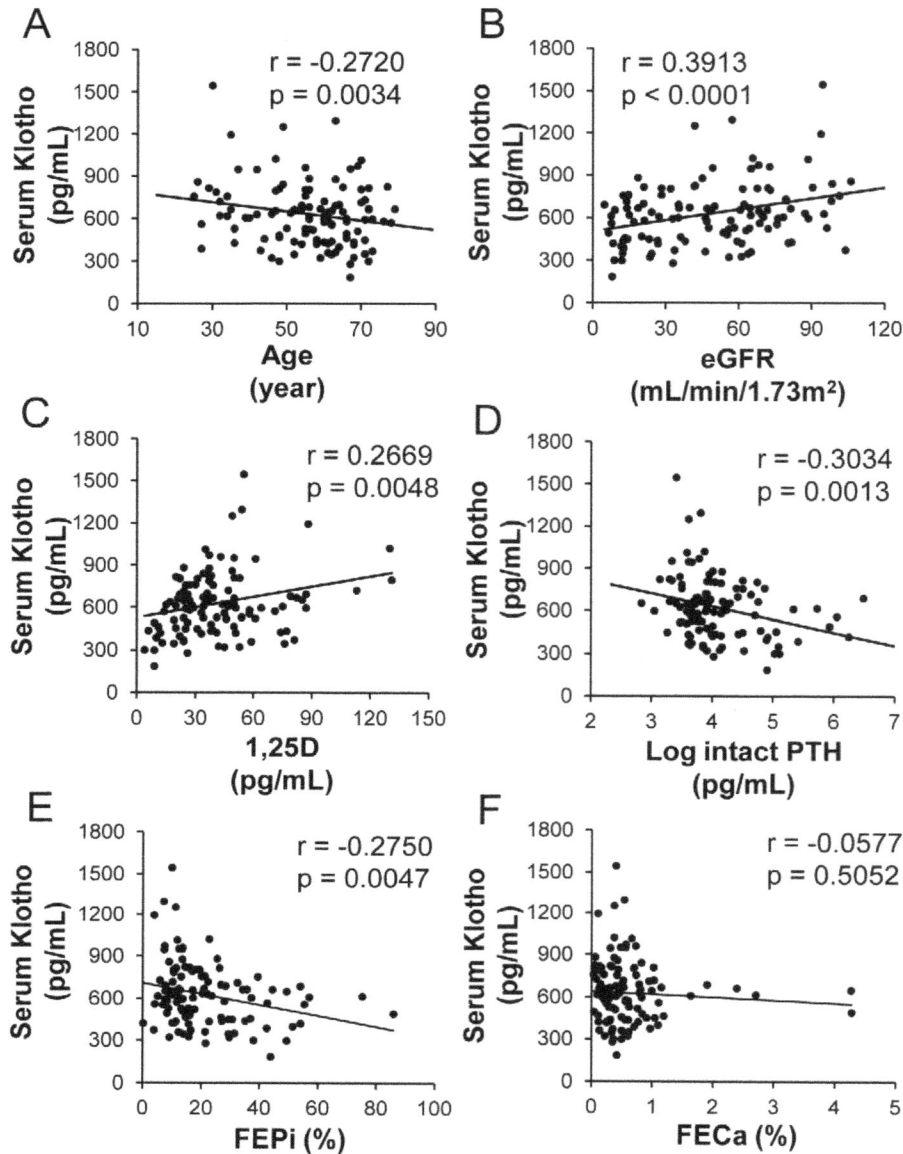

Figure 1. Correlation between the serum Klotho levels (pg/mL) and various parameters. The relationships between the serum Klotho levels and patient age (years) (A), estimated glomerular filtration rate (eGFR) (mL/min/1.73 m²) (B) and markers of chronic kidney disease-mineral and bone disorder (CKD-MBD), including 1,25-dihydroxyvitamin D (1,25D) (pg/mL) (C), log intact parathyroid hormone (PTH) (pg/mL) (D), fractional excretion of phosphate (FEPi) (%) (E) and fractional excretion of calcium (FECa) (%) (F) are shown. The serum Klotho levels were inversely correlated with age and positively correlated with eGFR (**A, B**). Regarding CKD-MBD markers, the serum Klotho levels were significantly correlated with 1,25D and negatively correlated with log intact PTH and FEPi; however, no significant correlation was observed with FECa (**C–F**). (**A–F**) N = 114.

blood pressure, use of antihypertensive drugs, drinking and smoking. In addition, serum Klotho was also a significant predictor of arterial stiffness in the full model including confounders such as age, MBP, diabetes mellitus, dyslipidemia, eGFR, albuminuria, phosphate, PTH, 1,25D and FGF23, and the adjusted odds ratio (OR) for serum Klotho (per 100 pg/mL increase) was 0.60 (95% CI: 0.39 to 0.98; p = 0.0075). There have been some reports discussing the associations between baPWV and CKD-MBD parameters such as phosphate [45], 1,25D [46], PTH [47,48] and FGF23 [49,50]; however, these associations are inconsistent. Several reports have shown that increases in aortic stiffness begin as early as CKD stage 2 and increase with the progression to stages 3 and 4 [51,52]. Conversely, improvements

in aortic stiffness have been associated with improved prognoses in patients with end-stage renal disease [53]. The role of serum Klotho in the progression of arterial stiffness has not yet been elucidated in human CKD; however, *in vivo* gene delivery of Klotho into skeletal muscle prevents medial hypertrophy of the aorta in an animal model of atherosclerotic disease [12]. It also improves endothelium-dependent relaxation of the aorta in response to acetylcholine in association with increases in nitric oxide production, suggesting that soluble Klotho plays a protective role against the development of vascular endothelial dysfunction. Although the receptor for soluble Klotho located in the vascular endothelium has not been identified, soluble Klotho regulates calcium influx to maintain the integrity of vascular endothelial

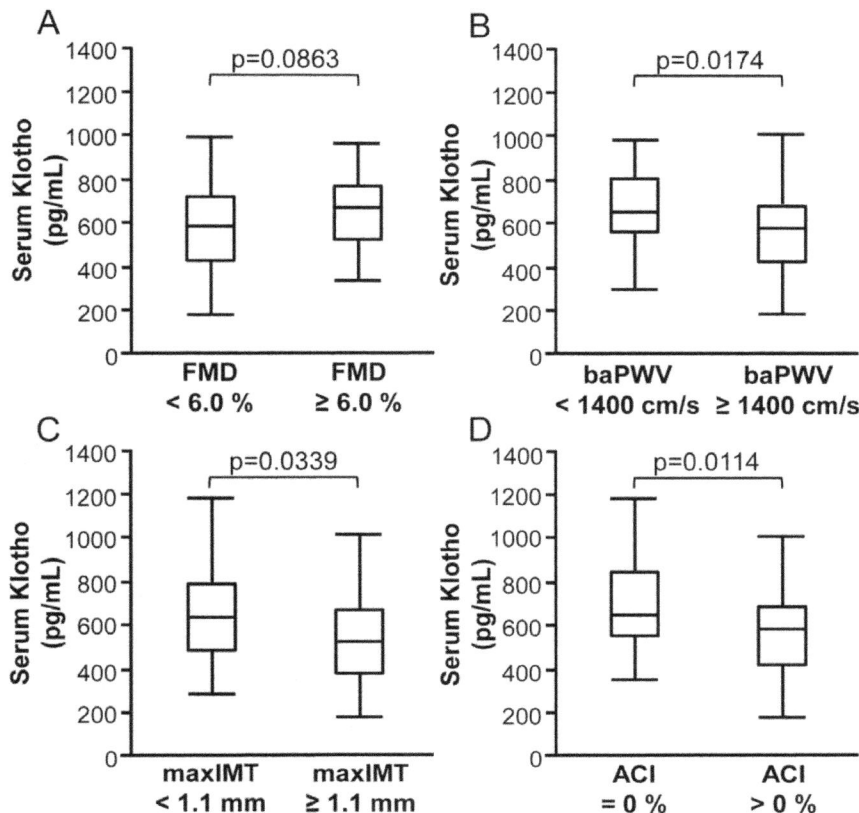

Figure 2. Box and line plots showing the levels of serum Klotho (pg/mL) according to the stratified levels of vascular dysfunction. They include flow-mediated dilatation (FMD) (%), a marker of endothelial dysfunction (A), ankle-brachial pulse wave velocity (baPWV) (cm/sec), a marker of arterial stiffness (B), maximum intima-media thickness (max IMT) (mm), a marker of atherosclerosis (C), and the aortic calcification index (ACI) (%), a marker of vascular calcification (D). The serum Klotho levels were significantly lower in patients with FMD<6.0%, PWV≥1400 cm/s, max IMT≥1.1 mm and ACI>0% compared to patients with FMD≥6.0%, PWV<1400 cm/s, max IMT<1.1 mm and ACI=0%, respectively (A–D). (A) N = 70 and n = 40 in FMD<6.0% and FMD≥6.0%, respectively. (B) N = 60 and n = 45 in PWV<1400 cm/s and PWV≥1400 cm/s, respectively. (C) N = 82 and n = 29 in max IMT<1.1 mm and max IMT≥1.1 mm, respectively. (D) N = 28 and n = 75 in ACI=0% and ACI>0%, respectively. The boxes denote the medians and 25th and 75th percentiles. The lines mark the 5th and 95th percentiles.

cells in a mouse model and in *in vitro* endothelial cell culture studies [22]. The 'local' vascular Klotho in human arteries may act as an endogenous inhibitor of vascular calcification and as a cofactor required for vascular FGF23 signaling [31]. Conducting further studies will therefore be necessary in order to investigate how 'systemic' serum Klotho interacts with the mechanisms of arterial stiffness in human CKD.

An association between Klotho deficiency and vascular calcification has been reported in aging mice and in a mouse model of CKD [10,16,24]. In the assessment of vascular calcification conducted in the current study, the levels of serum Klotho were decreased in CKD patients with ACI>0% compared to those in patients without aortic calcification (Figure 2D), although the levels of serum Klotho were not significantly correlated with the degree of ACI (Figure S2H) or were not independent determinants of ACI (Table S3). There are two possible reasons why the serum Klotho levels are not significantly correlated with the degree of aortic calcification in human CKD patients. First, soft tissue calcification in human CKD may progress more slowly than that observed in murine CKD [16], despite phosphorus and calcium playing major roles in the calcification process in CKD patients. The CKD cohort in our study comprised mostly patients with CKD of stages 1 to 3 (68.4%), which are the early to middle stages of CKD, rather than

patients with severe renal dysfunction or uremia that may induce a more procalcific CKD phenotype [54].

Increased serum phosphorus levels are associated with cardiovascular disease in both patients with chronic kidney disease (CKD) and in the general population. High phosphate levels may play a direct role in vascular dysfunction. In the current study, however, there were no significant correlations between the serum phosphate levels and the FMD (r = −0.0530, p = 0.5596), baPWV (r = 0.1217, p = 0.2778), max IMT (r = 0.1030, p = 0.2695) or ACI (r = 0.0245, p = 0.7988). Kestenbaum et al. reported a significant increase in the mortality risk in patients with CKD with phosphate levels higher than 3.5 mg/dL [55]. In our cohort, only 41.4% (46 out of 114) patients exhibited serum phosphate levels higher than 3.5 mg/dL, so the phosphate levels might not correlate with the vascular dysfunction in this study. A recent report demonstrated that a high phosphate level directly affects endothelial dysfunction [56]. Indeed, our data suggest that there is some relationship between the FEPi and FMD (r = −0.2520, p = 0.0077), although the correlation was not statistically significant. Another report using an animal model indicated that changes in extracellular phosphorus concentrations may directly modulate the vascular smooth muscle function [57]. Based on these findings, phosphate could still be a major direct player in the pathogenesis of the vascular dysfunctions observed in patients with CKD.

Multivariate odds ratio (95% CI) for baPWV

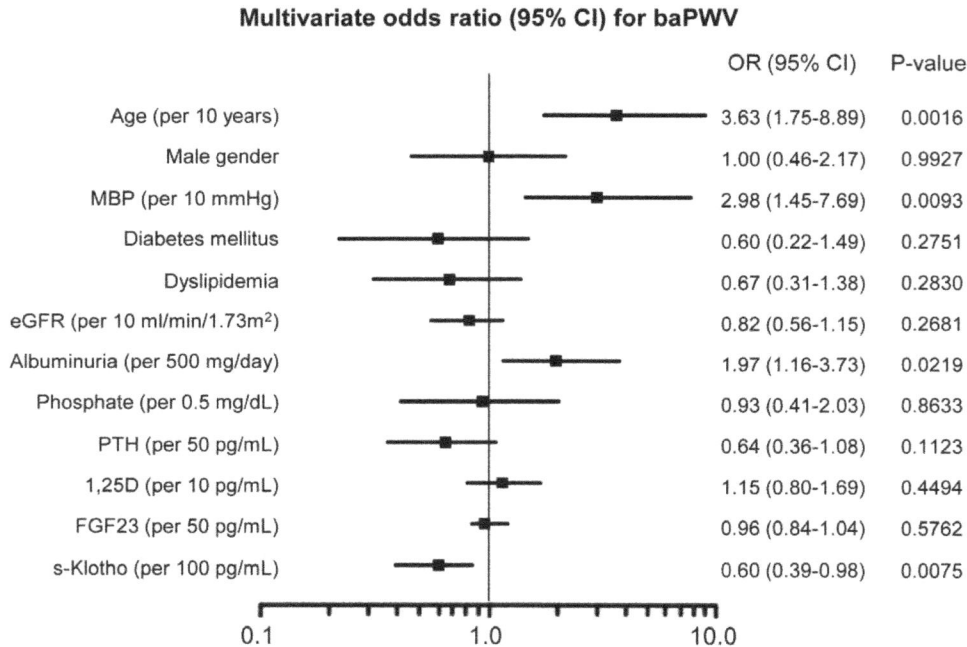

	OR (95% CI)	P-value
Age (per 10 years)	3.63 (1.75-8.89)	0.0016
Male gender	1.00 (0.46-2.17)	0.9927
MBP (per 10 mmHg)	2.98 (1.45-7.69)	0.0093
Diabetes mellitus	0.60 (0.22-1.49)	0.2751
Dyslipidemia	0.67 (0.31-1.38)	0.2830
eGFR (per 10 ml/min/1.73m²)	0.82 (0.56-1.15)	0.2681
Albuminuria (per 500 mg/day)	1.97 (1.16-3.73)	0.0219
Phosphate (per 0.5 mg/dL)	0.93 (0.41-2.03)	0.8633
PTH (per 50 pg/mL)	0.64 (0.36-1.08)	0.1123
1,25D (per 10 pg/mL)	1.15 (0.80-1.69)	0.4494
FGF23 (per 50 pg/mL)	0.96 (0.84-1.04)	0.5762
s-Klotho (per 100 pg/mL)	0.60 (0.39-0.98)	0.0075

Figure 3. Multivariate odds ratio for ankle-brachial pulse wave velocity (baPWV) among patients with CKD displayed as the odds ratio (OR) (solid boxes) with 95% confidence intervals (CIs) (horizontal limit lines). For continuous variables, the unit of change is given in parenthesis based on the multivariate model described in Table 2. MBP, mean blood pressure; eGFR, estimated glomerular filtration rate; PTH, parathyroid hormone; 1,25D, 1,25-dihydroxyvitamin D; FGF23, fibroblast growth factor 23.

Table 2. A multiple logistic regression analysis of predictors of PWV≥1400 cm/sec.

	β	p
Metabolic model		
serum Klotho	−0.00404	0.0315
non HDL	0.00226	0.8185
antihyperlipidemic drugs	0.42663	0.2660
HbA1c (NGSP)	0.43333	0.4369
antidiabetic drugs	0.43224	0.5107
CKD model		
serum Klotho	−0.00349	0.0431
eGFR	0.01367	0.3911
albuminuria	0.00062	0.1904
Hemoglobin	−0.01483	0.9467
CKD-MBD model		
serum Klotho	−0.00431	0.0368
serum calcium	−0.96331	0.4039
serum phosphate	−0.65510	0.4178
intact PTH	−0.00625	0.2903
1,25D	0.00367	0.8244
FGF23	−0.00052	0.6933

Adjusted for age, gender, mean blood pressure, antihypertensive drug use, drinking and current smoking. CKD, chronic kidney disease; 1,25D, 1,25-dihydroxyvitamin D; eGFR, estimated glomerular filtration rate; FGF23, fibroblast growth factor 23; HDL, high density lipoprotein; MBD, mineral and bone disorder; NGSP, national glycohemoglobin standardization program.

Membrane Klotho functions as a co-receptor for FGF23, a bone-derived hormone that induces phosphate excretion into the urine [19]. The presence of membrane Klotho determines the target organs of FGF23 and its signaling since most tissues express receptors for FGF. Nakano et al. recently reported that the serum intact FGF23 level is the earliest indicator among various CKD-MBD-related factors and that a high intact FGF23 level and a low 25-hydroxyvitamin D (25D) level independently predict poor renal outcomes, even after adjusting for other MBD-related factors, in patients with pre-dialysis CKD [58]. However, the serum Klotho level was not evaluated in that report, and the exact functions of serum soluble Klotho have yet to be defined [59]. Therefore, whether an excess level of FGF23 and the occurrence of adverse outcomes in patients with CKD are mediated by a deficiency of serum Klotho remains unclear [60].

There have been discrepancies among the study results concerning the correlation between the serum Klotho levels and GFR in patients with CKD [17,32,61]. One study found that the plasma Klotho level was not related to the kidney function in patients with CKD, but this study population included nearly 40% patients with diabetes mellitus (39.4%) [61]. In contrast, the serum levels of soluble Klotho were decreased in patients with early stages of CKD in a different study including 15.4% diabetes mellitus cases [17]. These discrepancies may be due to two possible causes. First, including diabetic patients in the CKD cohort may underestimate the level of serum Klotho, since the level of serum Klotho is lower in diabetic patients compared to non-diabetic patients [32]. Second, several ELISA kits to detect the level of soluble Klotho are commercially available, potentially leading to different results in terms of the association of serum Klotho with the renal function.

Our study has several limitations and strengths that should be kept in mind when interpreting the results. First, the cross-sectional nature of our observations precluded making any cause-effect inferences about the relationship between the serum Klotho level and arterial stiffness in CKD patients. Second, we lacked data regarding the patients' dietary phosphorus intake, a critical factor for CKD-MBD and the CKD-associated incidence of CVD, which may be related to the serum Klotho level. However, this weakness is, in part, offset by the criteria of our study because patients who were being treated with vitamin D or phosphate binders were excluded.

In conclusion, the serum Klotho level was found to significantly correlate with markers of CKD-MBD and is an independent biomarker of arterial stiffness in patients with CKD. Further studies are required to elucidate which intervention(s) can modulate the level of serum Klotho, as has been reported in rodents [13,62,63], and whether any interventions to increase or maintain the serum Klotho level can prevent cardiovascular events and mortality in CKD patients.

Subjects and Methods

Subjects

The subjects in this study were patients admitted to the Renal Unit of Okayama University Hospital. All patients were diagnosed with CKD according to their estimated glomerular filtration rate (eGFR) and the presence of kidney injury as defined by the National Kidney Foundation K/DOQI Guidelines [64,65]. Hypertension was defined as systolic blood pressure (SBP)$\geq$140 mmHg or diastolic blood pressure (DBP)$\geq$90 mmHg or the use of antihypertensive drugs. The eGFR was calculated according to the simplified version of the Modification of Diet in Renal Disease (MDRD) formula [eGFR = 194$\times$(sCr)$^{-1.094}\times$(age)$^{-0.287}$(if female$\times$0.739)] [66]. Smoking status (current smoker vs. non-smoker) was determined from a medical interview. Current drinking was defined as drinking alcohol at least two times per week in the last year. All procedures in the present study were carried out in accordance with institutional and national ethical guidelines for human studies, and guidelines proposed in the Declaration of Helsinki. The ethics committee of Okayama University Graduate School of Medicine, Dentistry and Pharmaceutical Sciences approved the study. Written informed consent was obtained from each subject. This study was registered with the Clinical Trial Registry of the University Hospital Medical Information Network (registration number UMIN000003614). According to the established protocol, we excluded any patients with established atherosclerotic complications (coronary artery disease, congestive heart failure or peripheral vascular disease). Patients with nephrotic syndrome and patients who were being treated with vitamin D or phosphate binders were excluded. None of the patients had an acute infection at the time of the study.

Laboratory measurements

Each subject's arterial blood pressure was measured by a physician after a 10 minute resting period to obtain the systolic and diastolic pressures. The mean blood pressure (MBP) was calculated as DBP+(SBP−DBP)/3. All samples were obtained from patients in the morning after 12 hours of fasting. The soluble α-Klotho (Klotho) concentrations in the serum were measured using an ELISA system (Immuno-Biological Laboratories, Gunma, Japan) [27]. The serum levels of intact FGF23 were determined using a commercial sandwich ELISA kit (Kainos Laboratories, Inc., Tokyo, Japan). The serum levels of total protein, albumin, creatinine, calcium, inorganic phosphate and glucose, as well as the urinary levels of albumin, creatinine, calcium and inorganic phosphate, were measured in all patients.

The serum levels of 1,25-dihydroxyvitamin D (1,25D) and 25-hydroxyvitamin D (25D) were measured using a radioimmunoassay and the serum intact PTH levels were measured using an immunoradiometric assay. The fractional excretion of phosphorus (FEPi) and calcium (FECa) were calculated as (urine mineral$\times$serum creatinine)/(serum mineral$\times$urine creatinine).

Vascular assessments

Endothelial dysfunction. Flow-mediated dilatation (FMD) and endothelium-independent vasodilatation (nitroglycerin-mediated dilatation; NMD) of the brachial artery were assessed noninvasively, as previously described [44]. The subjects were instructed to fast for at least 12 hours before testing and to abstain from smoking and ingesting alcohol, caffeine or antioxidant vitamins prior to testing. We obtained ultrasound measurements according to the guidelines for ultrasound assessment of the FMD of the brachial artery. Using a 10-MHz linear array transducer probe, the longitudinal image of the right brachial artery was recorded at baseline and then continuously from 30 seconds before to at least two minutes after the cuff deflation that followed suprasystolic compression (50 mmHg above systolic blood pressure (SBP)) of the right forearm for five minutes. The diastolic diameter of the brachial artery was determined semi-automatically using an instrument equipped with a software program for monitoring the brachial artery diameter (Unex Co. Ltd., Nagoya, Japan). The FMD was estimated as the percent change in the diameter over the baseline value at maximal dilation during reactive hyperemia. A total of 10 minutes were allowed to elapse for vessel recovery, after which a further resting scan was taken. Then, 0.3 mg of nitroglycerin was administered, and a final scan was performed five minutes later. We defined patients having endothelial dysfunction as those with FMD<6.0% in the current study based on previous reports [44,67,68].

Measurement of intima-media thickness (IMT). Ultrasonography of the carotid artery was performed using a high resolution real-time scanner with a 7.5 MHz transducer, as previously described [40]. The examination was performed with the subject in the supine position, and the carotid bifurcation, as well as the common carotid artery, were scanned on both sides. The maximum IMT value was measured as follows. The carotid artery was scanned in the longitudinal and transverse directions. The site of the most advanced atherosclerotic lesion that showed the greatest distance between the lumen-intima interface and the media-adventitia interface was located in both the right and left carotid arteries. When plaque was detected on ultrasonography, it was observed as localized thickening rather than a circumferential change in the vessel wall. The greatest thickness of the intima-media complex (including plaque) was used for the maximum IMT value. We identified patients having atherosclerosis based on atheromatous plaques of focal increases in IMT$\geq$1.1 mm in accordance with a prior study that showed the normal limit of IMT to be $\leq$1.0 mm [69].

Measurement of ankle-brachial pulse wave velocity (baPWV). Pulse wave velocity (PWV) measurements were obtained at the bedside of each subject using a volume plethysmographic apparatus (FORM/ABI; Colin, Komaki, Japan) after the subject had rested in the supine position for at least five minutes, as previously described [40]. This instrument allows simultaneous recording of the baPWV and the brachial and ankle BPs on both sides, in addition to recording an electrocardiogram and heart sounds. We defined patients having arterial stiffness as those with baPWV$\geq$1400 since a baPWV$\geq$1400 cm/sec is an independent variable of the risk stratification according to the

Framingham score and for the discrimination of patients with atherosclerotic cardiovascular disease [70].

Measurement and calculation of the aortic calcification index (ACI). The ACI was determined as previously described [42,43]. A non-contrast CT scan of the abdominal aorta was performed. Calcification of the abdominal aorta above the bifurcation of the common iliac arteries was evaluated semi-quantitatively in 10 CT slices at 1 cm intervals. Calcification was considered to be present if an area ≥ 1 mm^2 displayed a density ≥ 130 Hounsfield units. The cross-section of the abdominal aorta on each slice was divided into 12 segments radially. A segment containing an aortic wall with calcification in any section was defined as having aortic calcification. The number of calcified segments was counted in each slice and divided by 12. The values thus obtained for the 10 slices were added together, divided by 10 (the number of slices inspected) and then multiplied by 100 to express the result as a percentage: ACI (%) = (total score for calcification in all slices)/(12 [number of segments in each slice] $\times 10$ [number of slices]) $\times 100$. The ACI was used as a marker for the extent of aortic calcification. We defined CKD patients having abdominal calcification as those with ACI>0%, as described previously [42,43].

Statistical analysis

Non-normally distributed variables were expressed as the median (interquartile range) and normally distributed variables were expressed as the mean ± SD as appropriate. A value of P<0.05 was considered to be statistically significant. Differences between groups were analyzed using Student's *t*-test and the Mann-Whitney U-test as appropriate. The Spearman rank correlation was used to determine the correlations between two variables. A multiple logistic regression analysis was applied to test the independent links between the vascular function and potential functional correlates of the outcome variables [71,72]. A multivariable logistic regression analysis was performed to determine the predictors of baPWV. This multivariate model was built using pre-specified variables including age, gender, MBP, diabetes mellitus, dyslipidemia, eGFR, albuminuria, phosphate, PTH, 1,25D, FGF23 and serum Klotho. The P values, odds ratios (ORs) and corresponding two-sided 95% confidence intervals (CIs) for the predictors are presented. The statistical analyses were performed using the JMP software package release 8 (SAS Institute Inc., Cary, NC, USA).

Supporting Information

Figure S1   Box and line plots showing the levels of serum Klotho (pg/mL) according to the estimated glomerular filtration rate (eGFR) (mL/min/1.73 m^2) or the levels of serum log intact fibroblast growth factor 23 (FGF23) (pg/mL) according to the estimated glomerular filtration rate (eGFR) (mL/min/1.73 m^2). The serum soluble Klotho levels significantly decreased in association with declines in eGFR (**A**), while the log-transformed intact FGF23 levels significantly increased in association with declines in eGFR (**B**). (**A**) serum Klotho levels, eGFR$\geq$90 (stage 1), 799.0 (670.6–940.9); eGFR 60–89 (stage 2), 637.4 (546.2–637.4); eGFR 30–59 (stage 3), 595.4 (498.8–773.9); eGFR 15–29 (stage 4), 578.3 (425.9–751.0); eGFR 0–14 (stage 5), 525.1 (389.0–661.4) pg/mL. (**A, B**) eGFR$\geq$90, n = 11; 60–89, n = 36; 30–59, n = 31; 15–29, n = 16, 0–14, n = 20. *, **, *** and **** indicate p<0.05, p<0.01, p<0.005 and p<0.001, respectively. The boxes denote the medians and 25th and 75th percentiles. The lines mark the 5th and 95th percentiles.

Figure S2   Correlation between the serum Klotho levels (pg/mL) and the other markers of chronic kidney disease-mineral and bone disorder (CKD-MBD). They include calcium (mg/dL) (A), phosphate (mg/dL) (B), 25-hydroxyvitamin D (25D) (C) and log intact fibroblast growth factor 23 (FGF23) (D) and various markers of vascular dysfunction, including flow-mediated dilatation (FMD) (%) (E), ankle-brachial pulse wave velocity (baPWV) (cm/sec) (F), maximum intima-media thickness (max IMT) (mm) (G) and the aortic calcification index (ACI) (%) (H). The serum Klotho levels tended to be positively correlated with calcium and phosphate and negatively correlated with log intact FGF23, while no significant association was observed between the serum Klotho levels and 25D (**A–D**). Regarding markers of vascular dysfunction, the serum Klotho levels were positively correlated with FMD and negatively correlated with baPWV and max IMT, while the correlation between the serum Klotho levels and ACI was not significant (**E–H**). (**A, B, D, E–H**) N = 114. (**C**) N = 58.

Figure S3   Multivariate odds ratio for flow-mediated dilatation (FMD) among patients with CKD displayed as the odds ratio (OR) (solid boxes) with 95% confidence intervals (CIs) (horizontal limit lines). For continuous variables, the unit of change is given in parenthesis based on the multivariate model described in Table S1. MBP, mean blood pressure; eGFR, estimated glomerular filtration rate; PTH, parathyroid hormone; 1,25D, 1,25-dihydroxyvitamin D; FGF23, fibroblast growth factor 23.

Figure S4   Multivariate odds ratio for maximum intima-media thickness (max IMT) among patients with CKD, displayed as odds ratio (OR) (solid boxes) with 95% confidence intervals (CIs) (horizontal limit lines). For continuous variables, unit of change is given in parenthesis based on the multivariate model described in Table S2. MBP, mean blood pressure; eGFR, estimated glomerular filtration rate; PTH, parathyroid hormone; 1,25D, 1,25-dihydroxyvitamin D; FGF23, fibroblast growth factor 23.

Figure S5   Multivariate odds ratio for aortic calcification index (ACI) among patients with CKD displayed as the odds ratio (OR) (solid boxes) with 95% confidence intervals (CIs) (horizontal limit lines). For continuous variables, the unit of change is given in parenthesis based on the multivariate model described in Table S3. MBP, mean blood pressure; eGFR, estimated glomerular filtration rate; PTH, parathyroid hormone; 1,25D, 1,25-dihydroxyvitamin D; FGF23, fibroblast growth factor 23.

Table S1   A multiple logistic regression analysis of predictors of FMD$\geq$6.0%.

Table S2   A multiple logistic regression analysis of predictors of max IMT$\geq$1.1 mm.

Table S3   A multiple logistic regression analysis of predictors of ACI>0%.

Acknowledgments

We thank Ms. M. Hada, H. Tsuji and S. Kameshima for their technical assistance. We also extend our gratitude to the physicians in the Department of Medicine and Clinical Science, Okayama University Graduate School of Medicine, Dentistry and Pharmaceutical Sciences for the collection of blood samples.

Author Contributions

Conceived and designed the experiments: MK HS KN HI H. Makino. Performed the experiments: MK TI. Analyzed the data: MK HS H. Morinaga AO TY YK HAU SK YM. Contributed reagents/materials/analysis tools: H. Morinaga KT AO. Wrote the paper: MK HS.

References

1. Sarnak MJ, Levey AS, Schoolwerth AC, Coresh J, Culleton B, et al. (2003) Kidney disease as a risk factor for development of cardiovascular disease: a statement from the American Heart Association Councils on Kidney in Cardiovascular Disease, High Blood Pressure Research, Clinical Cardiology, and Epidemiology and Prevention. Circulation 108: 2154–2169.
2. Go AS, Chertow GM, Fan D, McCulloch CE, Hsu CY (2004) Chronic kidney disease and the risks of death, cardiovascular events, and hospitalization. N Engl J Med 351: 1296–1305.
3. Moe S, Drüeke T, Cunningham J, Goodman W, Martin K, et al. (2006) Definition, evaluation, and classification of renal osteodystrophy: A position statement from Kidney Disease: Improving Global Outcomes (KDIGO). Kidney Int 69: 1945–1953.
4. (2009) KDIGO clinical practice guideline for the diagnosis, evaluation, prevention, and treatment of Chronic Kidney Disease-Mineral and Bone Disorder (CKD-MBD). Kidney Int Suppl: S1–130.
5. Moe SM, Drueke T (2008) Improving global outcomes in mineral and bone disorders. Clin J Am Soc Nephrol 3 Suppl 3: S127–130.
6. Isakova T, Wahl P, Vargas GS, Gutierrez OM, Scialla J, et al. (2011) Fibroblast growth factor 23 is elevated before parathyroid hormone and phosphate in chronic kidney disease. Kidney Int 79: 1370–1378.
7. Yilmaz MI, Sonmez A, Saglam M, Yaman H, Kilic S, et al. (2010) FGF-23 and vascular dysfunction in patients with stage 3 and 4 chronic kidney disease. Kidney Int 78: 679–685.
8. Kuro-o M (2011) Phosphate and Klotho. Kidney Int Suppl 79: S20–S23.
9. John GB, Cheng CY, Kuro-o M (2011) Role of Klotho in aging, phosphate metabolism, and CKD. Am J Kidney Dis 58: 127–134.
10. Kuro-o M, Matsumura Y, Aizawa H, Kawaguchi H, Suga T, et al. (1997) Mutation of the mouse klotho gene leads to a syndrome resembling ageing. Nature 390: 45–51.
11. Kuro-o M (2009) Klotho and aging. Biochim Biophys Acta (BBA) - General Subjects 1790: 1049–1058.
12. Saito Y, Nakamura T, Ohyama Y, Suzuki T, Iida A, et al. (2000) In vivo klotho gene delivery protects against endothelial dysfunction in multiple risk factor syndrome. Biochem Biophys Res Commun 276: 767–772.
13. Kuwahara N, Sasaki S, Kobara M, Nakata T, Tatsumi T, et al. (2008) HMG-CoA reductase inhibition improves anti-aging klotho protein expression and arteriosclerosis in rats with chronic inhibition of nitric oxide synthesis. Int J Cardiol 123: 84–90.
14. Akimoto T, Shiizaki K, Sugase T, Watanabe Y, Yoshizawa H, et al. (2012) The relationship between the soluble Klotho protein and the residual renal function among peritoneal dialysis patients. Clin Exp Nephrol 16: 442–447.
15. Asai O, Nakatani K, Tanaka T, Sakan H, Imura A, et al. (2012) Decreased renal α-Klotho expression in early diabetic nephropathy in humans and mice and its possible role in urinary calcium excretion. Kidney Int 81: 539–547.
16. Hu MC, Shi M, Zhang J, Quinones H, Griffith C, et al. (2011) Klotho deficiency causes vascular calcification in chronic kidney disease. J Am Soc Nephrol 22: 124–136.
17. Shimamura Y, Hamada K, Inoue K, Ogata K, Ishihara M, et al. (2012) Serum levels of soluble secreted alpha-Klotho are decreased in the early stages of chronic kidney disease, making it a probable novel biomarker for early diagnosis. Clin Exp Nephrol 16: 722–729.
18. Hu M-C, Shi M, Zhang J, Quiñones H, Kuro-o M, et al. (2010) Klotho deficiency is an early biomarker of renal ischemia–reperfusion injury and its replacement is protective. Kidney Int 78: 1240–1251.
19. Urakawa I, Yamazaki Y, Shimada T, Iijima K, Hasegawa H, et al. (2006) Klotho converts canonical FGF receptor into a specific receptor for FGF23. Nature 444: 770–774.
20. Nagai R, Saito Y, Ohyama Y, Aizawa H, Suga T, et al. (2000) Endothelial dysfunction in the klotho mouse and downregulation of klotho gene expression in various animal models of vascular and metabolic diseases. Cell Mol Life Sci 57: 738–746.
21. Saito Y, Yamagishi T, Nakamura T, Ohyama Y, Aizawa H, et al. (1998) Klotho protein protects against endothelial dysfunction. Biochem Biophys Res Commun 248: 324–329.
22. Kusaba T, Okigaki M, Matui A, Murakami M, Ishikawa K, et al. (2010) Klotho is associated with VEGF receptor-2 and the transient receptor potential canonical-1 Ca2+ channel to maintain endothelial integrity. Proc Natl Acad Sci U S A 107: 19308–19313.
23. Imura A, Tsuji Y, Murata M, Maeda R, Kubota K, et al. (2007) alpha-Klotho as a regulator of calcium homeostasis. Science 316: 1615–1618.
24. Kurosu H, Yamamoto M, Clark JD, Pastor JV, Nandi A, et al. (2005) Suppression of aging in mice by the hormone Klotho. Science 309: 1829–1833.
25. Imura A, Iwano A, Tohyama O, Tsuji Y, Nozaki K, et al. (2004) Secreted Klotho protein in sera and CSF: implication for post-translational cleavage in release of Klotho protein from cell membrane. FEBS Lett 565: 143–147.
26. Chen CD, Podvin S, Gillespie E, Leeman SE, Abraham CR (2007) Insulin stimulates the cleavage and release of the extracellular domain of Klotho by ADAM10 and ADAM17. Proc Natl Acad Sci U S A 104: 19796–19801.
27. Yamazaki Y, Imura A, Urakawa I, Shimada T, Murakami J, et al. (2010) Establishment of sandwich ELISA for soluble alpha-Klotho measurement: Age-dependent change of soluble alpha-Klotho levels in healthy subjects. Biochem Biophys Res Commun 398: 513–518.
28. Semba RD, Cappola AR, Sun K, Bandinelli S, Dalal M, et al. (2012) Relationship of low plasma klotho with poor grip strength in older community-dwelling adults: the InCHIANTI study. Eur J Appl Physiol 112: 1215–1220.
29. Semba RD, Cappola AR, Sun K, Bandinelli S, Dalal M, et al. (2011) Plasma klotho and cardiovascular disease in adults. J Am Geriatr Soc 59: 1596–1601.
30. Semba RD, Cappola AR, Sun K, Bandinelli S, Dalal M, et al. (2011) Plasma klotho and mortality risk in older community-dwelling adults. J Gerontol A Biol Sci Med Sci 66: 794–800.
31. Lim K, Lu TS, Molostvov G, Lee C, Lam FT, et al. (2012) Vascular Klotho deficiency potentiates the development of human artery calcification and mediates resistance to fibroblast growth factor 23. Circulation 125: 2243–2255.
32. Devaraj S, Syed B, Chien A, Jialal I (2012) Validation of an immunoassay for soluble Klotho protein: decreased levels in diabetes and increased levels in chronic kidney disease. Am J Clin Pathol 137: 479–485.
33. Komaba H, Koizumi M, Tanaka H, Takahashi H, Sawada K, et al. (2012) Effects of cinacalcet treatment on serum soluble Klotho levels in haemodialysis patients with secondary hyperparathyroidism. Nephrol Dial Transplant 27: 1967–1969.
34. Yokoyama K, Imura A, Ohkido I, Maruyama Y, Yamazaki Y, et al. (2012) Serum soluble alpha-klotho in hemodialysis patients. Clin Nephrol 77: 347–351.
35. Koh N, Fujimori T, Nishiguchi S, Tamori A, Shiomi S, et al. (2001) Severely Reduced Production of Klotho in Human Chronic Renal Failure Kidney. Biochem Biophys Res Commun 280: 1015–1020.
36. Sun C-Y, Chang S-C, Wu M-S (2012) Suppression of Klotho expression by protein-bound uremic toxins is associated with increased DNA methyltransferase expression and DNA hypermethylation. Kidney Int 81: 640–650.
37. Barreto FC, Barreto DV, Liabeuf S, Meert N, Glorieux G, et al. (2009) Serum indoxyl sulfate is associated with vascular disease and mortality in chronic kidney disease patients. Clin J Am Soc Nephrol 4: 1551–1558.
38. Kurosu H, Ogawa Y, Miyoshi M, Yamamoto M, Nandi A, et al. (2006) Regulation of fibroblast growth factor-23 signaling by klotho. J Biol Chem 281: 6120–6123.
39. Hu MC, Shi M, Zhang J, Pastor J, Nakatani T, et al. (2010) Klotho: a novel phosphaturic substance acting as an autocrine enzyme in the renal proximal tubule. FASEB J 24: 3438–3450.
40. Nakamura A, Shikata K, Hiramatsu M, Nakatou T, Kitamura T, et al. (2005) Serum interleukin-18 levels are associated with nephropathy and atherosclerosis in Japanese patients with type 2 diabetes. Diabetes Care 28: 2890–2895.
41. Morimoto S, Yurugi T, Aota Y, Sakuma T, Jo F, et al. (2009) Prognostic significance of ankle-brachial index, brachial-ankle pulse wave velocity, flow-mediated dilation, and nitroglycerin-mediated dilation in end-stage renal disease. Am J Nephrol 30: 55–63.
42. Hanada S, Ando R, Naito S, Kobayashi N, Wakabayashi M, et al. (2010) Assessment and significance of abdominal aortic calcification in chronic kidney disease. Nephrol Dial Transplant 25: 1888–1895.
43. Ohya M, Otani H, Kimura K, Saika Y, Fujii R, et al. (2010) Improved Assessment of Aortic Calcification in Japanese Patients Undergoing Maintenance Hemodialysis. Intern Med 49: 2071–2075.
44. Yunoki T, Nakamura A, Miyoshi T, Enko K, Kohno K, et al. (2011) Ezetimibe improves postprandial hyperlipemia and its induced endothelial dysfunction. Atherosclerosis 217: 486–491.
45. Chue CD, Edwards NC, Moody WE, Steeds RP, Townend JN, et al. (2012) Serum phosphate is associated with left ventricular mass in patients with chronic kidney disease: a cardiac magnetic resonance study. Heart 98: 219–224.
46. London GM, Guerin AP, Verbeke FH, Pannier B, Boutouyrie P, et al. (2007) Mineral metabolism and arterial functions in end-stage renal disease: potential role of 25-hydroxyvitamin D deficiency. J Am Soc Nephrol 18: 613–620.
47. Schillaci G, Pucci G, Pirro M, Monacelli M, Scarponi AM, et al. (2011) Large-artery stiffness: a reversible marker of cardiovascular risk in primary hyperparathyroidism. Atherosclerosis 218: 96–101.
48. Rosa J, Raska I Jr, Wichterle D, Petrak O, Strauch B, et al. (2011) Pulse wave velocity in primary hyperparathyroidism and effect of surgical therapy. Hypertens Res 34: 296–300.

49. Desjardins L, Liabeuf S, Renard C, Lenglet A, Lemke HD, et al. (2012) FGF23 is independently associated with vascular calcification but not bone mineral density in patients at various CKD stages. Osteoporos Int 23: 2017–2025.

50. Ford ML, Smith ER, Tomlinson LA, Chatterjee PK, Rajkumar C, et al. (2012) FGF-23 and osteoprotegerin are independently associated with myocardial damage in chronic kidney disease stages 3 and 4. Another link between chronic kidney disease-mineral bone disorder and the heart. Nephrol Dial Transplant 27: 727–733.

51. Briet M, Bozec E, Laurent S, Fassot C, London GM, et al. (2006) Arterial stiffness and enlargement in mild-to-moderate chronic kidney disease. Kidney Int 69: 350–357.

52. Townsend RR, Wimmer NJ, Chirinos JA, Parsa A, Weir M, et al. (2010) Aortic PWV in chronic kidney disease: a CRIC ancillary study. Am J Hypertens 23: 282–289.

53. Guerin AP, Blacher J, Pannier B, Marchais SJ, Safar ME, et al. (2001) Impact of aortic stiffness attenuation on survival of patients in end-stage renal failure. Circulation 103: 987–992.

54. Kramann R, Couson SK, Neuss S, Kunter U, Bovi M, et al. (2011) Exposure to uremic serum induces a procalcific phenotype in human mesenchymal stem cells. Arterioscler Thromb Vasc Biol 31: e45–54.

55. Kestenbaum B, Sampson JN, Rudser KD, Patterson DJ, Seliger SL, et al. (2005) Serum phosphate levels and mortality risk among people with chronic kidney disease. J Am Soc Nephrol 16: 520–528.

56. Di Marco GS, Konig M, Stock C, Wiesinger A, Hillebrand U, et al. (2012) High phosphate directly affects endothelial function by downregulating annexin II. Kidney Int [Epub ahead of print]

57. Six I, Maizel J, Barreto FC, Rangrez AY, Dupont S, et al. (2012) Effects of phosphate on vascular function under normal conditions and influence of the uraemic state. Cardiovasc Res 96: 130–139.

58. Nakano C, Hamano T, Fujii N, Matsui I, Tomida K, et al. (2012) Combined use of vitamin D status and FGF23 for risk stratification of renal outcome. Clin J Am Soc Nephrol 7: 810–819.

59. Martin A, David V, Quarles LD (2012) Regulation and function of the FGF23/klotho endocrine pathways. Physiol Rev 92: 131–155.

60. Wolf M (2010) Forging Forward with 10 Burning Questions on FGF23 in Kidney Disease. J Am Soc Nephrol 21: 1427–1435.

61. Seiler S, Wen M, Roth HJ, Fehrenz M, Flugge F, et al. (2012) Plasma Klotho is not related to kidney function and does not predict adverse outcome in patients with chronic kidney disease. Kidney Int [Epub ahead of print]

62. Yoon HE, Ghee JY, Piao S, Song JH, Han DH, et al. (2011) Angiotensin II blockade upregulates the expression of Klotho, the anti-ageing gene, in an experimental model of chronic cyclosporine nephropathy. Nephrol Dial Transplant 26: 800–813.

63. Lau WL, Leaf EM, Hu MC, Takeno MM, Kuro OM, et al. (2012) Vitamin D receptor agonists increase klotho and osteopontin while decreasing aortic calcification in mice with chronic kidney disease fed a high phosphate diet. Kidney Int 82: 1261–1270.

64. (2004) K/DOQI clinical practice guidelines on hypertension and antihypertensive agents in chronic kidney disease. Am J Kidney Dis 43: S1–290.

65. Imai E, Horio M, Nitta K, Yamagata K, Iseki K, et al. (2007) Estimation of glomerular filtration rate by the MDRD study equation modified for Japanese patients with chronic kidney disease. Clin Exp Nephrol 11: 41–50.

66. Matsuo S, Imai E, Horio M, Yasuda Y, Tomita K, et al. (2009) Revised equations for estimated GFR from serum creatinine in Japan. Am J Kidney Dis 53: 982–992.

67. Teragawa H, Kato M, Kurokawa J, Yamagata T, Matsuura H, et al. (2001) Usefulness of flow-mediated dilation of the brachial artery and/or the intima-media thickness of the carotid artery in predicting coronary narrowing in patients suspected of having coronary artery disease. Am J Cardiol 88: 1147–1151.

68. Uchida HA, Nakamura Y, Kaihara M, Norii H, Hanayama Y, et al. (2006) Steroid pulse therapy impaired endothelial function while increasing plasma high molecule adiponectin concentration in patients with IgA nephropathy. Nephrol Dial Transplant 21: 3475–3480.

69. Handa N, Matsumoto M, Maeda H, Hougaku H, Ogawa S, et al. (1990) Ultrasonic evaluation of early carotid atherosclerosis. Stroke 21: 1567–1572.

70. Yamashina A, Tomiyama H, Arai T, Hirose K, Koji Y, et al. (2003) Brachial-ankle pulse wave velocity as a marker of atherosclerotic vascular damage and cardiovascular risk. Hypertens Res 26: 615–622.

71. Kitagawa M, Sugiyama H, Morinaga H, Inoue T, Takiue K, et al. (2011) Serum High-Sensitivity Cardiac Troponin T Is a Significant Biomarker of Left-Ventricular Diastolic Dysfunction in Subjects with Non-Diabetic Chronic Kidney Disease. Nephron Extra 1: 166–177.

72. Morinaga H, Sugiyama H, Inoue T, Takiue K, Kikumoto Y, et al. (2012) Effluent Free Radicals are Associated with Residual Renal Function and Predict Technique Failure in Peritoneal Dialysis Patients. Perit Dial Int 32: 453–461.

8

Increased Expression of Intranuclear Matrix Metalloproteinase 9 in Atrophic Renal Tubules is Associated with Renal Fibrosis

Jen-Pi Tsai[1,2], Jia-Hung Liou[1,3,4], Wei-Tse Kao[1], Shao-Chung Wang[1,5], Jong-Da Lian[6], Horng-Rong Chang[1,6]*

1 Institute of Medicine, Chung Shan Medical University, Taichung, Taiwan, 2 Department of Nephrology, Buddhist Dalin Tzu Chi General Hospital, Chiayi, Taiwan, 3 Department of Pathology, Changhua Christian Hospital, Changhua, Taiwan, 4 Department of Medical Technology, Jen-The Junior College of Medicine, Nursing and Management, Miaoli, Taiwan, 5 Department of Urology, Chung Shan Medical University Hospital, Taichung, Taiwan, 6 Division of Nephrology, Department of Internal Medicine, Chung Shan Medical University Hospital, Taichung, Taiwan

Abstract

Background: Reduced turnover of extracellular matrix has a role in renal fibrosis. Matrix metalloproteinases (MMPs) is associated with many glomerular diseases, but the histological association of MMPs and human renal fibrosis is unclear.

Methods: This is a retrospective study. Institutional Review Board approval was obtained for the review of patients' medical records, data analysis and pathological specimens staining with waiver of informed consents. Specimens of forty-six patients were examined by immunohistochemical stain of MMP-9 in nephrectomized kidneys, and the association of renal expression of MMP-9 and renal fibrosis was determined. MMP-9 expression in individual renal components and fibrosis was graded as high or low based on MMP-9 staining and fibrotic scores.

Results: Patients with high interstitial fibrosis scores (IFS) and glomerular fibrosis scores (GFS) had significantly higher serum creatinine, lower estimated glomerular filtration rate (eGFR), and were more likely to have chronic kidney disease (CKD) and urothelial cell carcinoma. Univariate analysis showed that IFS and GFS were negatively associated with normal and atrophic tubular cytoplasmic MMP-9 expression and IFS was positively correlated with atrophic tubular nuclear MMP-9 expression. Multivariate stepwise regression indicated that MMP-9 expression in atrophic tubular nuclei ($r = 0.4$, $p = 0.002$) was an independent predictor of IFS, and that MMP-9 expression in normal tubular cytoplasm ($r = -0.465$, $p < 0.001$) was an independent predictor of GFS.

Conclusions: Interstitial fibrosis correlated with MMP-9 expression in the atrophic tubular nuclei. Our results indicate that renal fibrosis is associated with a decline of MMP-9 expression in the cytoplasm of normal tubular cells and increased expression of MMP-9 in the nuclei of tubular atrophic renal tubules.

Editor: Nikos K. Karamanos, University of Patras, Greece

Funding: The authors have no funding or support to report.

Competing Interests: The authors have declared that no competing interests exist.

* E-mail: chr@csmu.edu.tw

Introduction

Scarring of renal tissue, which occurs in glomerulosclerosis, interstitial fibrosis, and tubular atrophy, is caused by a variety of primary insults, such as diabetes mellitus (DM), hypertension (HTN), primary glomerulopathies, autoimmune diseases, toxic injury, and congenital abnormalities [1]. The pathogenesis of renal fibrosis includes deposition of interstitial matrix, tubular cell loss, infiltration of inflammatory cells, fibroblast accumulation, rarefaction of peritubular microvasculature, and predisposition to renal progression in the presence of genetic polymorphisms [2]. Extracellular matrix (ECM) components accumulate during renal fibrosis resulting from an imbalance of ECM production and defective ECM degradation by proteolytic enzymes. Matrix metalloproteinases (MMPs) play a major role in ECM degradation.

MMPs are a family of zinc-dependent endopeptidases that are currently divided into six groups with varying substrate specificities modulated by tissue inhibitors of metalloproteinases (TIMPs). MMPs work synergistically to degrade ECM components and are involved in a variety of pathophysiological processes in which tissue remodeling is needed, such as embryonic development, angiogenesis, invasive cell behavior, inflammation, wound healing, and fibrosis [3,4]. Kidney tissue produces a number of proteases, and the MMP system and plasminogen/plasmin play major roles in degrading matrix proteins [3,5]. Changes in expression or activity of MMPs alter ECM turnover, and this can lead to glomerular sclerosis and other glomerulonephropathies (GNs) [6,7,8,9].

MMP-9 (gelatinase B), a 92 kDa type IV collagenase, is regulated through formation of proenzyme complexes with endogenous TIMP-1. MMP-9 can specifically degrade type IV and V collagens and gelatine [3]. The spatial expression of MMP-9 in the kidney is complex and species-specific. MMP-9 is mainly expressed in collecting duct cells and to a lesser extent in proximal tubule and podocytes of mice [10], in the proximal and distal tubules of monkeys [11], and in glomerular mesangial cells of humans [12]. MMP-9 is initially believed to be involved in the pathogenesis of chronic kidney disease (CKD). We recently reported that the circulating level of MMP-9 was inversely correlated with serum creatinine ($r = -0.344$, $p < 0.01$) [13].

Based on these previous studies and because MMP-9 is associated with ECM accumulation and tubulointerstitial fibrosis, we examined the relationship between histological renal expression of MMP-9 and renal fibrosis, including glomerular and interstitial fibrosis. We used human renal tissues which had various degrees of fibrosis that were remnants from previously nephrectomized kidneys.

Materials and Methods

From January 2006 to August 2009, pathological specimens from 90 patients who received unilateral or bilateral nephrectomy were retrospectively recruited. Institutional review board approval of Chung Shan Medical University Hospital was obtained for the review of patients' medical records, data analysis and pathological specimens staining with waiver of informed consents.

Of this study, forty-six patients who had stable renal function for more than 3 months before surgery were ultimately included. Patient age, gender, body mass index, status of cigarette smoking,

HTN, and DM were recorded. Estimated glomerular filtration rate (eGFR) was calculated by the abbreviated Modification of Diet in Renal Disease formula (aMDRD):

$$eGFR = 186 \times (serum\,Creatinine)^{-1.154} \times (age)^{-0.203} \times (0.742\,if\,female)$$

Chronic kidney disease (CKD) was defined by K/DOQI guidelines [14].

Tissue processing

Pathologic material was processed by conventional histological procedures. Representative sections were taken in the renal parenchyma at least 2 cm away from the tumor areas in cases with nephrectomy due to tumor. Each section was at least 2×2 cm^2. The formalin-fixed, paraffin-embedded tissues were cut into 4-mm hematoxylin- and eosin-stained sections and examined to evaluate the glomerular, renal tubular, and interstitial conditions. The scoring of fibrosis was based on Banff scoring for chronic lesions [15]. The low fibrosis group was defined by a score of 0 or 1 in the interstitium and glomeruli, and the high fibrosis group was defined by a score of 2 or 3 in these tissues.

Immunohistochemical staining

Paraffin embedded kidney tissue sections (4-mm) on poly-1-lysine-coated slides were deparaffinized. After treatment with 3% H$_2$O$_2$ in methanol, the sections were hydrated with gradient alcohol and PBS, incubated in 10 mM citrate buffer, and finally

Table 1. Demographic and clinical characteristics of patients divided by low and high renal interstitial fibrosis score (left) and glomerular fibrosis score (right).

	Fibrosis score (interstitium)			Fibrosis score (glomerulus)		
	low	high	P value	low	High	P value
Patient Number	28	18		34	12	
Gender (Male, %) Age (years)	13 (46.4) 56.1±14.8	10 (55.6) 60.2±10.3	0.546 0.431	17 (50) 57.2±14.6	6 (50) 59.2±8.8	1 0.783
CKD (n, %)	10 (35.7)	13 (72.2)	0.016	13 (38.2)	10 (83.3)	0.007
eGFR (ml/min)	74.2±22.7	42.2±27.5	0.001	72.2±22.3	32.1±25.8	<0.001
Creatinine (mg/dl)	1.04±0.32	3.59±3.93	0.001	1.07±0.32	4.78±4.38	<0.001
DM (n, %)	5 (18.5)	4 (22.2)	0.761	7 (21.2)	2 (16.7)	0.736
HTN (n, %)	10 (35.7)	10 (55.6)	0.185	12 (35.3)	8 (66.7)	0.059
BMI (kg/m²)	24.5±3.8	25.3±3.2	0.266	24.9±4	24.6±2.1	0.729
Smoker (n, %)	3 (11.1)	1 (5.6)	0.521	4 (12.1)	0 (0)	0.206
Glucose (mg/dl)	111.8±27.7	142.4±67.9	0.223	114.6±33.8	151.9±75.5	0.134
Hemoglobin (g/dl)	10.6±3.57	10.1±2.8	0.398	10.7±3.5	9.6±2.3	0.087
Albumin (mg/dl)	3.79±0.92	4.01±0.39	0.897	3.88±0.87	3.9±0.36	0.345
TCH (mg/dl)	176.6±32.1	195.9±49	0.18	181.6±36.4	199.8±54.5	0.432
Triglyceride (mg/dl)	143.0±75.5	165.6±84.6	0.487	146.8±82.9	175.9±72.9	0.485
Diagnosis (n, %)						
UCC	4 (14.3)	10 (55.6)	<0.001	8 (23.5)	6 (50)	<0.001
RCC	20 (71.4)	2 (11.1)		22 (64.7)	0 (0)	
Other	4 (14.3)	6 (33.3)		4 (11.8)	6 (50)	

BMI, body mass index; CKD, chronic kidney disease; DM, diabetes mellitus; eGFR, estimated glomerular filtration; HTN, hypertension; RCC, renal cell carcinoma; UCC, urothelial cell carcinoma, TCH, total cholesterol.
$p < 0.05$ indicates significance.

Table 2. Intensity of MMP-9 expression in different regions of renal tissues divided by low and high interstitial fibrosis score (left) and glomerular fibrosis score (right).

	Fibrosis score (interstitium)			Fibrosis score (glomerulus)		
	low	high	P value	low	high	P value
MMP-9 intensity						
NTn (n, %)						
Low	26 (92.9)	18 (100)	0.246	32 (94.1)	12 (100)	0.39
High	2 (7.1)	0 (0)		2 (5.9)	0 (0)	
NTc (n, %)						
Low	1 (3.6)	7 (38.9)	0.002	1 (2.9)	7 (58.3)	<0.001
High	27 (96.4)	11 (61.1)		33 (97.1)	5 (41.7)	
Gn (n, %)						
Low	28 (100)	18 (100)		34 (100)	12 (100)	
High						
Gc (n, %)						
Low	16 (57.1)	14 (77.8)	0.152	20 (58.8)	10 (83.3)	0.125
High	12 (42.9)	4 (22.2)		14 (41.2)	2 (16.7)	
ATn (n, %)						
Low	25 (89.3)	11 (61.1)	0.024	28 (82.4)	8 (66.7)	0.257
High	3 (10.7)	7 (38.9)		6 (17.6)	4 (33.3)	
ATc (n, %)						
Low	8 (28.6)	12 (70.6)	0.006	12 (35.3)	8 (72.7)	0.03
High	20 (71.4)	5 (29.4)		22 (64.7)	3 (27.3)	

NTn, normal tubular nucleus; NTc, normal tubular cytoplasm; Gn, glomerular nuclei; Gc, glomerular cytoplasm; ATn, atrophic tubular nuclei; ATc, atrophic tubular cytoplasm.
Data were analyzed by the chi-squared test and $p<0.05$ indicates significance.

Table 3. Associations between interstitial and glomerular fibrosis with clinicopathologic variables.

	Interstitial fibrosis		Glomerular fibrosis	
Variable	Beta	P value	Beta	P value
Age (year)	0.150	0.319	0.070	0.644
Sex (male, %))	0.089	0.556	0.000	1
Chronic kidney disease (n, %)	0.356	0.015	0.396	0.006
Creatinine (mg/dl)	0.461	0.001	0.603	<0.001
Estimated GFR (ml/min)	−0.544	<0.001	−0.612	<0.001
Body mass index (kg/m²)	0.009	0.436	−0.043	0.780
Smoker (n, %)	−0.096	0.532	−0.188	0.215
Diabetes mellitus (n, %)	0.045	0.767	−0.050	0.743
Hypertension (n, %)	0.195	0.193	0.278	0.061
Pathologic diagnosis	0.489	0.001	0.571	<0.001
Glucose (mg/dl)	0.302	0.062	0.333	0.038
Hemoglobin (g/dl)	−0.09	0.611	−0.161	0.362
Albumin (mg/dl)	0.157	0.444	0.012 0.012	0.954
Total cholesterol (mg/dl)	0.230	0.269	0.202	0.332
Triglyceride (mg/dl)	0.144	0.501	0.170	0.428
MMP-9 intensity (n, %)				
Glomerular cytoplasm	−0.211	0.158	−0.226	0.131
Atrophic tubular nucleus	0.333	0.024	0.167	0.267
Atrophic tubular cytoplasm	−0.410	0.005	−0.324	0.030
Normal tubular nucleus	−0.171	0.256	−0.127	0.402
Normal tubular cytoplasm	−0.455	0.001	−0.642	<0.001

Interstitial fibrosis scores were significantly correlated with glomerular fibrosis scores ($r=0.741$, $p<0.001$).
$p<0.05$ was considered statistically significant.

heated at $100°C$ for 20 min in PBS. Slides were incubated with the anti-MMP-9 antibody (Santa Cruz, CA) for 20 min at room temperature, and then with a horseradish peroxidase (HRP)/Fab polymer conjugate for another 30 min. Then, slides were thoroughly washed three times with PBS, and the sites of peroxidase activity were visualized using 3, 3-diamino-benzidine tetrahydrochloride as a substrate and hematoxylin as the counter stain. All immunohistochemical (IHC) data were independently scored by two blinded pathologists. Every slide was examined entirely for nuclear and cytoplasmic MMP-9 stains in the normal and atrophic renal tubules and in the normal and atrophic glomeruli. Each 2×2 cm² section contained at least 30 glomerular areas, and the actual number of examined glomeruli was based on the sectioned tissue size. The number of immunoreactive cells was calculated semi-quantitatively and evaluated as a percentage (0~100%) of positive cells in the observed tubules and glomeruli (normal and atrophic) as follows: intensity 0, negative; intensity 1+, 1~10%; 2+, 10~50%; and 3+, >50% [16]. The results of nuclear and cytoplasmic staining were recorded separately. The intensity of MMP-9 staining was classified as high (2 and 3) or low (0 and 1).

Statistical analysis

Continuous and categorical data were expressed as means ± standard deviations and as proportions, respectively. Categorical variables were analyzed by the chi-square test. The statistical significance between continuous variables was analyzed by the Mann-Whitney U test. Correlations of clinical variables with interstitial and glomerular fibrosis were evaluated by univariate linear regression analysis. Variables with p-values less than 0.1 in the univariate linear regression analysis were used for stepwise multivariate linear regression analysis to analyze the independent association of interstitial and glomerular fibrosis with clinical and pathological variables. A p-value less than 0.05 was considered statistically significant. All data were analyzed using SPSS version 14.0 statistical software.

Results

The mean age of the 46 patients at surgery was 57.7 ± 13.2 years. Nine patients (19.6%) had DM, 20 patients (43.5%) had HTN, and 23 patients (50%) had CKD. Fourteen patients (30.4%) were given nephrectomies due to urothelial cell carcinoma (UCC) and 22 patients (47.8%) were given nephrectomies due to renal cell carcinoma (RCC).

We classified the 46 patients based on high or low scores for interstitial and glomerular fibrosis. In particular, we compared the association between the interstitial fibrosis score (IFS) and glomerular fibrosis score (GFS) with the intensity of MMP-9 expression in each component of the specimen if both the compared components were on the same specimen. Our results

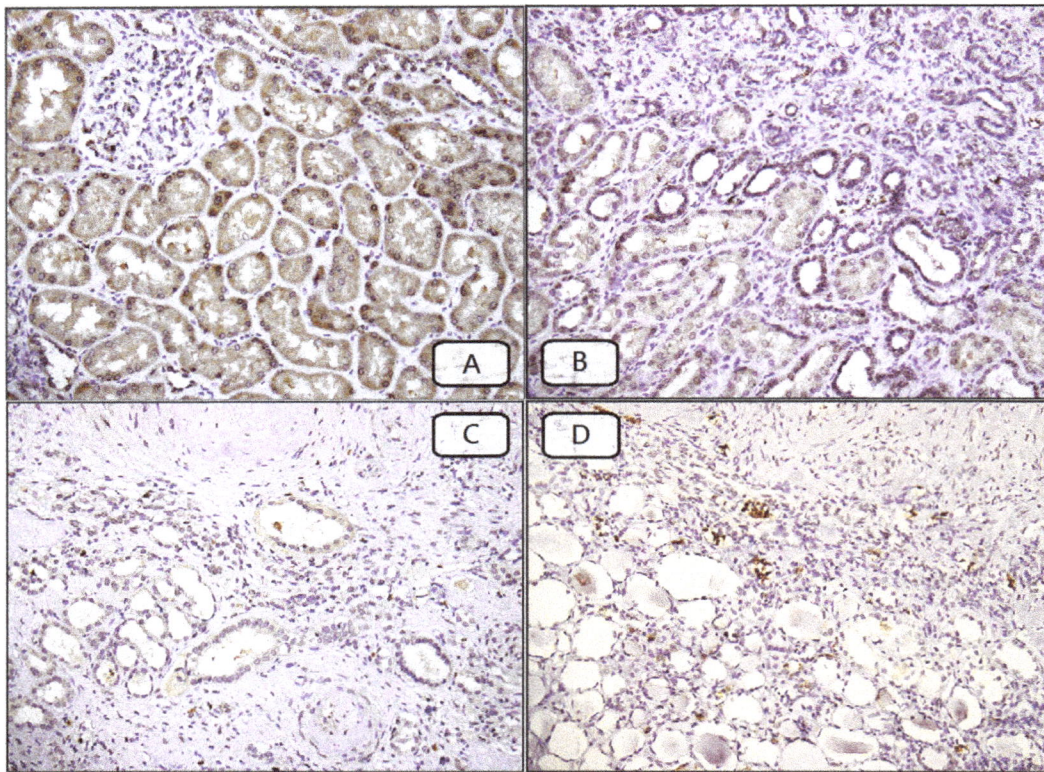

Figure 1. Representative panels showing different expression intensity of MMP-9 in atrophic tubular nuclear compared to normal tubular cytoplasm nearby fibrotic renal parenchyma. (A) no fibrosis with increased cytoplasm stain in normal tubules, (B) mild fibrosis with decreased cytoplasm stain in normal tubules and increased nuclear stain in atrophy tubules, (C) severe fibrosis with decreased cytoplasm stain in normal tubules, and (D) severe fibrosis with increased nuclear stain in atrophy tubules. (IHC stain, x 20).

indicate that IFS was inversely associated with eGFR (42.2±27.5 mL/min for high IFS, 74.2±22.7 mL/min for low IFS, $p = 0.001$), positively associated with CKD (72.2% for high IFS, 35.7% for low IFS, $p = 0.016$), and positively associated with UCC (55.6% for high IFS, 14.3% for low IFS, $p < 0.001$). Similarly, GFS was inversely associated with eGFR (32.1±25.8 mL/min for high GFS, 72.2±22.3 mL/min for low GFS, $p < 0.001$), positively associated with CKD (83.3% for high GFS, 38.2% for low GFS, $p < 0.007$), and positively associated with UCC (50% for high GFS, 23.5% for low GFS, $p < 0.001$) (Table 1).

Table 4. Multivariate analysis with stepwise linear regression of factors independently associated with interstitial and glomerular fibrosis.

Variable	Interstitial fibrosis		Glomerular fibrosis	
	Beta	P value	Beta	P value
Pathological diagnosis (n, %)	0.656	<0.001	0.511	<0.001
MMP-9 intensity (n, %)				
Atrophic tubular nucleus	0.400	0.002		
Normal tubular cytoplasm			−0.465	<0.001

Variables included p less than 0.1 in univariate linear regression analysis. $p < 0.05$ was considered statistically significant.

IFS was inversely associated with expression of MMP-9 in normal tubular cytoplasm (NTc) (61.1% for high IFS, 96.4% for low IFS, $p = 0.002$) and in atrophic tubular cytoplasm (ATc) (29.4% for high IFS, 71.4% for low IFS, $p = 0.006$), but positively associated with expression of MMP-9 in atrophic tubular nucleus (ATn) (38.9% for high IFS, 10.7% for low IFS, $p = 0.024$). GFS was inversely associated with expression of MMP-9 in normal tubular cytoplasm (NTc) (41.7% for high GFS, 97.1% for low GFS, $p < 0.001$) and in atrophic tubular cytoplasm (ATc) (27.3% for high GFS, 64.7% for low GFS, $p = 0.03$) (Table 2).

Table 3 showed the association between IFS and GFS and clinical and histological variables. Univariate analysis indicated that IFS was positively associated with serum creatinine (r = 0.461, $p = 0.001$), presence of CKD (r = 0.356, $p = 0.015$), and MMP-9 intensity in ATn (r = 0.333; $p = 0.024$), and negatively associated with eGFR (r = −0.544, $p < 0.001$), and MMP-9 expression in ATc (r = −0.410, $p = 0.005$) and NTc (r = −0.455, $p = 0.001$). GFS was positively associated with serum creatinine (r = 0.603, $p < 0.001$), presence of CKD (r = 0.396, $p = 0.006$), and blood glucose (r = 0.333, $p = 0.038$), and negatively associated with eGFR (r = −0.612, $p < 0.001$), and MMP-9 expression in ATc (r = −0.324, $p = 0.03$) and NTc (r = −0.642, $p < 0.001$). IFS and GSF were each associated with the pathological diagnosis of the nephrectomised kidney(s) (r = 0.498, $p = 0.001$; r = 0.571, $p < 0.001$, respectively). There was positive correlation between the expression of IFS and GFS (r = 0.741, $p < 0.001$).

Finally, we employed stepwise multivariate linear regression to identify the independent predictors of IFS and GFS. All variables

Table 5. Expression of MMP-9 in different renal tissues between patients with and without cancer.

	Cancer	Non-cancer	P value
MMP-9 intensity			
NTn (n, %)			1.0
Low	34 (94.4)	10 (100)	
High	2 (5.6)	0 (0)	
NTc (n, %)			0.344
Low	5 (13.9)	3 (30)	
High	31 (86.1)	7 (70)	
Gc (n, %)			0.72
Low	24 (66.7)	6 (60)	
High	12 (33.3)	4 (40)	
ATn (n, %)			0.089
Low	26 (72.2)	10 (100)	
High	10 (27.8)	0 (0)	
ATc (n, %)			0.083
Low	13 (37.1)	7 (70)	
High	22 (62.9)	3 (30)	

Abbreviation: Gc, glomerular cytoplasm; NTn, normal tubular nucleus; NTc, normal tubular cytoplasm; ATn, atrophic tubular nuclei; ATc, atrophic tubular cytoplasm.
Data were analyzed by the chi-squared test and Fisher's exact test accordingly and $p<0.05$ indicates significance.

Table 6. Associations between intensity of MMP-9 expression and cancer over different renal tissues.

	Cancer	
Variable	Beta	P value
MMP-9 intensity		
Glomerular cytoplasm	0.058	0.703
Atrophic tubular nucleus	−0.278	0.062
Atrophic tubular cytoplasm	−0.275	0.068
Normal tubular nucleus	−0.112	0.457
Normal tubular cytoplasm	−0.175	0.244

$p<0.05$ was considered statistically significant.

with p-values less than 0.1 in the univariate linear regression were included in this analysis (serum creatinine, status of HTN, fasting glucose, pathological diagnosis, and MMP-9 intensities in ATc, ATn and NTc). The results indicated that MMP-9 intensity in ATn ($r = 0.40$, $p = 0.002$) was an independent factor predicting IFS and that MMP-9 intensity in NTc ($r = -0.465$, $p<0.001$) was an independent factor predicting GFS (Table 4). Patients with different pathological diagnoses had significant correlation with IFS and GFS ($r = 0.656$, $p<0.001$; $r = 0.511$, $p<0.001$, respectively). Figure 1 showed a representative cross-section in which there was increased expression of MMP-9 in atrophic tubular nuclei (Panel B and D) and decreased in the normal tubular cytoplasm (Panel B and C) simultaneously.

In addition, we divided our patients into those without or with urinary tract cancers (included UCC and RCC) to evaluate the relationship between the intensity of MMP-9 expression and urinary tract cancers. Table 5 showed comparable percentage of MMP-9 expression over different renal tissues between groups. By univariate linear regression, there was no relationship between urinary tract cancer and intensity of MMP-9 expression over the renal tissues (Table 6).

Discussion

Our results demonstrated that the extent of interstitial fibrosis was associated with the intensity of MMP-9 expression in atrophic tubular nuclei, and that the extent of glomerular fibrosis was inversely associated with MMP-9 expression in normal tubular cytoplasm. In other words, the process of renal fibrosis involves a decline of MMP-9 expression in normal tubular cytoplasm and an increased expression of MMP-9 in the tubular nuclei of atrophic renal tubules. Although the molecular basis of increased intranuclear MMP-9 expression in renal fibrosis is still unknown, these

findings form a basis for further investigation of the role of MMP 9 in human renal injury.

Bengatta et al. reported that in a mouse model of acute kidney injury, MMP-9 expression was markedly increased in the S3 segment of the proximal tubule [17]. They postulated that MMP-9 had a protective role, because MMP-9 deficiency increased apoptosis and severity of renal lesions and substantially delayed recovery of renal function in their model. Previous studies of a rat model of tubulointerstitial fibrosis and glomerulosclerosis indicated reduced expression of MMP-9 [18,19]. Moreover, a study of diabetic nephropathy in a rat model indicated decreased MMP-9 expression and activity (mRNA and enzymatic activity of MMP-9: 21% and 51% respectively, $p<0.05$ vs. control), compatible with the increased ECM deposition associated with this disease [20]. Taken together, these data suggested that ECM turnover, which was modulated by MMPs, increases in the presence of acute kidney injury, but reduced degradation of MMPs ultimately resulted in development of renal fibrosis. Wang et al had reported that MMP-9 could modulate renal interstitial fibrosis in obstructive nephropathy by blocking tubular epithelial-to-myofibroblast, preserving tubular basement membrane and reducing ECM expression [21]. An angiotensin converting enzyme inhibitor, ramipril, had been investigated to find the contribution of MMP-9 in the process of glomerulosclerosis and chronic renal disease in hypertensive rats. MMP-9 mRNA expression was markedly suppressed to 10% of control levels independent of the treatment of ramipril, which suggested that the MMP-9 might play a role via other mechanisms other than inhibition of angiotensin converting enzyme inhibitor [19]. Similarly, our results with human tissue indicated decreased MMP-9 expression in NTc was associated with higher GFS. This indicated that the process of glomerulosclerosis involved intracellular degradation of cytosolic MMP-9.

Bauvois et al. evaluated the correlation between plasma MMP/TIMP expression and renal tissue fibrosis (glomerular sclerosis and interstitial fibrosis) in 83 patients [8]. They reported a relationship between the level of plasma MMP/TIMP and tissue fibrosis from these biopsy-proven cases of GN, but neither plasma MMPs nor TIMP-1 were significantly associated with risk of poor renal outcome (final serum creatinine <30 mL/min/1.73 m^2). The only significant risk factors were baseline creatinine clearance (odds ratio, 0.97; 95% confidence interval 0.95–0.99; $p = 0.0057$) and interstitial fibrosis (odds ratio, 1.46; 95% confidence interval 1.01–2.14; $p = 0.045$).

In addition to cleavage of the extracellular matrix by MMPs, proteolysis of nuclear matrix was implicated in numerous other cellular processes, such as apoptosis, cell cycle regulation, and DNA fragmentation [22]. Yang et al. had investigated the relationship of intracellular MMP-9 with plasma level of MMP-9 and tissue damage [22]. They designed an ischemic-reperfusion rat model, with a 90 min middle artery occlusion, and also used tissue from stroke patients to investigate the role of MMP-9 in ischemic brain neurons. Their results indicated an association of increased intranuclear MMP-9 activity in ischemic neurons at 3 h and increased DNA fragmentation at 24 h and 48 h after reperfusion. Nuclear MMPs had been reported to modulate cellular process by cleavage of the nuclear matrix protein poly-ADP-ribose-polymerase (PARP), an ATP-dependent DNA repair enzyme, and to inactivate PARP in a time-dependent manner. This was similar to the role of caspase-3, which played a protective role when PARP was over-activated and a detrimental effect by hindering repair of DNA strand breaks [23]. MMP inhibition also mediated increased activity of PARP-1 and decreased level of oxidized DNA in ischemic brain cells. In particular, Yang et al. [22] proposed that the increased intranuclear MMP-9 activity soon after stroke degraded PARP-1 and X-ray cross-complementary factor 1, contributing to a reduction of DNA base excision repair and accumulation of oxidized DNA bases in neurons, triggering neuronal death. Similarly, we noted increased MMP-9 expression in ATn was associated with greater IFS ($r = 0.40$, $p = 0.002$). Our results indicated that increased nuclear expression of MMP-9 in human atrophic renal tubular cells may play a role in the process of renal injury or fibrosis, although the molecular mechanism may differ from that proposed by Yang et al. for ischemic brain injury [22].

Although we found that the expression of MMP-9 correlated with tubulointerstitial fibrosis, there were reports showing that the MMP-9 expressions could be affected by upper urothelium carcinogenesis [24] and RCC [25]. In addition, Gialeli et al.

had reported that MMP-9 was capable to proteolytically modulate ECM which could promote tumor progression, and MMP inhibitors had been studied to control the enzyme activities to therapeutically intervene carcinogenesis [26]. Because 38 out of our 46 patients who received nephrectomies were due to urinary tract cancers (UCC and RCC). To reduce the possible impact of urinary tract cancers on the MMP-9 expression, we conducted this study by taking specimens at least 2 cm from the tumors. In addition, to test whether urinary tract cancers were associated with the intensity of MMP-9 expression in the adjacent renal tissues, we divided our patients into those without or with urinary tract cancers. The results showed that there were no significant association between the intensity of MMP-9 expression and various parts of renal tissues. Therefore, we considered that the intensity of MMP-9 expression in this study was independent of urinary tract cancers.

In summary, our analysis of the spatial expression of MMP-9 in human nephrectomized specimens indicates a novel role for MMP-9 in renal fibrosis. We postulate that increased intranuclear MMP-9 expression may reflect intranuclear gelatinase proteolysis, play a role in oxidative DNA damage by cleaving nuclear matrix proteins (PARP-1 and/or XRCC1), and contribute to cell death and fibrosis. Further experiments are needed to support this postulated mechanism.

Author Contributions

Conceived and designed the experiments: HRC JPT JHL WTK JDL SCW. Performed the experiments: JPT JHL WTK. Analyzed the data: JPT HRC. Contributed reagents/materials/analysis tools: JPT HRC SCW. Wrote the paper: JPT HRC.

References

1. Remuzzi G, Bertani T (1998) Pathophysiology of progressive nephropathies. N Engl J Med 339: 1448–1456.
2. Zeisberg M, Neilson EG (2010) Mechanisms of tubulointerstitial fibrosis. J Am Soc Nephrol 21: 1819–1834.
3. Lenz O, Elliot SJ, Stetler-Stevenson WG (2000) Matrix metalloproteinases in renal development and disease. J Am Soc Nephrol 11: 574–581.
4. Lelongt B, Legallicier B, Piedagnel R, Ronco PM (2001) Do matrix metalloproteinases MMP-2 and MMP-9 (gelatinases) play a role in renal development, physiology and glomerular diseases? Curr Opin Nephrol Hypertens 10: 7–12.
5. Liu Y (2006) Renal fibrosis: new insights into the pathogenesis and therapeutics. Kidney Int 69: 213–217.
6. Lods N, Ferrari P, Frey FJ, Kappeler A, Berthier C, et al. (2003) Angiotensin-converting enzyme inhibition but not angiotensin II receptor blockade regulates matrix metalloproteinase activity in patients with glomerulonephritis. J Am Soc Nephrol 14: 2861–2872.
7. Kunugi S, Shimizu A, Kuwahara N, Du X, Takahashi M, et al. (2011) Inhibition of matrix metalloproteinases reduces ischemia-reperfusion acute kidney injury. Lab Invest 91: 170–180.
8. Bauvois B, Mothu N, Nguyen J, Nguyen-Khoa T, Noel LH, et al. (2007) Specific changes in plasma concentrations of matrix metalloproteinase-2 and -9, TIMP-1 and TGF-beta1 in patients with distinct types of primary glomerulonephritis. Nephrol Dial Transplant 22: 1115–1122.
9. Urushihara M, Kagami S, Kuhara T, Tamaki T, Kuroda Y (2002) Glomerular distribution and gelatinolytic activity of matrix metalloproteinases in human glomerulonephritis. Nephrol Dial Transplant 17: 1189–1196.
10. Legallicier B, Trugnan G, Murphy G, Lelongt B, Ronco P (2001) Expression of the type IV collagenase system during mouse kidney development and tubule segmentation. J Am Soc Nephrol 12: 2358–2369.
11. Ogbureke KU, Fisher LW (2005) Renal expression of SIBLING proteins and their partner matrix metalloproteinases (MMPs). Kidney Int 68: 155–166.
12. Catania JM, Chen G, Parrish AR (2007) Role of matrix metalloproteinases in renal pathophysiologies. Am J Physiol Renal Physiol 292: F905–911.
13. Chang HR, Yang SF, Li ML, Lin CC, Hsieh YS, et al. (2006) Relationships between circulating matrix metalloproteinase-2 and renal function in patients with chronic kidney disease. Clin Chim Acta 366: 243–248.
14. (2002) K/DOQI clinical practice guidelines for chronic kidney disease: evaluation, classification, and stratification. Am J Kidney Dis 39: S1–266.
15. Solez K, Colvin RB, Racusen LC, Sis B, Halloran PF, et al. (2007) Banff '05 Meeting Report: differential diagnosis of chronic allograft injury and elimination of chronic allograft nephropathy ('CAN'). Am J Transplant 7: 518–526.
16. Tsai YY, Cheng YW, Lee H, Tsai FJ, Tseng SH, et al. (2005) Oxidative DNA damage in pterygium. Mol Vis 11: 71–75.
17. Bengatta S, Arnould C, Letavernier E, Monge M, de Preneuf HM, et al. (2009) MMP9 and SCF protect from apoptosis in acute kidney injury. J Am Soc Nephrol 20: 787–797.
18. Maric C, Sandberg K, Hinojosa-Laborde C (2004) Glomerulosclerosis and tubulointerstitial fibrosis are attenuated with 17beta-estradiol in the aging Dahl salt sensitive rat. J Am Soc Nephrol 15: 1546–1556.
19. Bolbrinker J, Markovic S, Wehland M, Melenhorst WB, van Goor H, et al. (2006) Expression and response to angiotensin-converting enzyme inhibition of matrix metalloproteinases 2 and 9 in renal glomerular damage in young transgenic rats with renin-dependent hypertension. J Pharmacol Exp Ther 316: 8–16.
20. McLennan SV, Kelly DJ, Cox AJ, Cao Z, Lyons JG, et al. (2002) Decreased matrix degradation in diabetic nephropathy: effects of ACE inhibition on the expression and activities of matrix metalloproteinases. Diabetologia 45: 268–275.
21. Wang X, Zhou Y, Tan R, Xiong M, He W, et al (2010) Mice lacking the matrix metalloproteinase-9 gene reduce renal interstitial fibrosis in obstructive nephropathy. Am J Physiol Physiol 299: F973–F982.
22. Yang Y, Candelario-Jalil E, Thompson JF, Cuadrado E, Estrada EY, et al. (2010) Increased intranuclear matrix metalloproteinase activity in neurons interferes with oxidative DNA repair in focal cerebral ischemia. J Neurochem 112: 134–149.
23. Mannello F, Luchetti F, Falcieri E, Papa S (2005) Multiple roles of matrix metalloproteinases during apoptosis. Apoptosis 10: 19–24.
24. Reis LO, Favaro WJ, Ferreira U, Billis A, Fazuoli GM, et al. (2010) Evolution on experimental animal model for upper urothelium carcinogenesis. World J Urol 28; 499–505.
25. Kawata N, Nagane Y, Hirakata H, Ichinose T, Okada Y et al. (2007) Significant relationship of matrix metalloproteinase 9 with nuclear grade and prognostic impact of tissue inhibitor of metalloproteinase 2 for incidental clear cell renal cell carcinoma. Urology 69; 1049–1053.
26. Gialeli C, Theocharis A, Karamanos N (2011) Role of matrix metalloproteinases in cancer progression and their pharmacological targeting. FEBS J 218; 16–27.

9

Multicenter Study of Creatinine- and/or Cystatin C-Based Equations for Estimation of Glomerular Filtration Rates in Chinese Patients with Chronic Kidney Disease

Jia-fu Feng[1]*[9], Ling Qiu[3][9], Lin Zhang[2], Xue-mei Li[4], Yu-wei Yang[1], Ping Zeng[1], Xiu-zhi Guo[3], Yan Qin[3], Hong-chun Liu[5], Xing-min Han[6], Yan-peng Li[6], Wei Xu[7], Shu-yan Sun[7], Li-qiang Wang[7], Hui Quan[8], Li-jun Xia[8], Hong-zhang Hu[8], Fang-cai Zhong[9], Rong Duan[10]

1 Laboratory Medicine, Mianyang Central Hospital, Mianyang, Sichuan Province, China, 2 Kidney Internal Medical Department, Mianyang Central Hospital, Mianyang, Sichuan Province, China, 3 Laboratory Medicine, Peking Union Medical College Hospital, Bejing, China, 4 Kidney Internal Medical Department, Peking Union Medical College Hospital, Bejing, China, 5 Laboratory Medicine, The First Affiliated Hospital of Zhengzhou University, Zhengzhou, Henan Province, China, 6 Department of Nuclear Medicine, The First Affiliated Hospital of Zhengzhou University, Zhengzhou, Henan Province, China, 7 Laboratory Medicine, The First Bethune Hospital of Jilin University, Jilin, Jilin Province, China, 8 Laboratory Department, Nuclear Industrial 416 Hospital, Chengdu, Sichuan Province, China, 9 Laboratory Department, The First People's Hospital of Neijiang, Neijiang, Sichuan Province, China, 10 Kidney Internal Medical Department, The First People's Hospital of Neijiang, Neijiang, Sichuan Province, China

Abstract

Objective: To establish equations for the estimation of glomerular filtration rates (eGFRs) based on serum creatinine (SCr) and/or serum cystatin C (SCysC) in Chinese patients with chronic kidney disease (CKD), and to compare the new equations with both the reference GFR (rGFR) and the literature equations to evaluate their applicability.

Methods: The 788 Chinese CKD patients were randomly divided into two groups, the training group and the testing group, to establish new eGFR-formulas based on serum CysC and to validate the established formulas, respectively. ^{99m}Tc-DTPA clearance (as the rGFR), serum Cr, and serum CysC were determined for all patients, and GFR was calculated using the Cockcroft-Gault equation (eGFR1), the MDRD formula (eGFR2), the CKD-EPI formulas (eGFR3, eGFR4), and the Chinese eGFR Investigation Collaboration formulas (eGFR5, eGFR6). The accuracy of each eGFR was compared with the rGFR.

Results: The training and testing groups' mean GFRs were 50.84±31.36 mL/min/1.73 m^2 and 54.16±29.45 mL/min/1.73 m^2, respectively. The two newly developed eGFR formulas were fitted using iterative computation: $eGFR7 = 173.9 \times CysC^{-0.725} \times Cr^{-0.184} \times age^{-0.193} \times 0.89(iffemale)(R^2 = 0.734)$ and $eGFR8 = 78.64 \times CysC^{-0.964}(R^2 = 0.764)$. Significant correlation was observed between each eGFR and the rGFR. However, proportional errors and constant errors were observed between rGFR and eGFR1, eGFR2, eGFR4, eGFR5 or eGFR6, and constant errors were observed between eGFR3 and rGFR, as revealed by the Passing & Bablok plot analysis. The Bland-Altman analysis illustrated that the 95% limits of agreement of all equations exceeded the previously accepted limits of <60 mL/min •1.73 m^2, except the equations of eGFR7 and eGFR8.

Conclusion: The newly developed formulas, eGFR7 and eGFR8, provide precise and accurate GFR estimation using serum CysC detection alone or in combination with serum Cr detection. Differences in detection methods should be carefully considered when choosing literature eGFR equations to avoid misdiagnosis and mistreatment.

Editor: Pal Bela Szecsi, Gentofte University Hospital, Denmark

Funding: This work was partially supported by the Science & Technology Department of Sichuan Province, China (2009SZ0066) (http://www.scst.gov.cn/info) and Sichuan Maker Biotechnology Co., Ltd. (http://makerbio.company.lookchem.cn/). The funders had no role in study design, data collection and analysis, decision to publish, or preparation of the manuscript.

Competing Interests: The study was supported by Sichuan Maker Biotechnology Co., Ltd., which provided a part of the funds, reagents and quality control materials. This does not alter the authors' adherence to all the PLOS ONE policies on sharing data and materials.

* E-mail: jiafufeng@yahoo.com.cn

[9] These authors contributed equally to this work.

Introduction

Chronic kidney disease (CKD) is a serious public health problem worldwide and is usually defined as kidney damage or decreased kidney function with glomerular filtration rates (GFRs) of less than 60 mL/min per 1.73 m^2 for 3 months or longer, regardless of cause [1–3]. Based on GFR, CKD is classified into different stages that require stage-specific management. Therefore, accurate measurement of GFR is critical to evaluate the patient's renal function. Currently, the "gold standard" for GFR determination is to measure the clearance of exogenous substances, such as inulin, iohexol, ^{51}Cr-EDTA, ^{99m}Tc-DTPA and ^{125}I-iothalamate [4]. However, these measurements are not only time-consuming, labor-intensive and expensive but also require the administration of rare substances; thus, these methods are not routinely used [5]. Therefore, serum or plasma creatinine levels have become the most commonly used markers for GFR determination because of the simplicity and lower costs of this method [6,7]. GFR can be calculated based on plasma or serum creatinine using the Cockcroft-Gault or the Modification of Diet in Renal Disease (MDRD) study equations [7,8]. However, using plasma or serum creatinine has significant disadvantages, such as the inability to measure renal function correctly when impairment is 50% or less [7]. Creatinine generation is proportional to muscle mass and related to an individual's age, sex, race and weight [4,7]. As a result, an increase in serum creatinine may not be observed until a substantial decrease in GFR has occurred.

Cystatin C (CysC) is a cysteine protease inhibitor with a molecular mass of 13 kDa [9]. It has been shown that cystatin C is a more sensitive marker of GFR changes than serum creatinine [10] because its levels are not affected by muscle mass, age, inflammation, fever or exogenous agents [11]. CysC is produced at a constant rate and cleared solely by glomerular filtration [11], and it can be measured easily with particle-enhanced nephelometric immunoassay (PENIA) [12] or particle-enhanced turbidimetric immunoassay (PETIA) [13]. Large amount of studies have shown that CysC is superior to SCr in predicting the function of kidney [14–18]. Therefore, CysC has been used as an alternative endogenous serum marker of GFR [19], and many formulas for GFR estimation have been developed based upon serum CysC determination [20,21]. However, these formulas were all established based on a small sample and outside of a laboratory, and the "gold standard" measurement of GFR and CysC is also very inconsistent. In addition, these equations have been established in Western populations and they may or may not be suitable for the Chinese population, which requires clinical validation.

The PETIA-CysC method is becoming more common in clinical practice because of its lower cost and more rapid detection than the PENIA-CysC method [22–25]. For creatinine measurement, the enzymatic method (enzymatic-Cr) is widely used in the clinical laboratory because of its low chance of cross-contamination and stable results [26–28]. In the present study, we applied enzymatic-Cr and PETIA-CysC to determine the creatinine levels and CysC levels, respectively. Following the measurements, we established the eGFR equations based on the levels of CysC and/or serum Cr(SCr) in Chinese CKD patients with multi-center cooperation and evaluated the applicability of these GFR estimating equations.

Materials and Methods

Subjects

A total of 788 CKD patients who were referred by nephrologists, diabetologists, cardiologists or general internists were selected from 6 general hospitals between October 2010 and December 2011 in different areas of China, including 421 males (aged 50.4±15.7 years) and 367 females (age,d 51.6±16.6 years). These were 355 patients from North China(Jilin and Beijing, China), 82 patients from Central China(Henan,China), and 351 patients from South China(Mianyang, Chendu and Neijiang, Sichuan, China).All patients met the diagnostic criteria of NKF-KDOQI CKD [1], and the following patients were excluded during the selection: (1) patients with acute kidney disease or acute renal insufficiency; (2) dialysis patients; (3) patients with merger edema, pleural effusion, ascites, thyroid disease, or viral hepatitis (carriers were exceptional); (4) malnourished patients (lower than normal protein, blood urea or urine conductivity); (5) disabled

patients; and (6) patients using antibacterial drugs, especially trimethoprim and cimetidine.

A total of 687 cases were chosen randomly for equation development (training group), which included 358 males (aged 50.2±15.6 years) and 329 females (aged 51.5±16.7 years). The remaining 101 cases were assigned to the equation validation (testing group), including 63 males (aged 51.7±16.1 years) and 38 females (aged 52.0±16.1 years).

The study was approved by the Medical Ethics Committee of Mianyang Central Hospital, Peking Union Medical College Hospital, The First Affiliated Hospital of Zhengzhou University, The First Bethune Hospital of Jilin University, Nuclear Industrial 416 Hospital, or The First people's Hospital of Neijiang, and written informed consent was obtained from all subjects.

Sample collection

Blood samples were collected at 8:00 AM. Approximately 5 ml of blood was collected into a BD Vacutainer® SST^{TM} II ADVANCE tube (Becton Dickinson, USA) for analysis of CysC and SCr concentrations. After one hour, blood samples were centrifuged at 3000 rpm for 15 min, and serum samples were collected and stored at −80°C until analysis within 480 hours.

Detection methods

Because of the distribution of subjects in different regions, reference GFR (rGFR) values can only be determined independently in each study institute. In order to make the inter-institutes variance as small as possible, a identical research program among study institutes was established, which including researcher training, ^{99m}Tc-DTPA drug selection (radiochemical purity greater than 95%, percentage of ^{99m}Tc-DTPA bound to plasma protein less than 5%), patients' preparation, intravenous injection, blood sampling time point and procedure, regular maintenance of instrument, and radioactivity measurement.

Reference GFR (rGFR) for each subject was measured when blood samples were collected. In all patients included in the six participating study institutes, ^{99m}Tc-DTPA clearance was measured as a rGFR. rGFR was measured by the dual plasma sampling method [29], standardized by body surface area (BSA), and resulted in the rGFR: rGFR (mL/min per 1.73 m^2) = [Dln (P1/P2)/(T2-T1)] exp {[(T1lnP2)−(T2lnP1)]/(T2−T1)}×0.93 ×1.73/BSA, where D is dosage of drug injected. P1 and P2 is plasma activity at T1(first blood sampling) and T2(second blood sampling,), respectively. Units for D, P1 and P2 were cpm/ml, for T1, T2 was minute.Unlike rGFR, SCr and CysC levels were measured in a single laboratory, using a 7600–020 Automatic Analyzer (Hitachi, Japan), CysC concentrations was measured by PETIA-CysC method and SCr concentrations were measured by an enzymatic method according to the determination of glycine after enzymatic conversion of creatinine to glycine that can be traced back to IDMS, which kits produced by Sichuan Maker Biotechnology Co., Ltd.(Sichuan, China), but CysC reagents are original equipment manufacture(OEM) products that were obtained from Gentian (Moss, Norway), its calibration can be traced back to ERM-DA471/IFCC. Serum CysC measurements were performed using the following instrument settings: Primary wavelength: 546 nm; Secondary wavelength: 700 nm. Temperature: 37°C; Read points: 19–34; sample blank position 16 and spline calibration method. 157 μL assay buffer (reagent 1), and 3.5 μL sample were mixed with 52 μL anti-cystatin C immunoparticles (reagent 2),. The sensitivity of the assay for CysC was 0.03 mg/L. The intra-assay CV was 2.25% (mean, 0.92 mg/L; n = 20), and the day-to-day CV was 3.18% (mean, 0.68 mg/L; n = 30). SCr measurements were performed using the following instrument settings: Primary wavelength: 546 nm; Secondary wavelength: 700 nm. Temperature: 37°C; Read points: 17–34; sample blank position 16 and linear calibration method. 155 μL enzyme working solution (reagent 1), and 2.0 μL sample were mixed with 26 μL chromogen solution (reagent 2),. The sensitivity of the assay for SCr was 2.40 μmol/L. The intra-assay CV was 1.12% (mean, 135.6 μmol/L; n = 20), and the day-to-day CV was 1.33% (mean, 382.5 μmol/L; n = 30).

eGFR calculation formula
Cockcroft-Gault formula [30]:

$$eGFR1 = [(140 - age) \times \text{body weight}]/(72 \times Cr)$$
$$\times 0.85(\text{if female}) \times 1.73/BSA$$

$$(BSA = 0.007184 \times \text{body weight}^{0.425} \times \text{height}^{0.725})$$

Simplified MDRD formula [31]:

$$eGFR2 = c\text{-}aGFR = 175 \times Cr^{-1.234} \times age^{-0.179} \times 0.79(\text{if female})$$

MDRD/CKD-EPI formula [32]:

$$eGFR3 = 76.7 \times CysC^{-1.19}$$

$$eGFR4 = 177.6 \times Cr^{-0.65} \times CysC^{-0.57} \times age^{-0.20}$$
$$\times 0.82(\text{if female}) \times 1.11(\text{if African})$$

eGFR formula of Chinese collaborative group [33]:

$$eGFR5 = 86 \times CysC^{-1.132}$$

$$eGFR6 =$$
$$169 \times Cr^{-0.608} \times CysC^{-0.63} \times age^{-0.157} \times 0.83(\text{if female})$$

Unified measurement units were used in the above 6 formulas and the following eGFR7 and eGFR8 formulas to facilitate comparative analyses: Cr: mg/dl; CysC: mg/L; BSA: m^2; age: years; body weight: kg; height: cm.

Statistical analyses

The measurement data are presented as the means±SD, median and range. The differences between genders were estimated by the student t-test for the normal distribution data or the Kolmogorov-Smirnov test for non-normally distribution data.The GFR estimation equations were established based on the Spearman correlation analysis and non-linear regression of parameters including rGFR, CysC, Cr and age. The differences between GFR estimates and rGFR were tested by ANOVA. The consistency was tested by correlation analysis and Bland-Altman analysis, and the previously accepted tolerances was defined as 60 mL/min •1.73 m^2 [34]. The differences between rGFR and eGFR were analyzed by Passing-Bablok regression analysis. The

difference distributions between eGFR and rGFR were performed by Mountain plot. The deviations are shown as the area between the Bland-Altman regression line of difference and the zero difference line. The precision is represented by the coefficient of repeatability (CR). The accuracies are shown as P$_{15}$, P$_{30}$, or P$_{50}$, which represented the proportion of eGFR within 15%, 30%, and 50% of rGFR ($\pm15\%$, $\pm30\%$, or $\pm50\%$). Kappa statistics were used to evaluate the agreement between stages classification from rGFR method and other eGFR methods. The K value can be interpreted as follows: poor agreement (<0.20), fair agreement (0.21–0.40), moderate agreement (0.41–0.60), good agreement (0.61–0.80) and very good agreement (0.81–1.0).The PASW Statistics 18.0 (SPSS Inc., Somers, NY, USA) and MedCalc11.5 (MedCalc Software, Mariakerke, Belguim) software products were used for these statistical analyses. Differences with $P<0.05$ are considered statistically significant.

Results

eGFR curve fitting based on the concentrations of serum CysC and serum Cr

The basic characteristics of the 788 patients are listed in Table 1. The datasets from the equation development group were tested by Spearman correlation analysis, which revealed negative correlations of rGFR with age, CysC and Cr (r = −0.212, −0.855 and −0.809, all $P = 0.000$). Further non-linear regression fitting was performed for rGFR with age, CysC and Cr, and iterative calculations were used to establish the equation:

$$eGFR7 = 173.9 \times CysC^{-0.725} \times Cr^{-0.184}$$
$$\times age^{-0.193} \times 0.89(\text{if female})(R^2 = 0.734)$$

In addition, the non-linear regression equation of rGFR was established using the CysC single index:

$$eGFR8 = 78.64 \times CysC^{-0.964}(R^2 = 0.764)$$

Analysis of the differences between the rGFR and eGFR values estimated by the equations

The aforementioned 8 equations were used to calculate the eGFRs of the 101 cases in the testing group, which were compared to the rGFR using ANOVA (Table 2). The calculated eGFR values were highly correlated ($P = 0.000$) with, but not significantly different (F = 0.812, $P = 0.592$) from, the rGFR values. Further Passing & Bablok analysis revealed that each eGFR value had no apparent linear deviation from the rGFR values (all $P>0.05$). However, among the eGFR values, eGFR1, eGFR2, eGFR4 and eGFR5 all showed significant proportional differences (the 95% CI of slopes did not include B = 1) and significant constant differences (the 95% CI of intercepts did not include A = 0) with eGFR6 (Fig 1-A, B, D-F); eGFR2 showed the most significant errors of both types (a = −21.267, b = 1.487), and eGFR3 also showed a highly significant constant error (Fig 1-C). Only two new equations of the eight did not show significant differences in the proportional errors and the constant errors.

Table 1. Demographic characteristics of the 788 Chinese CKD patients (up line: mean±SD, down line: median, range).

	Total	Male	Female	t/z	P
Training group (n = 687)					
n	687	358	329	-	-
Age (year)	50.8±16.1 51.0, 19.0–87.0	50.2±15.6 50.0, 19.0–87.0	51.5±16.7 52.0, 19.0–87.0	−1.056	0.293
Height (cm)	164.4±7.7 165.0, 148.0–184.0	168.8±6.6 170.0, 150.5–184.0	159.7±5.7 160.5, 148.0–175.0	19.514	0.000
Weight (kg)	63.5±11.7 63.0, 32.5–110.0	68.5±11.5 68.0, 46.0–110.5	59.2±9.4 57.0, 32.5–99.0	12.912	0.000
BSA (m²)	1.69±0.17 1.70, 1.18–2.28	1.78±0.16 1.79, 1.41–2.28	1.60±0.13 1.59, 1.18–2.05	16.470	0.000
rGFR(mL/min·1.73 m²)	50.84±31.36 44.19, 3.51,166.00	50.38±30.26 45.23, 3.51;147.91	51.33±32.56 43.50, 3.95;166.00	0.597	0.868
CysC (mg/L)	2.31±1.44 1.88, 0.59–8.62	2.39±1.50 1.95, 0.59–8.62	2.22±1.37 1.80, 0.60–7.44	−1.056	0.215
Cr(mg/dl)	2.78±2.78 1.73, 0.40–19.77	2.94±2.79 1.84, 0.46–19.77	2.60±2.78 1.69, 0.40–15.06	−1.585	0.113
Testing group (n = 101)					
n	101	63	38	–	–
Age (year)	51.8±16.0 51.0, 22.0–86.0	51.7±16.1 49.0, 22.0,86.0	52.0±16.1 56.5, 25.0,84.0	−0.101	0.920
Height (cm)	165.9±8.7 165.5, 150.0–182.0	170.0±7.5 170.0, 153.5–182.0	159.1±5.6 159.5, 150.0–174.0	8.331	0.000
Weight (kg)	65.6±14.0 63.0, 41.5–108.0	70.9±14.0 72.5, 47.0–108.0	56.8±8.9 55.0, 41.5–86.5	6.184	0.000
BSA (m²)	1.72±0.21 1.72, 1.34–2.27	1.81±0.19 1.82, 1.47–2.27	1.58±0.12 1.56, 1.34–1.88	7.517	0.000
rGFR(mL/min·1.73 m²)	54.16±29.45 47.85, 10.49–148.12	55.02±30.93 48.51, 10.49–148.12	52.73±27.16 44.52, 15.34–139.43	−0.284	0.776
CysC (mg/L)	2.13±1.41 1.79, 0.66–7.22	2.30±1.55 1.85, 0.66–7.22	1.85±1.09 1.74, 0.76–6.39	−0.964	0.335
Cr (mg/dl)	2.39±2.86 1.56, 0.48–23.34	2.46±2.25 1.63, 0.52–20.46	2.28±3.69 1.30, 0.48–23.34	−1.157	0.247

Note: training group vs. testing group; all measured indicators had P>0.05 (t represents t values of the student t-test. *z represents z values of Kolmogorov-Smirnov test.)

Consistency analysis of the estimated eGFR values and the rGFR values

As shown in Table 3, when the eGFR values were compared with the rGFR values, the most significant deviation was observed for eGFR2 (Figure 2-B, 3036 arbitrary units), followed by eGFR1 (Fig. 2-A, 2045 arbitrary units) and eGFR6 (Figure 2-C, 1435 arbitrary units). The deviations of the other 5 eGFR equations were similar to each other, and eGFR7 showed the smallest deviation (Figure 2D, 367 arbitrary units).

The performed accuracy showed significant differences in P_{30} and P_{50} among various eGFR equations ($\chi^2 = 28.341$ and 31.399, respectively; $P = 0.000$ for both). The highest performed accuracies in P_{30} and P_{50}, 74.26% and 95.05%, respectively, were observed for eGFR7, followed by eGFR8, with 72.28% and 93.07%, respectively. eGFR2 showed the lowest performed accuracies at 43.56% and 73.27%, respectively, followed by eGFR1 at 55.45% and 77.23%, respectively.

Overall, eGFR7 showed the highest performed accuracy for rGFR estimation (Figure 2-B, CR = 28.5 mL/min • 1.73 m²).

As shown in Table 2, the Bland-Altman analysis revealed that the percentage of each eGFR value falling outside the consistency limit was between 3.96 and 6.93%, which were not significantly different ($\chi^2 = 1.483$, $P = 0.983$). However, the eGFR3, eGFR4

Table 2. Overall limits of agreement between eGFR and rGFR (n = 101).

	mean±SD	correlation analysis		Bland-Altman analysis			
		r	P	Mean differences	95% AL	acceptable limits*	Out of limits n (%)
rGFR	54.16±29.45	-	-	-	-	-	-
eGFR1	56.60±29.70	0.7734	0.0000	−2.4	−51.8–46.9	98.7	6(5.94)
eGFR2	58.21±44.50	0.7774	0.0000	−4.1	−59.8–51.7	111.5	4(3.96)
eGFR3	48.44±±30.04	0.8600	0.0000	5.7	−25.2–36.6	61.8	5(4.95)
eGFR4	51.00±35.10	0.8510	0.0000	3.2	−33.0–39.3	72.3	6(5.94)
eGFR5	55.06±32.68	0.8600	0.0000	−0.9	−33.7–31.9	65.6	5(4.95)
eGFR6	56.96±39.07	0.8556	0.0000	−2.8	−43.2–37.6	80.8	5(4.95)
eGFR7	54.47±28.06	0.8729	0.0000	−0.3	−28.8–28.2	57.0	7(6.93)
eGFR8	52.59±27.07	0.8591	0.0000	1.6	−28.2–31.3	59.5	7(6.93)

Note: Units are mL/min·1.73 m²; 95% AL, 95% agreement limits. *Acceptable tolerance for the difference between rGFR and eGFR was defined as 60 mL/min/1.73 m². r is the Person's correlation coefficient between eGFR and rGFR.

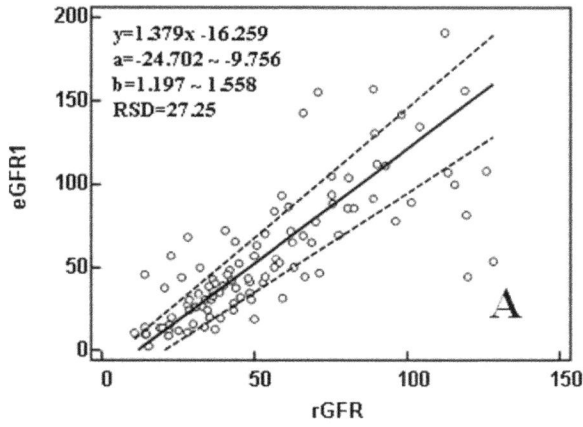

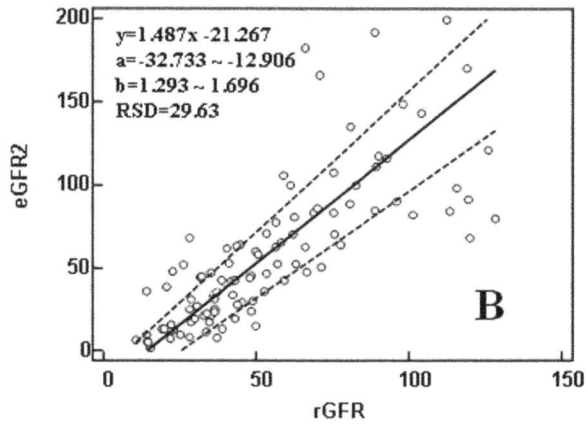

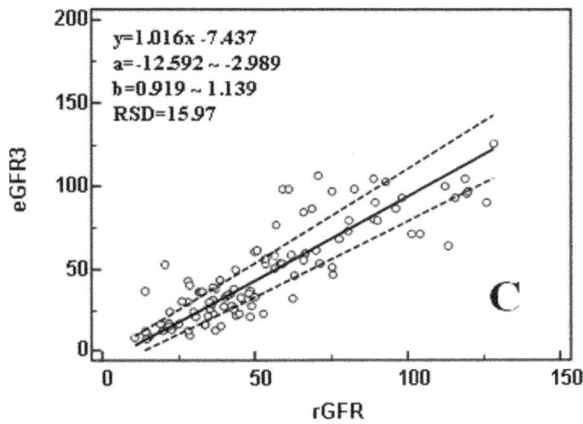

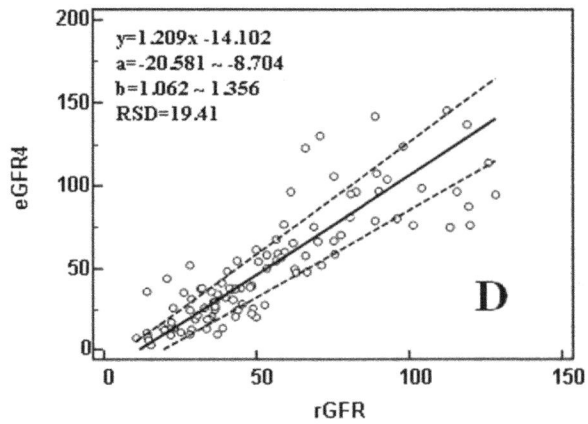

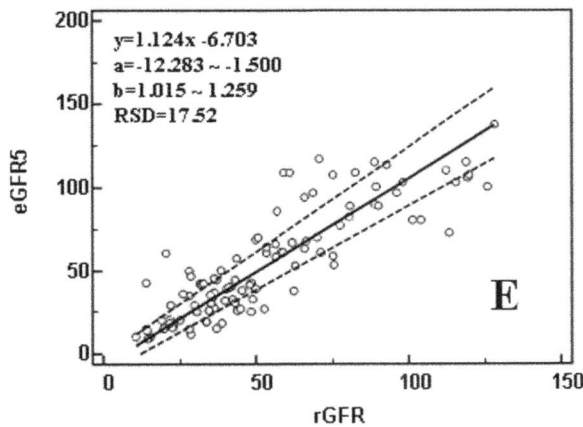

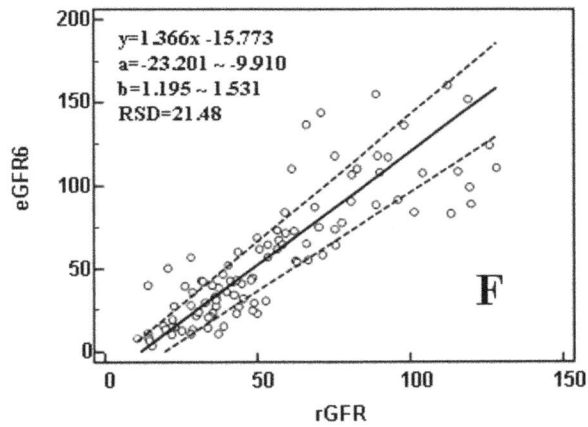

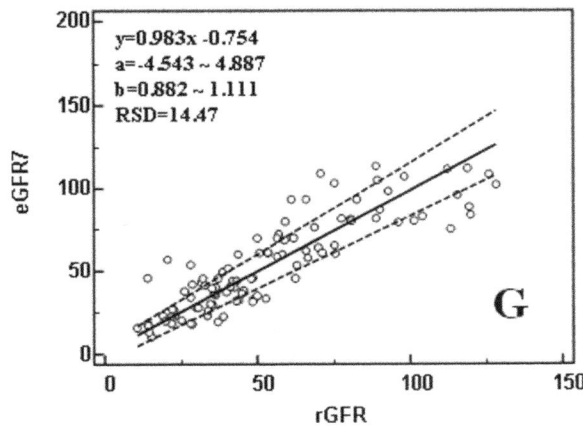

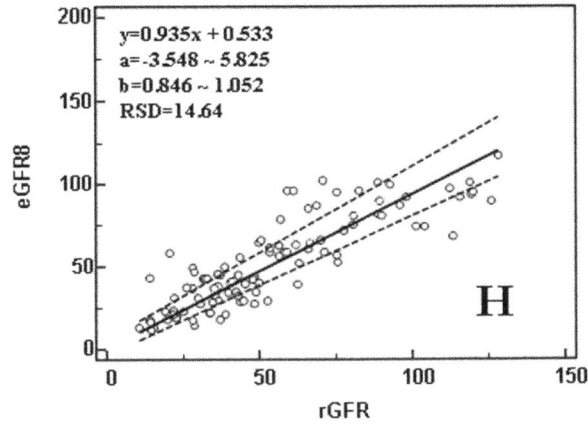

Figure 1. Passing-Bablok plot to analyze and compare eGFR with rGFR. (a: 95% confidence interval for the intercept; b: 95% confidence interval for the slope; RSD: residual standard deviation; Cusum test, all $P>0.05$)

and eGFR8 values were slightly lower than the rGFR values (positive deviation), while others were higher. The consistency limits of six equations were all higher than the previously accepted tolerances (<60 mL/min $\bullet$ 1.73 m^2), while those of eGFR7 and eGFR8 were within the previously accepted tolerances.

Using the Mountain chart, the newly developed formulas, eGFR7 and eGFR8, and 6 previously reported formulas in the literature were used to estimate the differences in the consistency between the estimated GFR values and the rGFR values (Figure 3). The median deviation of the distribution curve (M, i.e., P_{50}) was used to show their central tendency, with the range of P_5-P_{95} (R_{P5-P95}) representing the degree of dispersion (Table 4).

Compared with eGFR7 ($M=0.01$, $R_{P5-P95}=48.94$ mL/min $\bullet$ 1.73 m^2), eGFR1-6 all showed a larger M of deviation with rGFR (the M were 2.85, 3.77, 6.90, 6.63, 0.88 and 2.51 mL/min $\bullet$ 1.73 m^2, respectively) and wider curve distribution (the R_{P5-P95} were 68.43, 81.01, 52.09, 60.39, 54.04 and 69.09 mL/min $\bullet$ 1.73 m^2, respectively), indicating that their GFR estimation was worse than eGFR7 (Figure 3-A, B, and C-F). Among eGFR1-6, eGFR3 and eGFR4 showed an apparent rightward shift in their error distribution curves (P_5, M and P_{95} were all larger than eGFR7) (Figure 3-C and D), indicating overall underestimation of GFR by these two.

Similar results to those reported with eGFR7 were obtained with eGFR8 and all 6 previously reported equations (therefore, not shown, charted repeatedly). As shown in Figure 3-G, the deviation curves of eGFR7 and eGFR8 almost overlapped, indicating basically the same consistency in estimating the GFR.

Table 5 shows how many patients(percentage) were correctly classified for the different stages of CKD, according to GFR estimating equations based upon SCr and/or CysC. Overall a correct classification was achieved in 43.6% to 65.3% of the patients with the traditional eGFR equations and 73.3% to 74.3% with the new eGFR equations. The best percentage (74.3%) was achieved with the eGFR8, however, the eGFR7 gave a very close result 73.3%.

Discussion

GFR is traditionally considered to be the best overall index of the kidney function. Therefore, its accurate detection is critical for early diagnosis, proper staging, effective treatment and monitoring of CKD. The International Association of Nuclear Medicine has recommended the two-serum method to measure the clearance rate of ^{99m}Tc-DTPA as the reference method for GFR detection [35]. However, this method is difficult for clinical applications because of its complexity, high costs, high equipment requirement and radioactivity.

The PETIA-CysC is comparable with PENIA-CysC in accuracy, but PETIA-CysC can be detected using various types of automatic biochemical analyzers, so its detection speed is faster than PENIA-CysC and it can be easily and broadly applied in clinical laboratories. Therefore, many clinical laboratories have detected CysC using the PETIA-CysC method [36–40]. In addition, enzymatic detection of serum Cr shows less interference and low cross-contamination between samples [26–28]; therefore, it is also widely used by clinical laboratories.

In this study, we used the two-serum method ^{99m}Tc-DTPA clearance rate as the "gold standard" and determined serum Cr

with the enzyme-based method. We determined the serial CysC of 687 randomly selected Chinese CKD patients using the PETIA method. Two GFR estimating equations were established based on the top coefficient of the non-linear regression iterative calculation:

$$eGFR7 = 173.9 \times CysC^{-0.725} \times Cr^{-0.184} \times age^{-0.193}$$
$$\times 0.89(\text{if female})(R^2=0.734)$$

$$eGFR8 = 78.64 \times CysC^{-0.964}(R^2=0.764)$$

The R^2 of eGFR8 was higher than that of eGFR7, indicating that using both Cr and age for GFR estimation was not as effective as using CysC alone. Therefore, CysC has the potential to be a good substitute for Cr during the assessment of renal function.

The two equations developed in this study had limits of agreement (57.0 mL/min $\bullet$ 1.73 m^2 and 59.5 mL/min $\bullet$ 1.73 m^2, respectively) that were within the pre-set values of <60 mL/min $\bullet$ 1.73 m^2. They also showed only minor differences in their Mountain deviation distribution curves, with almost the same error (367 vs. 377 arbitrary units), precision (28.5 vs. 29.7 mL/min $\bullet$ 1.73 m^2), accuracy ($P>0.05$), and applicability in GFR estimation. When comparing the newly developed equations and the 6 previously reported ones, only eGFR7 and eGFR8 did not show apparent proportional errors (b's 95% CI contains B = 1) and constant errors (a's 95% CI contains A = 0) from rGFR. All equations showed high linear correlations (r>0.75, $P=0.000$) and acceptable Passing & Bablok regression linearity (Cusum test, $P>0.05$). Among these 6 previous equations, eGFR3 had only

Table 3. Bias, precision and accuracy of eGFR compared with rGFR (n = 101).

	Bias*	CR** mL/min·1.73 m²	Accuracy (%)		
			P_{15}	P_{30}	P_{50}
eGFR1	2045	49.3	36.63	55.45[a,d]	77.23[a,c]
eGFR2	3036	55.8	23.76[a,c]	43.56[a,c]	73.27[a,c]
eGFR3	628	30.9	34.65	63.37	86.14[b]
eGFR4	681	36.1	36.63	63.37	81.19[a,d]
eGFR5	490	32.8	39.60	65.35	89.11
eGFR6	1435	40.4	31.68	59.41[b]	82.18[a,d]
eGFR7	367	28.5	41.58	74.26	95.05
eGFR8	377	29.7	41.58	72.28	93.07
χ^2	–	–	10.812	28.341	31.399
P	–	–	0.147	0.000	0.000

*Bias, the area between the Bland-Altman regression line and the zero difference line; arbitrary unit, i.e., (mL/min·1.73 m²)². **CR, Coefficient of Repeatability, equal to the difference between the mean difference and the 95% upper limit of agreement. a: vs. eGFR7, by Pearson χ^2 test, $P<0.01$: b: vs. eGFR7, by Pearson χ^2 test, $P<0.05$; c: vs. eGFR8, by Pearson χ^2 test, $P<0.01$; d: vs. eGFR8, by Pearson χ^2 test, $P<0.05$.

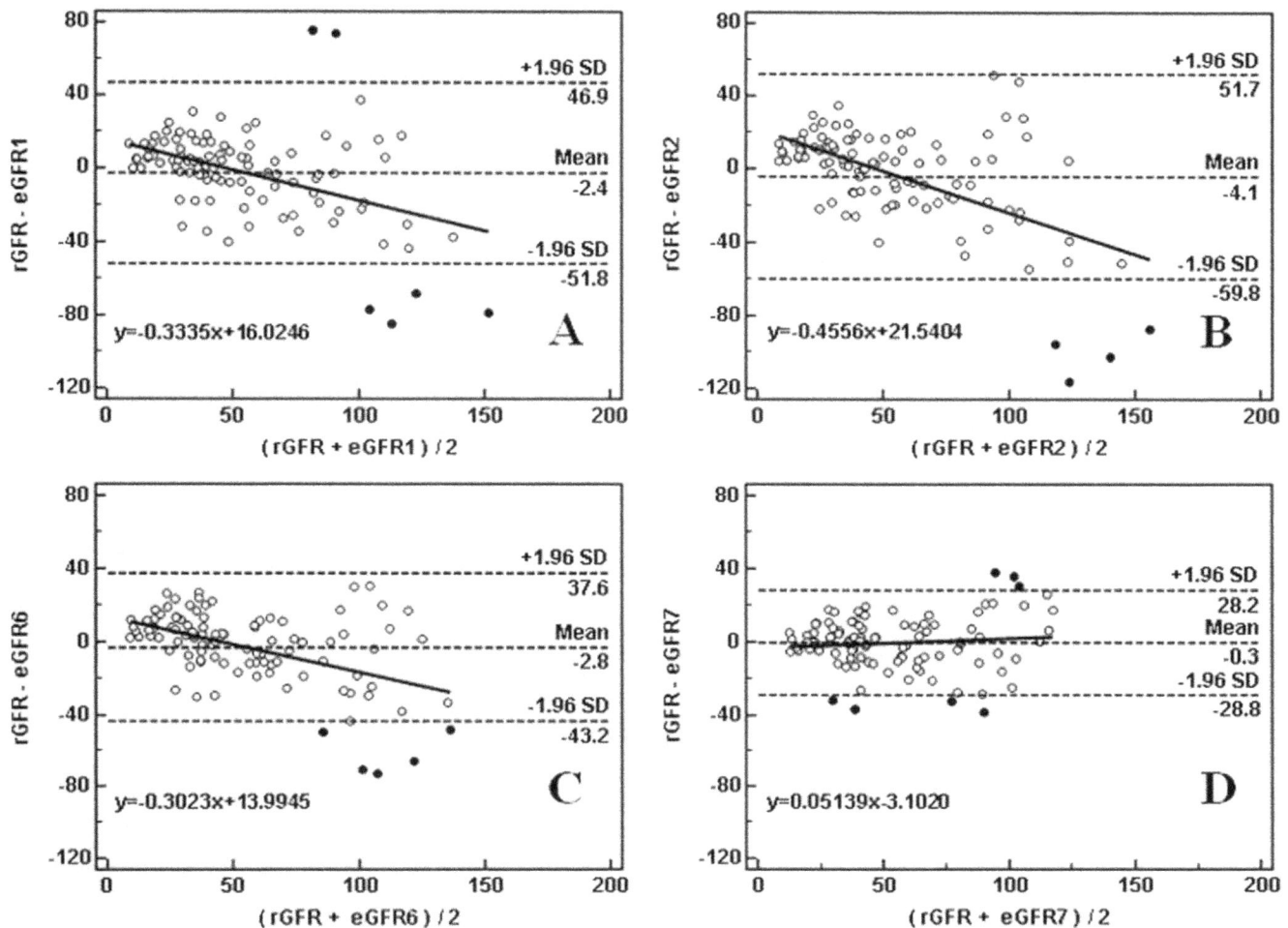

Figure 2. Altman-Bland plot: comparison between eGFR and rGFR (n = 101).

constant errors (a's 95% CI = −12.592 and −2.989, not containing 0) from rGFR, but all the other equations had both constant errors and proportional errors. These errors may have been caused by the differences in study subjects, GFR "gold standards", GFR markers, and GFR determination methods, which may be verified by the following comparisons of the newly developed equations and the literature equations.

In the estimation of GFR consistency, eGFR7 and eGFR8 were both better than eGFR1 and eGFR2 (limits of agreement = 57.0 and 59.5 vs. 98.7 and 111.5 mL/min • 1.73 m^2, respectively), and the limits of consistency for the latter two were both significantly higher than the pre-set professional cutoff value (<60 mL/min • 1.73 m^2). eGFR7 and eGFR8 also had smaller GFR estimating errors than eGFR1 and eGFR2 (367 and 377 vs. 2045 and 3036 arbitrary units, respectively). eGFR1 and eGFR2 also had worse estimation accuracy (CR = 49.3 and 55.8 vs. 28.5 and 29.7 mL/min • 1.73 m^2, respectively) and lower P_{30} and P_{50} than eGFR7 and eGFR8 (χ^2 test, P<0.05). The serum Cr can be easily affected by many factors, such as gender, age, muscle size, diet, medication and renal secretion and excretion (renal excretion becomes more apparent under pathological conditions), which may lead to the large errors and low accuracy of eGFR1 and eGFR2 in GFR estimation. In addition, the choice of Cr determination may also affect the applicability of eGFR1 and eGFR2. It was reported that

eGFR1 was better than eGFR2 when the enzyme-based measurement was selected [41]. A similar conclusion was reached in this study.

The two equations for MDRD/CKD-EPI, eGFR3 and eGFR4, with the limits of agreement being higher than the pre-set values of <60 mL/min • 1.73 m^2 at 61.8 and 72.3 mL/min • 1.73 m^2, respectively, were also worse than eGFR7 and eGFR8 in the GFR estimation for Chinese CKD patients. The Mountain deviation distribution curves of eGFR3 and eGFR4 both deviated to the right from the "0" point (M = 6.90 and 6.63 mL/min • 1.73 m^2, respectively,) with larger P_5, M and P_{95} than those of eGFR7 and eGFR8, indicating significant underestimation of GFR for Chinese CKD patients. Therefore, the MDRD/CKD-EPI equations may only have limited application in Chinese populations.

The two equations from the Chinese cooperative group, eGFR5 and eGFR6, did target the Chinese populations. However, their limits of agreement (65.6 and 80.8 mL/min • 1.73 m^2, respectively,) both exceeded the pre-set values of <60 mL/min • 1.73 m^2. Compared with eGFR7 and eGFR8, eGFR5 and eGFR6 showed broadening trends in the Mountain deviation distributions (P_5–P_{95} interval distribution width = 54.04 and 69.09 vs. 48.94 and 49.94 mL/min • 1.73 m^2, respectively,)), worse precision (CR = 32.8 and 40.4 vs. 28.5 and 29.7 mL/min • 1.73 m^2, respectively,)), and worse accuracy (P_{30}: eGFR6 vs.

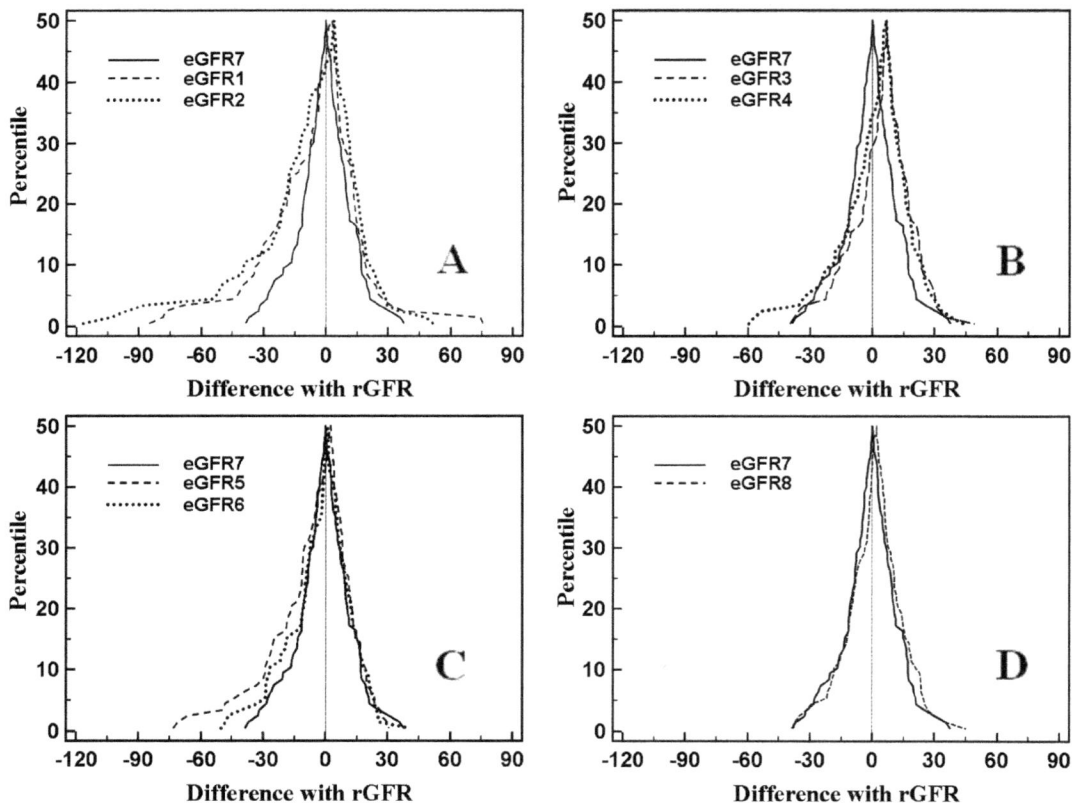

Figure 3. Mountain plot: comparison between newly developed eGFR formulas and various literature eGFR formulas.

eGFR7, χ^2 test, $P<0.05$; P_{50}: eGFR6 $vs.$ eGFR7 and eGFR8, χ^2 test, $P<0.05$), all of which indicate inferior consistency for rGFR.

In addition to the factor of race, differences in the determination methods for GFR markers, i.e., the different methods of detecting Cr and CysC, may also contribute to the deviation of the results between the newly developed equations and the previously reported ones. In the past, the picric acid assay was used to detect serum Cr (eGFR1-eGFR6 equations). Currently, many laboratories in China prefer the enzyme-based method to detect serum Cr in order to avoid cross contamination from picric acid. Routine CysC tests also include the PETIA and PENIA methods. Because it can be performed in an automatic biochemical analyzer and the

Table 4. Percentiles (P) of difference between eGFR and rGFR (mL/min • 1.73 m^2).

	P_5	P_{10}	P_{25}	$P_{50}(M)$	P_{75}	P_{90}	P_{95}
eGFR1	-42.52	-32.93	-14.24	2.85	12.12	19.06	25.91
eGFR2	-52.86	-39.34	-17.52	3.77	13.36	21.20	28.15
eGFR3	-22.21	-15.85	-2.06	6.90	14.67	23.74	29.88
eGFR4	-31.91	-19.84	-5.28	6.63	14.80	23.82	28.48
eGFR5	-30.58	-26.63	-9.25	0.88	9.42	18.96	23.46
eGFR6	-45.36	-29.05	-11.39	2.51	11.19	19.44	23.73
eGFR7	-27.94	-17.96	-8.31	0.01	8.89	17.13	21.00
eGFR8	-25.04	-18.27	-7.89	2.09	10.58	21.73	24.90

detection time can be as short as 5 minutes, PETIA has become the preferred method for CysC routine determinations. The MDRD/CKD-EPI and the Chinese collaboration group, however, used PENIA instead of PETIA to detect serum CysC (eGFR3-eGFR6 equations). In addition, the differences in CysC standards may also cause differences in detection results, which affect the applicability of eGFR equations. The first CysC certified reference material ERM-DA471/IFCC [42] was introduced in 2010, which allows CysC detection to be traced. As a result, studies on CysC-based GFR estimation equations may avoid matrix effects. Once serum CysC detection becomes standardized, its application in GFR evaluation will have greater advantages over Cr detection. In this study, we developed two eGFR equations based on the sole-indicator, CysC, in combination with serum creatinine levels and age, to evaluate renal functions precisely, accurately, simply and quickly with lower costs.

The difference of results between our new equation and traditional eGFR equations, largely may be due to different measured methods for the determination of SCr and CysC. That is, entered enzymatic-Cr results and/or PETIA-CysC results to traditional eGFR equations that were developed by Cr using the Jaffe's kinetic method and/or PENIA-CysC. It is this inadequate use that leads to the eGFR calculation resulting error. Of course, different choices of the "gold standard" in research programs, as well as technical proficiency of the same "gold standard" may also be the reasons of the error. In addition, the population differences in development group, such as the difference of the constituent ratio of the subjects age, sex, CKD stage, and complications, etc., may also be the reason that the results are not consistent between the traditional eGFR equations and this study equation. In this

Table 5. Classification of CKD by SCr- and/or CysC-based on eGFR equations(n = 101)*.

	CKD1	CKD2	CKD3	CKD4	CKD5	Total	κ(95%CI)
rGFR	13	22	44	17	5	101	
eGFR1	7(53.8)*	14(63.6)	28(63.6)	5(29.4)	2(40.0)	56(55.4)	0.403(0.280–0.526)
eGFR2	7(53.8)	15(68.2)	19(43.2)	3(17.6)	2(40.0)	44(43.6)	0.297(0.175–0.419)
eGFR3	10(76.9)	17(77.3)	26(59.1)	7(41.2)	3(60.0)	63(62.4)	0.504(0.382–0.626)
eGFR4	11(84.6)	17(77.3)	29(65.9)	5(29.4)	2(40.0)	64(63.4)	0.514(0.394–0.634)
eGFR5	12(92.3)	14(63.6)	28(63.6)	9(52.9)	3(60.0)	66(65.3)	0.536(0.413–0.659)
eGFR6	11(84.6)	14(63.6)	27(61.4)	7(41.2)	2(40.0)	61(60.4)	0.472(0.347–0.597)
eGFR7	12(92.3)	18(81.8)	32(72.7)	9(52.9)	3(60.0)	74(73.3)	0.641(0.527–0.755)
eGFR8	12(92.3)	18(81.8)	33(75.0)	10(58.8)	2(40.0)	75(74.3)	0.652(0.538–0.766)

*Accoding to the recommendations by K/DOQI. *Number of patients (%) correct classified. Reference method is plasma clearance of ^{99m}Tc-DTPA. Kappa analysis was used to evaluate the agreement between rGFR stages and each eGFR CKD stages.

study, there are statistical differences between gender for weight, height, and body surface area. It will worth considering whether they will cause the differences of the traditional eGFR results.

It is worth mentioning that although the meta-analysis demonstrated that CysC is superior to SCr in the determination of the GFR injuries [43,44]. However, most studies of CysC have focused on fields where the problems of SCr are most apparent, including specific population groups with malnutrition, extensive reduced body surface area, extremely low body mass, or a few comorbidities that have a large influence on the generation of creatinine. Nevertheless, Serum cystatin C may be influenced by factors other than renal function alone, including serum C-reactive protein [45], smoking [46], the subjects with very low GFR[47], thyroid function [48,49], immunosuppressive therapy [50], and occupational exposure to toxic agents such as lead, cadmium, and arsenic [51], etc. Thus, clinicians must be cautious when interpreting cystatin C levels alone if the subjects encounter these factors.In summary, different fitting eGFR equations with different estimation values can be developed based on different study subjects, different GFR "gold standards", and different detection

methods. The two newly established equations in this study showed effective but significantly different results from previously reported equations, most likely a result of the differences in detection methods and "gold standards". Currently, enzyme-based Cr detection and CysC PETIA detection are widely used in clinical laboratories. Our study demonstrated that the simple cystatin C formula could achieve a much better diagnostic performance than SCr formula containing more variables.Therefore, careful and complete consideration is required to choose the right eGFR equation for clinical applications to avoid misdiagnosis and errors in treatment.

Author Contributions

Read and approved the final manuscript: All authors. Conceived and designed the experiments: JFF LQ XML. Performed the experiments: XML PZ YQ XMH YPL HCL WX LJX FCZ. Analyzed the data: LQ YWY WX HQ FCZ. Contributed reagents/materials/analysis tools: LZ HCL XZG HZH LQW SYS RD. Wrote the paper: JFF LQ YWY.

References

1. Levey AS, Atkins R, Coresh J, Cohen EP, Collins AJ, et al. (2007) Chronic kidney disease as a global public health problem: approaches and initiatives- a position statement from Kidney Disease Improving Global Outcomes. Kidney Int 72: 247–259.

2. Levey AS, Eckardt KU, Tsukamoto Y, Levin A, Coresh J, et al. (2005) Definition and classification of chronic kidney disease: a position statement from Kidney Disease: Improving Global Outcomes (KDIGO). Kidney Int 67: 2089–2100.

3. National Kidney Foundation (2002) NFK-K/DOQI clinical practice guidelines for chronic kidney disease: evaluation, classification, and stratification. Am J Kidney Dis 39: S1–S266.

4. Florkowski CM, Chew-Harris JS (2011) Methods of Estimating GFR-Different Equations Including CKD-EPI. Clin Biochem Rev 32: 75–9.

5. Hojs R, Bevc S, Ekart R, Gorenjak M, Puklavec L. (2008) Serum cystatin C as an endogenous marker of renal function in patients with chronic kidney disease. Ren Fail 30: 181–6.

6. Inker LA, Schmid CH, Tighiouart H, Eckfeldt JH, Feldman HI, et al. (2012) CKD-EPI Investigators. Estimating glomerular filtration rate from serum creatinine and cystatin C. N Engl J Med 367: 20–9.

7. Slort PR, Ozden N, Pape L, Offner G, Tromp WF, et al. (2012) Comparing cystatin C and creatinine in the diagnosis of pediatric acute renal allograft dysfunction. Pediatr Nephrol 27: 843–9.

8. Larsson A, Flodin M, Hansson LO, Carlsson L (2008) Patient selection has a strong impact on cystatin C and Modification of Diet in Renal Disease (MDRD) estimated glomerular filtration rate. Clin Biochem 41: 1355–61.

9. Salgado JV, Neves FA, Bastos MG, França AK, Brito DJ, et al. (2010) Monitoring renal function: measured and estimated glomerular filtration rates- a review. Braz J Med Biol Res 43: 528–36.

10. Roos JF, Doust J, Tett SE, Kirkpatrick CM (2007) Diagnostic accuracy of cystatin C compared to serum creatinine for the estimation of renal dysfunction in adults and children- a meta-analysis. Clin Biochem 40: 383–391.

11. Ferguson MA, Waikar SS (2012) Established and emerging markers of kidney function. Clin Chem 58: 680–9.

12. Herget-Rosenthal S, Feldkamp T, Volbracht L, Kribben A (2004) Measurement of urinary cystatin C by particle-enhanced nephelometric immunoassay: precision, interferences, stability and reference range. Ann Clin Biochem 41(Pt 2): 111–8.

13. Voskoboev NV, Larson TS, Rule AD, Lieske JC (2012) Analytic and clinical validation of a standardized cystatin C particle enhanced turbidimetric assay (PETIA) to estimate glomerular filtration rate. Clin Chem Lab Med 50: 1591–6.

14. Liu J (2012) Evaluation of serum cystatin C for diagnosis of acute rejection after renal transplantation. Transplant Proc 44: 1250–3.

15. Cai X, Long Z, Lin L, Feng Y, Zhou N, et al. (2012) Serum cystatin C is an early biomarker for assessment of renal function in burn patients. Clin Chem Lab Med 50: 667–71.

16. Krishnamurthy N, Arumugasamy K, Anand U, Anand CV, Aruna V, et al. (2011) Serum cystatin C levels in renal transplant recipients. Indian J Clin Biochem 26: 120–4.

17. Kumaresan R, Giri P (2011) A comparison of serum cystatin C and creatinine with glomerular filtration rate in Indian patients with chronic kidney disease. Oman Med J 26: 421–5.

18. Yap M, Lamarche J, Peguero A, Courville C (2011) Serum cystatin C versus serum creatinine in the estimation of glomerular filtration rate in rhabdomyolysis,J Ren Care 37: 155–7.19.

19. Jaisuresh K, Sharma RK, Mehrotra S, Kaul A, Badauria DS, et al. (2012) Cystatin C as a marker of glomerular filtration rate in voluntary kidney donors. Exp Clin Transplant 10: 14–7.

20. Robles NR, Mena C, Cidoncha J (2012) Estimated Glomerular Filtration Rate from Serum Cystatin C: Significant Differences among Several Equations Results. Ren Fail 34: 871–5.

21. Hojs R, Bevc S, Ekart R, Gorenjak M, Puklavec L (2010) Serum cystatin C-based formulas for prediction of glomerular filtration rate in patients with chronic kidney disease. Nephron Clin Pract 114: c118–26.

22. Sohrabian A, Noraddin FH, Flodin M, Fredricsson A, Larsson A (2012) Particle enhanced turbidimetric immunoassay for the determination of urine cystatin C on Cobas c501. Clin Biochem 45: 339–44.

23. Bargnoux AS, Cavalier E, Cristol JP, Simon N, Dupuy AM, et al. (2011) Cystatin C is a reliable marker for estimation of glomerular filtration rate in renal transplantation: validation of a new turbidimetric assay using monospecific sheep antibodies. Clin Chem Lab Med 49: 265–70.

24. Bargnoux AS, Perrin M, Garrigue V, Badiou S, Dupuy AM, et al. (2011) Analytical performances of cystatin C turbidimetric assay: which impact on accuracy of glomerular filtration rate estimation in renal transplantation? Clin Chem Lab Med 50: 133–8.

25. Hansson LO, Grubb A, Lidén A, Flodin M, Berggren A, et al. (2010) Performance evaluation of a turbidimetric cystatin C assay on different high-throughput platforms. Scand J Clin Lab Invest 70: 347–53.

26. Greenberg N, Roberts WL, Bachmann LM, Wright EC, Dalton RN, et al. (2012) Clin Specificity characteristics of 7 commercial creatinine measurement procedures by enzymatic and Jaffe method principles. Chem 58: 391–401.

27. Liu WS, Chung YT, Yang CY, Lin CC, Tsai KH, et al. (2012) Serum creatinine determined by Jaffe, enzymatic method, and isotope dilution-liquid chromatography-mass spectrometry in patients under hemodialysis. J Clin Lab Anal 26: 206–14.

28. Wang X, Xu G, Li H, Liu Y, Wang F (2011) Reference intervals for serum creatinine with enzymatic assay and evaluation of four equations to estimate glomerular filtration rate in a healthy Chinese adult population. Clin Chim Acta 412: 1793–7.

29. Ma YC, Zuo L, Zhang CL, Wang M, Wang RF, et al. (2007) Comparison of ^{99m}Tc-DTPA renal dynamic imaging with modified MDRD equation for glomerular filtration rate estimation in Chinese patients in different stages of chronic kidney disease. Nephrol Dial Transplant 22: 417–23.

30. Cockcroft DW, Gault MH (1976) Prediction of creatinine clearance from serum creatinine. Nephron 16: 31–41.

31. Ma YC, Zuo L, Chen JH, Luo Q, Yu XQ, et al. (2006) Modified glomerular filtration rate estimating equation for Chinese patients with chronic kidney disease. J Am Soc Nephrol 17: 2937–44.

32. Stevens LA, Coresh J, Schmid CH, Feldman HI, Froissart M, et al. (2008) Estimating GFR using Serum Cystatin C Alone and in Combination with Serum

Creatinine: A Pooled Analysis of 3418 Individuals with CKD[J]. Am J Kidney Dis 51: 395–406.

33. Ma YC, Zuo L, Chen JH, Luo Q, Yu XQ, et al. (2007) Improved GFR estimation by combined creatinine and cystatin C measurements. Kidney Int 72: 1535–42.

34. Bland JM, Altman DG (1986) Statistical methods for assessing agreement between two methods of clinical measurement. Lancet 1: 307–10.

35. Blaufox MD, Aurell M, Bubeck B, Fommei E, Piepsz A, et al. (1996) Report of the Radionuclides in Nephrourology Committee on renal clearance. J Nucl Med 37: 1883–90.

36. Sohrabian A, Noraddin FH, Flodin M, Fredricsson A, Larsson A (2012) Particle enhanced turbidimetric immunoassay for the determination of urine cystatin C on Cobas c501. Clin Biochem 45: 339–44.

37. Al-Turkmani MR, Law T, Kellogg MD (2008) Performance evaluation of a particle-enhanced turbidimetric cystatin C assay on the Hitachi 917 analyzer. Clin Chim Acta 398: 75–7.

38. Conde-Sánchez M, Roldán-Fontana E, Chueca-Porcuna N, Pardo S, Porras-Gracia J (2010) Analytical performance evaluation of a particle-enhanced turbidimetric cystatin C assay on the Roche COBAS 6000 analyzer. Clin Biochem 43: 921–5.

39. Flodin M, Larsson A (2009) Performance evaluation of a particle-enhanced turbidimetric cystatin C assay on the Abbott ci8200 analyzer. Clin Biochem 42: 873–6.

40. Bargnoux AS, Servel AC, Piéroni L, Dupuy AM, Badiou S, et al. (2012) Accuracy of GFR predictive equations in renal transplantation: validation of a new turbidimetric cystatin C assay on Architect c8000. Clin Biochem 45: 151–3.

41. Liu X, Lv L, Wang C, Shi C, Cheng C (2012) Comparison of prediction equations to estimate glomerular filtration rate in Chinese patients with chronic kidney disease. Intern Med J 42: e59–67.

42. Grubb A, Blirup-Jensen S, Lindstrom V, Schmidt C, Althaus H, et al. (2010) First certified reference material for Cystatin C in human serum ERM-DA471/IFCC. Clin Chem Lab Med 48: 1619–21.

43. Dharnidharka VR, Kwon C, Stevens G (2002) Serum cystatin C is superior to serum creatinine as a marker of kidney function: a meta-analysis. Am J Kidney Dis 40: 221–6.

44. Roos JF, Doust J, Tett SE, Kirkpatrick CM (2007) Diagnostic accuracy of cystatin C compared to serum creatinine for the estimation of renal dysfunction in adults and children- A meta-analysis. Clin Biochem 40: 383–91.

45. Stevens LA, Coresh J, Greene T, Levey AS (2006) Assessing kidney function-measured and estimated glomerular filtration rate. N Engl J Med 354: 2473–83.

46. Sjostrom PA, Jones IL, Tidman MA (2009) Cystatin C as a filtration marker-haemodialysis patients expose its strengths and limitations. Scand J Clin Lab Invest 69: 65–72.

47. Horio M, Imai E, Yasuda Y, Watanabe T, Matsuo S (2011) Performance of serum cystatin C versus serum creatinine as a marker of glomerular filtration rate as measured by inulin renal clearance. Clin Exp Nephrol 15: 868–76.

48. Kotajima N, Yanagawa Y, Aoki T, Tsunekawa K, Morimura T (2010) Influence of thyroid hormones and transforming growth factor-b1 on cystatin C concentrations. J Int Med Res 38: 1365–73.

49. Fricker M, Wiesli P, Brandle M, Schwegler B, Schmid C (2003) Impact of thyroid dysfunction on serum cystatin C. Kidney Int 63: 1944–7.

50. Rule AD, Bergstralh EJ, Slezak JM, Bergert J, Larson TS (2006) Glomerular filtration rate estimated by cystatin C among different clinical presentations. Kidney Int 69: 399–405.

51. Poręba R, Gać P, Poręba M, Antonowicz-Juchniewicz J, Andrzejak R (2011) Relation between occupational exposure to lead, cadmium, arsenic and concentration of cystatin C. Toxicology283: 88–95.

10

Chinese Minimally Invasive Percutaneous Nephrolithotomy for Intrarenal Stones in Patients with Solitary Kidney: A Single-Center Experience

Zhichao Huang[1], Fajun Fu[2], Zhaohui Zhong[1], Lei Zhang[1], Ran Xu[1], Xiaokun Zhao[1]*

1 Department of Urology, Second Xiangya Hospital, Central South University, Changsha, Hunan, China, 2 Department of Urology, Changsha Central Hospital, Changsha, Hunan, China

Abstract

Objective: To report our experience with Chinese minimally invasive percutaneous nephrolithotomy (Chinese MPCNL) to manage patients with intrarenal stones in solitary kidney, and evaluate the safety, efficiency and feasibility of this technique.

Methods: Forty-one patients with intrarenal stones in solitary kidney underwent Chinese MPCNL in our department from March 2009 to February 2011. Demographic characteristics, operative parameters, number of tracts, stone-free rates (SFRs), stone analyses, hemoglobin levels, nephrostomy tube removal time, hospitalization time, and complications were evaluated. Serum creatinine (Scr) and glomerular filtration rate (GFR) were measured preoperatively, postoperatively at 1 month, and each follow-up visit. The 5-stage classification of chronic kidney disease (CKD) was used according to the National Kidney Foundation guidelines.

Results: The initial stone-free status was achieved in 35 (85.4%) patients after Chinese MPCNL. The mean follow-up time was 16.9±4.7 months (range: 12–24), and the final SFR improved to 97.6% after auxiliary procedures. Among all patients, complex stones were detected in 26 (63.4%) patients, and 9 (22.0%) required multiple tracts. The mean operative time and mean hospitalization time were 71.3±23.5 min (range: 40–139) and 6.1±0.5 days (range: 5–11), respectively. During preoperative period and postoperative period (1 month), Scr were 132.1±41.3 umol/L (range: 78.2–231.4) and 108.9±30.7 umol/L (range: 71.6–136.9), respectively ($P<0.05$), while GFR were 74.9±24.2 ml/min (range: 35–110) and 83.9±27.4 ml/min (range: 65–110), respectively ($P<0.05$). According to CKD classification, the renal function was stable, improved, and worse in 29 (70.7%), 11 (26.8%), and 1 (2.5%) patients, compared with the preoperative levels. No patient progressed to end-stage renal disease requiring dialysis.

Conclusions: Our experience with Chinese MPCNL demonstrates that it is safe, feasible and efficient for managing the intrarenal calculi in solitary kidney with a low complication rate. At long-term follow-up, renal function stabilized or even improved in the majority of patients with solitary kidney.

Editor: Emmanuel A. Burdmann, University of Sao Paulo Medical School, Brazil

Funding: The authors have no support or funding to report.

Competing Interests: The authors have declared that no competing interests exist.

* E-mail: hzc0305@163.com

Introduction

Percutaneous nephrolithotomy (PCNL) has become the first method of choice for patients with large and complex calculi since its introduction in 1976 [1]. The 2005 American Urological Association (AUA) Nephrolithiasis Clinical Guidelines recommend PCNL as the first-line treatment for calculi greater than 500 mm^2 [2]. The excellent stone-free rate (SFR) following PCNL is 78% to 95% [3]. However, PCNL can still be associated with significant complications, such as uncontrolled hemorrhage, injury to collecting system and surrounding viscera, urinary leakage, sepsis, loss of kidney, or even death [3]. Therefore, PCNL poses a significant risk, especially for patients with solitary kidney. Meanwhile, the standard size tract (26–30 F) may be too large for pediatric kidneys and some undilated adult kidneys. To

decrease morbidity, especially uncontrolled hemorrhage, some urologists have modified the technique of standard PCNL by performing it with a miniature endoscope by way of a small size tract (12–20 F) and named it as MPCNL [4,5,6]. Although MPCNL has exhibited advantages with respect to hemorrhage, injury to renal parenchyma, postoperative pain, and shortened hospitalization time [4,7,8], the disadvantages of need for specialized equipments and relatively low efficiency to fragment large stones than standard PCNL limited its indications. The indications of MPCNL are only limited to pediatric patients or adult patients with stone diameter less than 2 cm or as a secondary tract of standard PCNL [4,5,6].

In China, urologists have modified PCNL technique since the 1990s, using an 8/9.8 F rigid ureteroscope via the 14–18 F percutaneous tract provided by fascial dilator and matched peel-away sheath to manage the upper urinary tract calculi and termed it as Chinese MPCNL [9,10].

In this study, we evaluated the safety, efficiency and feasibility of Chinese MPCNL on management of intrarenal stones in solitary kidney and evaluated the long-term renal function. To our knowledge, few studies have been performed.

Materials and Methods

We obtained approval for this study from the ethics committee of our hospital. Meanwhile, we obtained informed consent from all participants in our study. The informed consent was written and specified in the operative consent. Between March 2009 and February 2011, 41 patients with intrarenal stones in solitary kidney (congenital in 4 patients, 9.8%; contralateral nephrectomy in 30 patients, 73.2%; and nonperfused kidney in 7 patients, 17.0%) underwent Chinese MPCNL in our department. Patient demographic characteristics, such as age, gender, previous renal intervention history were studied. Patients were evaluated preoperatively with blood routine tests, coagulation tests, urinalyses, urine cultures, and serum biochemistry. Before operation, computed tomography (CT) was performed routinely to assess the number, location, and size of the stone, identify the collecting system anatomy, and provide an anatomical proof for establishing percutaneous tract. Prophylactic preoperative wide-spectrum antibiotics were administered to patients with positive urine culture result according to the antibiotic susceptibility tests. Stone size was evaluated as the surface area and calculated according to the European Association of Urology (EAU) Guidelines [11]. Stones were classified as simple (isolated caliceal or renal pelvis stones) or complex (renal pelvis stones accompanying caliceal stones, complete or partial staghorn stones), regardless of its size.

A plain X-ray of the kidneys, ureters, and bladder (KUB) was performed 24 to 48 hours after operation to assess the effect of surgery and identify the position of D–J stent. In patients with complete stone-free or clinically insignificant residual fragments (CIRFs), the nephrostomy tube was clamped when the drainage was clear and subsequently removed. The D–J stent would be removed 2 to 3 weeks later. Otherwise, the flexible ureteroscopy and extracorporeal shock wave lithotripsy (ESWL) were performed as auxiliary procedures. All patients were assessed by CT one month after the final procedure to confirm the final SFR. Complete stone-free was defined as the absence of any fragments in kidney or had CIRFs, defined as ≤4 mm, nonsymptomatic, nonobstructive and noninfectious residual fragments [12].

Scr was measured before the operation, on the first postoperative day, and at each follow-up visit. GFR was determined preoperatively, postoperatively at 1 month and each follow-up visit. Calculated GFR was determined using the Cockroft and Gault formula, GFR = [(140-age)(weight in Kg)(0.85 for women)]/ $72 \times Cr$ (mg/100 ml) [13]. The CKD stages 1–5 were stratified as either normal, mild, moderately, severely decreased GFR, or those requiring dialysis or a kidney transplant (>90, 60–89, 30–59, 15–29, and <15 ml/min) according to the National Kidney Foundation guidelines [14]. The Scr, GFR, and CKD stage during preoperative period were compared with those at the follow-up visit.

All patients were followed for at least 12 months, especially patients with residual fragments. The first follow-up visit was performed 1 month after the final procedure and then patients were followed every 3 months during the first year and every 6 months thereafter. At each follow-up visit, urinalysis, urine culture, serum biochemistry, blood routine test, KUB+ intravenous urography (IVU), and renal ultrasound were performed to confirm the presence of urinary tract infection (UTI), hydronephrosis, fragments growth and stone recurrence.

Statistical analysis was performed using SPSS 17.0 (SPSS, Inc., Chicago, IL). The continuous variables were compared with student's t tests and Wilcoxon tests. Differences resulting in a P-value of <0.05 were considered significant.

Surgical Technique

All procedures were performed under continual epidural anesthesia or general anesthesia. Patient was firstly placed in a split lower limbs position, and a 5 F ureteral catheter was inserted into the target ureter under direct ureteroscopic vision. Then, the patient was turned into a prone position with a pack under the abdomen to minimize lumber lordosis. Access to the designed calyx was performed by the urologists with the help of fluoroscopy or ultrasonography using an 18-gauge needle (Cook Urological, Spencer, IN). A posterior middle calyx puncture via the 11th intercostal space between the posterior axillary line and scapula line was preferred. Tract dilation was serially performed using fascial dilator (Cook Urological, Spencer, IN) from 8 F to 18 F, and a matched peel-away sheath was placed. The stones were fragmented with a holmium laser or pneumatic lithotripter through an 8/9.8 F rigid ureteroscope (Richard Wolf, German) (Figure 1). The big fragments were removed with a forceps, while small fragments (<0.3 cm) were pushed out with an endoscopic pulsed perfusion pump. Flexible ureteroscopy was used to decrease the necessity of multiple tracts and determine the stone-free status. Finally, a 5 F D–J stent (Cook Urological, Spencer, IN) was inserted via the percutaneous tract with the assistance of guidewire, and a matched size nephrostomy tube was inserted in the collecting system. The operative time was calculated from the time of percutaneous puncture to the completion of nephrostomy tube placement.

Results

Our study identified 41 patients, including 27 (65.9%) men and 14 (34.1%) women. Patients' age was 16 to 69 years (mean: 51.4±14.7). Mean stone size was 912±517 mm^2 (range: 300–1800). Preoperative urine cultures were positive in 7 (17.1%) patients, including 4 patients with *E. coli*, 2 with *Pseudomonas aeruginosa* and 1 with *Enterococcus faecalis*. All these infections were treated with culture-specific antibiotics. Six (14.6%) patients had a previous renal intervention history in the same kidney (1 previous open surgery; 2 previous ESWL; 3 previous PCNL). Thirty-two (78.0%) patients managed with a single tract, and 9 (22.0%) required multiple tracts. The mean operative time was 71.3±23.5 min (range: 40–139). The initial SFR was 85.4% after the procedure of Chinese MPCNL, and 6 (14.6%) had significant residual calculi. Of these patients, four (9.8%) were performed with ESWL, and 2 (4.9%) needed a flexible ureteroscopy procedure. After all auxiliary procedures, forty (97.6%) patients achieved the stone-free status. Finally, there were 2 (4.9%) patients with CIRFs and one with significant residual calculi (7 mm). All of these 3 patients were followed up, and the size of the fragments was stable. During the long-term follow-up, spontaneous stone passage was noticed in 1 of 2 patients with CIRFs. The patient, stone and operative characteristics are shown in Table 1.

The mean Scr were 132.1±41.3 umol/L (range: 78.2–231.4), 108.9±40.7 umol/L (range: 71.6–136.9), and 107.1±35.6 umol/ L (range: 71.0–137.1) during the preoperative period, one month follow-up, and at the last follow-up visit (≥12 months). A statistical significance was detected in the one month follow-up period Scr when compared to the preoperative Scr (P<0.05). The same

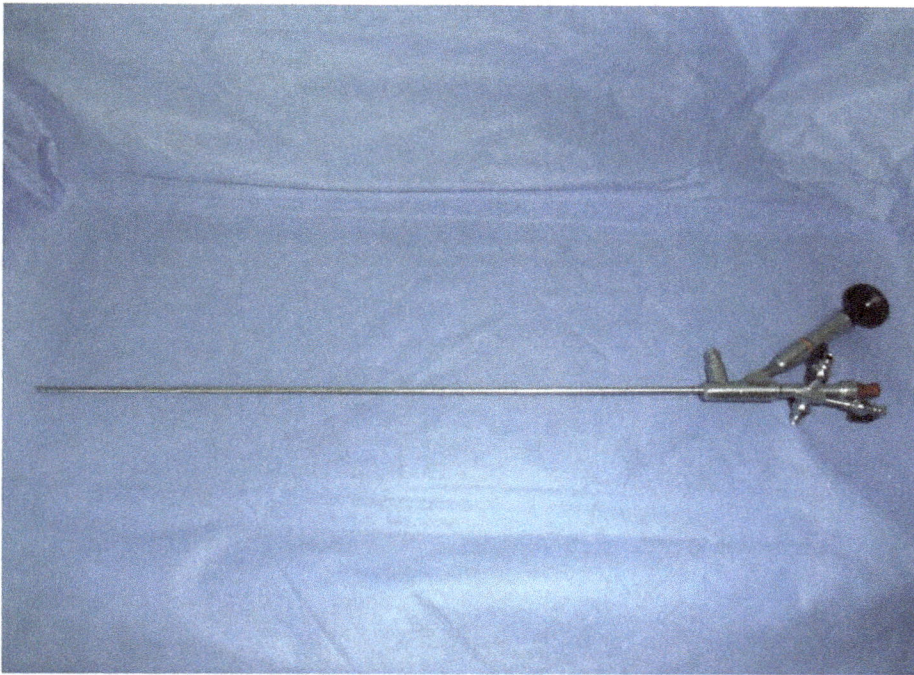

Figure 1. The 8/9.8 F rigid ureteroscope (Richard Wolf, German).

results were detected in GFR before operation it was 74.9±24.2 ml/min (range: 35.0–110.0) and by the end of one month follow-up it was 83.9±27.4 ml/min (range: 65.0–110.0) with statistical significance (P<0.05). However, our results showed no statistically significant difference both Scr and GFR from one month to the last follow-up visit. During the preoperative period, 11 (26.8%) patients had CKD stage 1, 15 (36.6%) had stage 2, 12 (29.3%) had stage 3, and 3 (7.3%) had stage 4, while CKD stage revealed stable, improved and worsening diseases in 29 (70.7%), 11 (26.8%) and 1 (2.5%) of patients at the last follow-up visit. During the whole follow-up period, no patient progressed to end-stage kidney disease requiring dialysis.

There were no intraoperative complications in all cases. Postoperative complications occurred in 5 (12.2%) patients. The details of complications are presented in Table 2. Five patients had postoperative fever (temperature of 38.5°C or greater), which was resolved spontaneously in one, while the remaining four patients (9.8%) with preoperative UTIs (E. coli in 2 patients, Pseudomonas aeruginosa in 1 patient and Enterococcus faecalis in 1 patient) were treated with a complete culture-specific antibiotics until body temperature, urinalysis and urine culture were normal. The stone composition in these 4 patients was struvite (3/4, 75%) and calcium oxalate (1/4, 25%). During the long term follow-up, the renal function remained stable in 3 of 4 patients. Only one patient had a decrease in renal function, but no one progressed to the end-stage kidney disease requiring dialysis. All postoperative urine culture results were coincident with the preoperative results. Although all preoperative UTIs were treated with culture-specific antibiotics, the UTIs were not eliminated thoroughly without removing the infectious stones in some cases. Four (9.8%) patients had hemorrhage, and only one required blood transfusion when the hemoglobin level dropped below 80 g/L. All patients with hemorrhage were cured conservatively, and no one received angioembolization. Two patients had prolonged hospitalization time because of urinary leakage from nephrostomy tract after

removal of the tube, which was resolved spontaneously without any specific intervention. No sepsis and other complications were detected in any patients after interventions.

Discussion

Treatment of patients with solitary kidney having intrarenal calculi is one of the most challenging problems in urology. An untreated intrarenal stone is likely to destroy the renal function and/or cause life-threatening sepsis [15]. The optimal goal of surgery is complete removal of the stone to prevent further stone formation and any correlative infection, and to preserve the renal function as far as possible [2]. For intrarenal stone, there are several alternative treatments, such as ESWL, PCNL, combination therapy, and open surgery [2,16,17]. Because of the relatively low SFR in managing large stone, risk of steinstrasse, and a high rate of retreatment, ESWL monotherapy has a very limited indication [17]. According to the AUA Guidelines, PCNL is characterized with a SFR of 74 to 83%, a blood transfusion rate of 14 to 24%, an acute complication rate of 15%, an auxiliary treatment rate of 18%, and has many advantages when compared with treatment alternatives such as ESWL monotherapy, combination therapy, and open surgery, especially in managing the complex or staghorn calculi [18]. Although standard PCNL is a well-recognized safe and efficient treatment for intrarenal calculi, it can still be associated with significant complications, such as uncontrolled hemorrhage, sepsis, injury to collecting system and surrounding viscera, even loss of kidney. The blood transfusion rates have been reported from 0.8% to 45% [19]. El-Nahas et al [20] demonstrated that the presence of solitary kidney was a significant risk factor of hemorrhage because compensatory hypertrophy of the renal parenchyma is a physiological response to solitary kidney. It is more likely to increase the risk of hemorrhage when urologists puncture and dilate the thick renal parenchyma because of damaging more renal tissue and blood vessel. Uncontrolled

Table 1. Patient, stone demographics and operative characteristics.

Age (Mean±SD, range) (year)	51.4±14.7 (16–69)
Gender (n, %)	
Male	27 (65.9%)
Female	14 (34.1%)
Cause of solitary kidney (n, %)	
Congential	4 (9.8%)
Previous nephrectomy	30 (73.2%)
Nonperfused kidney	7 (17.0%)
Stone side (n, %)	
Left	19 (46.3%)
Right	22 (53.7%)
Stone number (n, %)	
Single	30 (73.2%)
Multiple	11 (26.8%)
Stone type (n, %)	
Simple	15 (36.6%)
Complex	26 (63.4%)
Stone size (Mean±SD, range) (mm²)	912±517 (300–1800)
Previous renal intervention history (n, %)	
Open surgery	1 (2.4%)
ESWL	2 (4.9%)
PCNL	3 (7.3%)
Grade of hydronephrosis (n, %)	
None or mild	13 (31.7%)
Moderate or severe	28 (68.3%)
Positive preoperative urine culture (n, %)	7 (17.1%)
Preoperative serum hemoglobin (Mean±SD, range) (g/L)	114.7±26.9 (87–141)
Preoperative serum creatinine (Mean±SD, range) (umol/L)	132.1±41.3 (78.2–231.4)
Baseline GFR (Mean±SD, range) (ml/min)	74.9±24.2 (35.0–110.0)
Number of tract (n, %)	
Single	32 (78.0%)
Multiple	9 (22.0%)
Operative time (Mean±SD, range) (min)	71.3±23.5 (40–139)
Stone-free rate (n, %)	
Initial stone-free rate	35 (85.4%)
Final stone-free rate	40 (97.6%)
Auxiliary procedure requirement (n, %)	
ESWL	4 (9.8%)
Flexible ureteroscopy	2 (4.9%)
Nephrostomy tube removal time (Mean±SD, range) (day)	4.4±0.3 (4–7)
Hospitalization time (Mean±SD, range) (day)	6.1±0.5 (5–11)
Stone composition (n, %)	
Calcium oxalate	16 (39.0%)
Struvite	7 (17.1%)
Cystine	1 (2.4%)
Uric acid	2 (4.9%)
Mix	4 (9.8%)
Calcium oxalate and phosphate	11 (26.8%)

ESWL: extracorporeal shock wave lithotripsy.
PCNL: percutaneous nephrolithotomy.
GFR: glomerular filtration rate.
SD: standard deviation.

Table 2. Details of complications.

Postoperative fever	5 (12.2%)
Urinary tract infection	4 (9.8%)
Hemorrhage and hematuria	4 (9.8%)
Blood transfusion	1 (2.4%)
Prolonged tract leakage	2 (4.9%)

hemorrhage may require angioembolization or even nephrectomy [21]. Furthermore, major complications can lead to significant mortality, especially in patients with solitary kidney. Meanwhile, in clinical practice, the standard tract and endoscope may be too large for managing pediatric kidneys and some undilated adult kidneys.

To decrease the invasiveness and broaden the indication, Chinese urologists have modified the technique by using an 8/9.8 F rigid ureteroscope to manage the upper urinary tract calculi via 14–18 F percutaneous tract provided by fascial dilator and matched peer-away sheath. Compared with the tract of standard PCNL (26–30 F), the small tract (14–18 F) of Chinese MPCNL obviously reduced the damage of renal parenchyma and vessel. During the small tract dilation, the fascial dilator was pushed ahead with rotation, which pushed the vessels aside without injury. In our study, there was only one patient of hemorrhage that needed blood transfusion, and no uncontrolled hemorrhage was detected. The patient who needed blood transfusion, when the hemoglobin dropped below 80 g/L, had a complete staghorn stone with preoperative UTI (*E. coli*) and was treated conservatively with blood transfusion, hemostatic agents, bed rest and clamping the nephrostomy tube, which was resolved spontaneously without a super-selective embolization. The rates of transfusion and uncontrolled hemorrhage were significantly lower than those of standard PCNL previously reported in literature [22]. Meanwhile, approaching the collecting system through the posterior middle calyx provided the most direct and shortest tract from skin to collecting system, and may enable to access the majority of the collecting system even proximal ureter via the small endoscope with minimal deformity and torque on both the renal parenchyma and endoscope to manage the complex or staghorn stone through single tract [23]. Torquing the endoscope against the renal parenchyma to access calyx is one of the most important reasons of hemorrhage and has a positive correlation with high rates of blood transfusion and urinary leakage [24]. Taking all these factors into consideration, we believe that Chinese MPCNL has less invasiveness than standard PCNL. To shorten the operative time, small fragments were flushed out by forceful pulse stream produced by a pulse perfusion pump, and the big fragments were removed by forceps under direct vision of endoscope. Many researchers claimed that the small tract would obviously increase the intrapelvic pressure and result in backflow of irrigation fluid containing endotoxin or bacteria which would induce to bacteremia or even sepsis. Zhong W et al reported the mean intrapelvic pressures were 24.55, 16.49, 11.22, and 6.64 mmHg with the 14 F, 16 F, 18 F, and double-16 F tracts, which remained lower than the level causing backflow (30 mmHg) during Chinese MPCNL [8]. The low intrapelvic pressure is associated with the seldom possibility of postoperative fever and sepsis. In patients with staghorn or complex stones, it was usually hard to achieve complete stone-free with a single tract, especially when the residual calculi located in a calyx parallel to the previous

tract. Combined ESWL and flexible ureteroscopy can reduce the need of multiple tracts to manage complex or staghorn calculi. Furthermore, with the advancements in flexible ureteroscopic technology, the need of combined ESWL has been decreased [25]. Combined ESWL is considered for patients with small residual stone (≤2 cm) whose general medical condition prohibits the use of multiple tracts or flexible ureteroscopy. The combined PCNL and flexible ureteroscopy can effectively reduce the need of multiple tracts in complex or staghorn stones with a low rate of complication and discomfort, but does not significantly impact the final SFR and operative time [26]. For patients with a large residual stone burden, the multiple tracts Chinese MPCNL should be considered, because it not only decreased the intrapelvic pressure, but also flushed out the small fragments from the other tract, which obviously shortened the operative time and increased the SFR without increasing the potential morbidity [23]. In our opinion, Chinses MPCNL can broaden its indication for all kinds of upper urinary tract calculi that need standard PCNL intervention [27].

Controversy remains on the issue of whether Chinese MPCNL has the potential effect on renal function of solitary kidney. Traxer et al [28] investigated the extent of renal parenchyma injury in pigs underwent percutaneous puncture. They demonstrated a mean estimated parenchyma scar volume of the 30 F tract was 0.40 ml, which was equal to a mean parenchyma loss of 0.91%. Compared to the overall renal volume, the parenchyma scar resulting from the percutaneous tract is very small, so the influence of renal function induced by percutaneous tract can be ignored. Streem et al [29] reported Scr had no difference at one month in 5 patients who underwent PCNL with solitary kidney. Canes et al [30] reported that the renal function was preserved or even slightly improved, and the GFR level significantly increased one year after PCNL. In our study, a significant improvement in Scr and GFR was detected from preoperative period to one month follow-up. Mean Scr before Chinese MPCNL was 132.1±41.3 umol/L (range: 78.2–231.4) compared to 108.9±30.7 umol/L (range: 71.6–136.9) by the end of the one month follow-up period. The same results were observed in GFR. The mean preoperative GFR was 74.9±24.2 ml/min (range: 35.0–110.0) and calculated at 83.9±27.4 ml/min (range: 65.0–110.0) during the one month follow-up period. However, during the long-term follow-up, the renal function of some patients may gradually aggravate. The comorbidities in these patients such as hypertension, atherosclerosis, diabetes mellitus, and other diseases that could damage the kidney were the risk factors for worsening the renal function. In our study, one patient with decreasing renal function at the long term follow-up was diabetic.

Previous study has demonstrated that the patients with diabetes mellitus, large stone burden, UTI and impaired renal function (IRF) were more likely to require longer hospitalization time [31,32]. Patients with diabetes mellitus have a significantly higher incidence of perioperative complications, including uncontrolled hemorrhage requiring blood transfusion and severe UTI causing life-threatening sepsis. Meanwhile, the relationship between the hospitalization time and stone burden may be explained by longer operative time, higher complication rates of hemorrhage or urine extravasation, and increased requirements for auxiliary procedures in patients with a large stone burden. Furthermore, patients with IRF are usually anemic, and have coagulopathy. Therefore, the incidence of uncontrolled hemorrhage requiring blood transfusion or even super-selective embolization is higher in these patients. In our study, the mean hospitalization time was 6.1±0.5 days (range: 5–11 days), which was longer than previously reported by other authors. Mishra S et al prospectively compared 26 patients with MPCNL and 26 with standard PCNL. The results demonstrated that significant advantages of MPCNL over standard PCNL in terms of reduced hospitalization time (3.2 ± 0.8 vs 4.8 ± 0.6 days, $P\leq0.001$) [33]. Akman T et al retrospectively reported on 47 patients underwent PCNL with a solitary kidney. The mean hospitalization time was 2.87 ± 1.57 days [22]. China is a developing country, so Chinese MPCNL has been applied just in some major clinic. Because of the immature community medical system, patients are unwilling to discharge unless they can make a full recovery. What's more important, all preoperative examinations and preparations must be performed in the hospitalization according to the medical insurance system, which spends almost an extra 3 days and artificially increases the hospitalization time. Similarly, Zhong W et al reported on 29 Chinese patients with staghorn calculi ranging from 8.8 to 22.8 cm^2 (mean 11.7 cm^2) underwent Chinese MPCNL. Mean hospital stay was 9.8 days (range: 6–13 days) [34]. These reasons may explain why the hospitalization time in our study was longer than previously reported by other authors.

Recent interest in tubeless PCNL, in which a D–J stent is used in place of the nephrostomy tube, results from hopes of a shorter hospitalization time and a decrease in the discomfort associated with standard PCNL. Several studies have demonstrated that the use of tubeless procedure presents a shorter hospitalization time. Akman T et al retrospectively reviewed 1658 patients with renal calculi underwent PCNL. The mean hospitalization time was 2.89 ± 1.66 days (range: 1–21 days). Furthermore, the mean hospitalization time was 2.93 ± 1.70 days and 2.12 ± 0.53 days in patients underwent the standard PCNL and tubeless PCNL procedures, respectively ($P<0.0001$). According to their outcome of multivariate analysis, the tubeless procedure was variables diminishing the hospitalization time ($P = 0.0001$, $OR = 0.23$) [31]. Borges CF et al performed a systematic review with meta-analysis to compare tubeless versus conventional PCNL. Meta-analysis of data showed a benefit of shorter hospitalization time in tubeless PCNL group than conventional group (Mean difference: -1.11; CI 95% = -1.55 to -0.68; $P<0.00001$) [35]. However, tubeless PCNL was indicated in patients with mild-to-moderate stone burden, no perioperative complication, no residual stones needing auxiliary procedures, or depending on surgeon's experience [31]. Shoma AM et al reported on 100 patients with upper tract calculi randomized to tubeless and standard PCNL group using closed envelops. The results of their study showed that tubeless PCNL might be unsuitable for the patients with CKD or a supracostal approach [36]. In our study, most patients with solitary kidney underwent Chinese MPCNL via the 11th intercostal tract. Eleven patients had CKD stage 1, 15 had stage 2, 12 had stage 3, and 3 had stage 4. The associated coagulopathy in patients with CKD could increase the risk of hemorrhage, especially in the absence of

nephrostomy tube. The nephrostomy tube plays an important role in draining the urine, establishing hemostasis, avoiding obstruction resulting from blood clots and residual fragments, and retaining the access tract for a staged procedure. Furthermore, a good drainage is very important to patients with solitary kidney underwent Chinese MPCNL via supracostal tract for avoiding secondary infection resulting from hematomas or urine extravasation, and hemothorax if blood clots obstruct the collecting system. Meanwhile, most patients in our study underwent Chinese MPCNL with guidance of ultrasonography, and the flexible ureteroscopy was not widely applied because of economic condition and medical insurance. The certain stone-free status needed to be evaluated postoperatively by imaging examinations. So the D–J stent use together with nephrostomy tube can be explained by little confidence in intraoperative assessment of residual stones and potential requirements for auxiliary procedures, including second-look PCNL, ESWL and flexible ureteroscopy. In our opinion, adequate drainage is very important for patients with solitary kidney in order to prevent urine extravasation, perinephric hematomas, obstruction resulting from the blood clots and residual fragments, and to preserve the renal function as far as possible. Because of the relative harsh healthcare environment of our country, doctors must critically evaluate the interventions that we perform with an eye toward improving their safety. Therefore, we are not very optimistic with the use of a single D–J stent or nephrostomy tube in patients with solitary kidney. Further studies are required to evaluate the safety of single-use D–J stent or nephrostomy tube in such patients.

Our study has some limitations as well. Firstly, this was a study about a small group of patients from a single institution. Secondly, because of the small working channel of the ureteroscope, the vision might not be clear, especially when patient had bleeding in operation. Thirdly, since this is a retrospective study, stone culture and associated metabolic study were not performed.

In conclusion, our clinical experience with Chinese MPCNL demonstrates that it is safe, feasible, and efficient for managing intrarenal calculi in solitary kidney with a satisfactory SFR and morbidity compared with standard PCNL. The renal function remained stable or even improved in the majority of patients underwent Chinese MPCNL with solitary kidney at both short-term and long-term follow-up.

Author Contributions

Conceived and designed the experiments: ZH XZ. Performed the experiments: ZH XZ RX FF. Analyzed the data: ZH ZZ LZ. Contributed reagents/materials/analysis tools: ZH XZ FF. Wrote the paper: ZH XZ. Contribution type: ZH XZ FF.

References

1. Fernstrom I, Johansson B (1976) Percutaneous pyelolithotomy: a new extraction technique. Scand J Urol Nephrol 10: 257–259.

2. Preminger GM, Assimos DG, Lingeman JE, Nakada SY, Pearle MS, et al. (2005) CHAPTER 1: AUA GUIDELINE on management of staghorn calculi: diagnosis and treatment recommendations. J Urol 173: 1991–2000.

3. Michel MS, Trojan L, Rassweiler JJ (2007) Complications in percutaneous nephrolithotomy. Eur Urol 51: 899–906.

4. Jackman SV, Docimo SG, Cadeddu JA, Bishoff JT, Kavoussi LR, et al. (1998) The "mini-perc" technique: a less invasive alternative to percutaneous nephrolithotomy. World J Urol 16: 371–374.

5. Monga M, Oglevie S (2000) Minipercutaneous nephrolithotomy. J Endourol 14: 419–421.

6. Lahme S, Bichler KH, Strohmaier WL, Götz T (2001) Minimally invasive PCNL in patients with renal pelvic and calyceal stones. Eur Urol 40: 619–624.

7. Giusti G, Piccinelli A, Taverna G, Benetti A, Pasini L, et al. (2007) Miniperc? No, thank you! Eur Urol 51: 810–814; discussion 815.

8. Zhong W, Zeng G, WU K, Li X, Chen W, et al. (2008) Does a smaller tract in percutaneous nephrolithotomy contribute to high renal pelvic pressure and postoperative fever? J Endourol 22: 2147–2151.

9. Li X, Wu KJ (1998) Multiple channel percutaneous nephrolithotomy in the treatment of complex renal calculi. Chin J Urol 19: 469–470.

10. Li X, Zeng GH, Yuan J, Wu KJ, Shan CC, et al. (2004) Treatment of upper urinary calculi with the PCNL technique (Experience of 20 years). Beijing Da Xue Xue Bao 36: 124–126.

11. Tiselius HG, Alken P, Buck C, Gallucci M, Knoll T, et al. (2008) Guidelines on Urolithiasis. Eur Assoc Urol.

12. Rassweiler JJ, Renner C, Eisenberger F (2000) The management of complex renal stones. BJU Int 86: 919–928.

13. Cockcroft DW, Gault MH (1976) Prediction of creatinine clearance from serum creatinine. Nephron 16: 31–41.

14. Levey AS, Coresh J, Balk E, Kausz AT, Levin A, et al. (2003) National Kidney Foundation practice guidelines for chronic kidney disease: evaluation, classification, and stratification. Ann Intern Med 139: 137–147.

15. Ganpule AP, Desai M (2008) Management of the staghorn calculus: multiple-tract versus single-tract percutaneous nephrolithotomy. Curr Opin Urol 18: 220–223.

16. Chandhoke PS (1996) Cost-effectiveness of different treatment options for staghorn calculi. J Urol 156: 1567–1571.

17. Webb DR, Payne SR, Wickham JE (1986) Extracorporeal shock wave lithotripsy and percutaneous renal surgery. Comparisons, combinations and conclusions. Br J Urol 58: 1–5.

18. Singla M, Srivastava A, Kapoor R, Gupta N, Ansari MS, et al. (2008) Aggressive approach to staghorn calculi-safety and efficacy of multiple tracts percutaneous nephrolithotomy. Urology 71: 1039–1042.

19. Stoller ML, Wolf JS Jr, St Lezin MA (1994) Estimated blood loss and transfusion rates associated with percutaneous nephrolithotomy. J Urol 152 (6 Pt 1): 1977–1981.

20. El-Nahas AR, Shokeir AA, El-Assmy AM, Mohsen T, Shoma AM, et al. (2007) Post-percutaneous nephrolithotomy extensive hemorrhage: a study of risk factors. J Urol 177: 576–579.

21. Kessaris DN, Bellman GC, Pardalidis NP, Smith AG (1995) Management of hemorrhage after percutaneous renal surgery. J Urol 153 (3 Pt 1): 604–608.

22. Akman T, Binbay M, Tekinarslan E, Ozkuvanci U, Kezer C, et al. (2011) Outcomes of percutaneous nephrolithotomy in patients with solitary kidneys: a single-center experience. Urology 78: 272–276.

23. Guohua Z, Zhong W, Li X, Wu K, Chen W, et al. (2007) Minimally invasive percutaneous nephrolithotomy for staghorn calculi: a novel single session approach via multiple 14–18 Fr tracts. Surg Laparosc Endosc Percutan Tech 17: 124–128.

24. Aron M, Yadav R, Goel R (2005) Multi-tract percutaneous nephrolithotomy for large complete staghorn calculi. Urol Int 75: 327–332.

25. Desai M, Jain P, Ganpule A, Sabnis R, Patel S, et al. (2009) Developments in technique and technology: the effect on the results of percutaneous nephrolithotomy for staghorn calculi. BJU Int 104: 542–548; discussion 548.

26. Marguet CG, Springhart WP, Tan YH, Patel A, Undre S, et al. (2005) Simultaneous combined use of flexible ureteroscopy and percutaneous nephrolithotomy to reduce the number of access tracts in the management of complex renal calculi. BJU Int 96: 1097–1100.

27. He Z, Li X, Chen L, Zeng G, Yuan J (2007) Minimally invasive percutaneous nephrolithotomy for upper urinary tract calculi in transplanted kidneys. BJU Int 99: 1467–1471.

28. Traxer O, Smith TG 3rd, Pearle MS, Corwin TS, Saboorian H, et al. (2001) Renal parenchymal injury after standard and mini percutaneous nephrostolithotomy. J Urol 165: 1693–1695.

29. Streem SB, Zelch MG, Risius B, Geisinger MA (1986) Percutaneous extraction of renal calculi in patients with solitary kidneys. Urology 27: 247–252.

30. Canes D, Hegarty NJ, Kamoi K, Haber GP, Berger A, et al. (2009) Functional outcomes following percutaneous surgery in the solitary kidney. J Urol 181: 154–160.

31. Akman T, Binbay M, Yuruk E, Sari E, Seyrek M, et al. (2011) Tubeless procedure is most important factor in reducing length of hospitalization after percutaneous nephrolithotomy: results of univariable and multivariable models. Urology 77: 299–304.

32. Matlaga BR, Hodges SJ, Shah OD, Passmore L, Hart LJ, et al. (2004) Percutaneous nephrostolithotomy: predictors of length of stay. J Urol 172 (4 Pt 1): 1351–1354.

33. Mishra S, Sharma R, Garg C, Kurien A, Sabnis R, et al. (2011) Prospective comparative study of miniperc and standard PNL for treatment of 1 to 2 cm size renal stone. BJU Int 108: 896–899; discussion 899–900.

34. Zhong W, Zeng G, Wu W, Chen W, Wu K (2011) Minimally invasive percutaneous nephrolithotomy with multiple mini tracts in a single session in treating staghorn calculi. Urol Res 39: 117–122.

35. Borges CF, Fregonesi A, Silva DC, Sasse AD (2010) Systematic Review and Meta-Analysis of Nephrostomy Placement Versus Tubeless Percutaneous Nephrolithotomy. J Endourol 24: 1739–1746.

36. Shoma AM, Elshal AM (2012) Nephrostomy tube placement after percutaneous nephrolithotomy: critical evaluation through a prospective randomized study. Urology 79: 771–776.

11

Incidence and Outcome of Acute Phosphate Nephropathy in Iceland

Vala Kolbrún Pálmadóttir[1], Hjalti Gudmundsson[1], Sverrir Hardarson[2], Margrét Árnadóttir[3], Thorvaldur Magnússon[4], Margrét B. Andrésdóttir[3]*

1 Department of Internal Medicine, Landspitali University Hospital, Reykjavik, Iceland, 2 Department of Pathology, Landspitali University Hospital, Reykjavik, Iceland, 3 Division of Nephrology, Landspitali University Hospital, Reykjavik, Iceland, 4 Department of Internal Medicine, Akranes Hospital, Akranes, Iceland

Abstract

Background: Oral sodium phosphate solutions (OSPS) are widely used for bowel cleansing prior to colonoscopy and other procedures. Cases of renal failure due to acute phosphate nephropathy following OSPS ingestion have been documented in recent years, questioning the safety of OSPS. However, the magnitude of the problem remains unknown.

Methodology/Principal Findings: We conducted a population based, retrospective analysis of medical records and biopsies of all cases of acute phosphate nephropathy that were diagnosed in our country in the period from January 2005 to October 2008. Utilizing the complete official sales figures of OSPS, we calculated the incidence of acute phosphate nephropathy in our country. Fifteen cases of acute phosphate nephropathy were diagnosed per 17,651 sold doses of OSPS (0.085%). Nine (60%) were women and mean age 69 years (range 56–75 years). Thirteen patients had a history of hypertension (87%) all of whom were treated with either ACE-I or ARB and/or diuretics. One patient had underlying DM type I and an active colitis and one patient had no risk factor for the development of acute phosphate nephropathy. Average baseline creatinine was 81.7 µmol/L and 180.1 at the discovery of acute renal failure, mean 4.2 months after OSPS ingestion. No patient had a full recovery of renal function, and at the end of follow-up, 26.6 months after the OSPS ingestion, the average creatinine was 184.2 µmol/L. The average eGFR declined from 73.5 ml/min/1.73 m^2 at baseline to 37.3 ml/min/1.73 m^2 at the end of follow-up. One patient reached end-stage renal disease and one patient died with progressive renal failure.

Conclusion/Significance: Acute phosphate nephropathy developed in almost one out of thousand sold doses of OSPS. The consequences for kidney function were detrimental. This information can be used in other populations to estimate the impact of OSPS. Our data suggest that acute phosphate nephropathy may be greatly underreported worldwide.

Editor: Niels Olsen Saraiva Câmara, Universidade de Sao Paulo, Brazil

Funding: No direct funding was received for this study and no use was made of internal departmental funds. The authors were personally salaried by their institutions during the period of writing. No funding bodies had any role in the study design, data collection, analysis, decision to publish or preparation of the manuscript.

Competing Interests: The authors have declared that no competing interests exist.

* E-mail: mband@landspitali.is

Introduction

Acute kidney injury (AKI) and subsequent chronic kidney disease (CKD) have been reported after bowel cleansing with oral sodium phosphate solutions (OSPS) [1]. The clinical pathological entity has been termed "acute phosphate nephropathy" and is caused by deposition of calcium phosphate crystals in the renal tubules, resulting in acute tubular injury and eventual tubular atrophy and interstitial fibrosis [2]. The first biopsy proven case report of this toxic side effect on the kidneys was published in 2003 [3], 13 years after sodium phosphate solutions began to be used as a purgative for colonoscopy [4]. Subsequently, fewer than 40 cases of acute phosphate nephropathy have been reported worldwide, with risk factors of age (60+), female gender, hypertension, angiotensin converting enzyme inhibitors (ACE-I), angiotensin receptor blockade (ARB), diuretics and chronic kidney disease [5–7]. During the follow-up of patients with acute phosphate nephropathy, four progressed to end-stage renal disease while the remaining patients

manifested chronic kidney disease [7]. Thus, while an association between acute phosphate nephropathy and the ingestion of OSPS has been well documented, there are no clear indications of the global magnitude of this clinical problem. In fact, most clinicians assume that acute phosphate nephropathy is a rare but serious side effect of OSPS. In contrast, we hypothesize that the magnitude of the problem is highly underestimated and in fact that the majority of cases remain unrecognized. Most cases of acute phosphate nephropathy are clinically silent, and are often diagnosed by chance many months after the ingestion of the OSPS. Furthermore, elderly patients with an unexplained rise in creatinine without urinary abnormalities are not likely to undergo a renal biopsy. As OSPS has been a popular purgative for colonoscopy for almost 20 years in many countries it is possible that many individuals have suffered unrecognized acute and subsequent chronic kidney injury following ingestion of OSPS. A better knowledge of the incidence of acute phosphate nephropathy could help to elucidate the magnitude of this clinical problem.

Here we present a population based, retrospective analysis of all cases of acute phosphate nephropathy in Iceland. Furthermore, we are able to provide the minimum incidence rate of acute phosphate nephropathy in our country utilizing the complete official sales figures of OSPS in Iceland.

Materials and Methods

This is a retrospective analysis of medical records and biopsies of all cases of acute phosphate nephropathy that were diagnosed at Landspitali University Hospital in Reykjavik, during the period from January 2005 to October 2008. The study was approved by the Icelandic Data Protection Authority, the Bioethics Committee of Landspitali University Hospital and written consent was obtained from all living participants.

Diagnostic criteria were, as proposed by Markowitz et al. [8], (1) (acute) renal failure (2) pathologic findings of acute and/or chronic tubular injury with abundant tubular calcium phosphate deposition and (3) exposure to oral sodium phosphate bowel cleansing (Phosphoral (45 ml×2), Laboratories Casen-Fleet S.L.U.). Index cases were found by reviewing the pathological diagnosis of renal biopsies performed in the study period. Medical records were reviewed for age, gender, medical history, medication, the ingested dose of OSPS, indication for colonoscopy and symptoms after OSPS ingestion. The following serum creatinine values were documented: at baseline, at presentation of kidney injury, at the time of renal biopsy, the highest available, and the latest value. Estimated glomerular filtration rate (eGFR) was calculated according to the CKD-EPI (Chronic Kidney Disease Epidemiology Collaboration) equation [9]. Other laboratory results that were registered included haemoglobin level, s-calcium, s-phosphate and urinalysis, all were collected at or around the time of detection of renal failure. Patients were followed until September 30th 2009, date of starting renal replacement therapy or death, whichever came first.

Oral sodium phosphate solution (Phosphoral, 45 ml×2) was available without prescription in Iceland during the period March 1999 until May 2009, but since that time it has only been available by prescription. Yearly sales figures of Phosporal (45 ml×2) in Iceland were obtained from the Icelandic Medicines Control Agency (personal communication).

All renal biopsies were obtained and processed at Landspitali University Hospital in Reykjavík. Standard processing of renal biopsies included light microscopy and immunofluorescence. Light microscopy biopsies were stained with hematoxylin and eosin, periodic acid-Schiff, Massons's trichrome, and Jones methenamine silver. All cases were examined under polarized light and stained with von Kossa to differentiate calcium phosphate (nonpolarizable, von Kossa positive) from calcium oxalate (polarizable, von Kossa negative). For immunofluorescence, 3 μm cryostat sections sections were stained with polyclonal FITC-conjugated antibodies to IgG, IgA, IgM, C3, kappa, lambda, fibrinogen and albuminn (Dako). Calcium phosphate deposits were quantified on a scale from 1+ to 4+.

Statistical analysis

Descriptive summary statistics, including mean, median, standard deviation, and/or range were computed.

Results

Incidence rate

Fifteen cases of acute phosphate nephropathy were diagnosed between January 2005 and October 2008. They were preceded by OSPS (Phosphoral) bowel cleansing for colonoscopy in 14 cases and for preparation for colon operation in one. During this period, 17,651 doses of Phosphoral were sold in the country (incidence 0.085%).

Clinical characteristics of patients

The demographic data and clinical characteristics of the patients are shown in table 1. Sixty percent of the patients were women and the mean age at OSPS ingestion was 68.8 years (SD 7.0, range 56–77 years). Thirteen patients had a history of hypertension and all were treated with either ACE-I or ARB (N = 10) and/or diuretics (N = 8) at the time of OSPS bowel cleansing. One patient had DM type 1 and two patients had DM type 2. Two patients had a history of colitis ulcerosa. One patient had no concomitant illness (patient no 11). None of the patients had known hyperparathyroidism, heart failure or liver disease. At the presentation of kidney disease, 12 patients had s-calcium and phosphate levels within normal range, whereas three patients had low s-calcium and high s-phosphate. The majority of patients (73%) were anaemic at the time of presentation.

The indication for colonoscopy was anaemia in four cases, gastrointestinal discomfort (constipation, abdominal pain, diarrhea) in three, unknown in four patients and one each had unexplained weight loss, regular control of colitis ulcerosa (not active at the time of colonoscopy), control of incidental tumor finding on CT and preparation for colon operation. It was documented that all patients had used OSPS for bowel cleansing; four patients took 45 mL bottles ×2 and reported having definitely followed instructions. Patient no 3 threw up the first bottle so she ingested an extra bottle. Patient no 6 had bowel cleansing three times with OSPS in a three month period, two times for colonoscopy and once in preparation for radiography of the colon. The remaining nine patients all ingested OSPS for bowel cleansing, but it is not documented whether they followed the instructions closely or not. Most patients either denied any symptoms following the OSPS ingestion or symptoms were vague and non-specific (no symptoms (5), thirst (2), increased diuresis (1), persistent diarrhea and weight loss (1), malaise (1), cough (1), unknown (4)). One patient (no 4) had colonoscopy because of diarrhoea and was diagnosed with Clostridia difficile colitis. This patient was, unlike the other patients, hospitalized after the colonoscopy and more acutely ill.

Kidney function

An overview of kidney function before and after ingestion of OSPS is shown for each patient in table 2. Baseline creatinine was available in all patients at the average 4.4 months (SD 6.7 range 0–25.8 months) before the OSPS ingestion. Mean baseline creatinine was 81.7 μmol/L and mean eGFR was 73.5 ml/min/1.73 m². Four patients had an eGFR of <60 ml/min/1.73 m² at baseline. Deterioration of kidney function was diagnosed 4.2 months (mean, SD 4.5, range 1 day–16.3 months) after OSPS ingestion. The average creatinine at discovery of acute kidney injury was 180.1 μmol/L. The peak creatinine was on average 247.2 μmol/L and 217.8 when the biopsy was performed, which occurred at a median 6.2 months (range 0.4–39.8 months) after the ingestion of OSPS. After the initial rise in serum creatinine, it decreased with time in most patients (87%), but progressed in two, one of them received treatment for ESRD (no 8) and one died 17.8 months after OSPS ingestion from pneumonia (no 4). Patients have been followed for an average of 26.6 months after the OSPS ingestion, ranging from 5.3 to 65.9 months and at latest follow-up, the average creatinine was 184.3 μmol/L. The average eGFR declined from 73.5 ml/min/1.73 m² at baseline to 37.3 ml/min/

Table 1. Demographics and clinical characteristics of patients with acute phosphate nephropathy after OSPS ingestion.[a]

Patient	Age, sex	HT	DM	ACE-i/ARB	Diuretics	Proteinuria	Urinary sediment	S- calcium	S-phosphorus	Hemoglobin
1	59F	Y	N	Y	Y	Negative	10–25 wbc, 2–5 rbc	2.38	1.43	108
2	58M	Y	N	Y	Y	260 mg/24 hr	No abnormalities	2.25	1.17	109
3	75F	Y	N	Y	Y	0.13 g/24 hr	No abnormalities	1.05[b]	1.86	112
4	65M	N	Y type 1	N	N	Negative	2–5 wbc, 1–2 rbc[c]	1.97	1.66	126
5	71F	Y	N	Y	N	Negative	5–10 wbc, 1–2 rbc	1.32	1.19	84
6	74F	Y	N	Y	N	Negative	>100 wbc, 1–2 rbc, +++bacteria[d]	1.23	1.60	131
7	69F	Y	N	Y	N	Negative	5–10 wbc, 1–2 rbc	2.20	1.33	114
8	77M	Y	Y type 2	N	Y	Negative	No abnormalities	1.0[b]	2.31	111
9	56M	Y	N	Y	Y	Negative	No abnormalities	2.26	1.12	118
10	74F	Y	N	N	Y	Negative	10–25 wbc, 1–2 rbc	1.21[b]	1.33	114
11	62F	N	N	N	N	Negative	No abnormalities	1.30	1.02	150
12	71M	Y	Y type 2	Y	N	(+)	2–5 wbc, 5–10 rbc[c]	1.13[b]	0.99	135
13	71M	Y	N	Y	N	Negative	1–2 wbc	1.23[b]	1.41	116
14	75F	Y	N	N	Y	Negative	1–2 wbc, 2–5 rbc[c]	1.23[b]	1.21	85
15	75F	Y	N	Y	Y	Negative	25–50 wbc	1.25[b]	1.39	105

[a]Abbreviation used in table: HT, hypertension; DM, diabetes mellitus; ACE-i, Angiotensin convertive enzyme inhibitor; ARB, angiotensin receptor blockade; Y, yes; N, no; WNR, withing normal range; wbc, white blood cells; rbc, red blood cells. Normal values for s-calcium, 2.15–2.60 mmol/L; ionized calcium, 1.13–1.33 mmol/L; s-phosphorus, 0.75–1.65 mmol/L; Hemoglobin, 118–152 g/L (women), 134–171 g/L (men).
[b]Ionized s-calcium.
[c]In these sediments, hyaline, tubular cell, granular or Muddy Brown casts were also seen.
[d]After treatment of the UTI, urine analysis was normal.

1.73 m^2 at the end of follow-up and 13 patients had eGFR lower than $60 \text{ ml/min/}1.73 \text{ m}^2$.

The most frequent finding in the urinary sediment was sterile pyuria, with rare red blood cells. In some, hyaline, tubular cell or granular casts were seen. One patient had a urinary tract infection at the time of diagnosis. Urine dipstick was negative for protein in 12 patients and trace in one. Two patients had 24-hr urine protein measured, 260 and 130 mg/day, respectively (Table 1).

Renal biopsy findings

The renal biopsy findings in patients with acute phosphate nephropathy are shown in Table 3. As could be expected from this cohort of elderly people, global sclerosis of the glomeruli was seen in most biopsies (73%). Sampling for light microscopy included a mean of 20.2 glomeruli (range 5–44), and a mean of 3.7 (18.3%) glomeruli were sclerotic. Other glomeruli appeared normal. Vascular disease was mild or absent in most patient and considered to be moderate in one. The typical findings of acute phosphate nephropathy were present in all patients as shown in Figure 1. Calcium phosphate deposits were found mostly in distal tubules and collecting ducts, located within the cytoplasm of tubular epithelial cells, within tubular lumina, or in the interstitium. The calcifications did not polarize and stained intensely with von Kossa stain, which confirmed their composition as calcium phosphate. The quantity of calcium phosphate deposits was not associated with time after OSPS ingestion, increase in creatinine or the final outcome. Tubular injury was accompanied by interstitial oedema in particular in biopsies of two patients who had a biopsy taken at the earliest interval from OSPS ingestion, 12 and 30 days, respectively. Interstitial inflammation was seen in most biopsies (80%), but there did not seem to be a relationship between the length of time from OSPS ingestion to biopsy and the quantity of inflammation. Chronic, irreversible tubular injury in the form of tubular

atrophy and interstitial fibrosis was seen in all biopsies, ranging from 10 to 60% of the cortical area sampled.

Discussion

Acute phosphate nephropathy is an iatrogenic cause of kidney injury after bowel cleansing with OSPS. The relationship between ingestion of OSPS and the deposition of calcium and phosphate in the tubules, causing injury with subsequent interstitial scarring with concomitant loss of kidney function has been documented in 37 cases since 2003 [7]. The majority of the cases (21) come from a single-center study in the U.S. [2], single cases have been reported from other U.S. centers [3,10–12], Norway [13], Holland [14], Belgium [15], UK [16], Lebanon [17], Korea [18], New Zealand [19], and five from Israel [20], reflecting the widespread use of OSPS. We have diagnosed 15 additional patients with acute phosphate nephropathy since 2005, which are described in detail in this paper. Iceland has a population of 315,000 and one nephrology referral center which offers a unique opportunity to estimate the incidence of acute phosphate nephropathy following OSPS. Comparable estimation has not been possible to do in other countries [21]. Epidemiological studies, undertaken to assess the incidence of acute kidney injury after OSPS, have yielded conflicting results and have not fully elucidated this issue [22]. The largest study comprised 9799 individuals, 50 years of age or older, who had received either OSPS or polyethylene glycol (PEG) for bowel cleansing for colonoscopy. The incidence of acute kidney injury, defined by a ≥50% increase in serum creatinine, was 1.29% and 0.92%, for OSPS and PEG, respectively [23]. These studies are all hampered by the lack of renal biopsies for the diagnosis of acute phosphate nephropathy.

In total, 17,651 doses of Phosphoral (45 ml×2) were sold in Iceland during the study period. The incidence of acute phosphate nephropathy is thus 1/1177 doses of OSPS or

Table 2. Changes in kidney function before and after ingestion of oral sodium phosphate solutions.[a]

Patient	Age, sex	Kidney function -1[b]		Time -1[f]	Kidney function 1[c]	Time 1[g]	Kidney function 2[d]	Time 2[h]	Kidney function 3[e]		Time 3[i]
		SCr	eGFR	Days	SCr	Days	SCr	Months	SCr	eGFR	Months
1	59F	48	103	22	105	288	105	11.7	80	70	20.5
2	58M	67	101	93	170	95	166	9.6	116	59	22.9
3	75F	54	89	253	255	1	380	0.4	173	25	39.2
4	65M	73	93	61	120	0	312	1.0	440	11	17.8
5	71F	62	87	199	153	52	138	4.3	112	43	16.9
6	74F	66	79	10	310	104	308	3.5	121	38	7.7
7	69F	68	79	58	160	146	115	15.1	134	35	33.6
8	77M	92	69	7	131	2	555	39.8	554	8	46.4
9	56M	103	70	92	164	31	125	4.2	114	62	5.3
10	74F	81	62	775	194	45	198	6.2	170	25	27.2
11	62F	88	61	28	127	489	105	22.2	101	51	36
12	71M	110	58	3	144	275	132	18.3	144	41	33.8
13	71M	115	55	315	280	101	290	4.1	208	26	43.1
14	75F	98	49	0	239	185	221	6.6	194	21	23.1
15	75F	100	48	61	150	62	117	3.8	103	45	25.8

[a]Abbreviations used in table: SCr, s-creatinine in μmol/L; eGFR, estimated glomerular filtration rate in ml/min/1.73 m[2], calculated using CKD-EPI (Chronic Kidney Disease Epidemiology Collaboration) equation (see Methods).
[b]Kidney function -1, baseline value of SCr and eGFR (before ingestion of OSPS);
[c]Kidney function 1, SCr at presentation;
[d]Kidney function 2, SCr at the time of renal biopsy;
[e]Kidney function 3, SCr and eGFR at the time of last follow-up.
[f]Time -1, days between measurement of baseline creatinine and the ingestion of OSPS;
[g]Time 1, days between the ingestion of OSPS and the discovery of AKI;
[h]Time 2, months between the ingestion of OSPS and kidney biopsy;
[i]Time 3, months between ingestion of OSPS and the last follow-up.

1/2064 if all doses that have ever been sold in the country are taken into account (30,958). However, these numbers likely underestimate the magnitude of the problem, as sold doses of OSPS have not necessarily all been ingested and also because the diagnosis requires a kidney biopsy. Our study shows that the symptoms are frequently vague or even absent, and that the diagnosis of acute kidney injury is commonly found by chance. When these patients present with a rise in creatinine they are unlikely to undergo a renal biopsy for definite diagnosis for several reasons: Individuals at risk for developing acute phosphate nephropathy are elderly people (all above 55 years in our study), have a history of hypertension and are treated with medications that can cause fluctuations in the kidney function, i.e. diuretics and ACE-I or ARB and present with a bland urine sediment without clinically important proteinuria. The lag time between the marketing of the OSPS and the recognition of acute phosphate nephropathy as a side effect, which was six years in our country and up to 13 years in the U.S., emphasizes how latent and unexpected this condition is.

How do our results then compare with findings in other populations? Twenty-five cases of acute phosphate nephropathy have been reported in the medical literature coming from the U.S. [2,3,10–12]. However, based on our data we would expect 15,000 cases, in light of the proportional size differences of the U.S. and Icelandic populations (the U.S. has approximately thousand fold more inhabitants than Iceland). This striking difference is an obvious argument for the underreporting of acute phosphate nephropathy worldwide. Furthermore, we predict that the prevalence of acute phosphate nephropathy is even greater in the U.S., and the direct extrapolation based on number of

inhabitants may be a bias towards an underestimation of the problem. OSPS has been the preferred purgative in both countries; one U.S. center reported sodium phosphate purgatives to be used in up to 80–90% of patients for bowel preparation for colonoscopy [6]. It is, however, likely that colonoscopies are done more frequently in the U.S. compared to Iceland as routine screening for colon and rectal cancer with colonoscopy has not been put into practice in Iceland. In the U.S. the rate of screening colonoscopy increased dramatically after the introduction of full Medicare coverage of the procedure in 2002 [24,25].

The main limitation of the present study is its retrospective character and the lack of a control group. Our calculation of the national incidence of acute phosphate nephropathy is therefore crude, and most likely biased towards underestimation of the problem. Also there is incomplete information on the adherence to the prescribed hydration regimens and limited ability to find new risk factors. Despite these limitations, this is the only study available that is able to estimate the magnitude of the renal complication of OSPS use.

The large number of cases that have been diagnosed in Iceland compared to other countries is most likely due to the close collaboration of a small group of nephrologists (7) who receive all nephrology referrals in the country. They have been aware of acute phosphate nephropathy as a complication of OSPS use from the beginning of 2005. The nephrologists attend the meetings with a single pathologist and discuss all cases. Such setup can increase the awareness of both sides and may have lead to an increase in biopsies taken, especially when there was a history of exposure of OSPS (which has become a routine question in the case of an unexplained rise in s-creatinine). The pathologist may also have

Table 3. Biopsy results of 15 patients after ingestion of oral sodium phosphate solution.[a]

Patient	Glomeruli		Interstitium				Arteriolar hyalinosis	Other pathology
	Total number	Global sclerosis	Ca/P	TA/IF	Oedema	Inflammation		
1	32	2	4+	50%	-	++	none/mild	No
2	29	2	3+	40%	-	±	none/mild	No
3	5	0	3+	30%	++	-	none/mild	No
4	20	0	2+	30%	++	+	mild	No
5	24	4	3+	30%	-	+	none/mild	No
6	22	5	3+	30%	+	+	none/mild	No
7	22	9	2+	40%	-	+	mild	No
8	19	3	2+	60%	-	±	moderate	No
9	22	5	2+	40%	-	±	mild	No
10	10	0	3+	30%	-	±	none/mild	No
11	11	3	3+	10%	-	-	none/mild	No
12	10	4	1+	30%	+	+	mild	No
13	8	0	3+	50%	(+)	-	none/mild	No
14	25	5	3+	30%	-	+	mild	No
15	44	14	3+	50%	-	++	mild	No

[a]Abbreviations used in table: Ca, calcium; P, phosphate; TA, tubular atrophy; IF, interstitial fibrosis.

been more observant, especially when the clinician informs about OSPS use, although the diagnosis is rather straightforward and requires abundant tubular deposits of calcium phosphate (Figure 1). Alternatively, the Icelandic population may be more prone to develop acute phosphate nephropathy due to unknown genetic and environmental factors, but remarkable similarities between our patient group and the previously reported cases argues against that. The majority of our cases were women (60%) with an average age of 68.8 years and all patients were older than 55 years. This is comparable to the cases that have been diagnosed worldwide, 81% is female and their mean age was 66.1, ranging from 39–85 years and 70% older than 60 years [2,3,10–20]. The co-morbidities in our patients were also similar to the other cases,

87% of our patients had hypertension and all used either diuretics, and/or ACE-I or ARB, 20% had diabetes and 27% had e-GFR <60 ml/min per 1.73 m[2] at baseline. These risk factors have been reported with a similar rate before, 81% of previously reported cases have hypertension and most have been treated with the aforementioned drugs, 14% have diabetes and 22% have baseline e-GFR <60 ml/min per 1.73 m[2] [7]. In addition to this, inappropriate use of OSPS could be responsible for the high rate of cases in our country. The use of OSPS can be criticized in two of the patients, one who was exposed to repeated doses in a short period of time, and another who turned out to have an active colitis. We included all cases in this study, as clinical practice is clearly not always according to recommendations.

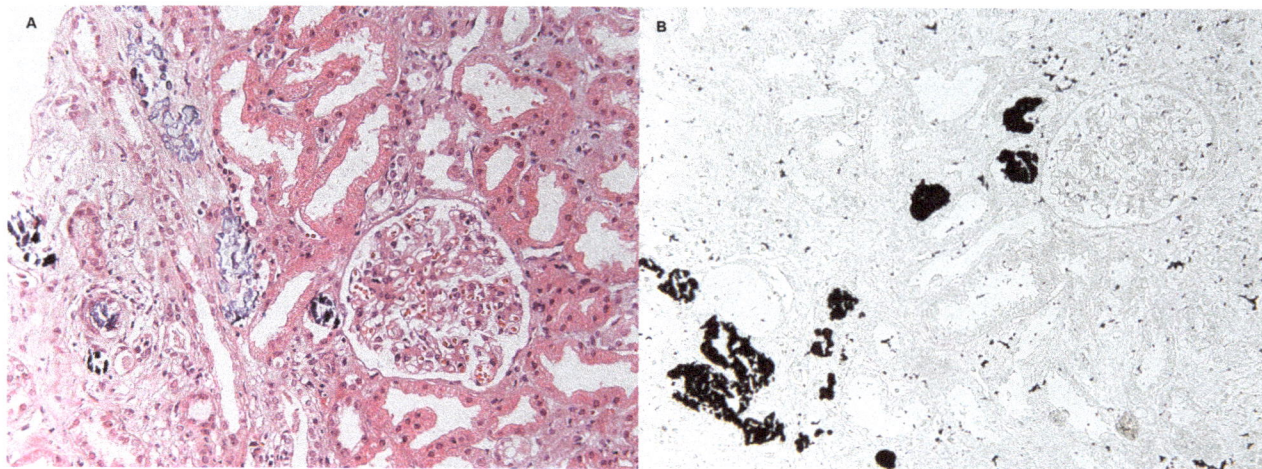

Figure 1. Renal biopsy findings in acute phosphate nephropathy. A) Abundant calcifications are seen within tubules and in the interstitium. Adjacent tubules are athrophic and there is interstitial fibrosis (Hematoxylin and eosin staining, original magnification x 400). B) Positive von Kossa staining in the same biopsy confirms that the calcifications are composed of calcium phosphate (original magnification x 400).

The consequences of acute phosphate nephropathy following OSPS on kidney function and future health of these patients is of major concern. Although the kidney function improved in most patients with time, one patient reached end-stage renal disease and one died with a pre-end-stage renal failure. At the end of follow-up, the eGFR had decreased by an average of 36 ml/min/1.73 m^2 from the baseline value. Studies have shown that acute kidney injury and chronic kidney disease are associated with an increased risk of cardiovascular disease and mortality [26–28].

This study is an important addition to the reported cases of acute phosphate nephropathy and confirms the risk factors that have been suggested in other studies. We were able to reveal the incidence of this complication due to the unique setting in our country. Approximately one out of every thousand sold doses of OSPS resulted in acute kidney injury and follow-up showed that the long-term consequences were not benign. This information can be used in other populations to estimate the impact of OSPS use. Our results suggest that acute phosphate nephropathy following OSPS is underestimated worldwide and that it may be an important iatrogenic cause of chronic kidney disease in the elderly now and in the near future.

Author Contributions

Conceived and designed the experiments: VKP HG SH MA TM MBA. Performed the experiments: VKP HG SH MBA. Analyzed the data: VKP SH MA MBA. Contributed reagents/materials/analysis tools: VKP HG SH MA TM MBA. Wrote the paper: VKP MBA.

References

1. Markowitz GS, Nasr SH, Klein P, Anderson H, Stack JI, et al. (2004) Renal failure due to acute nephrocalcinosis following oral sodium phosphate bowel cleansing. Hum Pathol 35: 675–684.
2. Markowitz GS, Stokes MB, Radhakrishnan J, D'Agati VD (2005) Acute phosphate nephropathy following oral sodium phosphate bowel purgative: an underrecognized cause of chronic renal failure. J Am Soc Nephrol 16: 3389–3396.
3. Desmeules S, Bergeron MJ, Isenring P (2003) Acute phosphate nephropathy and renal failure. N Engl J Med 349: 1006–1007.
4. Vanner SJ, MacDonald PH, Paterson WG, Prentice RS, Da Costa LR, et al. (1990) A randomized prospective trial comparing oral sodium phosphate with standard polyethylene glycol-based lavage solution (Golytely) in the preparation of patients for colonoscopy. Am J Gastroenterol 85: 422–427.
5. Brunelli SM, Lewis JD, Gupta M, Latif SM, Weiner MG, et al. (2007) Risk of kidney injury following oral phosphosoda bowel preparations. J Am Soc Nephrol 18: 3199–3205.
6. Russmann S, Lamerato L, Motsko SP, Pezzullo JC, Faber MD, et al. (2008) Risk of further decline in renal function after the use of oral sodium phosphate or polyethylene glycol in patients with a preexisting glomerular filtration rate below 60 ml/min. Am J Gastroenterol 103: 2707–2716.
7. Markowitz GS, Perazella MA (2009) Acute phosphate nephropathy. Kidney Int 76: 1027–1034.
8. Markowitz GS, Whelan J, D'Agati VD (2005) Renal failure following bowel cleansing with a sodium phosphate purgative. Nephrol Dial Transplant 20: 850–851.
9. Levey AS, Stevens LA, Schmid CH, Zhang YL, Castro AF, 3rd, et al. (2009) A new equation to estimate glomerular filtration rate. Ann Intern Med 150: 604–612.
10. Gonlusen G, Akgun H, Ertan A, Olivero J, Truong LD (2006) Renal failure and nephrocalcinosis associated with oral sodium phosphate bowel cleansing: clinical patterns and renal biopsy findings. Arch Pathol Lab Med 130: 101–106.
11. Steinman TI, Samir AE, Cornell LD (2008) Case records of the Massachusetts General Hospital. Case 27-2008. A 64-year-old man with abdominal pain, nausea, and an elevated level of serum creatinine. N Engl J Med 359: 951–960.
12. Rocuts AK, Waikar SS, Alexander MP, Rennke HG, Singh AK (2009) Acute phosphate nephropathy. Kidney Int 75: 987–991.
13. Aasebo W, Scott H, Ganss R (2007) Kidney biopsies taken before and after oral sodium phosphate bowel cleansing. Nephrol Dial Transplant 22: 920–922.
14. Slee TM, Vleming LJ, Valentijn RM (2008) Renal failure due to acute phosphate nephropathy. Neth J Med 66: 438–441.
15. Demoulin N, Jadoul M, Cosyns JP, Labriola L (2008) An easily overlooked iatrogenic cause of renal failure. Clin Nephrol 70: 176–177.
16. Connor A, Sykes L, Roberts IS, Weston CE (2008) Acute phosphate nephropathy after sodium phosphate preparations. Bmj 337: a182.
17. Beyea A, Block C, Schned A (2007) Acute phosphate nephropathy following oral sodium phosphate solution to cleanse the bowel for colonoscopy. Am J Kidney Dis 50: 151–154.
18. Kim HJ, Lee BH, Kwon SH (2008) A case of acute phosphate nephropathy after sodium phosphate preparation. Korean J Nephrol 27: 374–377.
19. Manley P, Somerfield J, Simpson I, Barber A, Zwi J (2006) Bilateral uraemic optic neuritis complicating acute nephrocalcinosis. Nephrol Dial Transplant 21: 2957–2958.
20. Ori Y, Herman M, Tobar A, Chernin G, Gafter U, et al. (2008) Acute phosphate nephropathy-an emerging threat. Am J Med Sci 336: 309–314.
21. Koretz RL (2006) The devil is in the denominator. Gastroenterology 130: 2240–2242; discussion 2242.
22. Brunelli SM (2009) Association between oral sodium phosphate bowel preparations and kidney injury: a systematic review and meta-analysis. Am J Kidney Dis 53: 448–456.
23. Hurst FP, Bohen EM, Osgard EM, Oliver DK, Das NP, et al. (2007) Association of oral sodium phosphate purgative use with acute kidney injury. J Am Soc Nephrol 18: 3192–3198.
24. Gross CP, Andersen MS, Krumholz HM, McAvay GJ, Proctor D, et al. (2006) Relation between Medicare screening reimbursement and stage at diagnosis for older patients with colon cancer. Jama 296: 2815–2822.
25. Seeff LC, Richards TB, Shapiro JA, Nadel MR, Manninen DL, et al. (2004) How many endoscopies are performed for colorectal cancer screening? Results from CDC's survey of endoscopic capacity. Gastroenterology 127: 1670–1677.
26. McCullough PA (2008) Radiocontrast-induced acute kidney injury. Nephron Physiol 109: p61–72.
27. Sarnak MJ, Levey AS, Schoolwerth AC, Coresh J, Culleton B, et al. (2003) Kidney disease as a risk factor for development of cardiovascular disease: a statement from the American Heart Association Councils on Kidney in Cardiovascular Disease, High Blood Pressure Research, Clinical Cardiology, and Epidemiology and Prevention. Circulation 108: 2154–2169.
28. Weiner DE, Tighiouart H, Amin MG, Stark PC, MacLeod B, et al. (2004) Chronic kidney disease as a risk factor for cardiovascular disease and all-cause mortality: a pooled analysis of community-based studies. J Am Soc Nephrol 15: 1307–1315.

12

Ultra Performance Liquid Chromatography-Based Metabonomic Study of Therapeutic Effect of the Surface Layer of *Poria cocos* on Adenine-Induced Chronic Kidney Disease Provides New Insight into Anti-Fibrosis Mechanism

Ying-Yong Zhao[1]*[⑨], Ya-Long Feng[1⑨], Xu Bai[2], Xiao-Jie Tan[2], Rui-Chao Lin[3], Qibing Mei[2]*

1 Key Laboratory of Resource Biology and Biotechnology in Western China, Ministry of Education, the College of Life Sciences, Northwest University, Xi'an, Shaanxi, P.R. China, **2** Solution Center, Waters Technologies (Shanghai) Ltd., Shanghai, P.R. China, **3** Research and Inspection Center of Traditional Chinese Medicine and Ethnomedicine, National Institutes for Food and Drug Control, State Food and Drug Administration, Beijing, P.R. China, **4** Department of Pharmacology, School of Pharmacy, the Fourth Military Medical University, Xi'an, Shaanxi, P.R. China

Abstract

The surface layer of *Poria cocos* (Fu-Ling-Pi, FLP) is commonly used in traditional Chinese medicine and its diuretic effect was confirmed in rat. Ultra performance liquid chromatography/quadrupole time-of-flight high-sensitivity mass spectrometry and a novel mass spectrometry^Elevated Energy data collection technique was employed to investigate metabonomic characteristics of chronic kidney disease (CKD) induced from adenine excess and the protective effects of FLP. Multiple metabolites are detected in the CKD and are correlated with progressive renal injury. Among these biomarkers, lysoPC(18:0), tetracosahexaenoic acid, lysoPC(18:2), creatinine, lysoPC (16:0) and lysoPE(22:0/0:0) in the FLP-treated group were completely reversed to levels in the control group which lacked CKD. Combined with biochemistry and histopathology results, the changes in serum metabolites indicate that the perturbations of phospholipids metabolism, energy metabolism and amino acid metabolism are related to adenine-induced CKD and to the interventions of FLP on all the three metabolic pathways. FLP may regulate the metabolism of these biomarkers, especially their efficient utilization within the context of CKD. Furthermore, these biomarkers might serve as characteristics to explain the mechanisms of FLP.

Editor: Wolf-Hagen Schunck, Max Delbrueck Center for Molecular Medicine, Germany

Funding: This study was supported in part by grants from the National Scientific Foundation of China (Nos. 81001622, 81073029) and China Postdoctoral Science Foundation (2012M521831) and Innovative Research Team in University of Ministry of Education of China (No. IRT1174). The funders had no role in study design, data collection and analysis, decision to publish, or preparation of the manuscript.

Competing Interests: In this work, two technological experts of Waters Technologies (Shanghai) Ltd, Xu Bai and Xiao-Jie Tan, have given great contribution to all the test and data analysis work on Waters AcquityTM Ultra Performance LC system (Waters, USA) equipped with a Waters XevoTM G2 QTof MS (Waters MS Technologies, Manchester, UK). The usage and publishing of the relative data were approved by Waters Technologies (Shanghai) Ltd. No conflicts of interest exist; all items are strictly in line with the regulation of PLOS ONE. This does not alter the authors' adherence to all the PLOS ONE policies on sharing data and materials.

* E-mail: zyy@nwu.edu.cn (YYZ); qbmei@fmmu.edu.cn (QM)

⑨ These authors contributed equally to this work.

Introduction

Kidney diseases are a serious and prevalent health problem, and manifestation includes changes in renal detoxification capacity, deregulation of salt and water balance and altered endocrine functions -overall, exerting a significant impact on the patient's short- or long-term survival. The prevalence of chronic kidney disease (CKD) continues to increase, mainly due to an increase in secondary disease as a consequence of diabetes and hypertension.

Metabonomics is a part of systems biology which refers to a holistic analytical approach to the low molecular mass organic endogenous metabolites in the tissue or bio-fluids [1]. Metabonomics provides variation of whole metabolic networks for characterizing pathological states in animals and human, as well giving diagnostic information and presenting mechanistic insight into the biochemical effects of the toxins and drugs [2]. Traditional Chinese medicines (TCM) are gaining more attention all over the world, due to their specific theory and long historical clinical practice. In the TCM research arena, this strategy has gained broad applications in many aspects, such as symptom subtyping, medicine quality control and therapeutic effect evaluation [3–5]. This research strategy is well coincident with the integrity and systemic feature of TCM. Mass spectrometry (MS) and nuclear magnetic resonance spectroscopy are two analytical tools commonly used in TCM metabonomics study [6]. In the MS-based metabonomics, ultra performance liquid chromatography-mass spectrometry (UPLC-MS) is considered to be suitable for large-scale untargeted metabolic profiling study due to its enhanced reproducibility of retention time [7,8]. In 2005, Wrona *et al* introduced MS^E (where E represents collision energy) technique for the first time [9]. MS^E can provide parallel alternating scans for acquisition at either low collision energy to obtain precursor ion information, or ramping of high collision energy to obtain full-scan accurate mass fragment, precursor ion and neutral loss information [10,11].

An adenine-induced CKD model provides valuable information of pathological mechanism for various complications in a persistent uremic state. In mammalian metabolism, excess adenine becomes a significant substrate for xanthine dehydrogenase, which oxidizes adenine to 2,8-dihydroxyadenine (DHA) via an 8-hydroxyadenine intermediate [12]. However, the very low solubility of DHA leads to precipitation in tubules of a kidney [13]. Long-term feeding of adenine to rats causes metabolic abnormalities similar to the CKD symptoms in humans. In our previous study, a metabonomic approach based on UPLC-MS was developed to characterize the metabolic profile associated with adenine-induced CKD and demonstrated that the utility of metabolic profiling combined with multivariate analysis was a powerful tool to investigate CKD pathogenesis [14–18].

Poria cocos (Schw.) Wolf (Polyporaceae) is a well-known traditional East-Asian medicinal plant that grows around the roots of pine trees in China, Japan, Korea and North America [19]. It has frequently been prescribed as one of the chief ingredients in composite prescriptions in TCM. Nearly 10% of the traditional Chinese medicinal preparations or prearations admitted to Chinese Pharmacopoeia (2010 edition) contain *Poria cocos* [20]. It is prepared from the dried sclerotia of *Poria cocos* Wolf as Fuling in China and Hoelen in Japan. The inner parts of the sclerotia of *P. cocos*, called "Fu-Ling" in Chinese, are used to treat chronic gastritis, acute gastroenteric catarrh, gastric atony, edema, nephrosis, dizziness, nausea and emesis [21].

As reported previously, the chemical constituents of *Poria cocos* mainly include triterpenes, polysaccharides and steroids [21–27]. However, the triterpenoid compounds is the main components of the epidermis ("Fu-Ling-Pi" in Chinese) of the sclerotia [28–30]. The Fu-Ling-Pi (FLP) it is believed to promote urination and to eliminate edema [20]. The diuretic effect of the ethanol and aqueous extracts of FLP has been evaluated in our recent study. The study confirmed that the not aqueous but ethanol extracts of the surface layer of *Poria cocos* presented a remarkable diuretic effect [31].

In the current study, metabonomics study based on ultra performance liquid chromatography/quadrupole time-of-flight high-sensitivity mass spectrometry (UPLC-Q-TOF/HSMS) and a novel mass spectrometry$^{\text{Elevated Energy}}$ (MS^E) data collection technique was applied to investigate the serum metabolite profiling of the renoprotective effect of FLP and its action mechanism. Potential biomarkers related with CKD were identified, and their metabolic pathways were also discussed. Furthermore, clinical biochemistry study were also carried out to ensure the success of the CKD model and to investigate the renoprotective effect of FLP. Therefore, metabonomics could be a promising scientific platform for therapeutic evaluation and action mechanism study of TCM.

Experimental

2.1 Chemicals and Reagents

Adenine (batch No.: A8626, Purity 99.0%) and formic acid solution (ref. BCBB6918, purity 50%) were purchased from Sigma-Aldrich (St. Louis, MO, USA). Creatinine (batch No.: 100877-200901, Purity 99.8%) was obtained from the National Institutes for Food and Drug Control (Beijing, China). L-tryptophan (batch No.: TB1991-25g, Purity 99.0%) and Valine

(batch No.: 1B1102-25g, Purity 99.0–101.5%) were purchased from Amresco Company (Amresco Inc., Solon, OH, USA). LC-grade methanol and acetonitrile were purchased from the Baker Company (Mallinckrodt Baker Inc., Phillipsburg, NJ, USA). Ultra high purity water was prepared using a Milli-Q water purification system (Millipore Corp., Billerica, MA, USA). Other chemicals were of analytical grade and their purity was above 99.5%.

2.2 Preparation of Ethanol of FLP

FLP was collected from Shaanxi Province in March 2012, and was identified by Prof. Y. Z. Wang (the College of Life Sciences, Northwest University, Xi'an, Shaanxi, P.R. China). A voucher specimen (120304) was deposited at Key Laboratory of Resource Biology and Biotechnology in Western China, Ministry of Education, Northwest University, Xi'an, Shaanxi. FLP was ground to powder (about 20 meshes) by a disintegrator, and the powder (2 kg) was extracted three times with 15 L 95% ethanol for 0.5 h by ultrasonic method. The extracts were combined together and filtrated, and then the filtrate was concentrated in vacuum using a rotary evaporator to give dried powder.

2.3 Animals

This study was carried out in strict accordance with the recommendations in the Guide for the Care and Use of Laboratory Animals of the State Committee of Science and Technology of the People's Republic of China. The protocol was approved by the Committee on the Ethics of Animal Experiments of the Northwest University (Permit Number: SYXK 2010-004). All surgery was performed under uretane anesthesia, and all efforts were made to minimize suffering. All procedures and care of the rats were in accordance with the institutional guidelines for animal use in research. Male Sprague-Dawley rats were obtained from the Central Animal Breeding House of the Fourth Military Medical University (Xi'an, China). The rats were maintained at a constant humidity (ca. 60%) and temperature (ca. 23°C) with a light/dark cycle of 12 h.

2.4 CKD Model and Drug Administration

Male rats underwent an adaptation period of several days, during which they were fed a commercial feed. Rats weighing 200 to 220 g were divided into 3 groups (n = 8/group): group 1(control group), group 2 (CKD model group) and group 3 (FLP-treated group with CKD). Groups 2 and 3 then were then given 200 mg/kg body weight of adenine dissolved in 1% (w/v) gum acacia solution by oral gavage once everyday continuously for 2 weeks, which produced experimental renal failure in the animal for two weeks. Group 1 was similarly provided an equal volume of gum acacia solution. During the adenine gastric gavage after 3 h, Group 3 was administered FLP (60 mg/ml) by gastric irrigation. The control group and model group were only administered by oral gavage with the 1% (w/v) gum acacia solution. Body weights were recorded daily.

2.5 Sample Collection

After two weeks, all the rats were anesthetized with 10% urethane, and blood samples were obtained by carotid artery cannula. Blood was centrifuged at 3000 rpm for 10 min and the supernatant was collected and stored at −80°C. The rats were killed and Kidneys were collected immediately after blood was drawn and the tissues were washed with saline buffer.

2.6 Determination of Body Weight, Kidney Index and Blood Sample

At the end of the experiment, rats were housed individually in metabolic cages for 24 h urinary collection and body weight was measured. Kidneys were weighed to determine the organ indexes (organ index = organ weight/terminal body weight×100%).

The levels of Serum creatinine (SCr), blood urea nitrogen (BUN), cholesterol and triglyceride were determined by Olympus AU640 automatic analyzer and the levels of white blood cell count (WBC), red blood cell (RBC), hemoglobin (HGB) and hematocrit (HCT) were determined by HF-3800 Routine blood analyzer.

2.7 Histopathology

A portion of kidney tissue was immersed in 10% neutral buffered formaldehyde solution, the tissues were dehydrated, embedded in paraffin, cut at 5 micrometer thickness and stained with hematoxylin and eosin (H&E) for histopathological examination.

2.8 Preparation of Metabonomic Samples

Prior to the analysis, the serum samples were thawed at room temperature. Acetonitrile (400 μl) was added to serum (200 μl) and vortex-mixed (IKA Instruments, Guangzhou, China) vigorously for 3 min. The mixture was settled at room temperature for 10 min, and then centrifuged (eppendorf Instruments, Hamburg, Germany) at 13000 rpm for 10 min at 4°C. The supernatant (400 μl) were pipetted out and lyophilized.

2.9 UPLC Conditions

The UPLC analysis was performed with a Waters Acquity™ Ultra Performance LC system (Waters, USA) equipped with a Waters Xevo™ G2 QTof MS (Waters MS Technologies, Manchester, UK). Chromatographic separation was carried out at 45°C on an ACQUITY UPLC HSS (high strength silica) T3 column (2.1 mm×100 mm, 1.8 μm, UK). The mobile phase consisted of water (A) and acetonitrile (B), each containing 0.1% formic acid. The optimized UPLC elution conditions were: 0–0.5 min, 1% B; 0.5–3.5 min, 1–35% B; 3.5–7.0 min, 35–99% B; 7.0–8.0 min, 99% B and 8.0–10.0 min, 99.0–1.0% B. The flow rate was 0.45 ml/min. The autosampler was maintained at 4°C. The lyophilized serum samples were dissolved in 100 μL of distilled acetonitrile/water (4:1). Every 2 μL sample solution was injected for each run.

2.10 Mass Spectrometry

Mass spectrometry was performed on a Xevo™ G2 QTof (Waters MS Technologies, Manchester, UK), a quadrupole and orthogonal acceleration time-of-flight tandem mass spectrometer. The scan range was from 50 to 1200 m/z. For both positive and negative electrospray modes, the capillary and cone voltage were set at 3.0 kV and 30 V, respectively. The desolvation gas was set to 800 L/h at a temperature of 450°C; the cone gas was set to 20 L/h and the source temperature was set to 150°C. The mass spectrometry was operated in W optics mode with 12,000 resolution using dynamic range extension. The data acquisition rate was set to 0.1 s, with a 0.1 s interscan delay. All analyses were acquired using the lockspray to ensure accuracy and reproducibility. Leucine–enkephalin was used as the lockmass at a concentration of 300 ng/mL and flow rate of 5 μL/min. Data were collected in continuum mode, the lockspray frequency was set at 10 s, and data were averaged over 10 scans. All the acquisition and analysis of data were controlled by Waters MassLynx v4.1 software.

2.11 Data Analysis

The mass data acquired were imported to Markerlynx XS (Waters Corporation, MA, USA) within the Masslynx software for peak detection and alignment. All of the data were normalized to the summed total ion intensity per chromatogram, and the resultant data matrices were introduced to the EZinfo 2.0 software for principal component analysis (PCA) and partial least squares-discriminate analysis (PLS-DA) analyses. Metabolite peaks were assigned by MS^E analysis or interpreted with available biochemical databases, such as HMDB (http: //www.hmdb.ca/), Chemspider (http: //www.chemspider.com) and KEGG (http: //www.kegg.com/). Other statistical analyses were used by one-way analysis of variance (ANOVA) and independent sample t-test. They were performed with SPSS 11.0 (SPSS Inc., Chicago, IL, USA). Significant differences were considered significant when test P values were less than 0.05.

Results and Discussion

3.1 Basic Physical Parameters

Figure 1 shows the parameters of body weight, urinary volume and kidney weight index among the studied groups. Body weight was decreased in the CKD group compared with that in the control group, but did not arrive at statistical significance. Similarly, compared with the CKD group, body weight was also slightly decreased in the FLP-treated group. Because FLP is used as a diuretic in clinic, decrease of weight body can be caused by FLP's diuretic effect. Urinary volume was markedly increased in the CKD group compared with that in the control group and arrived at statistical significance (P<0.01), but decrease of urinary volume was revealed in the FLP-treated group.

3.2 Biochemical Parameters

After day 14, blood samples were collected and BUN, Scr, cholesterol and triglyceride were determined. The results are given in Figure 2. BUN, Scr, cholesterol and triglyceride were all in higher concentrations in CKD group than in control group (P<0.01). These results demonstrate that the rat model exhibited typical pathologic features associated with CKD. Levels of BUN and Scr were significantly intervened by FLP (P<0.01).

The results of blood routine are given in Figure 3. A remarkable increase in WBC and a remarkable decrease in RBC, HGB and HCT were revealed in the blood parameters of the CKD group compared with the control group (P<0.01). These blood parameters showed that adenine can cause anemia symptom. FLP could increase RBC, HGB and HCT to the same extent although they could not increase RBC, HGB and HCT to the normal levels. These results demonstrate that the CKD was being prevented and alleviated, exhibiting a recovery via similarity to the healthy control group after taking FLP.

3.3 Histological Results

Figure 4 illustrates the histological findings obtained through the HE staining of transverse kidney sections from the adenine-induced rats. There was formation of foreign body granuloma in the renal tubules and interstitium and a marked fibrosis leading, in some extreme cases, to a contracted kidney (Figure 4B). These results demonstrate that the rat model exhibited the typical pathological features associated with CKD. In contrast, these pathological abnormalities were gradually ameliorated in the FLP-treated group (Figure 4C).

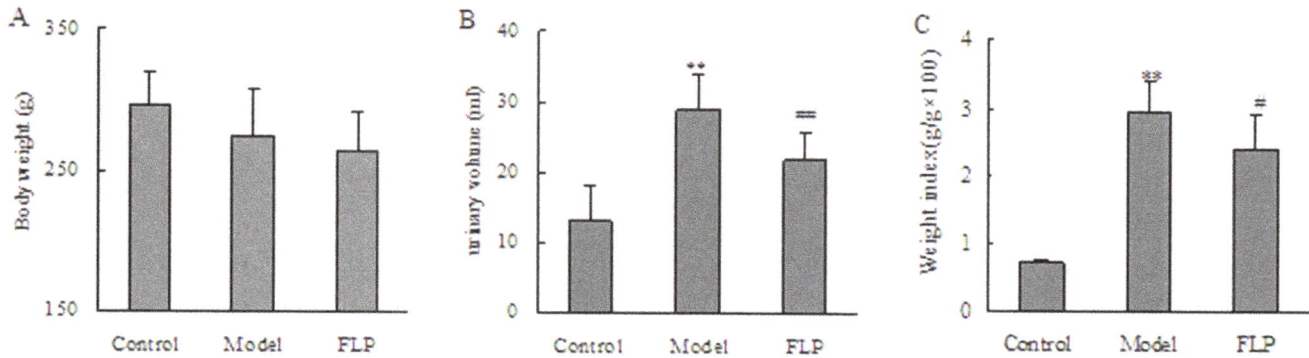

Figure 1. Physical parameter comparisons among the studied groups. (A) Body weight; (B) urinary volume and (C) kidney weight index. The data were expressed as mean ± SD. *$P<0.05$, **$P<0.01$ compared to the control groups and #$P<0.05$, ##$P<0.01$ compared to the CKD groups.

3.4 Method Development and Validation

High reproducibility is crucial for any analytical protocols, especially for metabonomics study which requires handling many samples. The precision and repeatability of the UPLC-MS method were validated by the reduplicate analysis of six injections of the same quality control samples and six parallel samples prepared using the same preparation method, respectively. The relative standard deviations (RSD) of retention time and peak area are below 0.45% and 3.4%, respectively. The resulting data showed that the precision and repeatability of the proposed method were satisfactory for metabonomic analysis. Metabolic profiling of serum samples was acquired using UPLC Q-TOF/MS system in the positive ion mode. The base peak intensity (BPI) chromato-

grams of serum samples from healthy control group, CKD group and FLP-treated group are shown in Figure 5.

3.5 Biomarker Elucidation

To determine whether the FLP was possibly to influence metabolic pattern of adenine-induced CKD rats and to find the metabolites with a significant concentration change (i.e. potential biomarkers), PLS-DA was carried out on the UPLC-MS data of serum samples. A PLS-DA model was built by 2112 variables. Figure 6 shows the score plot and the loading plot in the positive ion mode. The score plot shows that control, CKD and FLP-treated groups are classified clearly, which might suggest FLP has a protect effect on adenine-induced CKD model.

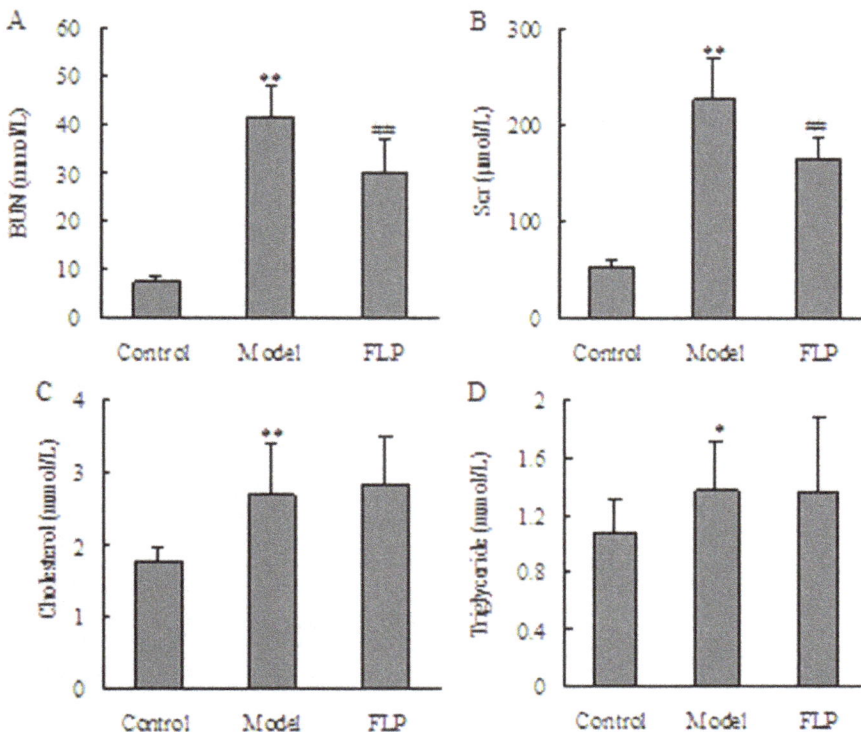

Figure 2. Basic serum biochemical parameter comparisons among the studied groups. (A) BUN; (B) Scr; (C) cholesterol; (D) triglyceride. The data were expressed as mean ± SD. *$P<0.05$, **$P<0.01$ compared to the control groups and #$P<0.05$, ##$P<0.01$ compared to the CKD groups.

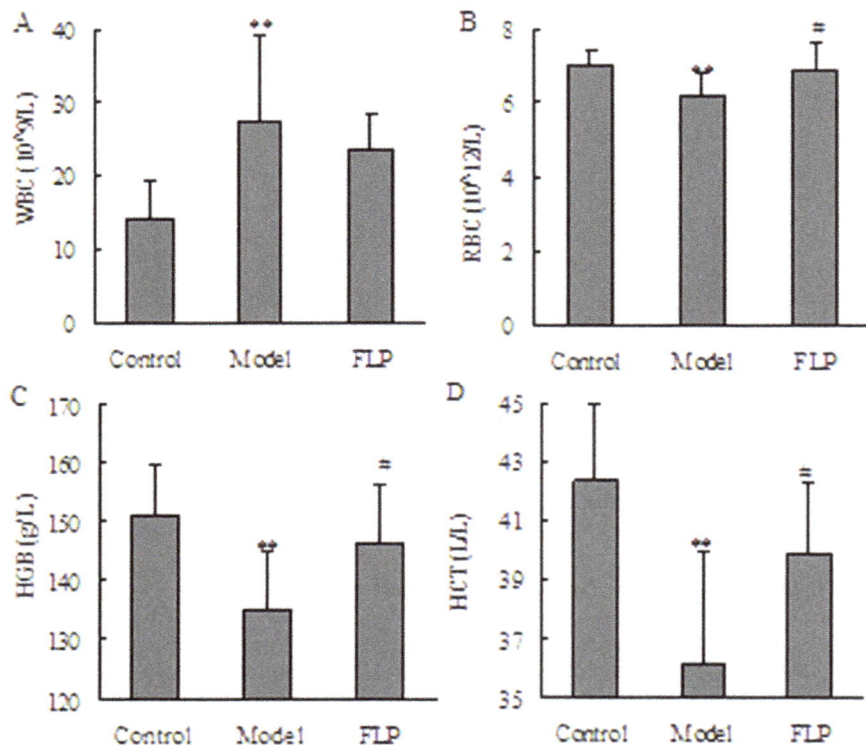

Figure 3. Basic blood routine parameters of the studied groups. (A) White blood cell count; (B) red blood cell; (C) hemoglobin and (D) hematocrit. The data were expressed as mean ± SD. *P<0.05, **P<0.01 compared to the control groups and #P<0.05, ##P<0.01 compared to the CKD groups.

In the score plot, scattered points of various samples were classified into three groups, which suggested that proper CKD-related patterns could be revealed by the proposed PLS-DA model and serum metabolic pattern significantly changed after the treatment of FLP. The loading plot displayed 20 potential CKD-related metabolites according to their VIP (Variable Importance in the Projection) values. To identify these metabolites, we first searched candidates from the databases of HMDB (http: //www. hmdb.ca/), Chemspider (http: //www.chemspider.com/) and KEGG (http: //www.kegg.com/) by masses and MS^E data, and due to the possible fragment mechanisms, items without the given mass fragment information were removed from the candidate list

and only the most probable items survived. MassLynx i-FIT algorithm is used to screen suggested elemental compositions by the likelihood that the isotopic pattern of the elemental composition matches a cluster of peaks in the spectrum, increasing confidence in identified compounds and simplifying results. The lower the i-FIT value, the better the fit. By comparing the retention times and mass spectra to the authentic chemicals, a part of the CKD-related metabolites were structurally confirmed.

Table 1 shows 14 compounds were tentatively identified on the basis of MS^E fragmentation data and i-FIT values, including phospholipid, amino acids and other compounds. The metabolites shown in Table 1 were ranked in the order of their VIP values,

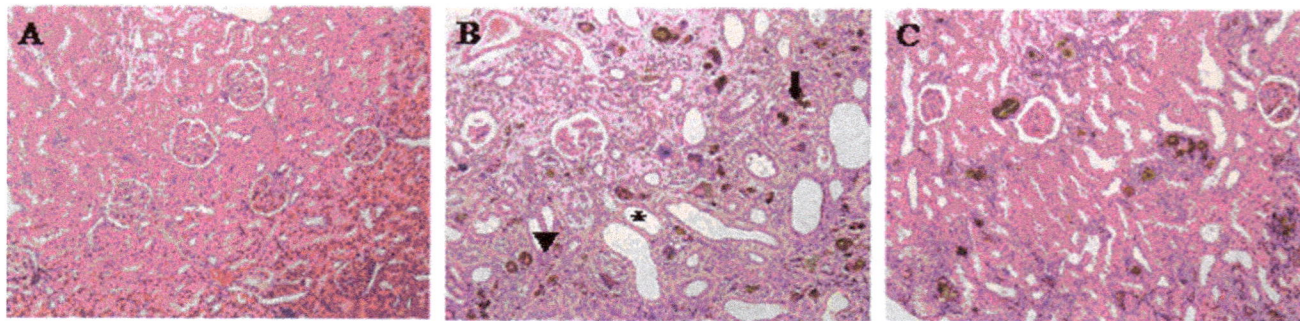

Figure 4. Histologic findings by HE-staining of transverse kidney sections. (A) normal control rats, (B) adenine-induced CKD rats and (C) FLP-treated group with CKD rats. Large dilated tubule (asterisk); lymphocytic infiltrate (arrowheads); 2,8-dihydroxyadenine crystal (arrows). There was formation of foreign body granuloma in the renal tubules and interstitium and a marked fibrosis leading, in some extreme cases, to a contracted kidney. These results demonstrate that the rat model exhibited the typical pathological features associated with CKD.

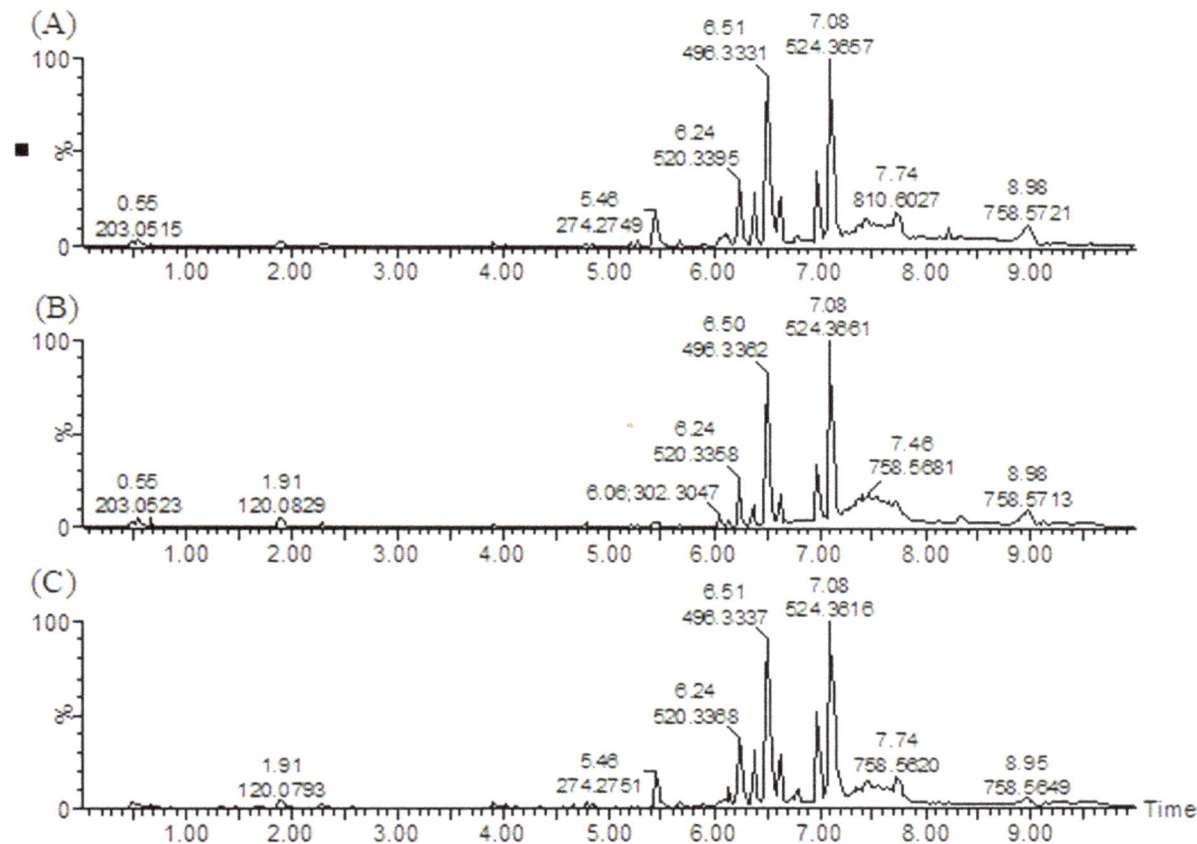

Figure 5. The UPLC-MS base peak intensity (BPI) chromatogram. (A) control group, (B) CKD group and (C) FLP-treated group.

such that metabolites listed in the front were more important than those in the rear. Most of these metabolites display CKD-related changes and the CKD-related changes are partly displayed in Figure 7. Many of these identified metabolites have also been reported in other CKD studies, such as phytosphingosine [16], PC(16:0/18:2) [16], tryptophan [16], lysoPC(16:1) [14], creatinine[14] and lysoPC (16:0) [14], while in the current study, the approach of metabonomics was employed and more CKD-related metabolites were discovered.

3.6 Biochemical Interpretation

In order to more clearly characterize treatment CKD effects of FLP, a correlation coefficient analysis was applied to investigate the connections between biomarkers and corresponding groups (Figure 7). Variables situated upper are positively correlated to group and those situated opposite are negatively correlated to the group. The markers 2, 3, 9, 11, 14 such as lysoPC(18:0), tetracosahexaenoic acid, lysoPC(18:2), creatinine, lysoPE(22:0/0:0) have negative correlation with the control group; others have positive correlation with the control group, indicating normal kidney function. Correlations between markers 1, 5, 6, 10, 13 with the control group while being relatively high when compared to the other variables, therefore the change in palmitic acid, PC(16:0/18:2), tryptophan, lysoPC(16:1), valine has the strongest association with normal kidney function and are enough to suggest that these markers can principally represent the CRF model in this study. The markers 2, 3, 7, 9, 11, 14 have positive correlation with the model group; others have negative correlation with the model group, shows the overall metabolic profile of adenine caused

a significant CKD. The markers 1, 2, 4, 6, 8, 10, 12, 13 have positive correlation with the FLP group; others have negative correlation with the FLP group, consistenting with the control group. The metabolism pathway of each biomarker was shown in Table 1 by searching the KEGG database. The 14 biomarkers were mainly distributed in related pathways of phospholipids metabolism, fatty acids metabolism and amino acids metabolism. In the FLP-treated rats, lysoPC(18:0), tetracosahexaenoic acid, prostaglandin PGE_2 glyceryl ester, lysoPC(18:2), creatinine and lysoPE(22:0/0:0) were up-regulated, but palmitic acid, phytosphingosine, PC(16:0/18:2), tryptophan, lysoPC(20:4), lysoPC(16:1), lysoPC (16:0) and valine were down-regulated compared with control rats. To evaluate protective effects of FLP, the intensity level of 14 biomarkers in the different groups was also analyzed (Figure 8). Except for PC(16:0/18:2), prostaglandin PGE_2 glyceryl ester, lysoPC(16:1) and valine, mean level of the key biomarkers was reversed to control at different degrees after oral administration (Figure 8). Among these biomarkers, lysoPC(18:0), tetracosahexaenoic acid, lysoPC(18:2), creatinine, lysoPC (16:0) and lysoPE(22:0/0:0) in the FLP-treated group were completed reversed to levels in the control group which lacked CKD. Thus, FLP may regulate the metabolism of these biomarkers, especially their efficient utilization within the context of CKD. Furthermore, these biomarkers might serve as characteristics to explain the mechanisms of FLP. Interestingly, the most important CKD-related metabolites were phospholipid and in total there were eight phospholipids, which accounts for 60% of all the identified biomarkers. Hereby, the pathway of phospholipids metabolism was discussed in the process of renal injury.

(A)

Scores Comp[1] vs. Comp[2] colored by Sample Group

(B)

Loadings Comp[1] vs. Comp[2]

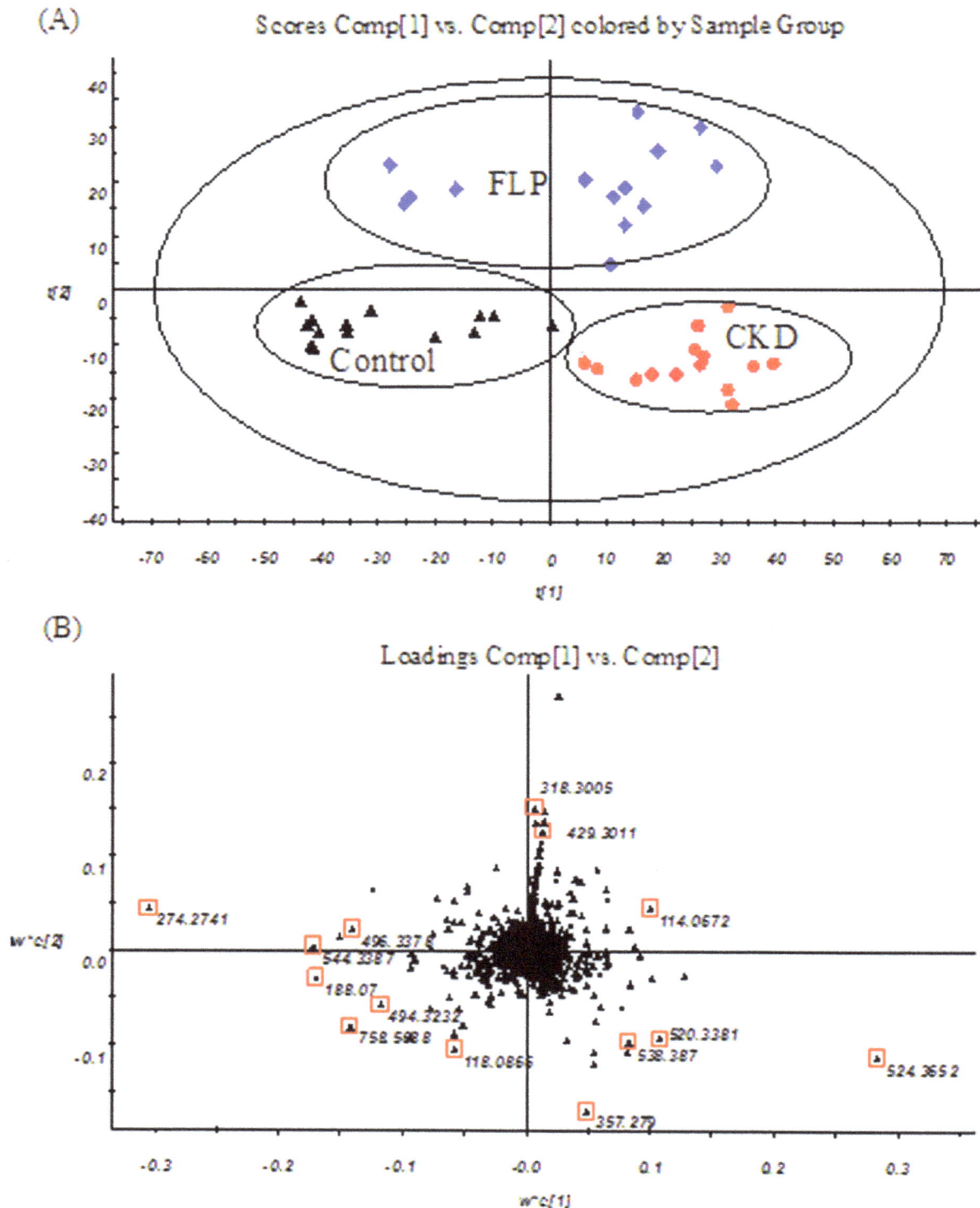

Figure 6. PLS-DA scores plots (A) and Loading plots (B) derived from UPLC-MS data of serum samples. (▲) control group, (●) CKD group and (◆) FLP-treated group. The variables marked (□) are the metabolites selected as potential biomarkers.

Lysophosphatidylcholines are a class of compounds that have a constant polar head, and fatty acyls of different chain lengths, position, degrees of saturation, and double bond location in plasma. Lysophosphatidylcholine level can be a clinical diagnostic indicator that reveals pathophysiological changes. Lysophosphati-

dylcholines are products or metabolites of phosphatidylcholines, which are structural components of animal cell membranes. The importance of plasma phospholipid abnormalities in renal damage is well recognized [32–34], but little attention has been paid to the study of some plasma phospholipid fractions, including lysopho-

Table 1. Identification of significantly differential endogenous metabolites in the rat kidney.

No	t_R	m/z	Scan mode	Qusi-molecular ion	Metabolite	Trend[a]	Trend[b]	Related pathway
1	5.47	274.2741	+	$[M+NH_4]^+$	Palmitic acid	↓***	↑***	Fatty acid metabolism
		255.2317	−	$[M-H]^-$				
2	7.09	524.3652	+	$[M+H]^+$	LysoPC(18:0)	↑***	↓***	Phospholipid metabolism
		522.3565	−	$[M-H]^-$				
3	5.27	357.2790	+	$[M+H]^+$	Tetracosahexaenoic acid	↑***	↓***	Fatty acid metabolism
		355.2641	−	$[M-H]^-$				
4	5.48	318.3005	+	$[M+H]^+$	Phytosphingosine	↓	↑**	Phospholipid metabolism
		316.2851	−	$[M-H]^-$				
5	7.70	758.5688	+	$[M+H]^+$	PC(16:0/18:2)	↓**	↑	Phospholipid metabolism
		756.5547	−	$[M-H]^-$				
6	2.30	188.0700	+	$[M+H-NH_3]^+$	Tryptophan	↓***	↑**	Phenylalanine, tyrosine, tryptophan bioaynthsis
		203.0795	−	$[M-H]^-$				
7	6.22	544.3387	+	$[M+H]^+$	LysoPC(20:4)	↓***	↑**	Phospholipid metabolism
		542.3250	−	$[M-H]^-$				
8	6.31	427.2848	+	$[M+H]^+$	Prostaglandin PGE$_2$ glyceryl ester	↑	↑***	arachidonic acid metabolism
		425.2544	−	$[M-H]^-$				
9	6.22	520.3381	+	$[M+H]^+$	LysoPC(18:2)	↑***	↓***	Phospholipid metabolism
		518.3251	−	$[M-H]^-$				
10	6.04	494.3232	+	$[M+H]^+$	LysoPC(16:1)	↓***	↑	Phospholipid metabolism
		492.3092	−	$[M-H]^-$				
11	0.58	114.0672	+	$[M+H]^+$	Creatinine	↑***	↓***	Arginie and proline metabolism
		112.0482	−	$[M-H]^-$				
12	6.36	496.3378	+	$[M+H]^+$	LysoPC (16:0)	↓***	↑**	Lipid metabolism
		494.3278	−	$[M-H]^-$				
13	0.58	118.0866	+	$[M+H]^+$	Valine	↓**	↓**	ABC transporters
		116.0717	−	$[M-H]^-$				
14	7.37	538.3870	+	$[M+H]^+$	LysoPE(22:0/0:0)	↑**	↓**	Lipid metabolism
		536.3768	−	$[M-H]^-$				

[a]Change trend of CRF rats vs control rats.
[b]Change trend of FLP rats vs CRF rats.
The levels of potential biomarkers were labeled with (↓) down-regulated and (↑) up-regulated (*$P<0.05$; **$P<0.01$; ***$P<0.001$).

sphatidylcholine, which might be expected to be important factors in the pathogenesis of the renal damage. This study indicated that up-regulated lysoPC(18:0), lysoPC(18:2) and lysoPE(22:0/0:0) and down-regulated lysoPC (16:0) were obviously observed in adenine-induced CKD group (Figure 8 and Table 1), and the reason is not completely clear. It is reported that oxidative stress is related to renal damage [35–37]. Clearly, patients with CKD undergo high oxidative stress because of decreasing antioxidant defenses and increasing prooxidant factors. Several pathophysiologic explanations were put forward. Some attribute the high oxidative stress to malnutrition and hypoalbuminemia, and others propose an association of comorbid factors such as advanced age, diabetes, and inflammatory and infectious phenomena [38,39]. When oxidative stress occurred, the generation of free radical can activate the phospholipase A2, which could hydrolyse phosphatidylcholine to produce lysophosphatidylcholine. This fact may explain the increasing trend of lysophosphatidylcholine in adenine-induced CKD group. Recent literature indicated that lysophosphatidylcholine, by activating protein kinase C signaling

pathways, stimulates epidermal growth factor receptor transactivation and down-stream mitogen-activated protein kinase signaling resulting in mesangial hypercellularity, which is a characteristic feature of diverse renal diseases [40].

Creatinine is another potential biomarker for the separation of CKD rats and FLP-treated group. Increase of creatinine was observed in serum metabolite profiles of CKD group compared with control group and decrease of creatinine was revealed in the serum metabolite profiles of FLP-treated group. Creatinine is an important biomarker to evaluate renal function. This finding corresponded to the results measured with biochemical method in clinical practice. It indicated that UPLC–MS technique and PLS-DA pattern classification are credible. Creatinine is a nonenzymatic breakdown product of creatine and phosphocreatine, and the creatine-phosphocreatine system is crucial for cellular energy transportation. It is reported that animal models with adenine-induced CRF is associated with progressive renal disturbances [16].

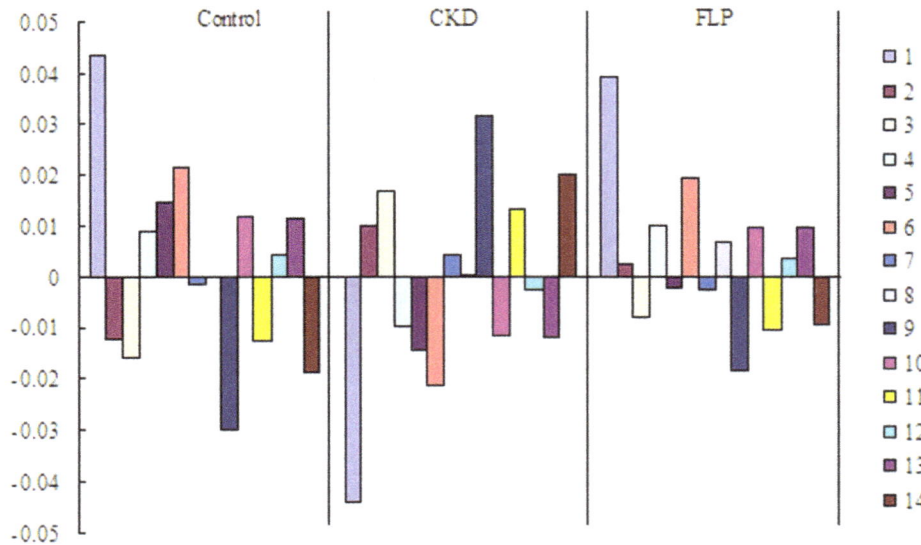

Figure 7. Correlation coefficient analysis between groups with corresponding markers in different groups. Variables are presented in control, CKD and FLP groups. Values of correlations are shown in the vertical axis (upper for positive correlations and low for negative correlations) and corresponding markers represented to the right of the bars. Numbers are consistent with Table 1.

Conclusions

A metabonomics method based on UPLC-MS has been developed to study the effects of FLP on adenine-induced CKD rats. Multivariate statistical analysis shows a clear separation among control group, CKD group and FLP-treated group. Some potential biomarkers like lysoPC(18:0), tetracosahexaenoic acid, lysoPC(18:2), creatinine, lysoPC (16:0) and lysoPE(22:0/0:0) have been identified. Combined with biochemistry and histopathology results, the changes in serum metabolites indicated pharmacological effects of FLP are related to phospholipids metabolism, energy

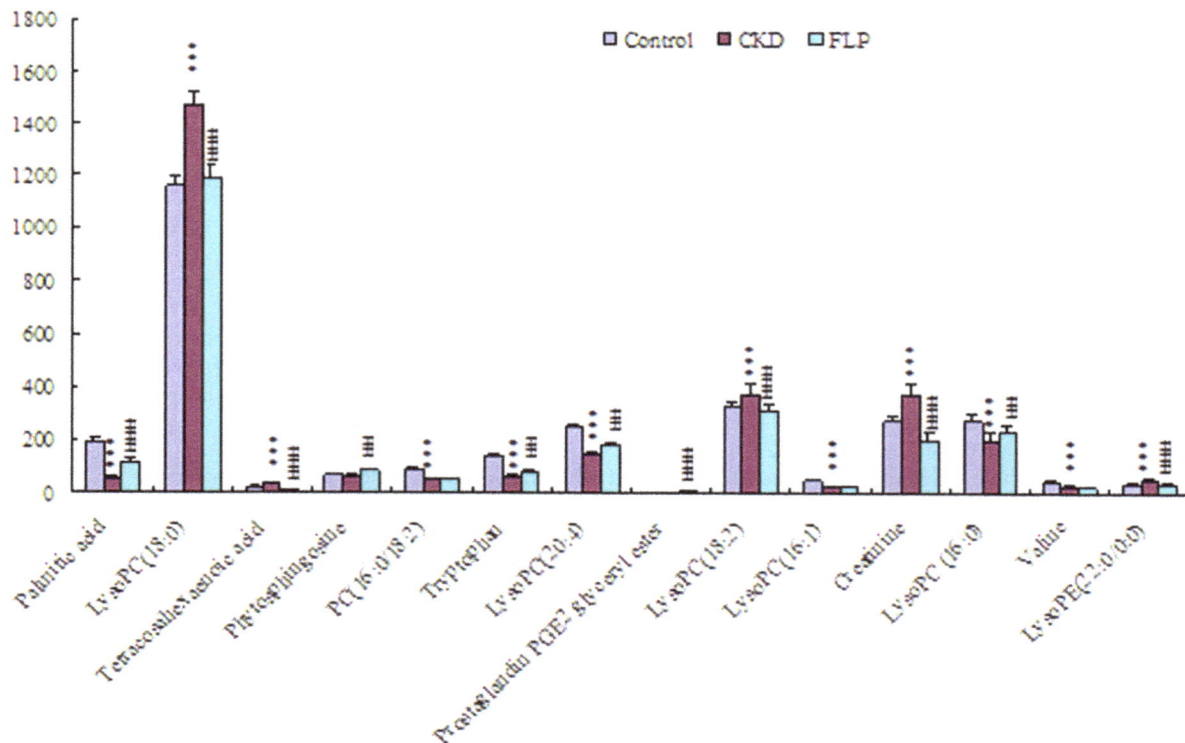

Figure 8. Differential expression levels (mean) of biomarkers in different groups. The "asterisk" indicated the statistical significance of the biomarkers changes by Student's t-test: *P<0.05, **P<0.01, ***P<0.001 significant difference compared with control group; #P<0.01, ##P<0.01, ###P<0.001 significant difference compared with CKD groups.

metabolism and amino acids metabolism. The work shows that the metabonomics method is a valuable tool in drug mechanism research.

References

1. Nicholson JK, Lindon JC, Holmes E (1999) "Metabonomics": understanding the metabolic responses of living systems to pathophysiological stimuli via multivariate statistical analysis of biological NMR spectroscopic data. Xenobiotica 29: 1181–1189.
2. Coen M, Holmes E, Lindon JC, Nicholson JK (2008) NMR-based metabolic profiling and metabonomic approaches to problems in molecular toxicology. Chem Res Toxicol 21: 9–27.
3. Van WH, Yuan K, Lu C, Gao P, Wang J, et al. (2009) Systems biology guided by Chinese medicine reveals new markers for sub-typing rheumatoid arthritis patients. J Clin Rheumatol 15: 330–337.
4. Xiang Z, Wang XQ, Cai XJ, Zeng S (2011) Metabolomics study on quality control and discrimination of three *Curcuma* species based on gas chromatograph-mass spectrometry. Phytochem Anal 22: 411–418.
5. Yang B, Zhang A, Sun H, Dong W, Yan G, et al (2012) Metabolomic study of insomnia and intervention effects of Suanzaoren decoction using ultra-performance liquid-chromatography/electrospray-ionization synapt high-definition mass spectrometry. J Pharmaceut Biomed 58: 113–124.
6. Lao YM, Jiang JG, Yan L (2009) Application of metabonomic analytical techniques in the modernization and toxicology research of traditional Chinese medicine. Brit J Pharmacol 157: 1128–1141.
7. Roux A, Lison D, Junot C, Heilier JF (2011) Applications of liquid chromatography coupled to mass spectrometry-based metabolomics in clinical chemistry and toxicology: A review. Clin Biochem 44: 119–135.
8. Wilson ID, Nicholson JK, Castro-Perez J, Granger JH, Johnson KA, et al (2005) High resolution "ultra performance" liquid chromatography coupled to oa-TOF mass spectrometry as a tool for differential metabolic pathway profiling in functional genomic studies. J Proteome Res 4: 591–598.
9. Wrona M, Mauriala T, Bateman KP, Mortishire-Smith RJ, O'Connor D, (2005) 'All-in-One' analysis for metabolite identification using liquid chromatography/hybrid quadrupole time-of-flight mass spectrometry with collision energy switching. Rapid Commun Mass Spectrom 19: 2597–2602.
10. Zhao YY, Cheng XL, Wei F, Bai X, Tan XJ, et al. (2013) Intrarenal metabolomic investigation of chronic kidney disease and its TGF-β1 mechanism in induced-adenine rats using UPLC Q-TOF/HSMS/MS^E. J Proteome Res 12: 692–703.
11. Zhao YY, Zhang L, Long FY, Cheng XL, Bai X, et al. (2013) UPLC-Q-TOF/HSMS/MS^E-based metabonomics for adenine-induced changes in metabolic profiles of rat faeces and intervention effects of ergosta-4,6,8(14), 22-tetraen-3-one. Chem Biol Interact 301: 31–38.
12. Wyngaarden JB, Dunn JT (1957) 8-hydroxyadenine as the metabolic intermediate in the oxidation of adenine to 2, 8-dihydroxyadenine by xanthine oxidase. Arch Biochem Biophys 70: 150–156.
13. Yokozawa T, Zheng PD, Oura H, Koizumi F (1986) Animal model of adenine-induced chronic renal failure in rats. Nephron 44: 230–234.
14. Zhao YY, Cheng XL, Wei F, Bai X, Lin RC (2012) Effect of ergosta-4,6,8(14), 22-tetraen-3-one (ergone) on adenine-induced chronic renal failure rat: A serum metabonomics study based on ultra performance liquid chromatography/high-sensitivity mass spectrometry coupled with MassLynx i-FIT algorithm. Clin Chim Acta 413: 1438–1445.
15. Zhao YY, Cheng XL, Wei F, Bai X, Lin RC (2012) Application of faecal metabonomics on an experimental model of tubulointerstitial fibrosis by ultra performance liquid chromatography/high-sensitivity mass spectrometry with MS^E data collection technique. Biomarkers 17: 721–729.
16. Zhao YY, Cheng XL, Wei F, Xiao XY, Sun WJ, et al (2012) Serum metabonomics study of adenine-induced chronic renal failure rat by ultra performance liquid chromatography coupled with quadrupole time-of-flight mass spectrometry. Biomarkers 17: 48–55.
17. Zhao YY, Liu J, Cheng XL, Bai X, Lin RC (2012) Urinary metabonomics study on biochemical changes in an experimental model of chronic renal failure by adenine based on UPLC Q-TOF/MS. Clin Chim Acta 413: 642–649.
18. Zhao YY, Shen X, Cheng XL, Wei F, Bai X, et al (2012) Urinary metabonomics study on the protective effects of ergosta-4,6,8(14), 22-tetraen-3-one on chronic renal failure in rats using UPLC Q-TOF/MS and a novel MS^E data collection technique. Process Biochem 47: 1980–1987.
19. Lee KY, Jeon YJ (2003) Polysaccharide isolated from *Poria cocos* sclerotium induces NF-jB/Rel activation and iNOS expression in murine macrophages. Int Immunopharmacol 3: 1353–1362.
20. Pharmacopoeia of People's Republic of China (Part I) (2010) Beijing: China Medical Science Press. 224–225 p.
21. Ríos JL (2011) Chemical constituents and pharmacological properties of *Poria cocos*. Planta Med 77: 681–691.
22. Sekiya N, Goto H, Shimada Y, Endo Y, Sakakibara I, et al (2003) Inhibitory effects of triterpenes isolated from hoelen on free radical-induced lysis of red blood cells. Phytother Res 17: 160–162.
23. Chen YY, Chang HM (2004) Antiproliferative and differentiating effects of polysaccharide fraction from fu-ling (*Poria cocos*) on human leukemic U937 and HL-60 cells. Food Chem Toxicol 42: 759–769.
24. Wang Y, Zhang M, Ruan D, Shashkov AS, Kilcoyne M, et al (2004) Chemical components and molecular mass of six polysaccharides isolated from the sclerotium of *Poria cocos*. Carbohyd Res 339: 327–334.
25. Akihisa T, Nakamura Y, Tokuda H, Uchiyama E, Suzuki T, et al (2007) Triterpene acids from *Poria cocos* and their anti-tumor-promoting effects. J Nat Prod 70: 948–953.
26. Zheng Y, Yang XW (2008) Two new lanostane triterpenoids from *Poria cocos*. J Asian Nat Prod Res 10: 289–292.
27. Zheng Y, Yang XW (2008) Poriacosones A and B: two new lanostane triterpenoids from *Poria cocos*. J Asian Nat Prod Res 10: 645–654.
28. Tai T, Akahori A, Shingu T (1993) Triterpenes of *Poria cocos*. Phytochemistry 32: 1239–1244.
29. Tai T, Shingu T, Kikuchi T, Tezuka Y, Akahor A (1995) Triterpenes from the surface layer of *Poria cocos*. Phytochemistry 39: 1165–1169.
30. Yang CH, Zhang SF, Liu WY, Zhang ZJ, Liu JH (2009) Two new triterpenes from the surface layer of *Poria cocos*. Helv Chim Acta 92: 660–667.
31. Zhao YY, Feng YL. Du X, Xi ZH. Cheng XL, et al (2012) Diuretic activity of the ethanol and aqueous extracts of the surface layer of *Poria cocos* in rat. J Ethnopharmacol 144: 775–778.
32. Otvos JD, Jeyarajah EJ, Bennett DW (1991) Quantification of plasma lipoproteins by proton nuclear magnetic resonance spectroscopy. Clin Chem 37: 377–386.
33. Ilcol YO, Dilek K, Yurtkuran MH, Ulus I (2002) Changes of plasma free choline and choline-containing compounds' concentrations and choline loss during hemodialysis in ESRD patients. Clin biochem 35: 233–239.
34. Ilcol YO, Dönmez O, Yavuz M, Dilek K, Yurtkuran M, et al (2002) Free choline and phospholipid-bound choline concentrations in serum and dialysate during peritoneal dialysis in children and adults. Clin biochem 35: 307–313.
35. Maldonado P, Barrera D, Rivero I, Mata R, Medina CO, et al (2003b) Antioxidant S-allylcysteine prevents gentamicin-induced oxidative stress and renal damage. Free Radical Biol Med 35: 317–324.
36. Maldonado P, Barrera D, Medina CO, Hernandez PR, Ibarra RM, et al (2003) Aged garlic extract attenuates gentamicin induced renal damage and oxidative stress in rats. Life Sci 73: 2543–2556.
37. Rahman A, Ahmed S, Vasenwala SM, Athar M (2003) Glyceryl trinitrate, a nitric oxide donor, abrogates ferric nitrilotriacetate-induced oxidative stress and renal damage. Arch Biochem Biophys 418: 71–79.
38. Miyata T, Kurokawa K, van Ypersele de SC (2000) Relevance of oxidative and carbonyl stress to long-term uremic complications. Kidney Int 76: S120–S125.
39. Shidfar F, Keshavarz A, Hosseyni S, Ameri A, Yarahmadi S (2008) Effects of omega-3 fatty acid supplements on serum lipids, apolipoproteins and malondialdehyde in type 2 diabetes patients. East Mediterran Health J 14: 305–315.
40. Bassa BV, Noh JW, Ganji SH, Shin MK, Roh DD, et al (2007) Lysophosphatidylcholine stimulates EGF receptor activation and mesangial cell proliferation: regulatory role of Src and PKC. Biochim Biophys Acta 1771: 1364–1371.

Author Contributions

Conceived and designed the experiments: YYZ QM. Performed the experiments: YLF. Analyzed the data: YYZ RCL. Contributed reagents/materials/analysis tools: XB XJT. Wrote the paper: YYZ RCL.

13

A Comparative Transcriptome Analysis Identifying FGF23 Regulated Genes in the Kidney of a Mouse CKD Model

Bing Dai[1,9,¤], Valentin David[1,9], Aline Martin[1], Jinsong Huang[1], Hua Li[1], Yan Jiao[2], Weikuan Gu[2], L. Darryl Quarles[1]*

1 University of Tennessee Health Science Center, Medicine-Nephrology, Memphis, Tennessee, United States of America, 2 University of Tennessee Health Science Center, Orthopaedic Surgery, Memphis, Tennessee, United States of America

Abstract

Elevations of circulating Fibroblast growth factor 23 (FGF23) are associated with adverse cardiovascular outcomes and progression of renal failure in chronic kidney disease (CKD). Efforts to identify gene products whose transcription is directly regulated by FGF23 stimulation of fibroblast growth factor receptors (FGFR)/α-Klotho complexes in the kidney is confounded by both systemic alterations in calcium, phosphorus and vitamin D metabolism and intrinsic alterations caused by the underlying renal pathology in CKD. To identify FGF23 responsive genes in the kidney that might explain the association between FGF23 and adverse outcomes in CKD, we performed comparative genome wide analysis of gene expression profiles in the kidney of the Collagen 4 alpha 3 null mice (Col4a3$^{-/-}$) model of progressive kidney disease with kidney expression profiles of Hypophosphatemic (Hyp) and FGF23 transgenic mouse models of elevated FGF23. The different complement of potentially confounding factors in these models allowed us to identify genes that are directly targeted by FGF23. This analysis found that α-Klotho, an anti-aging hormone and FGF23 co-receptor, was decreased by FGF23. We also identified additional FGF23-responsive transcripts and activation of networks associated with renal damage and chronic inflammation, including lipocalin 2 (Lcn2), transforming growth factor beta (TGF-β) and tumor necrosis factor-alpha (TNF-α) signaling pathways. Finally, we found that FGF23 suppresses angiotensin-converting enzyme 2 (ACE2) expression in the kidney, thereby providing a pathway for FGF23 regulation of the renin-angiotensin system. These gene products provide a possible mechanistic links between elevated FGF23 and pathways responsible for renal failure progression and cardiovascular diseases.

Editor: Niels Olsen Saraiva Câmara, Universidade de Sao Paulo, Brazil

Funding: Funding provided by National Institutes of Health Grant RO1-AR45955 from the National Institute of Arthritis and Musculoskeletal and Skin Diseases. The funders had no role in study design, data collection and analysis, decision to publish, or preparation of the manuscript.

Competing Interests: The authors have declared that no competing interests exist.

* E-mail: dquarles@uthsc.edu

9 These authors contributed equally to this work.

¤ Current address: Division of Nephrology, Shanghai Changzheng Hospital, Shanghai, China

Introduction

FGF23 is a bone-derived hormone that regulates phosphate and vitamin D metabolism through FGFR/α-Klotho co-receptors [1] that are expressed in a limited number of tissues, including the kidney [2]. In the kidney, FGF23 suppresses sodium-phosphate co-transporter function leading to phosphaturia and reduces 1,25(OH)$_2$D synthesis in the proximal tubule [3,4]. Physiologically, FGF23 is part of a bone-kidney feedback loop [4,5], where circulating 1,25(OH)$_2$D stimulates FGF23 production in bone and FGF23 suppresses 1,25(OH)$_2$D production in the kidney [5]. FGF23 expression is also regulated by local bone-derived factors that may link bone mineralization with renal phosphate handling [6,7,8].

FGF23 plays a pathological role in hereditary hypophosphatemic disorders [8] and tumor induced osteomalacia [9]. Elevations of circulating FGF23 also occur early in the course of chronic kidney disease (CKD), where it stimulates phosphaturia to maintain phosphate balance and contributes to the development of secondary hyperparathyroidism through suppression of 1,25(OH)$_2$D levels [10,11,12]. FGF23 is also markedly elevated in patients with end stage renal disease (ESRD) [13,14,15].

Elevated FGF23 levels are associated with left-ventricular hypertrophy and hypertension in patients with X-linked hypophosphatemia (XLH) [16]. FGF23 is also an independent risk factor for left ventricular hypertrophy [17] and cardiovascular disease [18] in the general population. In chronic kidney disease, FGF23 is one of the strongest predictors of mortality [19,20], and adverse cardiovascular outcomes [21,22]. In addition, elevated circulating FGF23 concentrations are independently associated with more rapid progression of kidney disease [23] and renal allograft loss [24].

There are many gaps in our knowledge of the molecular mechanisms whereby FGF23 regulates kidney function and leads to adverse outcomes in CKD. It is uncertain which tubular segment and FGF receptors mediate the effects of FGF23 on the kidney [25]. In addition, knowledge of the full complement of renal gene products regulated by FGF23 in the kidney that might mediate progressive renal damage or kidney processes affecting cardiovascular disease is largely unexplored. Without this information, it remains uncertain whether the associations between FGF23 and adverse outcomes represent cause-and-effect relationships or epiphenomena due to co-variance of FGF23 with other causative factors arising from the loss of renal function [26,27]. In addition, because of the limited number of organs that co-express FGFR/$-\alpha$-Klotho complexes [28], it is also possible that elevated circulating FGF23 are directly mediated by off-target effects of FGF23 to activate FGF receptors in non-renal tissues [22], rather than indirectly thru FGFR/α-Klotho-dependent modulation of systemic pathways affecting the cardiovascular system.

Determining the FGF23 responsive genes in the kidney in the setting of chronic kidney disease is challenging because of the systemic effects resulting from FGF23 regulation of phosphate and vitamin D homeostasis and the intrinsic abnormalities related to kidney disease process. To define FGF23 responsive genes in CKD, we performed a genome wide comparative analysis of kidney gene expression in the Col4a3$^{-/-}$ model of excess FGF23 [29] and CKD. We compared this CKD model to the kidney gene transcriptome of models of excess FGF23 without CKD that have different abnormalities of phosphate and vitamin D regulation [30,31]. Shared candidate FGF23 responsive genes in the kidney of these models were confirmed by assessing their expression in FGF23$^{-/-}$ mice and following the acute and chronic administration of recombinant FGF23 *in vivo*. Direct regulation of a subset of genes by FGF23 was assessed in distal tubule cells *ex vivo*. We identified several genes regulated by FGF23 that may link this hormone to processes responsible for progression of kidney disease as well as pathways responsible for adverse cardiovascular outcomes.

Results

Col4a3$^{-/-}$ Mice, a Model of FGF23 Excess

Col4a3$^{+/+}$(WT) Col4a3$^{+/-}$ and Col4a3$^{-/-}$ mice were found to be born with the expected Medelian frequency. Homozygous Col4a3$^{-/-}$ display are known to display a progressive decrease in kidney function [32]. By 12 weeks-of-age, we observed a decrease in body-weight in Col4a3$^{-/-}$ mice (**Figure 1A &B**) and the presence of kidney disease, as evidenced by reduced kidney size (**Figure 1C**) and histological evidence of glomerulosclerosis and interstitial cell infiltration (**Figure 1D**). A 3-fold increase in blood urea nitrogen (BUN) and 2-fold increase in creatinine were observed in Col4a3$^{-/-}$ mice (**Table 1**). Col4a3$^{-/-}$ mice had a 55-fold increase in serum PTH and a 9-fold increase in serum FGF23 concentrations along with an increase in fractional excretion of phosphate. Serum phosphate and calcium concentrations were also increased in Col4a3$^{-/-}$ mice (**Table 1**).

Identification of Additional Renal Signalization Pathways in Chronic Kidney Disease

Clustering of all the significant genes revealed two different patterns corresponding to increased and decreased expression of renal transcripts in Col4a3$^{-/-}$ mice as compared to their WT age-matched control animals (**Figure 2A**). Subsequent analysis revealed that chronic kidney disease led to a dramatic upregulation of gene transcripts, whereas the degree of downregulation was more limited. For instance, using a stringent, five-fold selection criteria to identify changes in gene transcripts, we found that only 4 transcripts were downregulated by this magnitude, whereas 500 genes were upregulated by at least 5-fold in Col4a3$^{-/-}$ mice (**Figure 2B**). This shows that kidney disease progression involves activation of gene transcription and that modifications in the renal transcriptiome is not simply a passive process caused by loss of functioning renal tissue.

The top 25 upregulated genes (**Table 2**) showed evidence of matrix protein replacement with increased collagen synthesis (Col1a1 and Col3a1) and cellular infiltration (Cxcl1, Lyzs, Ccl5, Lyz2, Lyz, C3 VCAM1 and Ear2), consistent with the histological presence of chronic kidney disease in the mice. In total, more than 30 transcripts of protein belonging to the collagen family were increased in the kidneys of Col4a3$^{-/-}$ mice, as well as proteins from the TNFα superfamilly (30 transcripts) and TGFβ superfamily (11 transcripts). Furthermore, TIMP1 was increased along with a substantial disregulation in proteases in the kidney of Col4a3$^{-/-}$ mice, with a total of 24 mettaloendopeptidases being overexpressed.

The top 25 down-regulated genes are shown in **Table 3**. Of note, we found evidence for reductions in DNAse1 and epidermal growth factor (EGF). In addition, we observed reductions in COP9 [33], which regulate ubiquitin-meidated proteoloysis of cullin that is cause of pseudohypoaldosteroinism type 2 and involved in distal tubular regulation of blood pressure and potasium homeostasis [34]. We also observed reduction in Cyp2c44, which important in producing compensatory renal artery vasodilation in response to salt-loading through the regulation of prostaglandin metabolism [35]. We also observed reduction in Slc6a19, which is a major luminal sodium-dependent neutral amino acid transporter in the proximal tubule [36] and parvalbumin, which is involved in distal convoluted sodium transport [37]. Higd1c, which belongs to hypoxia inducible genes that may play a role in protecting the kidney from hypoxic injury during progressive CKD [38], was also reduced in Col4a3$^{-/-}$ kidneys. Corin, a protease that activates atrial natriuretic peptide, was also reduced in the kidneys of Col4a3$^{-/-}$ mice [39].

A total of twelve up-regulated and twelve downregulated genes were randomly chosen from the renal Co4a3$^{-/-}$ transcriptome to be confirmed by RT-PCR as shown in **Table 4**. We also confirmed that the proteins encoded by the mRNAs of the most downregulated and upregulated genes, DNAse1 and Lcn2 respectively, were also altered, as shown in **Figure 3**.

FGF23-related Gene Transcripts in the Kidney

To establish that the Col4a3$^{-/-}$ microarray data set contained genes involved in FGF23 regulation of mineral metabolism, we initially focused on alterations in Cyp24a1, Cyp27b1, Npt2a, Npt2c and Klotho expression. We found that Col4a3$^{-/-}$ mice displayed an increase in the renal Cyp24a1 transcripts, (2.6 and 5.1 fold by microarray and RT-PCR, respectively) as well as marked increase in Cyp24a1 protein level (**Figure 4**). However, we failed to detect any significant changes in Cyp27b1 expression. Additionally, Npt2c (-2.0 and -2.3 fold by microarray and RT-PCR), but not Npt2a, was down-regulated in the kidney of Col4a3$^{-/-}$. Most importantly, α-Klotho, the FGF23 co-receptor, was down-regulated (-2 and -2.2 fold by microarray and RT-PCR) and α-Klotho protein levels in the kidney were reduced by immunohistochemical staining (**Figure 4**).

Comparative Analysis of FGF23 Excess Models

To determine additional FGF23-responsive genes in the kidney of Col4a3$^{-/-}$ mice, we compared microarray analysis of kidneys isolated from 12 week-old WT and Col4a3$^{-/-}$ mice with the renal transcriptome in Hyp mice, which have hypophosphatemia and elevated FGF23 caused by inactivating mutations of Phex in osteoblasts [40], and FGF23 transgenic mice [31]. We hypothesized that shared genes in these three data sets would be enriched with FGF23-responsive transcripts.

From 13694 transcripts present in all three datasets, 31 were found to be significantly altered in the kidney of two or more

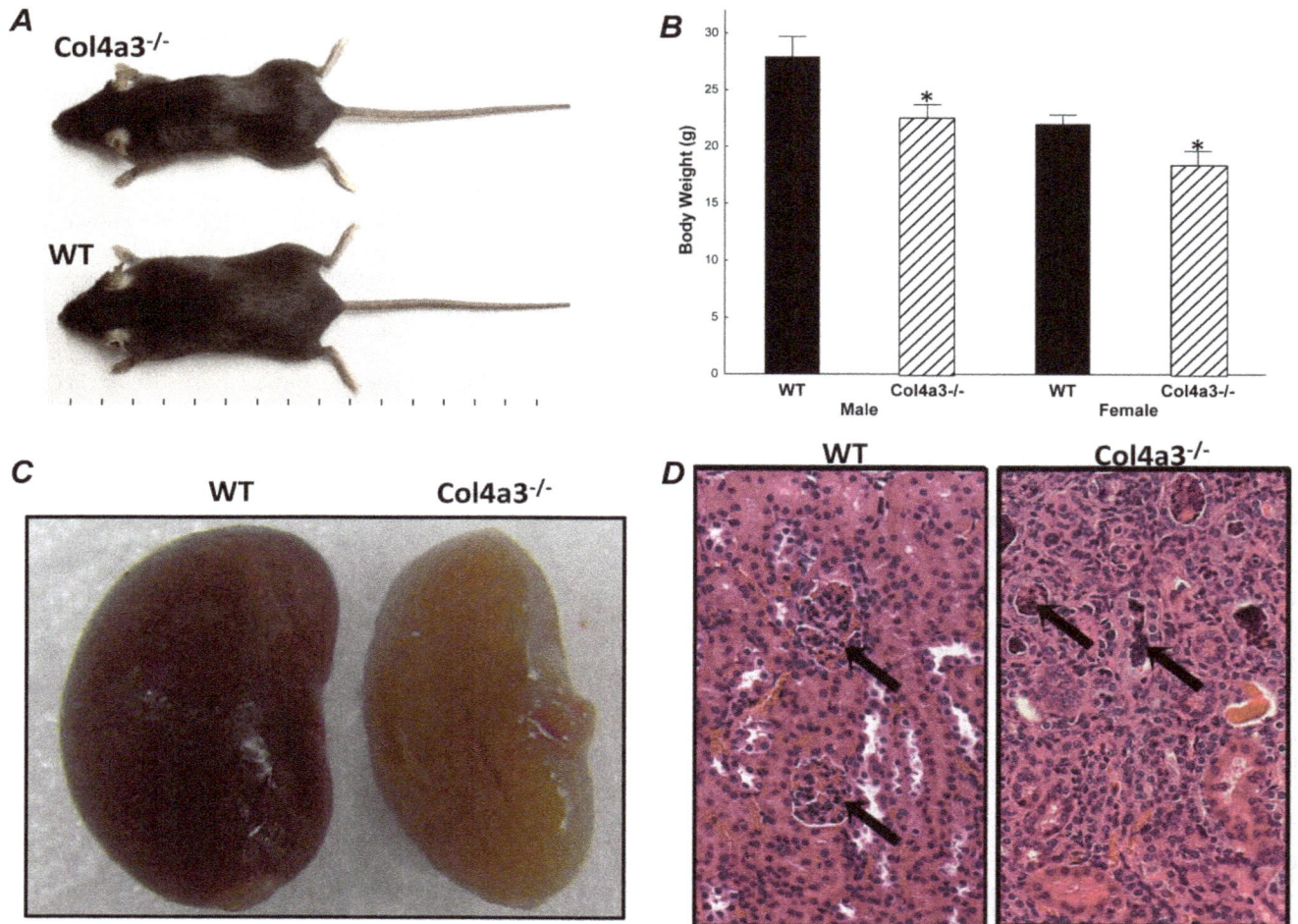

Figure 1. (A) Gross appearance and (B) body weight of 12 week-old wild-type (WT), and Col4a3−/− mice. (C) Kidney morphology showing reduced perfusion and (D) H&E renal histology showing glomerulosclerosis in the Col4a3$^{-/-}$ animals. Values are expressed as mean±SEM, P<0.05 vs: (*) WT, n≥13 mice/group.

mutant mice models compared to their respective WT control mice (**Figure 5**). We have identified 19 of these genes that were consistently (downregulated or upregulated compared to their

Table 1. Serum biochemistry of WT and Col4a3−/− mice.

	WT	Col4a3$^{-/-}$
BUN (mg/dL)	20.29±0.67	59.01±8.59*
Creatinine (mg/dL)	0.45±0.02	0.82±0.15*
FGF23 (pg/mL)	137.34±9.54	1248.29±188.50*
PTH (pg/mL)	32.28±3.81	1772.18±452.94*
FEPi (%)	4.66±1.62	14.82±2.65*
PO4$^-$ (mg/dL)	6.58±0.43	9.39±0.50*
Ca^{2+} (mg/dL)	8.88±0.33	9.38±0.29
ALP (IU/L)	67.16±7.52	87.79±10.56

Values are expressed as mean ± SEM from at least 13 mice per group. Comparisons were performed using one-way ANOVA and post-hoc Fisher test.BUN: Blood Urea Nitrogen; FEPi: Fractional Excretion of Phosphorus; PO4$^-$: phosphorus; Ca^{2+}: total calcium; ALP: Alkaline Phosphatase. (*) P<0.05 vs. WT.

respective controls in all three datasets) altered in Col4a3$^{-/-}$, Hyp and FGF23-transgenic mice (**Table 5**) by subsequently testing by PCR other populations of the same mice. Eleven gene transcripts were increased (**Table 5**), including lipocalin 2 (Lcn2), which was the most up-regulated transcript common to Col4a3$^{-/-}$ and FGF23tg databases (but not the Hyp data set). In addition, inflamatory markers, including VCAM1, which is expressed in proximal tubule cells in response to inflammatory renal diseases [41], complement factor I, a serine protease that regulates the complement cascacade, and galectin-3-binding protein (LGALS3BP), were increased in all data sets. Several genes related to cell signaling were also increased, including tumor-associated calcium signal transducer 2 (Tacstd2), Receptor activity modifying protein 2 (Ramp2), guanylate binding protein 2, immediate early response 3, (Ier3), phospholipase A2 (Pla2g7), phospholipid scramblase 1 (Plscr1). Lipoprotein-associated phospholipase A2 (Pla2g7), an enzyme mostly synthesized by plaque inflammatory cells (macrophages, T cells, mast cells) that hydrolyzes oxidized phospholipids in LDL was also upregulated.

With regards to down-regulated genes, 8 were reduced in all three data sets. Most interestingly, in addtion to reductions in α-Klotho described above, we also found that DNase1, a secreted nuclease that eliminates DNA from necrotic cells, was dramatically

A **B**

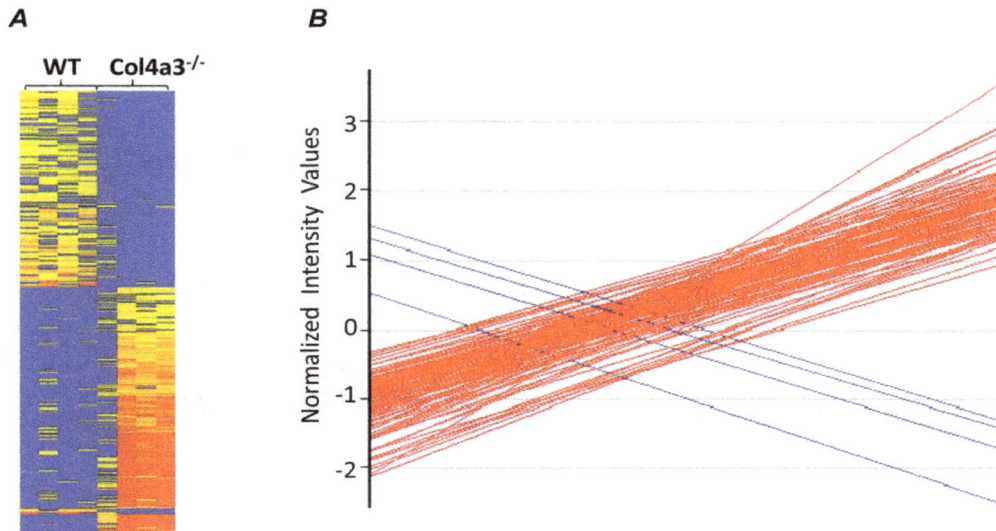

Figure 2. (A) Cluster analysis of microarray performed on Kidneys from 12 week-old wild-type (WT), and Col4a3$^{-/-}$ mice. Gene expression is represented on the heat map from the less expressed (blue) to the more expressed (red). **(B)** Graphic representation of transcripts expressed at least five fold in Col4a3$^{-/-}$ as compared to WT.

Table 2. Expression fold change of the top 25 kidney genes up-regulated in Col4a3$^{-/-}$ mice.

Gene Name	Symbol	Fold Change
lipocalin 2.	Lcn2	53.8
tissue inhibitor of metalloproteinase 1	Timp1	23.7
serine (or cysteine) peptidase inhibitor, clade A, member 3N.	Serpina3n	20.3
amiloride binding protein 1	Abp1	16.7
chemokine (C-X-C motif) ligand 1.	Cxcl1	14.4
lysozyme (Lyzs)	Lyzs	14.4
chemokine (C-C motif) ligand 5.	Ccl5	14.0
collagen, type I, alpha 1.	Col1a1	13.5
eosinophil-associated, ribonuclease A family, member 2.	Ear2	12.4
collagen, type III, alpha 1.	Col3a1	12.4
lysozyme 2	Lyz2	12.4
lysozyme.	Lyz	12.3
complement	C3	12.3
vascular cell adhesion molecule 1.	Vcam1	11.5
serine (or cysteine) peptidase inhibitor, clade A, member 10	Serpina10	9.3
chemokine (C-C motif) ligand 9	Ccl9	9.3
immunoglobulin lambda variable 1	Igl-V1	9.0
B-cell leukemia/lymphoma 2 related protein A1d	Bcl2a1d	8.4
CD44 antigen	Cd44	7.9
eosinophil-associated, ribonuclease A family, member 3	Ear3	7.8
matrix metallopeptidase 2.	Mmp2	7.7
CD14 antigen.	Cd14	7.6
ubiquitin D	Ubd	7.5
histone cluster 1, H2an	Hist1h2an	7.5
serine (or cysteine) peptidase inhibitor, clade A, member 3G	Serpina3g	7.3

Values were obtained after clustering analysis on microarray performed in kidney of *WT and Col4a3$^{-/-}$ mice* (cluster is represented in Figure 2). n = 4 samples/group. Values are expressed as fold change compared to the WT control value. Genes were selected based on a P value threshold of 0.05 and a minimum fold-change absolute value of 2.

A

B

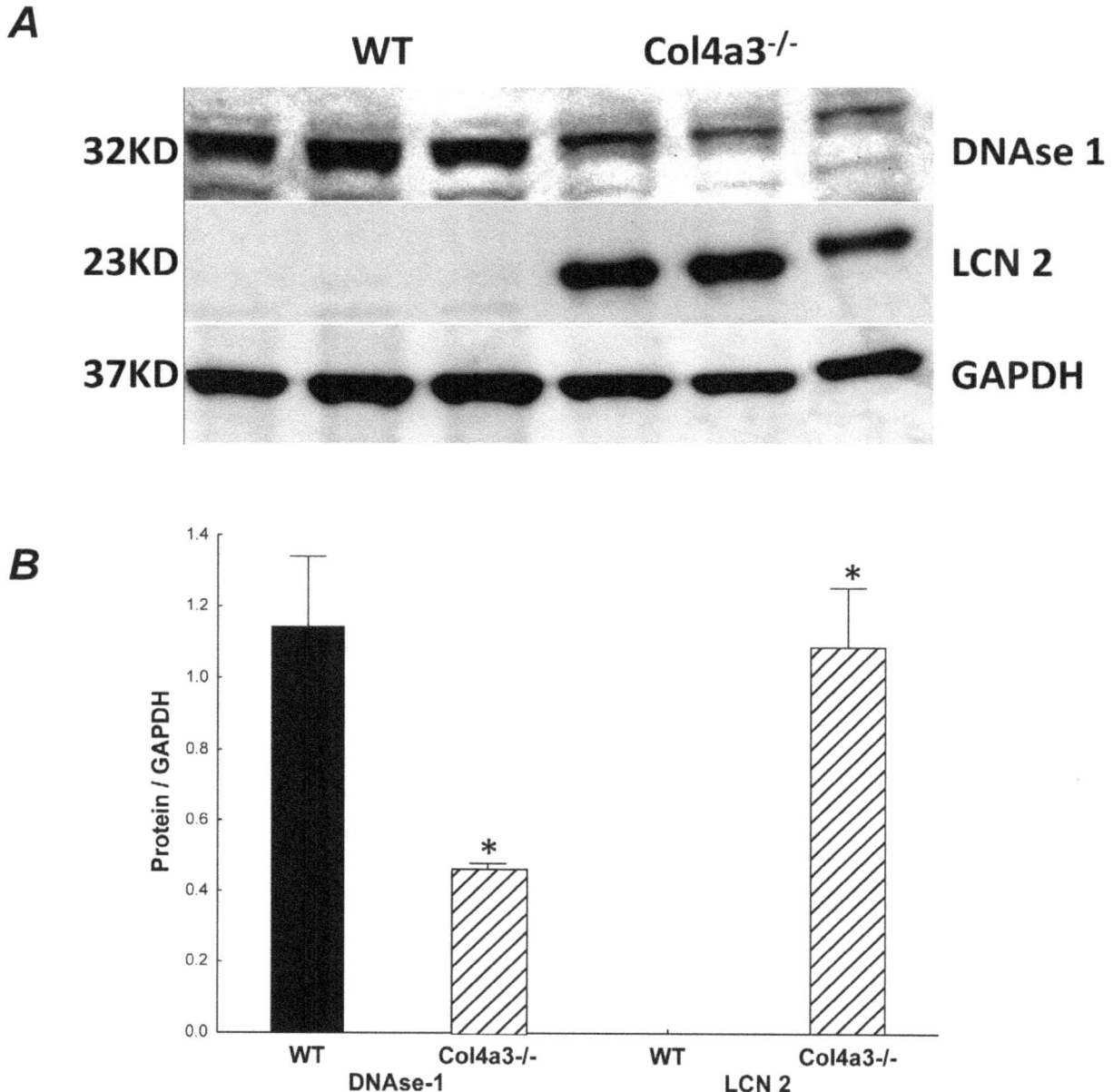

Figure 3. (A) Western blots and corresponding (B) quantification of the most upregulated and downregulated gene product in WT and Col4a3$^{-/-}$ mice.

reduced in all three data sets. Most interestingly, angiotensin-converting enzyme (ACE) 2, a homolog to the carboxypeptidase ACE, was decreased in all three data sets. Finally, Them2 (thioesterase superfamily member 2) a 140-amino-acid protein of unknown biological function was also decreased.

Finally, we performed an Ingenuity Pathway Analysis to identify molecular interactions networks (**Figure 6**) related to these newly identified transcripts. Consistent with the non-mineral metabolism pattern of the expanded set of FGF23-regulated genes, this analysis suggests a central role of activation of transforming growth factor beta and tumor necrosis factor alpha (TGF-beta and TNF-alpha), nuclear factor of kappa light polypeptide gene enhancer in B-cells 1 (NFkB), interleukin 1, beta (IL1B), interferon, platlet derived growth factor (PDGF), progesterone, protein kinase C,

epsilon (PRKCE), and Chemokine (C-C motif) ligand 13 (CCL13) pathways in the common genes regulated in the three data sets, consistent with activation of inflamatory and immunoregulatory processes.

Independent Confirmation of Newly Identified FGF23-responsive Genes

We have used complementary *in vivo* approaches to verify FGF23 regulated genes in the kidney. First, we tested the effects of chronic daily administration of rat recombinant rFGF23 on genes identified from the comparative microarray analysis, plus additional genes (Cyp24a1, Cyp27b1, Npt2a and Npt2c) in FGF23$^{-/-}$ and compound Col4a3$^{-/-}$ FGF23$^{-/-}$ mice. The FGF23 null background was used to minimize the effects of endogenous

Table 3. Fold-change of the top 25 down-regulated genes in Col4a3$^{-/-}$ mice.

Gene Name	Symbol	Fold Change
deoxyribonuclease I.	Dnase1	−8.4
minichromosome maintenance deficient 6	Mcm6	−7.2
hemoglobin, beta adult minor chain	Hbb-b2	−7.2
cytochrome P450, family 2, subfamily d, polypeptide 12	Cyp2d12	−6.8
COP9 (constitutive photomorphogenic) homolog, subunit 8.	COP9	−4.9
4-hydroxyphenylpyruvic acid dioxygenase.	Hpd	−4.8
hemoglobin, beta adult major chain	Hbb-b1	−4.6
cytochrome P450, family 2, subfamily c, polypeptide 44	Cyp2c44	−3.6
erythroid delta-aminolevulinate synthase 2	Alas2	−3.6
solute carrier family 6 (neurotransmitter transporter	Slc6a19	−3.5
epidermal growth factor	Egf	−3.3
parvalbumin	Pvalb	−3.2
camello-like 1	Cml1	−3.2
UDP glucuronosyltransferase 1 family, polypeptide A7C	Ugt1a7c	−3.0
G protein-coupled receptor 112	Gpr112	−3.0
ureidopropionase, beta	Upb1	−2.9
hypoxia inducible domain family, member 1C	Higd1c	−2.9
hydroxyacid oxidase (glycolate oxidase) 3.	Hao3	−2.8
bisphosphate 3'-nucleotidase 1	Bpnt1	−2.8
ureidopropionase, beta	Upb1	−2.8
sorbitol dehydrogenase	Sord	−2.7
endothelial cell-specific molecule 1	Esm1	−2.7
glycine N-methyltransferase	Gnmt	−2.7
adenylate kinase 3 alpha-like 1	Ak3l1	−2.7
corin	Corin	−2.7

Values were obtained after clustering analysis on microarray performed in kidney of *WT and Col4a3*$^{-/-}$ *mice* (cluster is represented in Figure 2). n = 4 samples/group. Values are expressed as fold change compared to the WT control value. Genes were selected based on a P value threshold of 0.05 and a minimum fold-change absolute value of 2.

FGF23 production peaks, as well as the amount of FGF23 injected to these animals. The administration of 50ng/g of rFGF23 twice daily to FGF23$^{-/-}$ and compound Col4a3$^{-/-}$ FGF23$^{-/-}$ mice resulted in a ~12-fold increase in Cyp24a1 and induced a decrease in Cyp27b1 expression (**Table 6**), consistent with known actions of FGF23 on these gene products. Additionally, we have found that chronic FGF23 administration induced elevations in 5 genes (lcn2, cfi, vcam1,gbp2 and plscr1) and decreased the expression of 4 genes (dnase1, car14 ace2 and slca2) in FGF23$^{-/-}$ mice.

Secondly, we have transferred FGF23$^{-/-}$ mice on the Col4a3$^{-/-}$ background, thus identifying genes that respond to CKD progression independently of FGF23. We found that lcn2, cfi, pla2g7, and ier3 were upregulated by kidney disease progression. In addition, we also administered rFGF23 to compound FGF23$^{-/-}$Col4a3$^{-/-}$ mice, to attempt separation of CKD effects from those mediated by FGF23, as well as possible interactions between FGF23 and CKD. The transfer of FGF23$^{-/-}$ on the CKD background, singled out genes that respond to FGF23 only with decline in renal function (upregulated: tacstd2, lgals3bp, ramp2; downregulated: afm, them2). Renal failure and FGF23 interacted to further increase FGF23 actions on lcn2, cfi and ier3, while CKD, although without independent regulatory actions per se, potentiated the effects of FGF23 on gbp2,,plscr1,

dnase1 and slc2a2. Interestingly, Klotho is upregulated by rFGF23 in FGF23$^{-/-}$ mice and normalized in animals with impaired renal function.

Since the chronic admnistaration of FGF23 may lead ot systemic changes, we also evualated the rapid, short-term response to rFGF23 admnistration. This was accomplished by examining the acute effects of rFGF23 administration in C57Bl6 mice after 1 and 12 h. We found that injection of rFGF23 resulted in a 10-fold increase in Cyp24a1 one hour after injection that persisted after 12 h. We also observed that rFGF23 induced a decrease in Cyp27b1 and Npt2c, but had no effect on Npt2a (**Table 7**). Lipocalin2 was confirmed to be increased in the kidney following rFGF23 administration. We also found that GBP2 Tacstd2 and Plscr1 were increased in response to acute FGF23 elevation. Furthermore, Dnase1 and Car14 were decreased by FGF23, consistent with the microarray data. However, we could not confirm FGF23 regulation of ACE2 and Them2 in these short-term FGF23 administration studies.

To investigate if FGF23 directly regulates these genes, we examined the effects of rFGF23 on distal 209 renal tubular cells *in vitro*. By real-time PCR, we found that 209 cells express α-klotho and FGFR4, and lesser amounts of FGFR1 or FGFR3 transcripts (data not shown). We found that 8 of 10 genes tested were directly modified by FGF23 *in vitro*, including FGF23 stimulation of

Table 4. Expression fold change of selected genes confirmed by RT-PCR in Col4a3$^{-/-}$ and WT mice.

Upregulated genes			Down regulated genes		
Gene Symbol	Microarray	RT-PCR	Gene Symbol	Microarray	RT-PCR
FGF23 regulated genes involved in mineral metabolism					
Cyp24a1	2.6	5.1	Npt2c	−2.0	−2.3
Cyp27b1	1.3 (NS)	1.1 (NS)	Npt2a	−1.4(NS)	−1.6(NS)
Genes significantly modified in microarray dataset					
Lcn2	53.8	313.3	Dnase1	−8.4	−7.8
Timp1	23.7	157.8	Hbb-b2	−7.2	−7.2
Vcam1	11.5	25.8	Cyp2d12	−6.8	−6.8
MGP	6.1	9.1	Hbb-b1	−4.6	−6.9
Adamts2	4.9	26.7	Cyp2c44	−3.6	−4.0
STAT3s1	2.4	4.6	Aqp 11	−2.4	−5.1
Slc34a2	4.0	7.9	Cyp 51	−2.3	−2.2
CFI	3.2	5.8	Car14	−2,5	−3.8
Pla2g7	1.7	6.5	Afm	−2.2	−1.9
Lgals3bp	2,1	18.7	Slca2	−1.6	−1.7

Values are expressed as fold change compared to the WT value. n = 4 samples/group. Comparisons were performed using Student T test. P<0.05 vs: WT.

increments in Cf1 and Ramp1 and decrements in α-Klotho, Car14, Slc2a2, ACE2, DNAse 1, and Afm in distal tubule cells after treatment with FGF23 (**Table 8**).

Discussion

Comparative analysis of gene expression profiles of the Col4a3$^{-/-}$ mice, a CKD model of elevated circulating levels of FGF23, and two other models of FGF23 excess and normal renal function [31,40,42,43], along with confirmation of FGF23 regulation of these transcripts in vivo and in vitro, identified novel genes not previously recognized to be regulated by FGF23 as well as confirmed the regulation of genes known to be regulated by FGF23 in the kidney.

The effects of FGF23 on phosphate and vitamin D metabolism are mediated by the regulation of Npt2a, Cyp27b1 and Cyp24a1 functions in the proximal tubule [9]. With the exception of Npt2a, we have evidence in Col4a$^{-/-}$ mice of alterations in Cyp24a1, Nap2a, Npt2c by FGF23, consistent with their known involvement in mediating FGF23 effects on kidney phosphate, calcium and vitamin D metabolism. The failure to observe changes in Npt2a gene transcripts likely points to the important role of post-translation regulation of brush border membrane insertion of this transporter in the regulation of phosphate transport [44]. Also, consistent with post-transcriptional regulation of Cyp27b1, FGF23 had only transient effects on Cyp27b1 gene transcription [45].

While serum soluble α-Klotho concentrations are inversely correlated with serum FGF23 [46] and reductions in α-Klotho mRNA levels in the kidney have been observed with CKD and other states of FGF23 excess FGF23 [47], direct regulation of α-Klotho by FGF23 has not been previously demonstrated. Rather, reductions in α-Klotho in CKD has been attributed to a primary decrement α-Klotho caused by loss of renal tubular cells in the diseased kidney, leading to secondary increments in FGF23 [48]. Both α-Klotho message and protein were decreased in kidneys of Col4a3$^{-/-}$ mice, and the administration of rFGF23 results in

decrements in α-Klotho expression in the kidney of wild-type mice and in cultured distal tubular cells. Interestingly however, chronic administration of rFGF23 to both Fgf23$^{-/-}$ and Col4a3$^{-/-}$Fgf23$^{-/-}$ mice, failed to suppress α-Klotho message levels, which may be due to offsetting effects of 1,25(OH)$_2$D, which is known to stimulate α-Klotho gene transcription [49], in this model. Regardless, FGF23 suppression of α-Klotho might have several physiological effects, including providing a mechanism to desensitize FGF23 signaling responses through FGFR [50] as well as regulate circulating forms of α-Klotho produced by the distal tubule that potential act as a hormone and/or paracrine co-factor for several growth factor receptors [28,48] [48,51].

We identified other gene products that could potentially account for the associations between elevated circulating FGF23 concentrations renal failure progression and cardiovascular mortality that have been found in clinical association studies. At present it is not certain if these untoward effects associated with elevations in FGF23 are due to direct effects of FGF23 on FGFR/α-Klotho complexes in the kidney, off "target effects" of high levels of FGF23 to directly activate FGFRs in the absence of α-Kotho in the heart [22], or represent epiphenomena caused by effects of CKD to increase FGF23 levels. In support of on-target actions, we identified FGF23-regulated renal genes with mechanistic linkages to cardiovascular diseases. In this regard, we found that ACE2 is reduced by excess FGF23 in all three models and found that FGF23 suppresses ACE2 expression in the distal tubule cultures. ACE2 is a negative regulator of the rennin-angiotensin system (RAS) that has vasodilator and natriuretic effects, leading to reduced blood pressure [52]. A direct effect of FGF23 to suppress ACE2 provides an alternative explanation for the recently proposed associations between vitamin D deficiency, activation of the renin-angiotensin system and regulation of α-Klotho expression [53]. FGF23 direct suppression of ACE2 expression could lead to activation of RAS, establishing a linkage between increased FGF23 and increased mortality.

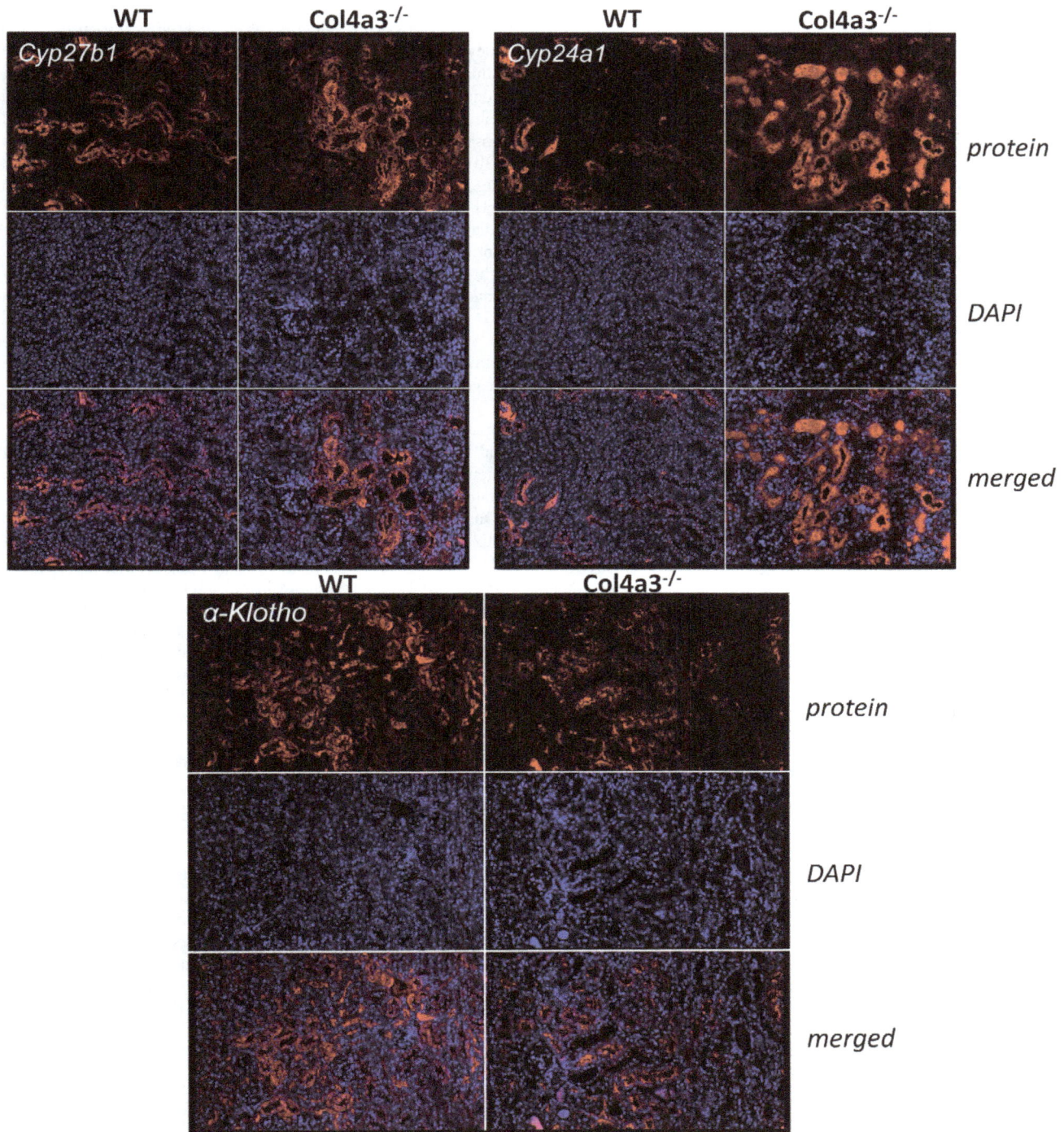

Figure 4. Immunohistochemistry of Cyp27b1, Cyp24a1 and α-klotho in the kidneys of WT and Col4a3$^{-/-}$ mice.

We also identified renal gene products that may mediate a direct effect of FGF23 to accelerate the progression of chronic kidney disease. In addtion to α-Klotho, which has been shown to modulate renal damage [54], we also observed FGF23 regulation of several other genes associated with renal injury, including, Cfi, which has been shown to contribute to inflammatory and acute renal injury [55,56], and suggesting an effect of FGF23-mediated complement activation; DNase1, which is associated with systemic lupus erythematosus (SLE) [57,58], implicating a role of FGF23 in stimulating inflamatory responses in the kidney; carbonic anhydrase 14 (car14), whose inactivation in transgenic mice leads to progressive renal injury [59,60]. Additionally, both slc2a2 and afamin were found to be downregulated in the distal tubular cell line by Fgf23. Slc2a2 (also known as the glucose transporter gene GLUT2) is a disease causing gene for Fanconi-Bickel syndrome, which has systemic as well as characteristic tubular nephropathy

A

B

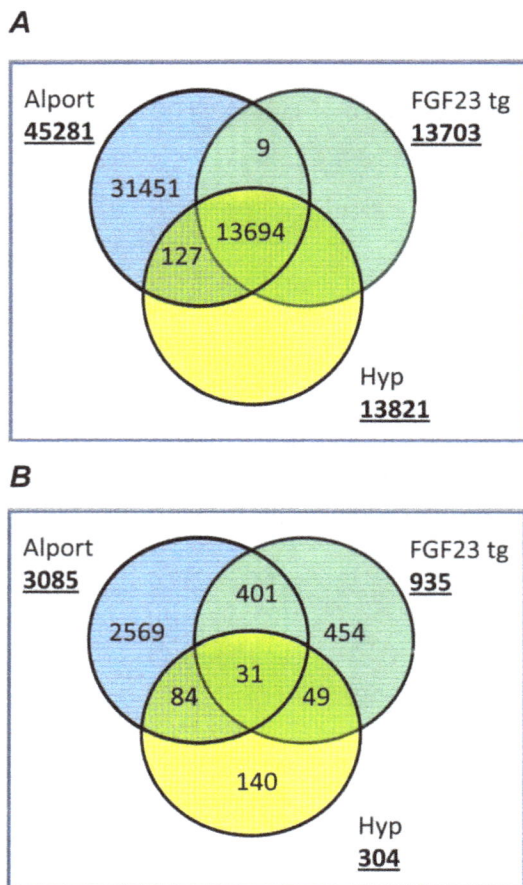

Figure 5. Venn diagram of (A) the total number of genes detected in all 3 data sets and (B) significantly regulated genes in all 3 models.

abnormalities [61]. Decrements in afamin (Afm), a vitamin E-binding protein, related to vitamin D binding protein [62], are observed in early acute renal allograft rejection [63].

Regarding additional genes involved in renal injury, we found that lcn2 (or NGAL) was markedly increased in the Col4a3^{-}/- and the FGF23Tg data set as well as in Fgf23$^{-/-}$ and Col4a3^{-} Fgf23$^{-/-}$ mice receiving rFGF23. Lcn2 mRNA is normally expressed in the kidney [64] where it promotes epithelial differentiation of the mesenchymal progenitors, leading to the generation of glomeruli, proximal tubules, Henle's loop and distal tubules [65,66]. Lcn2 expression is markedly induced in injured epithelial cells through NF-κB dependent pathways [67], and plays a central role in controlling cell survival and proliferation [68–69]. Lcn2 has been shown to contribute to CKD progression both in mice and humans [70]. The magnitude of the increase in Lcn2 as a response to FGF23 was greater in animals with CKD, suggesting that other factors other than FGF23 are also stimulating transcription of this gene. Additionally, 8 other genes which are significantly expressed during the repair stage in AKI were also increased in the kidneys of Col4a3$^{-/-}$ mice, including C3, Vcam1, Serpin10 m C3, Lyz, Col3a1, Col1a1, and abp1 [71]. Finally, Them2, which belongs to a family of enzymes that play an important role in lipid metabolism and might contribute to tubular toxicity [72] was also increased in models of FGF23 excess.

Finally, pathway analysis identified TGF- β and TNF- α signaling pathways as being involved in FGF23 responses in the kidney. The TGF-β pathway are increased in most forms of CKD in humans and experimental animals and controls including fibrogenesis, apoptosis, epithelial-to-mesenchymal transition, and inflammation leading to glomerulosclerosis and tubulointerstitial fibrosis [73]. Three additional genes observed to be altered in a Tgf-β1 Tg mouse model of CKD, were also in the top modified genes in the Col4a3$^{-/-}$ kidneys, including Timp1, Lcn2 and Cxcl1 [73]. TNF alpha is a central proinflammatory agonist mediator that is generated in a wide variety of innate and adaptive immune responses inflammatory mechanisms regulated by TNF might contribute to renal disease progression and cardiovascular events [74,75,76], and even in non-calcified aortas in patients with CKD display increased TNF immunoreactivity [77]. The central role of these pathways, together with IL1-beta, another pro-inflammatory cytokine, demonstrate that the inflammatory state that correlates with kidney disease may be modified by FGF23. We also found FGF23 associated increases in VCAM1, which is expressed in proximal tubule cells in response to inflammatory renal diseases [41], and interferon-induced guanylate-binding protein 2 (GBP2), which regulates cell growth and matrix metalloproteinase expression [78].

Our analysis has several limitations. Data sets from Hyp and FGF23Tg mice have fewer number of genes analyzed than the Col4a3$^{-/-}$ (~13,000 vs. ~45,000, respectively), with the resulting possibility that some genes may have been missed. The presence of CKD could mask FGF23-responsive genes since both FGF receptors and klotho expression and function are altered. However, this appears to be an minor issue, since we confirmed that the known FGF23 regulated genes were still altered in this model. In addition, the microarray analysis was performed in whole tissues, which gives a composite read out of all cell types. We also did not define the specific tubular segments or the role of Klotho/FGFR complexes in the FGF23-mediated changes in gene expression in the kidney. Further studies will be needed to determine the cell-type specific alterations in gene expression. Age difference between the animals of all three databases may also confound the interpretation. The functional significance of FGF23 regulation of these genes remains to be established.

Regardless, we have discovered novel and potentially important FGF23 regulated genes involved in inflammation and progressive renal fibrosis as well as alterations in factors with systemic effects, such as ACE2, which might impact on cardiovascular function. Further studies are needed to test the role of these factors in linking FGF23 to mortality and progressive renal dysfuction.

Materials and Methods

Animals and Genotyping

All mice were maintained on a standard diet (7912, Harlan Teklad, Madison, WI, USA). Animal care and protocols were in accordance with the guidelines established by the University of Tennessee Institutional Animal Care and Use Committee as detailed in the "Guide for Care and Use of Laboratory Animals," prepared by the Institute on Laboratory Animal Resources, National Research Council (Department of Health & Human Services Publication NIH 86–23, National Academy Press, 1996) and UTHSC IACUC specifically approved this study (protocol 1884). Animals were anesthetized before serum collection and sacrifice by ip injection of ketamin (120 mg/Kg) and xylazin (20 mg/Kg), followed by cervical dislocation. During the entire period of the study, activity, respiratory rate, muscle strength via grip strength, feeding and drinking, fur loss were the major signs

Table 5. Expression fold change of 19 renal genes modified in models of excess FGF23.

Gene Name	Symbol	Col4a3−/−	Hyp	FGF23tg
Increased				
lipocalin 2	Lcn2	53.8	NM	2.0
vascular cell adhesion molecule 1	Vcam1	11.5	1.4	1.4
complement component factor i	Cfi	3.2	3.2	1.6
tumor-associated calcium signal transducer 2	Tacstd2	2.5	1.3	1.4
lectin, galactoside-binding, soluble, 3 binding protein	Lgals3bp	2.1	1.3	1.3
phospholipase A2, group VII	Pla2g7	1.7	1.9	2.0
immediate early response 3	Ier3	1.6	1.8	2.2
transporter 1, ATP-binding cassette, sub-family B	Tap1	1.6	1.5	1.2
receptor (calcitonin) activity modifying protein 2	Ramp2	1.5	1.5	1.6
phospholipid scramblase 1	Plscr1	1.4	1.4	1.3
guanylate binding protein 2	Gbp2	1.3	1.6	1.3
Decreased				
deoxyribonuclease I	Dnase1	−8.4	−4.3	−5.0
carbonic anhydrase 14	Car14	−2.5	−1.6	−1.7
Afamin	Afm	−2.2	−1.6	−1.5
Klotho	Kl	−2.0	−1.4	−1.6
abhydrolase domain containing 14A	Abhd14a	−1.9	−1.5	−1.3
angiotensin I converting enzyme 2	Ace2	−1.8	−2.3	−1.9
solute carrier family 2, member 2	Slc2a2	−1.6	−1.4	−1.3
thioesterase superfamily member 2	Them2	−1.6	−1.4	−1.2

Values are expressed as mean±SEM and as a relative percentage of the respective WT control value. Comparisons were performed using Student T test. P<0.05 vs: WT. NM, gene not present in the dataset.

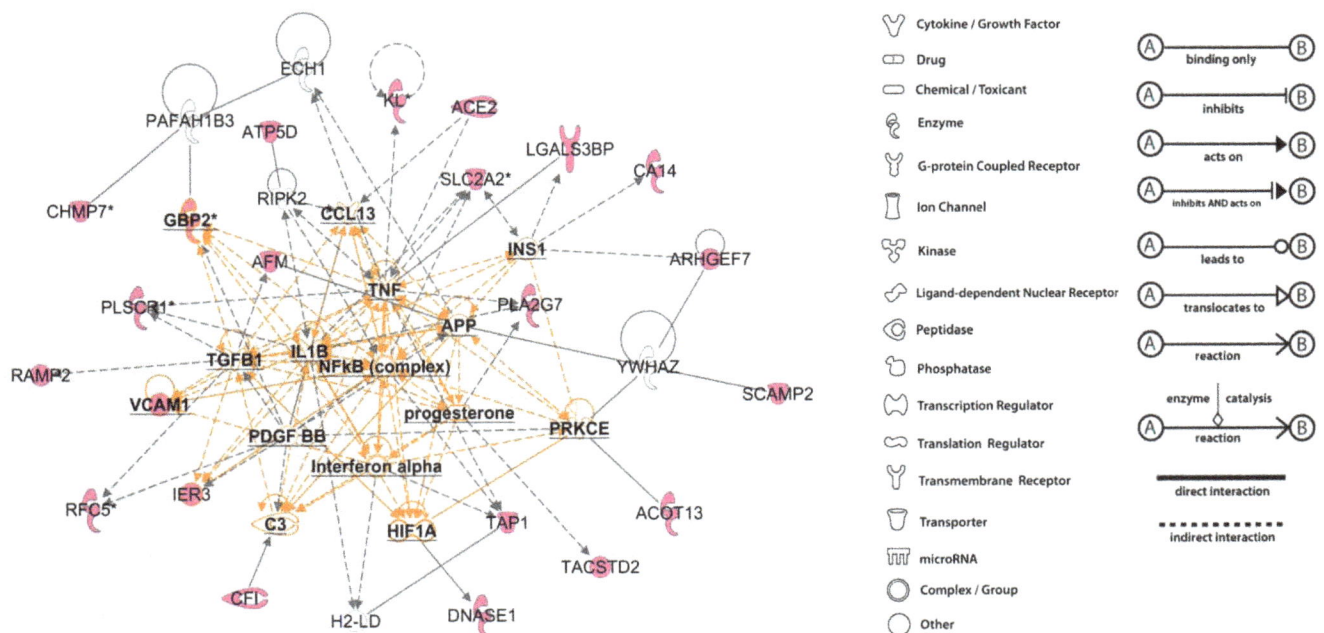

Figure 6. Ingenuity Pathway analysis (IPA) performed on 31 listed genes. The network is built according the identified interconnected pathways involving the highest majority of genes. Genes represented in pink color belong to the cluster. Genes represented in bold font are central regulators of the identified pathways that do not belong to the cluster. Genes represented in white color are other intermediary regulators that do not belong to the cluster.

Table 6. Expression fold change of renal genes modified after injection during 8 weeks of rFGF23.

Gene Name	Symbol	Fgf23$^{-/-}$	Col4a3$^{-/-}$ Fgf23$^{-/-}$	Col4a3$^{-/-}$ Fgf23$^{-/-}$
		+ rFGF23		+ rFGF23
FGF23 regulated genes involved in mineral metabolism				
cytochrome P450, family 24, subfamily A, polypeptide 1	Cyp24a1	+12.6	+1.5	+12.5
cytochrome P450, family 27, subfamily B, polypeptide 1	Cyp27b1	−7.7	+1.3	−3.9
solute carrier family 34 (sodium phosphate), member 3	Npt2c	−1.2 (NS)	−1.8	−2.6
solute carrier family 34 (sodium phosphate), member 1	Npt2a	−1.2 (NS)	1.0 (NS)	−1.2 (NS)
Increased in microarray comparative analysis				
Lipocalin-2	Lcn2	+1.9	+2.6	+6.3
complement component factor i	Cfi	+2.3	+1.3	+2.9
vascular cell adhesion molecule 1	Vcam1	+2.9	−1.1 (NS)	+4.5
guanylate binding protein 2	Gbp2	+2.1	+1.2 (NS)	+3.4
tumor-associated calcium signal transducer 2	Tacstd2	−2.4	−1.2 (NS)	+1.6
lectin, galactoside-binding, soluble, 3 binding protein	Lgals3bp	−3.4	−1.5	+1.8
phospholipase A2, group VII	Pla2g7	−1.1 (NS)	+1.4	−1.2 (NS)
immediate early response 3	Ier3	−1.2 (NS)	+2.0	+2.5
transporter 1, ATP-binding cassette, sub-family B	Tap1	−1.2 (NS)	−1.2 (NS)	+1.1 (NS)
receptor (calcitonin) activity modifying protein 2	Ramp2	−1.7	+1.1 (NS)	+1.5
phospholipid scramblase 1	Plscr1	+1.5	−1.2 (NS)	+2.1
Decreased in microarray comparative analysis				
deoxyribonuclease I	Dnase1	−2.4	+1.5	−8.1
carbonic anhydrase 14	Car14	−1.4	+1.3	−1.9
Afamin	Afm	+1.0 (NS)	+1.0 (NS)	−2.5
αKlotho	α-Kl	+1.9	+1.5	+1.0 (NS)
angiotensin I converting enzyme 2	Ace2	−16.7	(−1.3) NS	−15.6
solute carrier family 2, member 2	Slc2a2	−2.2	−1.1 (NS)	−4.5
thioesterase superfamily member 2	Them2	−1.1 (NS)	−1.2 (NS)	−1.9

Values are expressed as mean ± SEM and as a relative fold change of the non injected Fgf23$^{-/-}$ mice control value. Single (Fgf23$^{-/-}$) and compound (Col4a3$^{-/-}$ Fgf23$^{-/-}$) mice were injected (+rFGF23) or not twice a day with 50 ng/g of recombinant rat FGF23 during 8 weeks. Comparisons were performed using Student T test. P<0.05 vs. Ctr. N≥3/group. NS, gene is present but is not significantly different.

and symptoms that have been monitored.three times a week by the investigator team and daily by the Comparative Medicine employees. If any signs of discomfort or infection were observed, the animal was euthanized by CO2 inhalation followed by cervical dislocation and excluded from the study.

Heterozygous Col4a3$^{+/-}$ mice were initially obtained from Jackson Laboratories (Westgrove, PA, USA). To obtain the compound Col4a3$^{-/-}$ Fgf23 mice $^{-/-}$ we first crossed heterozygous Col4a3$^{+/-}$ females to Fgf23 mice $^{+/-}$ males to obtain Col4a3$^{+/-}$/Fgf23$^{+/-}$ mice and then crossed Col4a3$^{+/-}$/Fgf23$^{+/-}$ males to Col4a3$^{+/-}$/Fgf23$^{+/-}$.

Tail or ear biopsies were collected to genotype the mice. REDExtract-N-Amp Tissue PCR Kit (Sigma-Aldrich, St. Louis, MO, USA) was used for DNA extraction and PCR amplification. Mice were genotyped for col4a3 mutation and PCR was repeated in all mice after sacrifice to exclude artifacts and ensure the correct genotype [30,79].

Administration of Rat Recombinant FGF23

Rat recombinant FGF23 (rFGF23) was administered intraperitoneally (ip) to WT, Fgf23$^{-/-}$ and Col4a3$^{-/-}$/Fgf23$^{-/-}$ mice. To test the chronic effects of FGF23, FGF23$^{-/-}$ and compound Col4a3$^{-/-}$ FGF23$^{-/-}$ mice were administered twice daily (every 12 hours) with 50 ng/g rFGF23 during eight weeks. Kidneys were collected 12 hours after the last rFGF23 administration. This procedure partially corrected the circulating FGF23 levels in serum samples collected 6 and 12 hours after the last injection (69±22 and 47±16 in FGF23$^{-/-}$ mice and 65±14 and 41±12 in Col4a3$^{-/-}$FGF23$^{-/-}$). To test the acute effects of excess FGF23, C57Bl6 mice were given a single injection of 50ng/g rFGF23 and the kidneys were collected 1 and 12 hours after the injection. Experimental animals were compared to animals of the same genotype receiving 0.9% NaCl vehicle.

Serum Biochemistry

Serum samples were collected by intracardiac exsanguination. Serum calcium was measured using a Calcium CPC Liquicolor Kit (Stanbio Laboratories, Boerne, TX, USA) and serum phosphorus was measured using the phosphomolybdylate-ascorbic acid method, as previously described [80]. Serum parathyroid hormone (PTH) levels were measured using the Mouse Intact PTH ELISA kit (Immutopics, Carlsbad, CA, USA). Serum 1,25(OH)$_2$D and 25OHD levels were measured using the vitamin D EIA Kits (Immunodiagnostic Systems, Fountain Hills, AZ,

Table 7. Expression fold change of renal genes modified 1 and 12 h after injection or rFGF23.

Gene Name	Symbol	1 h	12 h
FGF23 regulated genes involved in mineral metabolism			
cytochrome P450, family 24, subfamily A, polypeptide 1	Cyp24a1	10.8	3.5
cytochrome P450, family 27, subfamily B, polypeptide 1	Cyp27b1	−3	NS
solute carrier family 34 (sodium phosphate), member 3	Npt2c	−1.3	−1.5
solute carrier family 34 (sodium phosphate), member 1	Npt2a	NS	NS
Increased in microarray comparative analysis			
Lipocalin-2	Lcn2	3.3	NS
complement component factor i	Cfi	2.2	3.1
vascular cell adhesion molecule 1	Vcam1	NS	NS
guanylate binding protein 2	Gbp2	2.2	NS
tumor-associated calcium signal transducer 2	Tacstd2	1.5	2.3
lectin, galactoside-binding, soluble, 3 binding protein	Lgals3bp	NS	2.3
phospholipase A2, group VII	Pla2g7	1.4	−1.5
immediate early response 3	Ier3	NS	NS
transporter 1, ATP-binding cassette, sub-family B	Tap1	NS	NS
receptor (calcitonin) activity modifying protein 2	Ramp2	NS	NS
phospholipid scramblase 1	Plscr1	NS	2
Decreased in microarray comparative analysis			
deoxyribonuclease I	Dnase1	NS	−2.0
carbonic anhydrase 14	Car14	NS	−2.2
Afamin	Afm	NS	NS
αKlotho	α-Kl	−1.5	1.7
angiotensin I converting enzyme 2	Ace2	NS	NS
solute carrier family 2, member 2	Slc2a2	1.3	1.5
thioesterase superfamily member 2	Them2	NS	NS

Values are expressed as mean±SEM and as a relative fold change of the non injected control WT mice (Ctr)value. Comparisons were performed using Student T test. P<0.05 vs. Ctr. N≥ 4/group. NS, gene is present but is not significantly different.

Table 8. Expression fold change of selected genes confirmed by RT-PCR in a distal cell culture model, after 12 h of rFGF23 treatment.

Gene Symbol	Distal (209) Cells
Vcam1	NS
Cfi	2.0
Pla2g7	NS
Ramp2	1.3
αKl	−1.8
Car14	−3.7
Slc2a2	−2.2
Ace2	−1.7
Dnase1	−1.4
Afm	−1.4

Distal (209) tubular cell lines were cultured during 1 week and treated with 2 µg of rFGF23 per well. Values are expressed as mean±SEM and as a relative fold change of the untreated control. Comparisons were performed using Student T test. N≥ 4; P<0.05 vs: untreated control.

USA). Serum FGF23 levels were measured using the FGF23 ELISA kit (Kainos Laboratories, Tokyo, Japan).

RT-PCR and Microarray

RT-PCR and microarray analysis were performed on kidneys from 12 week-old mice. Total RNAs were isolated using TRI-reagent (Molecular Research Center, Cincinnati, OH, USA) according to previously published method [81]. First-strand cDNA was synthesized from the kidney RNAs using iScript cDNA Synthesis kit (Bio-Rad, Hercules, CA, USA). The 20µL reverse transcriptase reaction was based on 1µg total RNA. The iCycler iQ Real-Time PCR Detection System and iQ SYBR Green Supermix (Bio-Rad, Hercules, CA, USA) were used for real-time quantitative PCR analysis. The expression was normalized by glyceraldehyde-3-phosphate dehydrogenase (*Gapdh*) in the same sample and expressed as 100% of the control (WT). Sequences of primers used for real-time quantitative RT-PCR are listed in **Table 9**. The expression of 45,000 genes was tested on the kidney samples using the Illumina.SingleColor.MouseWG-6_V2_0_R1_11278593_A chip (Illumina, San Diego, CA, USA) at the DNA Discovery Core of University of Tennessee Health Science Center on 4 male mice per group. The resulting data were compared with previously published data reflecting the renal transcriptome in Hyp [40] and FGF23 transgenic mice [31].

Table 9. Sequences of primers used for RT-PCR.

Target Gene	Forward Primer	Reverse Primer
Ace2	CTTCTCTTCTCAGTGCCCAACCCA	CCCGTGCGCCAAGATCCCAT
Adamts2	CTGACGCCCAGGGCCGCTT	CGCCGTGAGCTGTTGATGCG
Afm	AGT GAC GAG TTC GCC TGC GT	CTG GCA CTG GCT TTG GTC GGT
Aqp 11	GTC CCC CGA AAT GGG TGC CG	GGC TCC CTC CTG CAT AGG CCA
Car14	TTG GAT CCT GGC TGC AGA TGG G	TGG CCA ATG GTC CTG ACC GTG
Cfi	AGA CTT GGC CCC GCA CTC CT	CAC ACA CTG GGG TGC CAG CC
Cyp 51	CCC TCA GAC GGT GGC AGG GT	GTC CAA GCG CTC TGC CCA GG
Cyp24a1	GTT CTG TCC ACG GTA GGC	CCA GTC TTC GCA GTT GTC C
Cyp27b1	ACA CTT CGC ACA GTT TAC G	TTA GCA ATC CGC AAG CAC
Cyp2c44	CCC AAG GGC ACC GCT GTG TT	AGC TCC ATG CGG GCC AAA CC
Cyp2d12	AGC CCA GAT CCC AAG GGC AGT	GGT GAC TGG GCA GGG TCC CA
Dnase1	TGC CTG GAC AGC GAC CCT GA	TGA GCC CCC GAG TCT GCA CT
Gbp2	ACA GTG CCT GTG AGA GAG GAC AGA	CTG TGC GGT AGA GGC CCA CGA
Hbb-b1	GCT TCT GAT TCT GTT GTG TTG ACT TGC	GAC AAC CAG CAG CCT GCC CA
Hbb-b2	AGG CCC TGG GCA GGT TGG TA	GCC ATG GGC CTT CAC CTT GGG
Ier3	GGC GCC AGC TAC CAA CCG AG	GAC CGG GGG CGC AGT AAT GG
Lcn2	TGG CAG GCA ATG CGG TCC AG	CCG TGG TGG CCA CTT GCA CA
Lgals3bp	AAG TGG TGG GCA GCA GCG TC	GCT CGA ACA GCT CCT GGG GC
Mgp	GCAGCGCCGAGGAGCCAAATA	AGGAAGGAGTGGGCCAGCCAG
αKlotho	AGC GAT AGT TAC AAC AAC	GCA TTC TCT GAT ATT ATA GTC
Npt2a	ATG CTG GCT TTC CTT TAC	CCA CAA TGT TCA TGC CTT CT
Npt2c	CGT GCG GAC TGT TAT CAA TG	TAC TGG GCA GTC AGG TTT CC
Pla2g7	TGC TGC CTC CCA TGG GTC CA	AGC CGG CAG CAG ACA TCA CC
Plscr1	GAG TCC CCT CTG CGA GGG AAA GC	CCC CGG TGG ACA GTT CAG TGG A
Ramp2	GAC AGC GTT GTG CCT CCC TCC	GCT GCA CCA GGG AGC AGT TCG
Slc2a2	CCA GCT TTG CAG TGG GCG GA	CCC AGG GCA CCC CTG AGT GT
Slc34a2	AAA TGC CCA GCC CAA CCC CG	GTC CGG CCA CTT TGC CTC CA
STAT3s1	CCCCGAAGCCGACCCAGGTA	TGCTGCAGGTCGTTGGTGTCA
Tacstd2	GCG ATG GCG ACC CGC TTT TG	GAC CCC GCC TGG GCC ATT TG
Tap1	GCC CTT GAG GCC TTA TCG GCG	ATG AGA CAA GGT TGC CGC TGC TG
Them2	TTT CTC CCG AGC ACG ACG CG	GGA GCA GCC GAG ACA AGC GT
Timp1	CAC GGG CCG CCT AAG GAA CG	TCC GTG GCA GGC AAG CAA AGT
Vcam1	TGT CAA CGT TGC CCC CAA GGA	GGC ATC CTG CAG CTG TGC CT

Western Blotting and Immunohistochemistry

These techniques were performed as previously described [8,82,83]. Briefly, total proteins from kidneys were extracted in 1ml lysis buffer of T-PER Tissue protein extraction reagent (Pierce, IL, USA). supplemented with protease inhibitors (Roche Applied Science, IN, USA). Protein lysates (25 µg/sample) were reduced and extracted in LDS Sample buffer (Invitrogen, CA, USA) heated for 10 min at 70°C, migrated on NuPAGE Novex 10% Bis-Tris Gels (Invitrogen, CA, USA), and then analyzed by Western blotting using the ECL Advance WB Detection Kit (GE Healthcare, UK). The immunoreactive bands were visualized using enhanced chemiluminescence detection reagents (GE Healthcare, UK) on a Fluor-S Multi Imager (BioRad, CA, USA). Band intensities were determined by densitometry using ImageJ (NIH, USA).

For immunohistochemistry, left kidneys were dehydrated in absolute ethanol and embedded in paraffin. 5µm thick sections were cut on a rotary microtome. Sections were dried overnight on pre-charged pre-cleaned slides (VWR Scientific, PA, USA), deparaffinized and rehydrated. Nonspecific sites were blocked with 1X animal free blocker (Vector Laboratories Inc., CA, USA) and then sections were incubated with specific primary antibodies for 1 hour. An Immunohistological Vectastain ABC kit (Vector Laboratories Inc., CA, USA) was subsequently used for detection of the target protein and slides counterstained with DAPI, dehydrated and mounted with entellan. The following primary antibodies have been used: goat-raised anti-human Klotho (sc-22218), goat-raised anti-human Cyp27b1 (sc-49642), goat-raised anti-human Cyp24a1 (sc-32165), goat-raised anti-mouse lipocalin2 (sc-18698), goat-raised anti-mouse DNase1 (sc-19269) from Santa Cruz Biotechnology (Santa Cruz, CA).

Cell Culture

Immortalized renal tubular cells were kindly donated by Peter Friedman [84]. Cells were plated in standard 25 cm^2 flasks and allowed to grow until confluence. Cells were removed with 0.25% trypsin solution containing 0.02% EDTA (Sigma- Aldrich, St. Louis, MO, USA) and plated on 6-well plates for 7 days, then treated with 2 μg/well of rFGF23 or vehicle for 24 hours.

Statistics

Differences among the two groups were tested by Student T test using the Statistica software (Statsoft, Tulsa, OK, USA). The differences were considered statistically significant at p<0.05.

Microarray analysis and filtering was performed as previously described [8]. Briefly, microarray data were analyzed using GeneSpring GX7.3 software (Agilent Technologies, Santa Clara, CA, USA). The Robust Multichip Averaging probe summarization algorithm was used to perform background correction, normalization, and probe summarization. Data were normalized per chip and per gene to the median. Genes were filtered to include only those that were expressed in at least one of the eight samples. The statistical analysis was performed using a one-way ANOVA followed by Benjamini-Hochberg multiple test correction assuming variances were equals to minimize the false positive discovery. P value was set at 0.05. Cluster analysis using a gene tree classification, Pearson correlation and average linkage was then performed to identify groups of genes for which the patterns of expression were similar. Pathway analysis was performed using the Ingenuity program (Ingenuity Systems, Redwood City, CA, USA) to match the identified genes of interest to already known broader networks of genes contained in the literature database.

Acknowledgments

The authors thank Drs. Ivan Gerling, for his help and advice on microarray analysis.

Author Contributions

Conceived and designed the experiments: VD DQ. Performed the experiments: BD VD YJ. Analyzed the data: VD DQ AM BD. Contributed reagents/materials/analysis tools: AM HL JH YJ WG. Wrote the paper: VD DQ.

References

1. Martin A, David V, Quarles LD (2012) Regulation and function of the FGF23/klotho endocrine pathways. Physiol Rev 92: 131–155.
2. Kurosu H, Ogawa Y, Miyoshi M, Yamamoto M, Nandi A, et al. (2006) Regulation of fibroblast growth factor-23 signaling by klotho. J Biol Chem 281: 6120–6123.
3. Li H, Martin A, David V, Quarles LD (2011) Compound deletion of Fgfr3 and Fgfr4 partially rescues the Hyp mouse phenotype. Am J Physiol Endocrinol Metab 300: E508–517.
4. Liu S, Quarles LD (2007) How fibroblast growth factor 23 works. J Am Soc Nephrol 18: 1637–1647.
5. Liu S, Tang W, Zhou J, Stubbs JR, Luo Q, et al. (2006) Fibroblast growth factor 23 is a counter-regulatory phosphaturic hormone for vitamin D. J Am Soc Nephrol 17: 1305–1315.
6. Mirams M, Robinson BG, Mason RS, Nelson AE (2004) Bone as a source of FGF23: regulation by phosphate? Bone 35: 1192–1199.
7. Liu S, Guo R, Simpson LG, Xiao ZS, Burnham CE, et al. (2003) Regulation of fibroblastic growth factor 23 expression but not degradation by PHEX. J Biol Chem 278: 37419–37426.
8. Martin A, Liu S, David V, Li H, Karydis A, et al. (2011) Bone proteins PHEX and DMP1 regulate fibroblastic growth factor Fgf23 expression in osteocytes through a common pathway involving FGF receptor (FGFR) signaling. Faseb J 25: 2551–2562.
9. Quarles LD (2008) Endocrine functions of bone in mineral metabolism regulation. J Clin Invest 118: 3820–3828.
10. Hasegawa H, Nagano N, Urakawa I, Yamazaki Y, Iijima K, et al. (2010) Direct evidence for a causative role of FGF23 in the abnormal renal phosphate handling and vitamin D metabolism in rats with early-stage chronic kidney disease. Kidney Int 78: 975–980.
11. Isakova T, Wolf MS (2010) FGF23 or PTH: which comes first in CKD ? Kidney Int 78: 947–949.
12. Wetmore JB, Quarles LD (2009) Calcimimetics or vitamin D analogs for suppressing parathyroid hormone in end-stage renal disease: time for a paradigm shift? Nat Clin Pract Nephrol 5: 24–33.
13. Weber TJ, Liu S, Indridason OS, Quarles LD (2003) Serum FGF23 levels in normal and disordered phosphorus homeostasis. J Bone Miner Res 18: 1227–1234.
14. Imanishi Y, Inaba M, Nakatsuka K, Nagasue K, Okuno S, et al. (2004) FGF-23 in patients with end-stage renal disease on hemodialysis. Kidney Int 65: 1943–1946.
15. Komaba H, Fukagawa M (2010) FGF23-parathyroid interaction: implications in chronic kidney disease. Kidney Int 77: 292–298.
16. Nehgme R, Fahey JT, Smith C, Carpenter TO (1997) Cardiovascular abnormalities in patients with X-linked hypophosphatemia. J Clin Endocrinol Metab 82: 2450–2454.
17. Hsu HJ, Wu MS (2009) Fibroblast growth factor 23: a possible cause of left ventricular hypertrophy in hemodialysis patients. Am J Med Sci 337: 116–122.
18. Parker BD, Schurgers LJ, Brandenburg VM, Christenson RH, Vermeer C, et al. (2010) The associations of fibroblast growth factor 23 and uncarboxylated matrix Gla protein with mortality in coronary artery disease: the Heart and Soul Study. Ann Intern Med 152: 640–648.
19. Stubbs JR, Quarles LD (2009) Fibroblast growth factor 23: uremic toxin or innocent bystander in chronic kidney disease? Nephrol News Issues 23: 33–34, 36–37.
20. Gutierrez OM, Mannstadt M, Isakova T, Rauh-Hain JA, Tamez H, et al. (2008) Fibroblast growth factor 23 and mortality among patients undergoing hemodialysis. N Engl J Med 359: 584–592.
21. Isakova T, Xie H, Yang W, Xie D, Anderson AH, et al. (2011) Fibroblast growth factor 23 and risks of mortality and end-stage renal disease in patients with chronic kidney disease. JAMA 305: 2432–2439.
22. Faul C, Amaral AP, Oskouei B, Hu MC, Sloan A, et al. (2011) FGF23 induces left ventricular hypertrophy. J Clin Invest 121: 4393–4408.
23. Fliser D, Kollerits B, Neyer U, Ankerst DP, Lhotta K, et al. (2007) Fibroblast growth factor 23 (FGF23) predicts progression of chronic kidney disease: the Mild to Moderate Kidney Disease (MMKD) Study. J Am Soc Nephrol 18: 2600–2608.
24. Wolf M, Molnar MZ, Amaral AP, Czira ME, Rudas A, et al. (2011) Elevated fibroblast growth factor 23 is a risk factor for kidney transplant loss and mortality. J Am Soc Nephrol 22: 956–966.
25. Liu S, Vierthaler L, Tang W, Zhou J, Quarles LD (2008) FGFR3 and FGFR4 do not mediate renal effects of FGF23. J Am Soc Nephrol 19: 2342–2350.
26. Fukumoto S, Araya K, Backenroth R, Takeuchi Y, Nakayama K, et al. (2005) A novel mutation in fibroblast growth factor 23 gene as a cause of tumoral calcinosis. Journal of Clinical Endocrinology & Metabolism 90: 5523–5527.
27. Stubbs JR, Liu S, Tang W, Zhou J, Wang Y, et al. (2007) Role of hyperphosphatemia and 1,25-dihydroxyvitamin D in vascular calcification and mortality in fibroblastic growth factor 23 null mice. J Am Soc Nephrol 18: 2116–2124.
28. Kuro-o M, Matsumura Y, Aizawa H, Kawaguchi H, Suga T, et al. (1997) Mutation of the mouse klotho gene leads to a syndrome resembling ageing. Nature 390: 45–51.
29. Stubbs JR, He N, Idicula A, Gillihan R, Liu S, et al. (2011) Longitudinal evaluation of FGF23 changes and mineral metabolism abnormalities in a mouse model of chronic kidney disease. J Bone Miner Res 27: 38–46.
30. Liu S, Zhou J, Tang W, Jiang X, Rowe DW, et al. (2006) Pathogenic role of Fgf23 in Hyp mice. Am J Physiol Endocrinol Metab 291: E38–49.
31. Marsell R, Krajisnik T, Goransson H, Ohlsson C, Ljunggren O, et al. (2008) Gene expression analysis of kidneys from transgenic mice expressing fibroblast growth factor-23. Nephrol Dial Transplant 23: 827–833.
32. Stubbs JR, He N, Idicula A, Gillihan R, Liu S, et al. (2011) Longitudinal evaluation of FGF23 changes and mineral metabolism abnormalities in a mouse model of chronic kidney disease. J Bone Miner Res.
33. Wolf DA, Zhou C, Wee S (2003) The COP9 signalosome: an assembly and maintenance platform for cullin ubiquitin ligases? Nat Cell Biol 5: 1029–1033.
34. Boyden LM, Choi M, Choate KA, Nelson-Williams CJ, Farhi A, et al. (2012) Mutations in kelch-like 3 and cullin 3 cause hypertension and electrolyte abnormalities. Nature 482: 98–102.
35. DeLozier TC, Tsao CC, Coulter SJ, Foley J, Bradbury JA, et al. (2004) CYP2C44, a new murine CYP2C that metabolizes arachidonic acid to unique stereospecific products. J Pharmacol Exp Ther 310: 845–854.
36. Camargo SM, Singer D, Makrides V, Huggel K, Pos KM, et al. (2009) Tissue-specific amino acid transporter partners ACE2 and collectrin differentially interact with hartnup mutations. Gastroenterology 136: 872–882.
37. Belge H, Devuyst O (2010) [Parvalbumin and regulation of ion transport in the distal convoluted tubule of the kidney]. Med Sci (Paris) 26: 566–568.

38. Song YR, You SJ, Lee YM, Chin HJ, Chae DW, et al. (2010) Activation of hypoxia-inducible factor attenuates renal injury in rat remnant kidney. Nephrol Dial Transplant 25: 77–85.

39. Wang W, Shen J, Cui Y, Jiang J, Chen S, et al. (2012) Impaired sodium excretion and salt-sensitive hypertension in corin-deficient mice. Kidney Int 82: 26–33.

40. Meyer MH, Dulde E, Meyer RA, Jr. (2004) The genomic response of the mouse kidney to low-phosphate diet is altered in X-linked hypophosphatemia. Physiol Genomics 18: 4–11.

41. Tu Z, Kelley VR, Collins T, Lee FS (2001) I kappa B kinase is critical for TNF-alpha-induced VCAM1 gene expression in renal tubular epithelial cells. J Immunol 166: 6839–6846.

42. Machuca E, Benoit G, Antignac C (2009) Genetics of nephrotic syndrome: connecting molecular genetics to podocyte physiology. Hum Mol Genet 18: R185–194.

43. Yoder BK, Mulroy S, Eustace H, Boucher C, Sandford R (2006) Molecular pathogenesis of autosomal dominant polycystic kidney disease. Expert Rev Mol Med 8: 1–22.

44. Weinman EJ, Steplock D, Shenolikar S, Biswas R (2011) Fibroblast growth factor-23-mediated inhibition of renal phosphate transport in mice requires sodium-hydrogen exchanger regulatory factor-1 (NHERF-1) and synergizes with parathyroid hormone. J Biol Chem 286: 37216–37221.

45. Yuan B, Xing Y, Horst RL, Drezner MK (2004) Evidence for abnormal translational regulation of renal 25-hydroxyvitamin D-1alpha-hydroxylase activity in the hyp-mouse. Endocrinology 145: 3804–3812.

46. Yamazaki Y, Imura A, Urakawa I, Shimada T, Murakami J, et al. (2010) Establishment of sandwich ELISA for soluble alpha-Klotho measurement: Age-dependent change of soluble alpha-Klotho levels in healthy subjects. Biochem Biophys Res Commun 398: 513–518.

47. Koh N, Fujimori T, Nishiguchi S, Tamori A, Shiomi S, et al. (2001) Severely reduced production of klotho in human chronic renal failure kidney. Biochem Biophys Res Commun 280: 1015–1020.

48. Kuro-o M (2011) Phosphate and Klotho. Kidney Int Suppl 121: S20–23.

49. Haussler MR, Haussler CA, Whitfield GK, Hsieh JC, Thompson PD, et al. (2010) The nuclear vitamin D receptor controls the expression of genes encoding factors which feed the "Fountain of Youth" to mediate healthful aging. J Steroid Biochem Mol Biol 121: 88–97.

50. Freedman NJ, Kim LK, Murray JP, Exum ST, Brian L, et al. (2002) Phosphorylation of the platelet-derived growth factor receptor-beta and epidermal growth factor receptor by G protein-coupled receptor kinase-2. Mechanisms for selectivity of desensitization. J Biol Chem 277: 48261–48269.

51. Haruna Y, Kashihara N, Satoh M, Tomita N, Namikoshi T, et al. (2007) Amelioration of progressive renal injury by genetic manipulation of Klotho gene. Proc Natl Acad Sci U S A 104: 2331–2336.

52. Gurley SB, Allred A, Le TH, Griffiths R, Mao L, et al. (2006) Altered blood pressure responses and normal cardiac phenotype in ACE2-null mice. J Clin Invest 116: 2218–2225.

53. de Borst MH, Vervloet MG, ter Wee PM, Navis G (2011) Cross talk between the renin-angiotensin-aldosterone system and vitamin D-FGF-23-klotho in chronic kidney disease. J Am Soc Nephrol 22: 1603–1609.

54. Mitani H, Ishizaka N, Aizawa T, Ohno M, Usui S, et al. (2002) In vivo klotho gene transfer ameliorates angiotensin II-induced renal damage. Hypertension 39: 838–843.

55. Chan MR, Thomas CP, Torrealba JR, Djamali A, Fernandez LA, et al. (2009) Recurrent atypical hemolytic uremic syndrome associated with factor I mutation in a living related renal transplant recipient. Am J Kidney Dis 53: 321–326.

56. Thurman JM, Ljubanovic D, Royer PA, Kraus DM, Molina H, et al. (2006) Altered renal tubular expression of the complement inhibitor Crry permits complement activation after ischemia/reperfusion. J Clin Invest 116: 357–368.

57. Hakkim A, Furnrohr BG, Amann K, Laube B, Abed UA, et al. (2010) Impairment of neutrophil extracellular trap degradation is associated with lupus nephritis. Proc Natl Acad Sci U S A 107: 9813–9818.

58. Yasutomo K, Horiuchi T, Kagami S, Tsukamoto H, Hashimura C, et al. (2001) Mutation of DNASE1 in people with systemic lupus erythematosus. Nat Genet 28: 313–314.

59. Datta R, Shah GN, Rubbelke TS, Waheed A, Rauchman M, et al. (2010) Progressive renal injury from transgenic expression of human carbonic anhydrase IV folding mutants is enhanced by deficiency of p58IPK. Proc Natl Acad Sci U S A 107: 6448–6452.

60. Kaunisto K, Parkkila S, Rajaniemi H, Waheed A, Grubb J, et al. (2002) Carbonic anhydrase XIV: luminal expression suggests key role in renal acidification. Kidney Int 61: 2111–2118.

61. Santer R, Groth S, Kinner M, Dombrowski A, Berry GT, et al. (2002) The mutation spectrum of the facilitative glucose transporter gene SLC2A2 (GLUT2) in patients with Fanconi-Bickel syndrome. Hum Genet 110: 21–29.

62. Voegele AF, Jerkovic L, Wellenzohn B, Eller P, Kronenberg F, et al. (2002) Characterization of the vitamin E-binding properties of human plasma afamin. Biochemistry 41: 14532–14538.

63. Freue GV, Sasaki M, Meredith A, Gunther OP, Bergman A, et al. (2010) Proteomic signatures in plasma during early acute renal allograft rejection. Mol Cell Proteomics 9: 1954–1967.

64. Cowland JB, Borregaard N (1997) Molecular characterization and pattern of tissue expression of the gene for neutrophil gelatinase-associated lipocalin from humans. Genomics 45: 17–23.

65. Yang J, Goetz D, Li JY, Wang W, Mori K, et al. (2002) An iron delivery pathway mediated by a lipocalin. Mol Cell 10: 1045–1056.

66. Yang J, Blum A, Novak T, Levinson R, Lai E, et al. (2002) An epithelial precursor is regulated by the ureteric bud and by the renal stroma. Dev Biol 246: 296–310.

67. Meldrum KK, Hile K, Meldrum DR, Crone JA, Gearhart JP, et al. (2002) Simulated ischemia induces renal tubular cell apoptosis through a nuclear factor-kappaB dependent mechanism. J Urol 168: 248–252.

68. Haussler U, von Wichert G, Schmid RM, Keller F, Schneider G (2005) Epidermal growth factor activates nuclear factor-kappaB in human proximal tubule cells. Am J Physiol Renal Physiol 289: F808–815.

69. Mishra J, Mori K, Ma Q, Kelly C, Yang J, et al. (2004) Amelioration of ischemic acute renal injury by neutrophil gelatinase-associated lipocalin. J Am Soc Nephrol 15: 3073–3082.

70. Viau A, El Karoui K, Laouari D, Burtin M, Nguyen C, et al. (2010) Lipocalin 2 is essential for chronic kidney disease progression in mice and humans. J Clin Invest 120: 4065–4076.

71. Holman RR, Haffner SM, McMurray JJ, Bethel MA, Holzhauer B, et al. (2010) Effect of nateglinide on the incidence of diabetes and cardiovascular events. N Engl J Med 362: 1463–1476.

72. Hunt MC, Rautanen A, Westin MA, Svensson LT, Alexson SE (2006) Analysis of the mouse and human acyl-CoA thioesterase (ACOT) gene clusters shows that convergent, functional evolution results in a reduced number of human peroxisomal ACOTs. FASEB J 20: 1855–1864.

73. Ju W, Eichinger F, Bitzer M, Oh J, McWeeney S, et al. (2009) Renal gene and protein expression signatures for prediction of kidney disease progression. Am J Pathol 174: 2073–2085.

74. Bolton CH, Downs LG, Victory JG, Dwight JF, Tomson CR, et al. (2001) Endothelial dysfunction in chronic renal failure: roles of lipoprotein oxidation and pro-inflammatory cytokines. Nephrol Dial Transplant 16: 1189–1197.

75. Pereira BJ, Shapiro L, King AJ, Falagas ME, Strom JA, et al. (1994) Plasma levels of IL-1 beta, TNF alpha and their specific inhibitors in undialyzed chronic renal failure, CAPD and hemodialysis patients. Kidney Int 45: 890–896.

76. Knight EL, Rimm EB, Pai JK, Rexrode KM, Cannuscio CC, et al. (2004) Kidney dysfunction, inflammation, and coronary events: a prospective study. J Am Soc Nephrol 15: 1897–1903.

77. Koleganova N, Piecha G, Ritz E, Schirmacher P, Muller A, et al. (2009) Arterial calcification in patients with chronic kidney disease. Nephrol Dial Transplant 24: 2488–2496.

78. Kresse A, Konermann C, Degrandi D, Beuter-Gunia C, Wuerthner J, et al. (2008) Analyses of murine GBP homology clusters based on in silico, in vitro and in vivo studies. BMC Genomics 9: 158.

79. Feng JQ, Huang H, Lu Y, Ye L, Xie Y, et al. (2003) The Dentin matrix protein 1 (Dmp1) is specifically expressed in mineralized, but not soft, tissues during development. J Dent Res 82: 776–780.

80. David V, Martin A, Hedge AM, Drezner MK, Rowe PS (2011) ASARM peptides: PHEX-dependent and -independent regulation of serum phosphate. Am J Physiol Renal Physiol 300: F783–791.

81. Liu S, Zhou J, Tang W, Menard R, Feng JQ, et al. (2008) Pathogenic role of Fgf23 in Dmp1-null mice. Am J Physiol Endocrinol Metab 295: E254–261.

82. David V, Martin A, Hedge AM, Rowe PS (2009) Matrix extracellular phosphoglycoprotein (MEPE) is a new bone renal hormone and vascularization modulator. Endocrinology 150: 4012–4023.

83. Martin A, David V, Laurence JS, Schwarz PM, Lafer EM, et al. (2008) Degradation of MEPE, DMP1, and release of SIBLING ASARM-peptides (minhibins): ASARM-peptide(s) are directly responsible for defective mineralization in HYP. Endocrinology 149: 1757–1772.

84. Gesek FA, Friedman PA (1995) Sodium entry mechanisms in distal convoluted tubule cells. Am J Physiol 268: F89–98.

14

A miR-1207-5p Binding Site Polymorphism Abolishes Regulation of *HBEGF* and is Associated with Disease Severity in CFHR5 Nephropathy

Gregory Papagregoriou[1], Kamil Erguler[1], Harsh Dweep[2], Konstantinos Voskarides[1], Panayiota Koupepidou[1], Yiannis Athanasiou[3], Alkis Pierides[4], Norbert Gretz[2], Kyriacos N. Felekkis[5]*[☉], Constantinos Deltas[1]*[☉]

1 Molecular Medicine Research Center and Laboratory of Molecular and Medical Genetics, Department of Biological Sciences, University of Cyprus, Nicosia, Cyprus, 2 Medical Research Center, University of Heidelberg, Mannheim, Germany, 3 Department of Nephrology, Nicosia General Hospital, Nicosia, Cyprus, 4 Department of Nephrology, Hippocrateon Hospital, Nicosia, Cyprus, 5 Department of Life and Health Sciences, University of Nicosia, Nicosia, Cyprus

Abstract

Heparin binding epidermal growth factor (HBEGF) is expressed in podocytes and was shown to play a role in glomerular physiology. MicroRNA binding sites on the 3′UTR of *HBEGF* were predicted using miRWalk algorithm and followed by DNA sequencing in 103 patients diagnosed with mild or severe glomerulopathy. A single nucleotide polymorphism, miRSNP C1936T (rs13385), was identified at the 3′UTR of *HBEGF* that corresponds to the second base of the hsa-miR-1207-5p seed region. When AB8/13 undifferentiated podocytes were transfected with miRNA mimics of hsa-miR-1207-5p, the HBEGF protein levels were reduced by about 50%. A DNA fragment containing the miRSNP allele-1936C was cloned into the pMIR-Report Luciferase vector and co-transfected with miRNA mimics of hsa-miR-1207-5p into AB8/13 podocytes. In agreement with western blot data, this resulted in reduced luciferase expression demonstrating the ability of hsa-miR-1207-5p to directly regulate HBEGF expression. On the contrary, in the presence of the miRSNP 1936T allele, this regulation was abolished. Collectively, these results demonstrate that variant 1936T of this miRSNP prevents hsa-miR-1207-5p from down-regulating HBEGF in podocytes. We hypothesized that this variant has a functional role as a genetic modifier. To this end, we showed that in a cohort of 78 patients diagnosed with CFHR5 nephropathy (also known as C3-glomerulopathy), inheritance of miRSNP 1936T allele was significantly increased in the group demonstrating progression to chronic renal failure on long follow-up. No similar association was detected in a cohort of patients with thin basement membrane nephropathy. This is the first report associating a miRSNP as genetic modifier to a monogenic renal disorder.

Editor: Niels Olsen Saraiva Câmara, Universidade de Sao Paulo, Brazil

Funding: This work was supported mainly by the George & Maria Tyrimos endowment through a grant to CD by the Pancyprian Gymnasium, Nicosia, as a scholarship to support GP and by a grant NEW INFRASTRUCTURE/STRATEGIC/0308/24 by the Cyprus Research Promotion Foundation (www.research.org.cy) to CD. The funders had no role in study design, data collection and analysis, decision to publish, or preparation of the manuscript.

Competing Interests: The authors have declared that no competing interests exist.

* E-mail: Deltas@ucy.ac.cy (CD); felekkis.k@unic.ac.cy (KNF)

☉ These authors contributed equally to this work.

Introduction

The inherited monogenic glomerulopathies is a genetically and phenotypically highly heterogeneous group of conditions. Even in specific monogenic diseases, the exact molecular pathomechanism underlying the variable expressivity is rarely well understood. This heterogeneity is exemplified by the observation that not all patients who develop chronic kidney disease (CKD) due to a primary genetic cause will proceed to end-stage kidney disease (ESKD). In such diseases, glomerular defects that include but are not limited to the glomerular basement membrane, the glomerular endothelium and the podocytes can alter the kidney's filtration barrier integrity and lead to an adverse outcome in patients. A subset of glomerular defects emerging from germinal mutations in specific genes or are acquired are directly reflected on podocytes, which may lose their structural integrity and functional properties [1,2].

Microscopic hematuria (MH) of glomerular origin can be a benign condition persisting for life or can be the starting point of a progressive process that may lead many years later to proteinuria and decline of renal function resulting in CKD or ESKD [3]. A prime example is thin basement membrane nephropathy (TBMN), where patients in the same family who bear an identical heterozygous mutation in either the *COL4A3* or *COL4A4* gene that encodes for the α3 or α4 chain of collagen type IV respectively, may follow a quite diverse disease course. In recent studies on a large cohort of patients we showed that a small percentage of patients will remain for life with benign isolated MH; however a larger fraction of patients will proceed to proteinuria and CKD. Overall 15–20% of patients will have an even worse course and reach ESKD at ages after 50 years of age. In fact, nearly 50% of patients after 50 years will require hemodialysis or a renal transplant [4].

Similarly, in another recently revisited C3 glomerulopathy that is caused by mutations in the *CFHR5* gene which plays a role in the regulation of the alternative pathway of complement activation, nearly all patients present with MH since childhood while they may also develop macroscopic hematuria as a response to infections of the upper respiratory tract. A subset of patients will remain stable but about 15%, predominantly males will develop proteinuria and CKD or ESKD [5]. Female patients appear to have a milder disease progression and according to our recently published work, 14/18 patients who reached ESKD were males. This variable expressivity might be explained by a host of factors including genetic modifiers through yet unknown molecular mechanisms. MicroRNA (miRNA) regulation of gene expression could be one of these factors.

The role of miRNAs in processes such as maturation of the mammalian kidney was recently established by the podocyte-specific inactivation of Dicer, the RNAse III endonuclease responsible for miRNA maturation, in mice [6,7,8]. Podocyte foot processes were consequently depleted, while apoptosis commenced. The affected animals initially developed albuminuria followed by glomerular sclerosis and tubulo-interstitial fibrosis with acute renal disease progression and eventually death of mice by 6–8 weeks. The pathological phenotype was completed by proteinuria, glomerular basement membrane abnormalities and mesangial expansion, assimilating a congenital glomerulopathy. This proves that miRNAs have a fundamental role in regulating kidney physiological development; hence they must have a role in renal disease as well.

miRNAs belong to the most abundant class of small RNAs in animals. It is a recently discovered class of eukaryotic, endogenous, non-coding RNAs that play a key role in the regulation of gene expression. When mature they are short, single-stranded RNA molecules approximately 21–23 nucleotides in length, and they are partially complementary to one or more messenger RNA (mRNA) molecules [9]. Their main function is to down-regulate gene expression by inhibiting translation or by targeting the mRNA for degradation or deadenylation [10]. The mature miRNA mainly acts by targeting a miRNA recognition element (MRE) on an mRNA's 3'UTR and binding on it through a Watson-Crick base-pairing manner [11]. miRNA target recognition properties depend on its 'seed region', which includes nucleotides 2–8 from the 5'-end of each miRNA [12]. Base-pairing between the 3'-segment of the miRNA and the mRNA target is not always essential for repression, but strong base-pairing within this region can partially compensate for weaker seed matches or enhance repression [13].

In general there are two main mechanisms by which miRNAs can be involved in disease pathogenesis. A mutation on the miRNA itself can render it the primary causative gene. On the other hand, a miRNA can be indirectly involved in disease expression if the gene it targets is defined as the causative gene. The only evidence of a miRNA itself being the primary causative gene came from the work of Mencia et al., in which they identified a point mutation in the seed region of miR-96 which causes autosomal dominant non-syndromic hearing loss [14]. An engineered mouse model with a mutation in the seed region of miR-96, presented a phenotype similar to the human disease confirming the primary role of miR-96 [15]. In contrast, a miRNA can be considered as secondary cause to the disease when a genetic variation alters the binding of that miRNA to a causal gene. Evidence for such mechanism was shown for miR-24 when a point mutation that altered its binding to SLITRK1 gene was identified in patients with Tourette syndrome [16]. Similarly, point mutations on REEP1 which is a causative gene for hereditary spastic paraplegia were found on the binding sites of two miRNAs (miR-140 and miR-691) [17,18].

Involvement of miRNAs in inherited diseases is not limited to those two mechanisms. Evidence suggests that miRNAs can act as disease modifiers as a result of genetic variations on the precursor molecules or the miRNA-target binding sites. Single nucleotide polymorphisms (SNPs) can affect all states of the miRNAs' synthesis (pri-, pre-, and mature) and alter the miRNA biogenesis or function. Variations that alter the biogenesis of miRNAs were associated with predispositions to various diseases including congenital heart disease [19], schizophrenia [20], papillary thyroid carcinoma [21] and others. Despite that, it should be noted that genetic variations within the pre-miRNAs and specifically within the seed-region are rare and comprise less than 1% of the miRNA-related SNPs [22].

MicroRNA associated single nucleotide polymorphisms (miRSNPs) found on miRNA target sites within 3'UTRs of mRNAs, are relatively common. A miRSNP can eliminate or weaken the binding of a miRNA to its target site or increase the binding by creating a perfect sequence match to the seed of a miRNA that normally is not associated with the given mRNA, provided that both miRNA and mRNA share the same tissue of expression. In both cases the result will be a significant alteration in protein levels. There are currently three databases available (Patrocles, dbSMR and PolymiRTS) that compile SNPs on the mRNA 3'UTR region of human and mouse genes that create or destroy miRNA binding sites [23,24,25].

Here we hypothesized that miRSNPs might act as genetic modifiers predisposing to a milder or more severe disease on the background of a primary inherited glomerulopathy, such as TBMN and/or CFHR5 nephropathy. The initial bioinformatics *in silico* analysis that was followed by extensive DNA re-sequencing revealed one such polymorphism, SNP C1936T in the 3'UTR of *HBEGF* (rs13385, 3'UTR+1006), that corresponds to the second position of the seed region of miRNA hsa-miR-1207-5p. Its significance was demonstrated by functional studies in undifferentiated cultured podocytes and by association studies in two cohorts of patients. Specifically, in the presence of a mimic for miRNA hsa-miR-1207-5p there was down regulation of the HBEGF expression, judged by western blot analysis. This was corroborated by the use of luciferase sensor constructs of both alleles, where the 1936T allele demonstrated abrogation of miRNA binding. Most interestingly, the 1936T allele was shown to act as a genetic modifier, as it was genetically associated with a higher risk for progression to severe renal disease in the presence of a primary glomerulopathy, C3 glomerulonephritis.

Methods

Patients

Patients who participated in this study were diagnosed with TBMN or CFHR5 nephropathy and were all shown to have inherited mutations in either the *COL4A3/COL4A4* genes or the *CFHR5* gene respectively, in heterozygosity. All participants were informed by the clinicians and signed a consent form. The project is approved by the Cyprus National Bioethics Committee. A total of 232 anonymous DNA samples from our DNA bank served as controls.

TBMN patients originate from 16 large Cypriot families. Seventy-eight of 103 patients are heterozygous for the G1334E–*COL4A3* mutation, 19 of 103 are heterozygous for the G871C–*COL4A3* mutation and 6 of 103 are heterozygous for the c.3854delG–*COL4A4* mutation [26]. Due to the slow disease progression patients with "mild disease" (see below) and younger than 48-yo (born before January 1963) were excluded. The CFHR5 nephropathy group was comprised of 45 male and 33 female patients (born before January 1975), all sharing a common exons 2–3 heterozygous duplication in *CFHR5* gene [5]. Pedigrees and analytical clinical data have been published in detail elsewhere [26,27]. For both, TBMN and CFHR5 cohorts, "mildly" affected patients are those having only microscopic or macroscopic hematuria episodes (but no CKD) or hematuria plus low grade proteinuria (<400 mg/24 hrs, but no CKD). "Severely" affected patients are those having hematuria plus proteinuria >500 mg/24 hrs or hematuria plus proteinuria plus CKD or ESKD. CKD was defined as an elevated serum creatinine over 1.5 mg/dl. Patients with remittent or borderline proteinuria were excluded. Patients with a concomitant renal disease (*e.g.*, over five years diabetes, diabetic nephropathy, vesicoureteral reflux) or at the extreme of body weights (outside ±2 SD of the cohort mean) were also excluded.

Gene selection

In accordance with our hypothesis we searched for SNPs in the 3′UTR region of genes and specifically around the putative target regions of respective miRNAs. Eighty five genes were selected based on a wide spectrum of criteria. Candidate genes belong to four general categories based on their glomerular expression, their involvement in monogenic glomerular diseases, whether they were previously associated with a polygenic disease that presents secondary glomerulopathy and other genes expressed in the kidney or elsewhere that were found to be important for renal function or are closely related to genes selected in other categories. Podocyte specific genes, such as NPHS1, NPHS2 or PDPN are considered as good candidates, while polygenic diseases include diabetes, systemic lupus erythematosus, IgA nephropathy, glomerulonephritis and hypertensive nephrosclerosis. Published data regarding kidney or glomerulus specific gene expression microarray experiments enriched the candidate gene list, thus including genes coding for transcription factors, activators, structural proteins etc. In addition, genes implicated in tubular disease like *PKD1* and *PKD2* were also included.

miRNA target prediction analysis

Candidate gene names were imported into miRWalk algorithm (www.ma.uni-heidelberg.de/apps/zmf/mirwalk) and prediction of miRNA target sequences on their mRNA 3′UTR was performed using 7 nucleotides as the minimum seed number. A multiple comparison using 4 additional algorithms was performed for filtering purposes, each one working based on different sets of properties among mRNA-miRNA targeting; TargetScan, miRanda, miRDB and RNA22. In search for polymorphic variants by DNA sequencing around the miRNA target sequences, our attention was restricted only to pairs of miRNA-mRNA targets that were predicted by all five algorithms and gave a p-value<0.05. This p-value was automatically calculated by the miRWalk algorithm by using Poisson distribution and depicts the distribution of the probability of a miRNA 5′-end sequence to be randomly paired with a given 3′UTR mRNA sequence.

DNA sequencing analysis of target regions

DNA sequencing of predicted target regions was performed using BigDye™ V3.1 chemistry on an ABI Prism™ Genetic Analyzer (Applied Biosystems, California USA). Sequencing primers (all supplied by MWG, Ebersberg, Germany) were designed to flank the target region but also included an additional 300 bp on average on each side. Sequence electropherograms were obtained from the ABI Sequencing Analysis™ V5.2 software

(Applied Biosystems, California, USA) and sequences were imported into BioEdit™ Software to be aligned against a reference sequence with ClustalW algorithm [28]. SNPs that were identified in positions other than the predicted ones were evaluated using the miRanda tool (http://www.microrna.org) and cross-referenced with initial predictions.

Expression reporter system constructs

To evaluate the binding efficiency of miRNAs onto predicted target sequences, the pMiR-REPORT™ miRNA Expression Reporter Vector System (AMBION, Texas, USA) was used. For the case where we identified a SNP in the 3′UTR region, each allele was obtained with a polymerase chain reaction (PCR) amplification from two patients, each one homozygous for either allele and primers were designed to introduce a *Spe*I and a *Hind*III restriction enzyme sites to be cloned into the pMiR-REPORT™ Luciferase vector. For rs13385, the insert included 297 bp of *HBEGF* 3′UTR that flanked the SNP. Ligation products were transformed into competent DH5a *E. coli* cells (Takara, Japan). Insert verification included a restriction reaction with *Spe*I and *Hind*III and sequencing using 100 ng of DNA.

Transfection of AB8/13 podocytes

The AB8/13 undifferentiated podocyte cells, supplied by Dr Moin A. Saleem [29], were incubated at 33°C at 5% CO_2 and cultured in RPMI medium, supplemented with 10% Fetal Bovine Serum (FBS) (Invitrogen, California, USA), 1% of 100 units/ml Penicillin/Streptomycin (Invitrogen, California, USA) and 1% Insulin-Transferrin-Selenium (Invitrogen, California, USA). For the luciferase reporter system experiments, AB8/13 cells were triply transfected with equal amounts of the pMIR-REPORT™ Luciferase and β-gal vectors and 25 nM of miScript™ hsa-miR-1207-5p mimic (QIAGEN, West Sussex, UK) or the AllStars™ Negative Control scrambled sequence LNA (QIAGEN, West Sussex, UK), using Lipofectamine 2000 (Invitrogen, California, USA). The β-gal vector was used for normalization. Every experiment was performed in triplicates in 6-well cell culture plates with the appropriate controls. Cells were harvested 12 h after transfection. The Dual-Light Assay™ Kit (Applied Biosystems, Caifornia USA) was used for the quantification of both luciferase and β-gal in an automated luminometer (Sirius, Berthold Detection Systems, Pforzheim, Germany). For western blot experiments, AB8/13 cells were transfected with 25 nM of miScript™ hsa-mir-1207-5p mimics and inhibitors, as well as with AllStars™ Negative Control scrambled sequence LNA (QIAGEN, West Sussex, UK) for 16 hours.

Western blot experiments

AB8/13 cells were lysed in equal volumes of pre-heated 2xSDS loading buffer (Sodium Dodecyl Sulphate–125 mM Tris-HCl pH 6.8, 20% Glycerol, 2% SDS, 2% β-mercaptoethanol and bromophenol blue) and homogenized using a 2 ml syringe. Whole cell lysates were subsequently electrophoresed in a 12% SDS-Polyacrylamide gel. Gel transfer was held in a wet transfer system on Hybond Polyvinylidene Fluoride (PVDF–Millipore, Massachusetts, USA) membranes. Membranes were blocked with 5% non-fat dry milk in PBS/0.01% Tween20 for 1 hour at room temperature. Primary antibody was diluted in milk and added to the membrane for one hour. HBEGF protein was detected with the murine primary monoclonal antibody G-11 (SantaCruz Biotechnology, California, USA) at around 24 kDa. β-Tubulin was used as loading control by using the T-4026 primary antibody (SIGMA, Taufkirchen, Germany). As secondary antibody we used the rabbit anti-mouse antibody (SantaCruz Biotechnology,

California, USA), conjugated with Horseradish Peroxidase (HRP). Proteins were detected using the Enhanced ChemiLuminescence (ECL) Plus Blotting Detection system (Amersham Biosciences, Buckinghamshire, UK) and were visualized by autoradiography on photographic film (KODAK X-OMAT, New York, USA). Band density was defined by ImageJ Software (http://imagej.nih.gov/ij).

Real-Time PCR for miRNA detection

To examine the endogenously expressed levels of hsa-miR-1207-5p, total RNA enriched in small RNAs was isolated from AB8/13, HEK293 and SHSY-5Y neuroblastoma cells using the miRNeasy Mini Kit (QIAGEN, West Sussex, UK). MiRNA specific reverse transcription was performed with the miScript^{TM} Reverse Transcription Kit (QIAGEN, West Sussex, UK). Real-Time PCR was performed on a Roche Lightcycler (Roche Diagnostics, Indianapolis, USA) using the miScript^{TM} SYBR® Green PCR Kit (QIAGEN, West Sussex, UK), according to the manufacturers protocol. Detection of mature hsa-miR-1207-5p was accomplished using miScript^{TM} Assay primers, supplied by QIAGEN. MiRNA enriched total RNA from human renal epithelial cells (HREpiC) was supplied by ScienCell (California, USA). Each experiment was performed twice in duplicates and miScript^{TM} Hs_SNORA73A_1 small RNA was used as reference, with primers supplied from QIAGEN.

Genotyping of miRSNP C1936T

Genotyping for the C1936T SNP was performed in all samples, either by direct re-sequencing (TBMN samples) or by restriction reaction analysis (CFHR5 and healthy control samples). For this purpose, a restriction recognition site for BsrI was engineered in the forward PCR primer, by substituting the penultimate T by an **A** (Forward primer: 5′- CAA AGT GTA ACA GAT ATC AGT GTC TCC CCG TGT CCT CTC CC**A** G – 3′, Reverse Primer: 5′- GCT TTG CTA ATA CCT TCT CCA GAC TGT CCT CTG CTG CAC TGA -3′). The recognition site is created upon PCR amplification of the T allele. Subsequent sequencing analysis of selected samples confirmed the validity of this test. In addition, C1936T was also analyzed in the AB8/13 cell line by sequencing analysis, demonstrating a CC homozygous genotype.

Statistical analysis

Genotyping results were statistically evaluated using two-sided Barnard's unconditional test of superiority, as it was shown that it is more powerful for 2×2 contingency tables with limited observations than conventional conditional tests [30,31,32]. The reported Wald statistic is the standardized difference between the two binomial proportions of each category [30]. For the analysis of contingency tables we used StatXact 9 (Cystat, Cambridge, MA, USA) [33], as suggested in a publication by Ludbrook J. (2008) [34]. In order to provide an open-source alternative for performing the Barnard's test, the "Barnard" package has been developed for the statistical scripting language R. The Barnard package is included in the Comprehensive R Archive Network (http://cran.r-project.org/web/packages/Barnard), where it is freely available for download and immediate use by anyone. C1936T was tested for Hardy-Weinberg equilibrium using Pearson's chi-square test in controls. Luciferase expression levels were analyzed using one-way non-parametric ANOVA after being normalized against β-gal expression levels. One-way ANOVA was also used to test densitometry results from western blot analyses, followed by Tukey post-testing.

Results

Bioinformatic analysis for identification of miRNAs as modifiers of glomerulopathies

Heritable monogenic glomerulopathies that present with MH display interfamilial and intrafamilial phenotypic heterogeneity, thereby suggesting the involvement of modifier genes in disease progression [35]. We herewith hypothesized the putative role of miRNAs as disease modifiers and we searched for functional polymorphic variants in the predicted target sites of miRNAs for genes expressed or located in the glomerulus. To this end, we guided our search for SNPs within the miRNA target sites of genes selected as described in Methods. Expression in podocytes, localization in the slit diaphragm and the glomerulus basement membrane rendered genes as good candidates for our study.

With the use of miRWalk (http://www.ma.uni-heidelberg.de/apps/zmf/mirwalk) and four other prediction algorithms (miR-Base, TargetScan, miRDB and RNA22), we looked for validated miRNAs that target the candidate genes. We narrowed down the candidates of interest by selecting only miRNA-mRNA pairs that were predicted by all five algorithms (Table 1).

Identification of candidate SNPs by sequence analysis

A segment of about 500–600 nts encompassing the miRNA binding site in the 3′UTR of selected genes, was re-sequenced in 103 patients with TBMN, classified as severe or mild. Table 2 summarizes the results of the sequencing analysis depicting the gene sequenced, the miRNA predicted to bind to the 3′UTR of that gene and the SNPs identified. Although various SNPs were identified in the group of patients sequenced, none was located on the predicted miRNA binding sites. However, a SNP was identified in the binding site of another miRNA that was originally excluded due to a lower significance compared to top candidates. Specifically, while sequencing around the hsa-miR-379 target site in the HBEGF 3′UTR, we identified a biallelic variation of C or T at position 1936 (C1936T) in the target region of hsa-miR-1207-5p which is also predicted to target HBEGF. The C1936T SNP is found at what corresponds to position 2 of the 'seed' region of hsa-miR-1207-5p (Fig. 1A) suggesting a possible elimination or severe compromise of the ability of this miRNA to bind on HBEGF mRNA.

Verification of functional significance by in vitro experimentation

In order to verify whether HBEGF is a true target of hsa-miR-1207-5p and that the presence of C1936T SNP alters the binding and regulation incurred by the miRNA, we performed luciferase 'sensor' assays. A segment of the HBEGF 3′UTR containing the 1936C (pMIR-REPORT-HBEGF-1936C) or 1936T (pMIR-REPORT-HBEGF-1936T) variant was cloned into the 3′UTR of the luciferase gene in pMIR-REPORT plasmid. Reporter plasmids and β-gal reference plasmid were co-transfected in AB8/13 podocyte cell line with either hsa-miR-1207-5p mimic or negative control mimics for 12 hours followed by luciferase and β-gal measurement. Co-transfection of hsa-miR-1207-5p mimics with the pMIR-REPORT-HBEGF-1936**C** resulted in significant reduction in luciferase expression (47.14%+/−0.42 SEM of normalized RLU relative to control) demonstrating that this miRNA directly binds on HBEGF 3′UTR region (Fig. 1B). In agreement, transfection of hsa-miR-1207-5p mimics in AB8/13 cells significantly reduced the endogenous levels of HBEGF protein as demonstrated by Western blot analysis at about 20% of total expression, while hsa-miR-1207-5p inhibitors boosted HBEGF levels by reducing the endogenously expressed miRNA

Table 1. Prediction results using five different miRNA-target prediction tools.

GENE	miRNA	RNA22	miRANDA	miRDB	miRWalk	TargetScan	SEED LENGTH	START	SEQUENCE	END	p-VALUE
PDPN	hsa-mir-485-5p	✓	✓	✓	✓	✓	8	1453	AGAGGCUG	1446	0.031
HBEGF	hsa-mir-212	✓	✓	✓	✓	✓	9	1584	UAACAGUCU	1576	0.0056
HBEGF	hsa-mir-132	✓	✓	✓	✓	✓	10	1584	UAACAGUCUA	1575	0.0014
HBEGF	hsa-mir-379	✓	✓	✓	✓	✓	8	1833	UGGUAGAC	1826	0.0223
FN1	hsa-mir-96	✓	✓	✓	✓	✓	8	8340	UUUGGCAC	8333	0.0169
FN1	hsa-mir-144	✓	✓	✓	✓	✓	9	8331	UACAGUAUA	8323	0.0042
GJA1	hsa-mir-495	✓	✓	✓	✓	✓	8	2244	AAACAAAC	2237	0.0261
PKD2	hsa-mir-183	✓	✓	✓	✓	✓	8	4768	UAUGGCAC	4761	0.0315
PKD2	hsa-mir-372	✓	✓	✓	✓	✓	9	4022	AAAGUGCUG	4014	0.008
PPARA	hsa-mir-223	✓	✓	✓	✓	✓	9	5877	UGUCAGUUU	5869	0.0314
SP1	hsa-mir-24	✓	✓	✓	✓	✓	7	5240	UGGCUCA	5240	0.2725
SP1	hsa-mir-31	✓	✓	✓	✓	✓	9	6960	AGGCAAGAU	6952	0.0197
SP1	hsa-mir-105	✓	✓	✓	✓	✓	7	5548	UCAAAUG	5542	0.2725
SP1	hsa-mir-155	✓	✓	✓	✓	✓	8	2560	UUAAUGCU	2553	0.0764
TJP1	hsa-mir-144	✓	✓	✓	✓	✓	8	6469	UACAGUAU	6462	0.0218

Ticks under algorithm names indicate the successful prediction of each miRNA-mRNA pair per prediction tool. "Start" and "end" columns state the exact position of the putative miRNA target region on the 3′UTR of the respective mRNA. Numbering refers to position from the start of the mRNA 3′UTR. For sequencing analysis, pairs that had p-values of less than 0.05 were selected.

levels (Fig. 1C). Densitometry of western blots revealed a significant decrease or increase of HBEGF levels on mimic or inhibitor transfection respectively. (Fig. 1C, lower panel).

On the contrary, in the presence of pMIR-REPORT-HBEGF-1936**T**, transfection of hsa-miR-1207-5p mimics did not significantly alter luciferase expression (90.56%+/−3.8 SEM of normalized RLU relative to control) in AB8/13 cells (Fig. 1B). Combined these results demonstrate that hsa-miR-1207-5p can directly regulate *HBEGF* expression and this regulation is abolished if there is a T nucleotide at position 1936 of *HBEFG's* 3′UTR.

Table 2. Results after re-sequencing of 103 samples with mutations in *COL4A3* or *COL4A4* genes and thin basement membrane nephropathy.

GENE	miRNAs	miRNA POSITION	PCR AND SEQUENCING PRIMERS	PREDICTION HITS	SNPs FOUND	NOTES
PDPN	hsa-mir-485-5p	1453-1446	5′- GTTAGGGCAGGTGGGATG -3′ 5′- TGTATGCGGCTGGTAAGTAG -3′	5/5	T1226A G1545A G1262A 1251DEL-G	SNPs not on miRNA target sites
HBEGF	hsa-mir-132 hsa-mir-212	1584-1575 1584-1576	5′- TGAACTGGAAGAAAGCAACA -3′ 5′- ACCCCTACATCCTGACCATAC -3′	5/5	None	No SNPs found
HBEGF	hsa-mir-379	1833-1826	5′- ACTCCTCATCCCCACAATCT -3′ 5′- CCCACCTCCAACCTTCTC -3′	5/5	C1936T	SNP found at neighboring position, which is target for hsa-miR-1207-5p
FN1	hsa-mir-96 hsa-mir-144	8340-8332 8331-8322	5′- TTGGGATCAATAGGAAAGCA -3′ 5′- GAAGAGATGAAGTGACAAAACC -3′	5/5	None	No SNPs found
PKD2	hsa-mir-183	4768-4760	5′- TCCAGGTTGAAAGTGAAAC -3′ 5′- CAGGGAAAGATAATAGGGAAGA -3′	5/5	None	No SNPs found
PKD2	hsa-mir-372	4022-4014	5′- TTCCCATGTGGCTCTACTCA -3′ 5′- AGACCCTCTCGTAAAGAAAACA -3′	5/5	G4003A G4210A	SNPs not on miRNA target sites
PPARA	hsa-mir-223	5877-5868	5′- GTTAGGGCAGGTGGGATG -3′ 5′- TGTATGCGGCTGGTAAGTAG -3′	5/5	None	No SNPs found
SP1	hsa-mir-31	6960-6951	5′- GACTTCCCCAAACCCAGA -3′ 5′- CACCCATCCCTTCCAGAG -3′	5/5	None	No SNPs found
TJP1	hsa-mir-144	6469-6462	5′- GGAGGGTGAAGTGAAGACAA -3′ 5′- GCATAGCCAGAAAGAACAGAA -3′	5/5	A6485C	SNPs not on miRNA target sites

Sequencing primers were designed to flank the predicted target sites and also include about 300 bp on either side. Prediction hits represent the number of tools that successfully predicted the miRNA-mRNA binding.

A

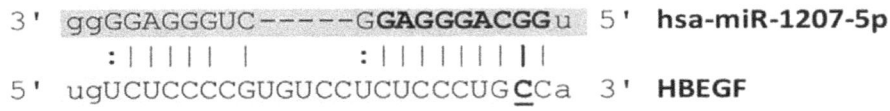

3' ggGGAGGGUC-----G**GAGGGACGG**u 5' **hsa-miR-1207-5p**

    :|||||| | :||||||| ||

5' ugUCUCCCCGUGUCCUCUCCCUG<u>**C**</u>Ca 3' **HBEGF**

B

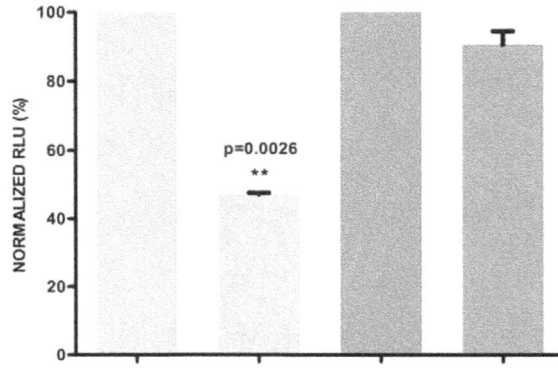

pMIR-REPORT-HBEGF-1936C	+	+	-	-
pMIR-REPORT-HBEGF-1936T	-	-	+	+
hsa-miR-1207-5p MIMIC	-	+	-	+
NEGATIVE CONTROL MIMIC	+	-	+	-

C

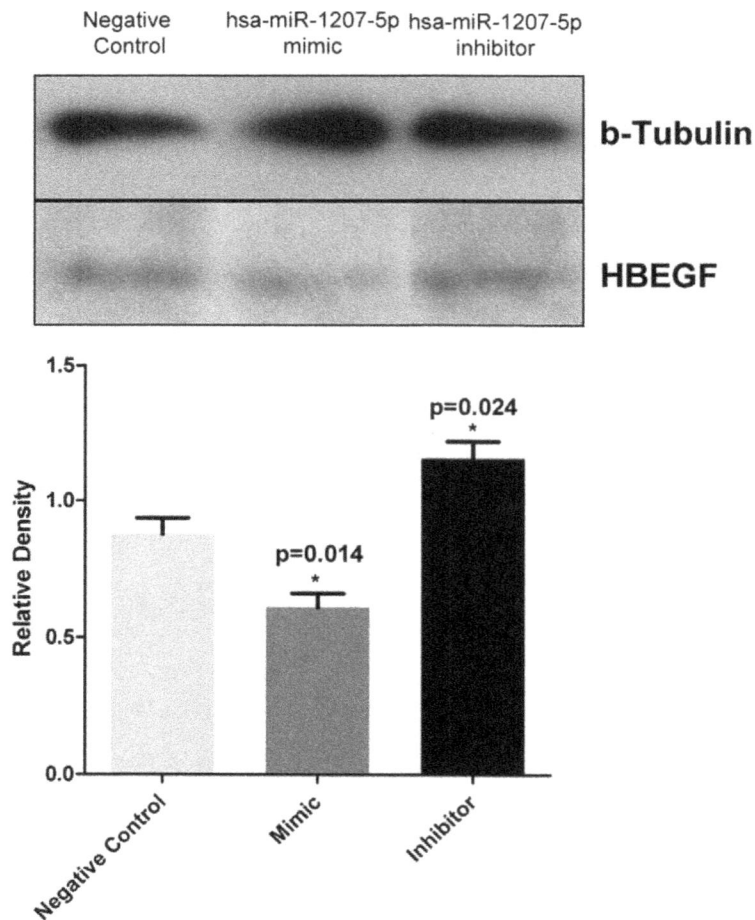

Figure 1. Effect of C1936T miRSNP in _HBEGF_ gene on regulation by hsa-miR-1207-5p, in a podocyte culture system. A) Schematic depicting the position of miRSNP C1936T on the target region of hsa-miR-1207-5p on _HBEGF_. This miRSNP corresponds to the second base of the seed region of hsa-miR-1207-5p, underlined C. B) Normalized luciferase relative light units (RLUs) in AB8/13 cell lysates after transfection with sensor constructs. Co-transfection of the pMIR-REPORT-HBEGF-1936C with hsa-miR-1207-5p miRNA LNA mimics resulted in significant reduction of luciferase expression, with a p-value of 0.0026 using one-way non-parametric ANOVA test. In contrast, the pMIR-REPORT construct bearing the 1936T allele (pMIR-REPORT-HBEGF-1936T) abolished the hsa-miR-1207-5p binding site as demonstrated from the loss of RLU reduction. Results represent mean values of triplicates ± SEM. C) Western blot of HBEGF from AB8/13 cells after transient transfection with hsa-miR-1207-5p miRNA LNA mimics, inhibitors and the AllStars™ Negative Control scrambled sequence LNA. This is a representative of six experiments. Lower panel presents the statistical analysis of western blot densitometry results, normalized against the Negative Control. Values represent the mean ± SEM. Results illustrate the reduction of HBEGF protein levels at the presence of hsa-miR-1207-5p mimics (p = 0.014), while miRNA inhibitors significantly increased HBEGF levels (p = 0.024).

The hsa-miR-1207-5p is highly enriched in podocytes as demonstrated by miRNA specific Real-Time PCR experiments. Specifically, miR-1207-5p is expressed 2-fold higher in differentiated AB8/13 podocytes, compared to undifferentiated cells (Fig. 2). In addition, human renal epithelial cells express 4-fold higher miR-1207-5p than differentiated AB8/13 cells. Other cell lines, such as HEK293 and SHSY-5Y demonstrate limited expression levels of miR-1207-5p when compared to podocytes.

Genotyping results

We then tested the hypothesis that this variant may act as a genetic modifier in two cohorts of patients with inherited monogenic glomerulopathies. From 232 control subjects that were genotyped, 70% were CC homozygotes, 27% CT heterozygotes and 3% TT homozygotes. The control population obeys the Hardy-Weinberg equilibrium (p = 0.812), as tested by the Pearson's chi-square test. Sequencing analysis showed that 68.2% of patients having mild TBMN are homozygous for the C allele, 6.8% are homozygous for the T allele and 25% CT heterozygotes (Table 3). As regards patients with severe TBMN disease, 76.3% were CC homozygotes, 1.7% TT homozygotes and 22% CT heterozygotes. There was no statistical significance between the two groups, upon two-sided Barnard's testing (p-value = 0.368). We then tested a separate cohort of 78 patients diagnosed with CFHR5 nephropathy. Among 45 CHFR5 patients with milder disease progression, 86.6% are homozygous for the C allele, while the remaining are CT heterozygotes. In contrast, 63.6% of the 33 severely affected CFHR5 patients are CC homozygotes and 36.4% are CT heterozygotes. Barnard's test with a 95% confidence interval revealed an association between mild CFHR5 and the CC genotype, with a p-value of 0.018 and Wald statistic of −2.385 (Fig. 3).

Further grouping of TT homozygotes and CT heterozygotes, indicated a significant difference between mild CFHR5 patients and mild TBMN patients with a p = 0.0.038 after Barnard's test with a Wald statistic of 2.089. The corresponding frequencies did not differ significantly between severe CFHR5 and severe TBMN patients. Collectively, evidence suggests that the CT/TT genotype has no significant effect on the severity of TBMN, but it increases the risk for a severe outcome in patients with CFHR5 nephropathy, by 3.7 times.

A separate evaluation of women in our CFHR5 cohort, revealed significance between mildly and severely affected women with a p-value of 0.035 and a Wald statistic of −2.234 (Fig. 4). As women are known to have a milder course of the disease, it is 8 times more likely to have a severe phenotype if the patient is a female and a carrier of a CT/TT genotype.

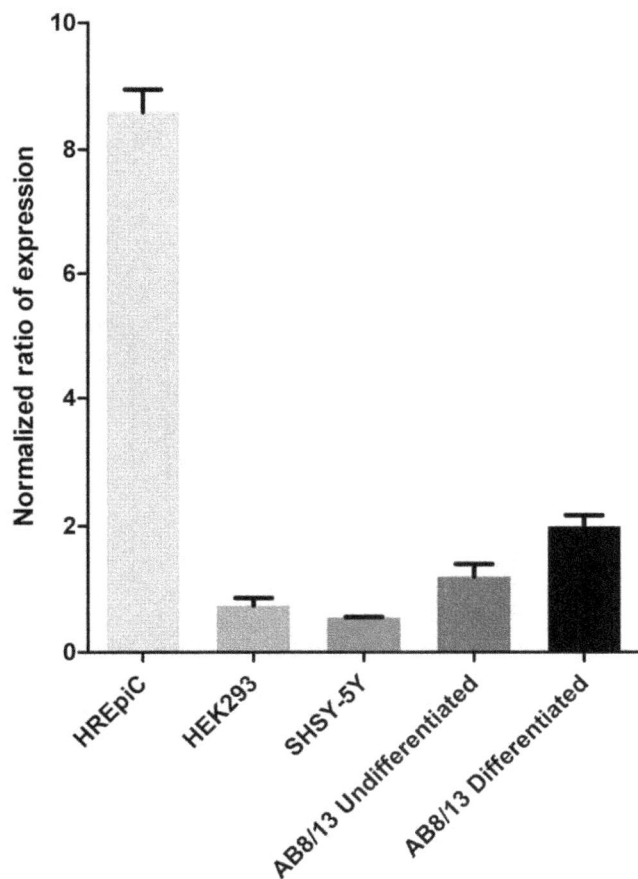

Figure 2. Expression analysis of miR-1207-5p in various cell lines. Relative expression analysis of mature hsa-miR-1207-5p levels in various cell types, as tested by miRNA specific Real-Time PCR experiments. Both AB8/13 differentiated and undifferentiated podocytes revealed significantly high expression levels of miR-1207-5p, compared to HEK293 and SHSY-5Y neuroblastoma cells. Further examination of miR-1207-5p levels in human renal epithelial cells (HREpiC), recorded 4-fold higher mature miRNA than the AB8/13 differentiated podocyte cell line. Results represent the mean of quadruplicate values ± SEM.

Discussion

The phenotypic heterogeneity and variable expression, exemplified as a broad spectrum of symptoms in a cohort of patients, is the norm in many monogenic disorders including renal conditions, such as glomerulopathies. The role of genetic modifiers, at least partly, is frequently invoked as they are hypothesized to act in symphony with a validated mutation in a single gene. For example, recent publications have reported several occasions

Table 3. Genotype and allele frequencies in all study groups.

GENOTYPE/ALLELE	MILD TBMN (COL4A3/COL4A4 MUTATIONS)		SEVERE TBMN (COL4A3/COL4A4 MUTATIONS)		MILD CFHR5 NEPHROPATHY		SEVERE CFHR5 NEPHROPATHY	
CC	30	68.2%	45	76.3%	39	86.6%	21	63.6%
CT	11	25%	13	22%	6	13.4%	12	36.4%
TT	3	6.8%	1	1.7%	0	0%	0	0%
CT/TT	14	31.8%	14	23.7%	6	13.4%	12	36.4%

Under each group label, left columns demonstrate the number of subjects for each genotype and allele, while right columns the respective percentages.

where SNPs in genes confer a higher risk for progression of pathology, for example a SNP in the DKK3 gene or in the eNOS gene in polycystic kidney disease [36,37,38].

Having in mind recent advances in our understanding of molecular pathogenetic mechanisms, it is reasonable to expect that one other class of modifiers, among others, could be sequence variations on the target sites of miRNAs, in genes whose function relates to the disease under study. Inheritance of such variants is not expected to cause a disease in a Mendelian fashion; however their stochastic co-segregation with a primary disease-causing mutation may affect the risk for slower or faster progression of the

phenotype. A mutation in a miRNA gene itself that is responsible for a Mendelian phenotype has been reported once, to our knowledge, whereas several publications report on the presence of pathology-associated variants in the target sites of known miRNAs. At the same time miRNAs can act as disease modifiers as a result of genetic variations on the precursor molecules. Specifically,

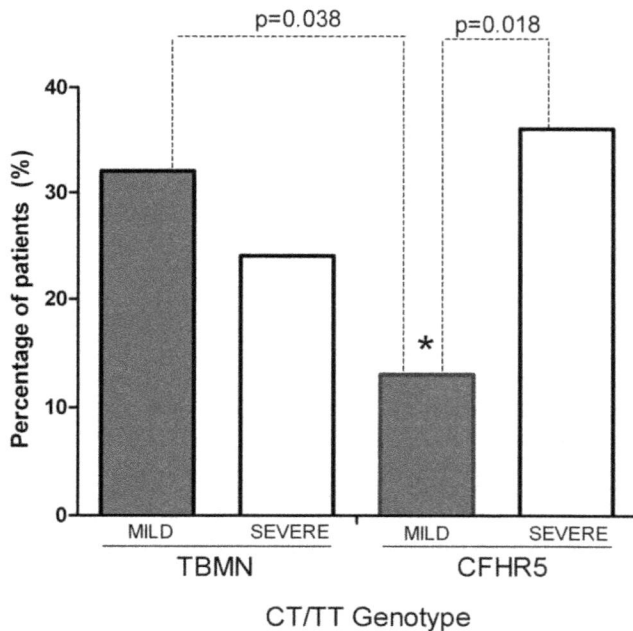

Figure 3. Mildly affected CFHR5 patients have lower occurrence of the 1936T allele. Graphical representation of both TBMN and CFHR5 nephropathy cohorts used in this study in relation to the number of CT and TT patients. Nephropathy patients with mild CFHR5 have significantly lower percentage of the CT genotype when compared with severe CFHR5 patients (p = 0.018), indicating a protective effect of the CC genotype. Statistical comparison between mild TBMN and mild CFHR5 patients demonstrated a significant underrepresentation of the 1936T allele in mild CFHR5 patients (p = 0.038). Mild TBMN patients did not differ from severe TBMN patients (p = 0.368). All statistical analyses were performed using two-sided Barnard's test.

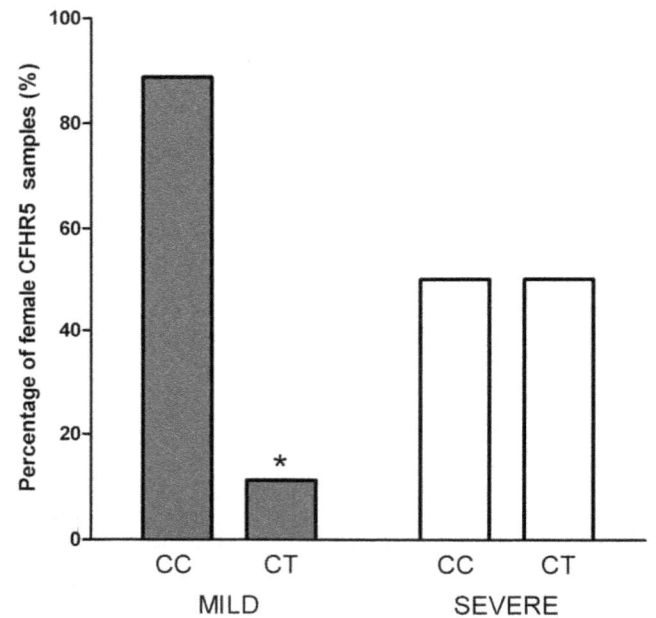

Figure 4. The 1936C/T HBEGF genotype is overrepresented in women affected with severe CFHR5. Comparison of C1936T genotypes in women manifesting CFHR5 nephropathy. Women are known to have a milder course of the disease when compared to men and this is also demonstrated when they are statistically compared with severe CFHR5 women as regards the C1936T SNP. The 1936C allele has a significantly lower representation in severe CFHR5 women, compared to mild women, thus suggesting a protective effect for this allele (p = 0.035).

SNPs may occur at the level of the pri-miRNA, pre-miRNA or mature miRNA. Such SNPs may affect either the biogenesis or the action of the mature miRNA, contributing to deregulation of target gene expression and consequently to disease development [39]. Notwithstanding this situation, most common are the miRNA-associated single nucleotide polymorphisms (miRSNPs) that are located in the miRNA target sites within the 3′UTRs of corresponding mRNAs. Several studies have identified associations of miRSNPs with complex trait diseases such as diabetes [40], asthma [41], Parkinson [42], hypertension [43], breast cancer with early age at onset [44] and others.

In this report, we show data according to which a reduction of hsa-mir-1207-5p binding ability on its target site in the 3′UTR of *HBEGF* due to the presence of C1936T SNP is associated with the severity of CFHR5 nephropathy in patients inheriting the pathogenic *CFHR5* gene duplication of exons 2–3. To our knowledge this is the first time a miRSNP is shown to be correlated with the phenotypic manifestation of a monogenic glomerular disease. Specifically, we showed that in a cohort of patients inheriting this CFHR5 nephropathy, the 1936C allele at the binding site for miRNA hsa-miR-1207-5p is associated with a less severe phenotype, as this is exemplified in patients who are protected from the development of high grade proteinuria and CKD (p = 0.018, Fig. 3). When concentrating on the subgroup of women, only three of 27 with mild disease inherited the T allele, compared to three of six women with severe disease (Fig. 4). This finding obtains particular significance in view of the fact that women follow a much milder course of disease compared to men, according to a previous work of our group [5,27]. The exact mechanism by which *HBEGF* can alter disease phenotype is currently unknown and under investigation. However, we hypothesize that the role of *HBEGF* in proliferation and fibrosis of mesangial cells is very critical to this end. In support of its functional significance, we showed in cell culture experiments that the presence of the T allele eliminates the binding of the miRNA, thus resulting in higher HBEGF protein levels (Fig. 1).

We undertook a rather difficult approach to identify such a SNP, by collecting genes from the literature that are known to be involved in glomerular structure and function. In order to narrow down our search we utilized prediction algorithms in an attempt to extract the best candidate genes for sequence. In our case, the hsa-miR-1207-5p was predicted by two out of five algorithms to target *HBEGF*. Although not a top candidate, luckily enough hsa-miR-1207-5p target site is positioned nearby a site for an alleged good candidate miRNA (hsa-miR-379). As a result, we managed to prove the functional interaction of hsa-miR-1207-5p with *HBEGF*, because the cell culture experiments as well as the statistical evaluation in our cohort of patients supported its implication in gene regulation at post-transcription level. This case is a prime example where despite the improvement in bioinformatics tools and methods for predicting miRNA targets, some valuable information can still escape. The systematic approach we used however, along with the flexibility of our tools, enabled us to identify a functional SNP that otherwise would have been missed.

HBEGF belongs to the epidermal growth factor superfamily. It is also known as the Diphtheria toxin receptor since it is required for the surface binding of diphtheria toxin and entry into the cell [45]. This growth factor is expressed at high levels in podocytes, tubular epithelial cells and mesangial cells [46]. Several studies have emphasized the role of HBEGF in kidney function under normal or pathologic conditions. Ischemia/reperfusion (IR) injury was shown to be mediated by HBEGF, as reduction in expression of this protein had a protective effect in various IR models [45,47]. As a member of a growth factor family, HBEGF can promote cellular proliferation in both mesangial and renal epithelial cells. Specifically, studies using renal proximal tubular cells revealed that proliferation in this cell type is mediated by HBEGF through an autocrine/paracrine mechanism which antagonizes the action of Src kinases [48]. In addition, *HBEGF* is expressed in mesangial cells and is involved in mesangial cells proliferation in glomerulonephritis and contributes to lesion formation in focal glomerular sclerosis through stimulation of mitogens at those sites [49,50]. Similarly, HBEGF participates in renal fibrosis by regulating both TGF-β-mediated fibronectin expression and collagen expression in mesangial cells [51].

In humans, the miR-1207-5p is transcribed from the PVT1 locus on chromosome 8q24 [52]. The PVT1 gene is encoding for a non-translated RNA and has been found to be implicated in diabetic nephropathy and breast and colon cancer, in translocations related to Burkitt's lymphoma and associated with Hodgin's lymphoma [53,54,55,56]. Interestingly, end-stage renal disease occurring in patients with diabetes type 2 has been associated with PVT1, while variants in the same gene were associated with ESKD in patients with type 1 diabetes [57,58]. A recent study by Alvarez and DiStefano investigated PVT1 properties in depth and confirmed its high expression in mesangial cells, as well as proposed an up-regulation in the levels of the miRNAs emerging from PVT1 by elevated glucose in the mesangium [53]. These findings can supplement the results of our study and together are suggestive of novel roles for PVT1 influenced miR-1207-5p expression and translational regulation of HBEGF in terms of maintaining the physiological function of the mesangium or the glomerulus in general.

In conclusion, we presented evidence for the novel genetic modifier role of miRNA hsa-miR-1207-5p in predisposing patients with a monogenic recently described CFHR5 nephropathy, to more severe phenotype. The fact that all our patients shared the same exact germinal mutation probably was a factor that facilitated the identification of this modifier, as there was no confounding allelic heterogeneity. At the same time our data implicate *HBEGF* as the gene through which this miRNA exerts its effect. Further work at the cellular level and perhaps with the use of animal models will help elucidate in more detail the exact mechanism by which this hsa-miR-1207-5p/*HBEGF* pair plays its role. Notwithstanding our positive results and conclusions, it does not escape our attention that our cohorts are somewhat small. At this point in time it is impossible to enlarge the relevant cohort or to derive a new one before the passage of many years. Also, to our knowledge no patients have been diagnosed yet, of a different ethnic origin, as the C3 glomerulonephritis caused by a CFHR5 mutation appears endemic to Cyprus.

Acknowledgments

We thank Dr Moin A. Saleem for supplying the AB8/13 cell line and Dr Ilia Vonta for assistance on statistical evaluations.

Author Contributions

Conceived and designed the experiments: GP KNF CD. Performed the experiments: GP PK KV. Analyzed the data: GP KE HD NG KNF CD. Contributed reagents/materials/analysis tools: NG YA AP. Wrote the paper: KNF CD GP.

References

1. Wiggins RC (2007) The spectrum of podocytopathies: a unifying view of glomerular diseases. Kidney Int 71: 1205–1214.

2. Barisoni L, Schnaper HW, Kopp JB (2007) A proposed taxonomy for the podocytopathies: a reassessment of the primary nephrotic diseases. Clin J Am Soc Nephrol 2: 529–542.

3. Cohen RA, Brown RS (2003) Clinical practice. Microscopic hematuria. N Engl J Med 348: 2330–2338.

4. Voskarides K, Damianou L, Neocleous V, Zouvani I, Christodoulidou S, et al. (2007) COL4A3/COL4A4 mutations producing focal segmental glomerulosclerosis and renal failure in thin basement membrane nephropathy. J Am Soc Nephrol 18: 3004–3016.

5. Gale DP, de Jorge EG, Cook HT, Martinez-Barricarte R, Hadjisavvas A, et al. (2010) Identification of a mutation in complement factor H-related protein 5 in patients of Cypriot origin with glomerulonephritis. Lancet 376: 794–801.

6. Harvey SJ, Jarad G, Cunningham J, Goldberg S, Schermer B, et al. (2008) Podocyte-specific deletion of dicer alters cytoskeletal dynamics and causes glomerular disease. J Am Soc Nephrol 19: 2150–2158.

7. Shi S, Yu L, Chiu C, Sun Y, Chen J, et al. (2008) Podocyte-selective deletion of dicer induces proteinuria and glomerulosclerosis. J Am Soc Nephrol 19: 2159–2169.

8. Ho J, Ng KH, Rosen S, Dostal A, Gregory RI, et al. (2008) Podocyte-specific loss of functional microRNAs leads to rapid glomerular and tubular injury. J Am Soc Nephrol 19: 2069–2075.

9. Farazi TA, Juranek SA, Tuschl T (2008) The growing catalog of small RNAs and their association with distinct Argonaute/Piwi family members. Development 135: 1201–1214.

10. Wu L, Fa J, Belasco GJ (2006) MicroRNAs direct rapid deadenylation of mRNA. PNAS Vol. 103. pp 4034–4039.

11. Reinhart BJ, Slack FJ, Basson M, Pasquinelli AE, Bettinger JC, et al. (2000) The 21-nucleotide let-7 RNA regulates developmental timing in Caenorhabditis elegans. Nature 403: 901–906.

12. Chen K, Song F, Calin GA, Wei Q, Hao X, et al. (2008) Polymorphisms in microRNA targets: a gold mine for molecular epidemiology. Carcinogenesis 29: 1306–1311.

13. Lal A, Navarro F, Maher CA, Maliszewski LE, Yan N, et al. (2009) miR-24 Inhibits cell proliferation by targeting E2F2, MYC, and other cell-cycle genes via binding to "seedless" 3′UTR microRNA recognition elements. Mol Cell 35: 610–625.

14. Mencia A, Modamio-Hoybjor S, Redshaw N, Morin M, Mayo-Merino F, et al. (2009) Mutations in the seed region of human miR-96 are responsible for nonsyndromic progressive hearing loss. Nat Genet 41: 609–613.

15. Lewis MA, Quint E, Glazier AM, Fuchs H, De Angelis MH, et al. (2009) An ENU-induced mutation of miR-96 associated with progressive hearing loss in mice. Nat Genet 41: 614–618.

16. Abelson JF, Kwan KY, O'Roak BJ, Baek DY, Stillman AA, et al. (2005) Sequence variants in SLITRK1 are associated with Tourette's syndrome. Science 310: 317–320.

17. Beetz C, Schule R, Deconinck T, Tran-Viet KN, Zhu H, et al. (2008) REEP1 mutation spectrum and genotype/phenotype correlation in hereditary spastic paraplegia type 31. Brain 131: 1078–1086.

18. Zuchner S, Wang G, Tran-Viet KN, Nance MA, Gaskell PC, et al. (2006) Mutations in the novel mitochondrial protein REEP1 cause hereditary spastic paraplegia type 31. Am J Hum Genet 79: 365–369.

19. Xu J, Hu Z, Xu Z, Gu H, Yi L, et al. (2009) Functional variant in microRNA-196a2 contributes to the susceptibility of congenital heart disease in a Chinese population. Hum Mutat 30: 1231–1236.

20. Sun G, Yan J, Noltner K, Feng J, Li H, et al. (2009) SNPs in human miRNA genes affect biogenesis and function. RNA 15: 1640–1651.

21. Jazdzewski K, Liyanarachchi S, Swierniak M, Pachucki J, Ringel MD, et al. (2009) Polymorphic mature microRNAs from passenger strand of pre-miR-146a contribute to thyroid cancer. Proc Natl Acad Sci U S A 106: 1502–1505.

22. Saunders MA, Liang H, Li WH (2007) Human polymorphism at microRNAs and microRNA target sites. Proc Natl Acad Sci U S A 104: 3300–3305.

23. Georges M, Clop A, Marcq F, Takeda H, Pirottin D, et al. (2006) Polymorphic microRNA-target interactions: a novel source of phenotypic variation. Cold Spring Harb Symp Quant Biol 71: 343–350.

24. Hariharan M, Scaria V, Brahmachari SK (2009) dbSMR: a novel resource of genome-wide SNPs affecting microRNA mediated regulation. BMC Bioinformatics 10: 108.

25. Bao L, Zhou M, Wu L, Lu L, Goldowitz D, et al. (2007) PolymiRTS Database: linking polymorphisms in microRNA target sites with complex traits. Nucleic Acids Res 35: D51–54.

26. Pierides A, Voskarides K, Athanasiou Y, Ioannou K, Damianou L, et al. (2009) Clinico-pathological correlations in 127 patients in 11 large pedigrees, segregating one of three heterozygous mutations in the COL4A3/COL4A4 genes associated with familial haematuria and significant late progression to proteinuria and chronic kidney disease from focal segmental glomerulosclerosis. Nephrol Dial Transplant 24: 2721–2729.

27. Athanasiou Y, Voskarides K, Gale DP, Damianou L, Patsias C, et al. (2011) Familial C3 Glomerulopathy Associated with CFHR5 Mutations: Clinical Characteristics of 91 Patients in 16 Pedigrees. CJASN In Press.

28. Hall TA (1999) BioEdit: a user-friendly biological sequence alignment editor and analysis program for Windows 95/98/NT. Nucl Acids Symp Ser 41: 95–98.

29. Saleem MA, O'Hare MJ, Reiser J, Coward RJ, Inward CD, et al. (2002) A conditionally immortalized human podocyte cell line demonstrating nephrin and podocin expression. J Am Soc Nephrol 13: 630–638.

30. Lydersen S, Fagerland MW, Laake P (2009) Recommended tests for association in 2×2 tables. Stat Med 28: 1159–1175.

31. Barnard GA (1947) Significance tests for 2×2 tables. Biometrika 34: 123–138.

32. Mehta CR, Hilton LF (1993) Exact power of conditional and unconditional tests: Going beyond the 2×2 contingency table. Am Stat 47: 91–98.

33. Mehta CR (1991) StatXact: A Statistical Package for Exact Nonparametric Inference. Am Stat 45: 74–75.

34. Ludbrook J (2008) Analysis of 2×2 tables of frequencies: matching test to experimental design. Int J Epidemiol 37: 1430–1435.

35. Deltas C, Pierides A, Voskarides K (2011) The role of molecular genetics in diagnosing familial hematuria(s). Pediatr Nephrol Epub 21 Jun 2011 - DOI: 10.1007/s00467-011-1935-5.

36. Liu M, Shi S, Senthilnathan S, Yu J, Wu E, et al. (2010) Genetic variation of DKK3 may modify renal disease severity in ADPKD. J Am Soc Nephrol 21: 1510–1520.

37. Persu A, Stoenoiu MS, Messiaen T, Davila S, Robino C, et al. (2002) Modifier effect of ENOS in autosomal dominant polycystic kidney disease. Hum Mol Genet 11: 229–241.

38. Lamnissou K, Zirogiannis P, Trygonis S, Demetriou K, Pierides A, et al. (2004) Evidence for association of endothelial cell nitric oxide synthase gene polymorphism with earlier progression to end-stage renal disease in a cohort of Hellens from Greece and Cyprus. Genet Test 8: 319–324.

39. Iwai N, Naraba H (2005) Polymorphisms in human pre-miRNAs. Biochem Biophys Res Commun 331: 1439–1444.

40. Lv K, Guo Y, Zhang Y, Wang K, Jia Y, et al. (2008) Allele-specific targeting of hsa-miR-657 to human IGF2R creates a potential mechanism underlying the association of ACAA-insertion/deletion polymorphism with type 2 diabetes. Biochem Biophys Res Commun 374: 101–105.

41. Tan Z, Randall G, Fan J, Camoretti-Mercado B, Brockman-Schneider R, et al. (2007) Allele-specific targeting of microRNAs to HLA-G and risk of asthma. Am J Hum Genet 81: 829–834.

42. Wang G, van der Walt JM, Mayhew G, Li YJ, Zuchner S, et al. (2008) Variation in the miRNA-433 binding site of FGF20 confers risk for Parkinson disease by overexpression of alpha-synuclein. Am J Hum Genet 82: 283–289.

43. Martin MM, Buckenberger JA, Jiang J, Malana GE, Nuovo GJ, et al. (2007) The human angiotensin II type 1 receptor+1166 A/C polymorphism attenuates microrna-155 binding. J Biol Chem 282: 24262–24269.

44. Song F, Zheng H, Liu B, Wei S, Dai H, et al. (2009) An miR-502-binding site single-nucleotide polymorphism in the 3′-untranslated region of the SET8 gene is associated with early age of breast cancer onset. Clin Cancer Res 15: 6292–6300.

45. Mulder GM, Nijboer WN, Seelen MA, Sandovici M, Bos EM, et al. (2010) Heparin binding epidermal growth factor in renal ischaemia/reperfusion injury. J Pathol 221: 183–192.

46. Smith JP, Pozzi A, Dhawan P, Singh AB, Harris RC (2009) Soluble HB-EGF induces epithelial-to-mesenchymal transition in inner medullary collecting duct cells by upregulating Snail-2. Am J Physiol Renal Physiol 296: F957–965.

47. Luo CC, Ming YC, Chao HC, Chu SM, Pang ST (2011) Heparin-Binding Epidermal Growth Factor-Like Growth Factor Downregulates Expression of Activator Protein-1 Transcription Factor after Intestinal Ischemia-Reperfusion Injury. Neonatology 99: 241–246.

48. Zhuang S, Kinsey GR, Rasbach K, Schnellmann RG (2008) Heparin-binding epidermal growth factor and Src family kinases in proliferation of renal epithelial cells. Am J Physiol Renal Physiol 294: F459–468.

49. Takemura T, Murata Y, Hino S, Okada M, Yanagida H, et al. (1999) Heparin-binding EGF-like growth factor is expressed by mesangial cells and is involved in mesangial proliferation in glomerulonephritis. J Pathol 189: 431–438.

50. Paizis K, Kirkland G, Khong T, Katerelos M, Fraser S, et al. (1999) Heparin-binding epidermal growth factor-like growth factor is expressed in the adhesive lesions of experimental focal glomerular sclerosis. Kidney Int 55: 2310–2321.

51. Uchiyama-Tanaka Y, Matsubara H, Mori Y, Kosaki A, Kishimoto N, et al. (2002) Involvement of HB-EGF and EGF receptor transactivation in TGF-beta-mediated fibronectin expression in mesangial cells. Kidney Int 62: 799–808.

52. Huppi K, Volfovsky N, Runfola T, Jones TL, Mackiewicz M, et al. (2008) The identification of microRNAs in a genomically unstable region of human chromosome 8q24. Mol Cancer Res 6: 212–221.

53. Alvarez ML, DiStefano JK (2011) Functional characterization of the plasmacytoma variant translocation 1 gene (PVT1) in diabetic nephropathy. PLoS One 6: e18671.

54. Guan Y, Kuo WL, Stilwell JL, Takano H, Lapuk AV, et al. (2007) Amplification of PVT1 contributes to the pathophysiology of ovarian and breast cancer. Clin Cancer Res 13: 5745–5755.

55. Graham M, Adams JM (1986) Chromosome 8 breakpoint far 3′ of the c-myc oncogene in a Burkitt's lymphoma 2;8 variant translocation is equivalent to the murine pvt-1 locus. EMBO J 5: 2845–2851.

15

When Health Systems are Barriers to Health Care: Challenges Faced by Uninsured Mexican Kidney Patients

Ciara Kierans[1]*, Cesar Padilla-Altamira[1], Guillermo Garcia-Garcia[2], Margarita Ibarra-Hernandez[2], Francisco J. Mercado[3]

1 Department of Public Health and Policy, The University of Liverpool, Liverpool, United Kingdom, 2 Division of Nephrology, Hospital Civil de Guadalajara, University of Guadalajara Health Sciences Centre, Hospital 278, Jalisco, Mexico, 3 Depto Salud Pública, CUCS, Universidad Guadalajara, Guadalajara, Jalisco, Mexico

Abstract

Background: Chronic Kidney Disease disproportionately affects the poor in Low and Middle Income Countries (LMICs). Mexico exemplifies the difficulties faced in supporting Renal Replacement Therapy (RRT) and providing equitable patient care, despite recent attempts at health reform. The objective of this study is to document the challenges faced by uninsured, poor Mexican families when attempting to access RRT.

Methods: The article takes an ethnographic approach, using interviewing and observation to generate detailed accounts of the problems that accompany attempts to secure care. The study, based in the state of Jalisco, comprised interviews with patients, their caregivers, health and social care professionals, among others. Observations were carried out in both clinical and social settings.

Results: In the absence of organised health information and stable pathways to renal care, patients and their families work extraordinarily hard and at great expense to secure care in a mixed public-private healthcare system. As part of this work, they must navigate challenging health and social care environments, negotiate treatments and costs, resource and finance healthcare and manage a wide range of formal and informal health information.

Conclusions: Examining commonalities across pathways to adequate healthcare reveals major failings in the Mexican system. These systemic problems serve to reproduce and deepen health inequalities. A system, in which the costs of renal care are disproportionately borne by those who can least afford them, faces major difficulties around the sustainability and resourcing of RRTs. Attempts to increase access to renal therapies, therefore, need to take into account the complex social and economic demands this places on those who need access most. This paper further shows that ethnographic studies of the concrete ways in which healthcare is accessed in practice provide important insights into the plight of CKD patients and so constitute an important source of evidence in that effort.

Editor: Emmanuel A. Burdmann, University of Sao Paulo Medical School, Brazil

Funding: This work was supported by grants from The Darwin Initiative (14-032), The Cambridge Conservation Initiative (CCI 05/10/006) and The Leverhulme Trust (F/01 503/B). The funders had no role in study design, data collection and analysis, decision to publish, or preparation of the manuscript.

Competing Interests: The authors have declared that no competing interests exist.

* E-mail: c.kierans@liv.ac.uk

Introduction

Chronic Kidney Disease (CKD) is a global public health concern. CKD is the 12th leading cause of death worldwide [1], its incidence growing by approximately 8% annually [2]. Low and middle-income countries are facing increasing difficulties supporting resource-intensive Renal Replacement Therapy (RRT) and providing equitable patient care [3,4]. In countries characterised by extreme health inequalities, unregulated medical environments [1] and an absence of comprehensive kidney registries, the true burden of CKD remains difficult to assess [5]. Furthermore, CKD has a more complex aetiology than in industrialised countries. In addition to the established risk factors of diabetes and hypertension, infectious and environmental causes create challenges for prevention monitoring and treatment [6,7,1]. The scale of the problem and the difficulties associated with its management have generated intense scientific debate about how to deliver cost-effective treatment through targeted health reform in under-resourced contexts [8,1]. Mexico, the focus of this article, is one country which exemplifies the challenges faced by low and middle-income countries in managing CKD.

CKD in Mexico

The prevalence of CKD in Mexico is similar to industrialised nations, while the resources for its treatments lag significantly behind [9,7]. With close to 9% of the population diagnosed with CKD [9,11,12], and 60,000 patients on RRT [13,10], the condition is rapidly becoming a major national concern, particularly with regard to inequalities of access to treatment [12,10].

Health inequalities in Mexico are commonly linked to its fragmented, state-corporatist system of health care provision. This system generates problematic distinctions between insured and uninsured populations. Workers in the formal economy, approximately 55–60% of the population, are covered by an insurance infrastructure administered by social security institutes. IMSS (Instituto Mexicano del Seguro Social (Mexican Institute of Social Security)), is the largest, accounting for 82% of those with health insurance [14]. The remainder of the Mexican population has no coverage and relies on subsidised services and programmes provided by clinics, hospitals and various programmes run by the Health Secretariat. These services are run at a significant out-of-pocket cost to the poor who use them [15,16]. Reforms designed to alleviate the catastrophic poverty produced by an inadequate public health infrastructure have been pursued, most recently through the development of *Seguro Popular* (Popular Health Insurance). Advanced in 2001 as an integrated health insurance programme for the poor, Seguro Popular was to be funded by federal and state subsidies and a means-tested premium paid by families, who were to enrol on the programme on a voluntary basis. It aimed to develop an explicit package of services, facilitate greater market competition and shift the federal budget to demand-based allocation of services [17,18]. The underlying assumption was that access to medical care would be enhanced through market discipline and a greater distribution of costs [19–23]. Seguro Popular's development, implementation and evaluation received extensive coverage by the Lancet in 2006, and again most recently in July 2012, where it has been presented as *the* route to universal health coverage and social protection, an evidenced example, one that other low and middle-income countries can learn from [24–29]. While Seguro Popular has increased access to care for some conditions (though not for CKD, End Stage Renal Disease or their treatments), its critics argue it has not reduced inequalities in access, but is serving to further fragment and stratify Mexico's health system, exacerbating inefficiencies in delivery [17,20,21,30,31,32].

One of the difficulties researchers and analysts currently face in assessing the merits and limits of reforms such as Seguro Popular, is the absence of evidence around their translation into practice. Existing evaluations have tended towards broad health systems analysis, provided in the main by quantitative overviews, and often conducted by those also charged with implementing reform [33,34]. They tell us little about the challenges faced by patients and their families in trying to access health care, or indeed by health professionals in attempting to ensure equity and quality of service provision. In order to develop equitable access strategically, it is imperative that researchers fully account for the situated experiences of health care in addition to synoptic overviews, when attempting to understand how health systems perform in practice [35].

By drawing on the contributions of ethnographic approaches, we aim to provide an account of this kind. Ethnographic research is a form of "social research based on the close-up, on-the-ground observation of people and institutions in real time and space in which the investigator embeds herself near (or within) the phenomenon, so as to detect how and why agents on the scene think and act the way they do" [36].

The paper, therefore, has two aims: (1) to put forward an ethnographic framework for analysing patterns of healthcare access at local levels and (2) to demonstrate the challenges and barriers encountered by uninsured CKD patients when attempting to access health services.

Methods

Setting

The setting for the research was Hospital Civil de Guadalajara in the State of Jalisco, Mexico. It is a large tertiary facility which has served Jalisco's poor since 1792. The hospital operates from state and federal funds, private donations from individuals and contributions from non-governmental organizations. However, it functions as an independent health care provider, with its own budget and board of directors. The hospital is unique in Mexico. It is the country's largest dialysis and kidney transplant centre for those without health insurance, and it is the only facility which subsidises both haemo- and peritoneal dialysis for the poor. Outside of that, patients are charged according to their level of income. The hospital has been home to a transplantation programme since 1990. It runs a large peritoneal dialysis programme – the main modality of renal care in Mexico [37] – and a haemodialysis unit which, due to limited resources, is used as a back-up to the peritoneal programme [38].

The decision to locate the study here was due to the hospital's stated commitment to patients without health insurance, but also because the city, more generally, is home to a number of successful renal care and transplantation programmes. Nephrologists based here established the Jalisco State Dialysis and Transplantation Registry in 1993 the only one of its kind in Mexico [9]. This has helped to keep CKD, particularly End State Renal Disease under epidemiologic surveillance and generate data that index CKD and its treatment nationally and internationally [39]. All public, social security institutions participate, such as IMSS, ISSSTE (Instituto de Seguridad y Servicios Sociales de los Trabajadores del Estado (Institute for Social Security and Services for State Workers)), the Hospital Civil, Guadalajara and institutions belonging to the Health Secretariat. This generates data on approximately 90% of the dialysis and transplant state population. All patients who started on renal replacement therapy between January 1998 and December 2010 at these social security facilities are included. At the start of dialysis, patients' social security or insurance institution is registered along with age, gender, aetiology of renal disease and treatment modality. Unadjusted incidence and prevalence rates are reported and data on the number of nephrologists and dialysis and transplant facilities are annually updated (information on the methods used by the registry are in the public domain [40] and the quantitative data collected by the registry has provided an important statistical backdrop to the ethnographic, qualitative methods used in this study).

Inequalities of outcome between CKD patients with and without insurance in Jalisco are, as a result, well-evidenced and have provided impetus for a series of strategic interventions aimed at reducing inequity and supporting improvements in screening and prevention [40,12]. In Jalisco, those without insurance suffer high mortality when end-stage renal disease develops, with approximately half dying within 6 months of dialysis therapy initiation [37]. For insured patients, acceptance and prevalence rates are considerably higher (478 per million population (pmp) and 1211 pmp, respectively) than the uninsured (231 pmp and 286 pmp); for rate of kidney transplantation, this is 82 pmp versus 20 pmp; for provision of dialysis units 21 versus 3; and for number of nephrologists 12.1 pmp versus 3.4 pmp [12]. Social Security covers 44.2% of the population in the state and a further 3.5% are covered by civil service and private schemes. While 15.6% are identified as having *Seguro Popular*, 36.6% are left without any coverage or benefits [41]. These latter figures, however, only relate to those who have chosen to enrol in Seguro Popular. As Seguro

Popular provides no coverage for renal replacement therapies, not all patients will register.

Ethnographic Approach

Data for this paper was collected between June and September 2011 and again during July and August 2012 as part of a collaborative ethnographic study carried out by researchers at the University of Guadalajara and the University of Liverpool, UK with support from clinicians at the Hospital Civil de Guadalajara. The advantage of approaching the problem of inequalities ethnographically was threefold: (1) Ethnographic research, is dependent (though not exclusively) on in-depth qualitative interviewing and forms of observation. This facilitates a clear focus on what people do, how people understand what they do and how such practices are embedded in particular cultural, social, economic and political contexts. (2) It pays attention to the connections between different areas of social life (like illness, the family and work) rather than separating them off as domains to be studied discretely. In the case of CKD, it concentrates on the contexts within which patients and their families attempt to access health care and traces the work families do vis-a-vis other related health and social care agents, such as health care professionals, policy makers, social security administrators, charitable and voluntary associations. (3) Ethnography, finally, takes into consideration socio-economic and political structures which play an integral role in healthcare. In this case, adopting an ethnographic approach made it possible to follow the problem of CKD to show how health care is navigated from below as well as administered from above. It thus describes how these systems operated in practice [42].

Data Collection

The study comprised 105 interviews incorporating 138 respondents, 32 of which were in-depth narrative style interviews and 73 were semi-structured. They included 51 renal patients across all modalities of treatment, 34 caregivers, donors and family members and 53 interviews distributed between health and social care professionals, patient support groups/charitable organisations and medical suppliers as well as Mexican scholars writing on this subject area (please see table 1). The respondents were purposely selected to obtain a maximum variation sample. In addition to interviews, observational research was carried out in the hospital: at medical consultations, in hospital wards and in related settings, such as patients' homes and patient support meetings and events. Approximately 200 pages of field notes were written, providing contextual information to ground the analysis of the qualitative interviews, as well as documenting the fieldwork process. The research strictly adhered to the ethical codes of practice set out in the requirements of the American Anthropological Association and the Association of Social Anthropologists, UK, which reflect the particularities of conducting ethnographic fieldwork. Both written and verbal consent were taken. Consent was verbal in cases where participants were uncomfortable providing a signature on forms, suspicious of bureaucratic processes or during informal ethnographic interviewing where it was not always appropriate to request written consent. In every case, we took time to explain the objectives, procedures and possible outcomes of our research. We asked permission to record the interviews, gave clear assurances on anonymity, confidentiality and the right to withdraw at any stage. Participants' queries and questions were answered before and after interviews. Both written and verbal consent procedures complemented each other in the process of ensuring an ethically robust study and were documented through the writing of field notes, a process, in this case, overseen collectively by the researchers

Table 1. Study Participants.

Participants	Total
Patients	51
Caregivers, donors and family members	34
Physicians	16
Social workers	7
Nurses	7
Psychologists	1
Nutritionists	1
Organ donor coordinators	1
Patient support associations	7
Health decision makers	4
Pharmaceutical and laboratory representatives	5
Pharmacists	1
Academic scholars	3
Total participants	138

involved. Ethics approvals for ethnographic fieldwork, which incorporates both formal and informal interviewing and written and verbal consent recorded in this way, were awarded by the University of Liverpool and the Hospital Civil de Guadalajara research ethics committees.

Analysis

This mix of interviewing and observation, which was carried out across different settings and across all our participants - patients, caregivers, health professionals and so on - yielded highly detailed and complex accounts of the process of accessing renal care. While these accounts are characterised by a diversity of patient and family experiences and histories, we were particularly interested in identifying 'structural' commonalities among the types of processes found across all cases: including the 'built-in' constraints on the kinds of pathways patients had to follow through the system and the kinds of demands placed on them as well as the resources they were required to expend as they did so. As a result, and for the purpose of this particular paper, we focused our attention on these commonalities, concentrating on the trajectories or journeys of healthcare seeking for CKD patients in Mexico. This has enabled us to effectively demonstrate the profound challenges poor families face, and the strategies they employ, in accessing renal care and managing CKD [43]. As part of reading through and analysing all our data, we identified the recurrence of various kinds of steps and actions taken by patients and their families, such as the forms of exchange underpinning access to health care, interactions with various personnel within pertinent clinical sites, as well as the wide range of resources that patients draw on to secure care. The three cases that were finally chosen were selected for their typicality, in that they usefully exemplified the kinds of structural problem which emerged across our data as a whole. The value in taking an ethnographic approach to the problem of accessing care is not to abstract away from the richness of real world cases but to show, with reference to them, what can be drawn out in order to help us make sense of further cases. More conventional approaches which rely on the use of interview quotations would not help us to achieve this. In fact, it would carve up the process of seeking care much more idiosyncratically, making it difficult to extrapolate beyond individuals' perspectives or subjective experiences. It is also very important to add that while we do not specifically draw out individual points-of-view from the rest of our informants, such as health professionals or members of charitable organisations, our analysis has been informed and developed in relation to their input: our many discussions with them and observations of the work they do. Their input has served to strengthen our analysis, as we have not simply relied on one constituency of informant. Developing a robust account of processes which are complex, messy and discontinuous in practice has, thus, relied on an analysis of the structural features of each 'case'. Our analysis was also informed by the rich legacy of 'interactional approaches' [44] to studies of health care and owes much to the well established concept of the patient 'career' [45] which has helped us develop our understanding of the significance of recurrent or 'typical' characteristics within the experience of healthcare.

Results

The cases relate to three transplant recipients (Elena, Emilio and Gabriel), all aged between 18–22. They provide insight into how families access care within the distributed and complex Mexican system, across public and private institutions, while attempting to find the appropriate financial, human and moral resources to do so. All were interviewed with family members, in the hospital and in their homes. All were from large working class families, with average annual incomes well below the average in Jalisco of approximately 81,430 pesos (approx 6,000 US dollars). None had a medical explanation as to why they had CKD. Emilio and Gabriel received their kidneys from their mothers, Elena from her older sister. Elena and Emilio had been on haemodialysis and Gabriel was on peritoneal dialysis. All had attempted to use Seguro Popular for different aspects of their health care, but learned in the course of seeking support, that it did not cover CKD or its treatments. All had come to Hospital Civil because of its reputation for quality care for poor patients. Descriptions of these cases can be found in tables 2, 3, 4.

Discussion

Exemplified by these cases and the wider interviews, four key practices within the trajectories of health care seeking have been identified as underpinning the 'work' families in Mexico must do to secure health care. These are described in table 5.

Taken together these practices constitute responses to the disintegrated character of care for the uninsured CKD patient in Mexico, drawing attention to its lack of structure and clear pathways to treatment. From the point of diagnosis, there is little information and no clearly defined administrative infrastructure. This means that families have to find their own routes through various public and private health care providers, laboratories, pharmacies, social support organisations and so on. In effect, each family has to 'make' a health care system for themselves, connecting together treatment as they go. That there is no financial coverage for this condition, despite the rhetoric of Seguro Popular's increasing coverage for the poor, means that every aspect of renal care has to be resourced by the family. Not only does this serve to make poor families poorer, it entrenches social and health inequalities, particularly gender inequalities, as the burden of care is disproportionately taken on by women as organ donors and carers as well as financial negotiators for health care.

What is evident in the work families do to negotiate access to health care is that the rhetorical distinctions between insured and uninsured break down and conflict in practice. This is demonstrated by the ways in which patients move between public and private providers and their associated insurance systems, depending on need, waiting times, quality of care and cost. For patients relying on renal replacement therapy, the consequences of this 'zigzagging' are inconsistency of care, difficulties in maintaining drug regimens, and making routine check-ups and monitoring. This profoundly threatens the sustainability of transplanted organs, due to infections, graft rejection and the haphazard taking of immunosuppressants.

Given efforts to increase access to renal replacement therapy for Mexico's poor at Hospital Civil, integrated care is of vital importance. In 2011, Hospital Civil had approximately 240 patients on peritoneal dialysis, 70 patients on haemodialysis and performed 53 transplants. This reflected an increase in capacity by

Table 2. Elena, her mother and sister Rita.

Elena was an 18 year old transplant recipient. She received a kidney from her older sister Rita in March 2011. She had been diagnosed with CKD in Hospital Civil in 2009, after attending three private physicians and another public hospital. Unsuitable for peritoneal dialysis, she was put on haemodialysis. Because her parents had IMSS insurance, the family were initially sent to IMSS facilities, only to find that Elena, no longer formally at school, was not covered.

On medical advice, she went to a private hospital, known for providing low-cost dialysis ($84 USD/session). To help finance, the family were given a letter by a doctor to go to DIF Jalisco (Desarrollo Integral de La Familia – a national public assistance organisation with Federal, State and Municipal offices). Support was provided for four free sessions, after which the family went to Caritas Mexico, (the international Catholic social welfare provider), followed by the DIF Zapopan municipal office, then by DIF in Guadalajara. Each provided payment for a few dialysis sessions. Elena's mother took on the role of sourcing financial support, while her sister negotiated her treatments and care. After three months of dialysis, they moved to another private clinic run in conjunction with a pharmaceutical company, with support from DIF Guadalajara and a philanthropic organisation.

One year into dialysis, the family made an 'informal' arrangement with a cleaning company to 'hire' Elena, so that she could qualify for IMSS insurance. Taking advantage of such slippages in an overburdened insurance system was not uncommon among patients. The family, in turn, agreed to pay the employer and employee's insurance contribution, however this lasted only as long as they could afford the premiums. With this in place, Elena received the remainder of her dialysis (two more months) free of charge at an IMSS affiliated hospital.

Attempts to secure a transplant were particularly difficult. IMSS could not transplant her due to long waiting times and after much negotiation, Hospital Civil agreed. The family would have to pay for all required pre-transplant tests, many out-sourced to private laboratories (approx $1,400 USD). To meet the costs, the family sold their land; appealed to everyone they knew; requested money from relatives in the US and petitioned local TV stations and businesses.

Elena was transplanted at a cost of approximately $1,241 USD (surgery only). The family, now penniless, went to a money lender to borrow money for immunosuppressants. They were finding it increasingly difficult to find the $37 USD for post-transplant monitoring and checkups, not to mention the $15 USD extra charges for taxi fares. Elena had complications post-transplant and had to be rushed back into hospital. With her family stripped of all resources, her sister said: "We are now between the sword and the wall, we don't have money for Elena's post-transplantation care or to pay the money lender. We don't know what we are going to do".

Table 3. Emilio and his mother Ana.

Emilio was 20 years old and unemployed. He was diagnosed with CKD at 14, his condition managed at a public hospital near his home, until kidney functioning reached 'end stage'. He then moved to Hospital Civil. He spent ten months on haemodialysis there, paid for by money raised by his family, while the necessary protocols prior to transplantation were conducted.

Emilio received a kidney donated by his mother, three months prior to interview. Since then he had been sick. His doctors weren't sure whether he was experiencing toxicity, rejection or a virus, and requested a biopsy. His mother was asked to purchase a biopsy needle ($146 USD), while Emilio was hospitalised, waiting for the biopsy. After this his mother was expected to bring the biopsied sample and Emilio's medical files for private clinical analysis ($365 USD). The biopsy had to be re-scheduled. The family were charged $132 for hospitalisation, Emilio's mother complained, and they secured a renegotiated price of $44.

Without insurance, the family relied financially on relatives working as cleaners and labourers in the US; on more immediate family to provide blood donations and smaller amounts of money; on a range of charitable donations and on fellow patients for advice for obtaining discounts on medications and sourcing less expensive laboratories for analysis. Since his transplant, Emilio's family have made an 'arrangement' with a neighbour who owns a corner shop to formally employ Emilio so that he qualifies for IMSS insurance which covers the cost of immunosuppressants.

Ana, his mother explained that resources are difficult to find morally and economically. Aside from being Emilo's donor and carer, she also looks after her husband, a labourer, who has prostate cancer. She says, "There are no rights for kidney patients ... it is a tragedy because lots of young people are getting sick with this condition .... Seguro Popular doesn't cover us. They send you to the gutter. They don't want to know – they will give you some drugs but not the expensive ones."

the hospital, which had in May of 2011 opened a new, modern haemodialysis facility. Despite its limited resources, Hospital Civil remains one of the few centres in Mexico providing comprehensive renal care to the uninsured. However, in a context where families have become responsible for their own health care, ensuring access to renal therapy is not enough, particularly when sustainability and continuity of treatment cannot be guaranteed. This raises critical questions about the importance of resourcing, not only in Mexico, but across low and middle-income countries. In particular, it raises questions about the manner in which costs are currently distributed between state, industry and society, and how these costs could be better borne by these parties to ensure greater equity and justice in health care.

A potential limitation of this study may reflect the fact that the experiences of our participants may not be representative of the specific experiences of individuals who seek renal care at other public institutions in other states. Nevertheless, due to the ways in which treatment is configured in Mexico, we can point to wider lessons to be learned. Our approach has attempted to provide an account of the structure of interactions with the public health system and to focus on commonalities across the variable trajectories of individual patients. Given that Seguro Popular is supported by federal government and that this form of health care delivery is reflective of the Mexican system as a whole, it is

reasonable, therefore, to suggest that the structuring of access to health care and the types of practices we have documented will be found in other states, and potentially across other conditions.

Conclusion

CKD disproportionately affects the poor and the socially disadvantaged, particularly in low and middle-income countries. Its burden is not limited to access to renal replacement therapy but to overall population health [46]. It is known to exacerbate other chronic conditions and impacts profoundly on mental health, working capacity and family life. All predictions show that CKD and its impacts are set to worsen over the coming decades [2]. In the interest of enhancing equity in health care, this has given rise to discussions about the importance of prevention [2], the necessity of low cost drugs [1] and the different roles to be played by the state, private sector, charitable organisations and citizens in the work of healthcare [46,47]. However, in order to gauge the effects on the most vulnerable, we cannot rely solely on synoptic views of health systems, medical interventions and outcomes to draw conclusions about equity or, indeed, as the basis for evaluations. This is of particular concern in low and middle-income countries engaging in health reform, as processes which may be planned to simplify and rationalise healthcare provision

Table 4. Gabriel and his mother Maria.

Gabriel is a college-level teacher from Chapala (62 kilometers from Guadalajara). He was diagnosed with kidney disease in 2008 and put on peritoneal dialysis (PD). For this, his family constructed an extra room from plywood within the existing space of their living room, at great personal cost. This had to be specially painted, kept immaculately clean and equipped with microwave, weighing scales and countless boxes of dialysate solution.

Gabriel's teaching job should guarantee IMSS insurance but he was told he would not be covered as his CKD was pre-existing. This, however, was not correctly communicated, but instead reflected a failure within his school to understand and explain adequately his level of social protection. To assist with the ensuing costs, support was provided by a relative who ran a local clinical laboratory, and gave them credit on medical tests. Further help was given by families, who had lost a member due to CKD, by establishing an informal distribution network of unused solution, disinfectant and medications.

After three years on PD, in June 2011, Gabriel received a kidney from his mother, but rejected the graft only a few weeks prior to our interview. He was back on PD and awaiting a cadaveric organ. Rejection was explained as a result of a miscommunication regarding the amount and type of immunosuppressants he would need. The family had, previously, raised the money for the transplant from fundraisers and family in the US, but were not prepared for the cost of immunosuppression. His mother, who cried when she talked of the kidney rejecting, explained that travelling to the hospital leaves no money to buy food as everything went to pay for routine check-ups, consultations and the bus fare. A few weeks prior, they were offered the chance of a cadaveric kidney. His mother explained:

"They (doctors) said come today, you can pay tomorrow, but I explained it isn't that easy. He (doctor) said you need only $365 USD for the cross-match tests. I said, but we know how much everything really costs, so we said no, we will wait until we have the money. He said, are you going to waste the opportunity, and we said, yes. A transplant ... for everything ... is somewhere between $3,600–4,380 USD. Everything has to be bought, even the material for stitching the wound. It is too much for a family. ... And Seguro Popular, we don't have it. For us, it only covers consultations and one or two pills. Even the doctors complain about it. It doesn't make sense, there is no point in it. It's just a government lie".

Table 5. The Practical Work done by Mexican CKD Patients and their Families.

Practices	Description
Navigating health and social care structures	Without any synoptic overview of health care provision or any established patient pathway, families must identify appropriate healthcare institutions in order to acquire a diagnosis, form of dialysis and secure a transplant. This routinely involves an unscripted set of journeys or zigzagging between various public and private health care providers, clinics and laboratories.
Negotiating treatments and costs	Without health insurance, families must pay for all aspects of their medical care – hospitalisation, surgeries, consultation, routine check-ups and tests, dialysis, pre-transplantation protocols, biopsy needles, stitching for wounds, disinfectant, antibodies, surgical procedures, among a wide range of medications e.g., erythropoietin and immunosuppressants. In addition, there are travel costs, dietary costs, structural housing costs for peritoneal dialysis patients, informal care giving and the loss of formal earnings. Some of these costs are negotiable as a result of lobbying social workers and medical staff, or partially covered by ad hoc insurance coverage.
Financing and resourcing health care	Financing CKD and its treatments requires ingenuity and hard work and involves appeals to family and neighbours, fund raising, negotiating with charitable and voluntary associations, selling land and inheritances, begging, appealing to local business or the media.
Managing formal and informal health information	Due to a lack of integrated administrative systems within and between hospitals, patients carry their own medical files and test-results to all appointments. This produces a burden of information that has to be understood, processed and disseminated regularly. Furthermore, it serves to shift the burden of responsibility onto the patient, making them the principal agent in the management of their health care, rather than the state or any 'sited' health care provider.

may actually massively complicate the processes of accessing care for those who need it most. On paper, current developments in Mexico are opening up CKD treatment to the poor. In practice, these developments are caught within a system which is leading to further impoverishment, as patients are caught in a 'medical poverty trap' [48]. In order to respond to the problems the poorest face in practice, we must attend to how systems of healthcare work in practice. This means tracing the impacts of healthcare reform, medical interventions and patient outcomes in local contexts.

Acknowledgments

We would like to thank all those who reviewed and provided critical comment and advice on previous drafts of this paper. They include Dr. Michael Mair, Professor Ann Jacoby, Professor Simon Capewell and Professor Margaret Whitehead (all, University of Liverpool) and Dr. Fergus Caskey (Renal Unit, Southmead Hospital, Bristol. We would particularly like to express our sincere gratitude to all the staff at the Hospital Civil, the patients and their families, without whose generosity and support, this research would not have been possible.

Author Contributions

Editing, critical reading of drafts: CK CPA FM MIH GGG. Conceived and designed the experiments: CK FM. Performed the experiments: CK FM CPA. Analyzed the data: CK FM CPA. Contributed reagents/materials/analysis tools: CK FM CPA GGG MIH. Wrote the paper: CK.

References

1. White S, Chadban S, Jan S, Chapman J, Cass A (2008) How can we achieve global equity in provision of renal replacement therapy? Bulletin World Health Org 86 3: 229–237.
2. Couser WG, Remuzzi G, Mendis S, Tonelli M (2011) The contribution of chronic kidney disease to the global burden of major noncommunicable diseases. Kidney Int 80:1258–1270.
3. Barsoum RS (2002) Overview: end-stage renal disease in the developing world. Artif Organs 26 9:737–746
4. Moosa MR, Kidd M (2006) The dangers of rationing dialysis treatment: the dilemma facing a developing country. Kidney Int 70:1107–1114.
5. Ayodele O, Alebiosu O (2010) Burden of Chronic Kidney Disease: An International Perspective. Advances Chronic Kid Dis 17 3:215–224.
6. Barsoum RS (2003) End-stage renal disease in North Africa. Kidney Int 63: S111–S114.
7. Kher V (2002) End-stage renal disease in developing countries. Kidney Int 62:350–62.
8. Aviles-Gomez R, Luquin-Arellano VH, Garcia-Garcia G, Ibarra-Hernandez M, Briseño-Renteria G (2006) Is renal replacement therapy for all possible in developing countries? Ethn Dis 16:S2-70-72.
9. Amato D, Álvarez-Aguilar C, Castañeda-Limones R, Rodriguez E, Avila-Diaz M, et al. (2005) Prevalence of chronic kidney disease in an urban Mexican population. Kidney Int Suppl 97:S11–17.
10. Paniagua R, Ramos A, Fabian R, Lagunas J, Amato D (2007) Chronic Kidney Disease and Dialysis in Mexico. Pert Dial Int 27 4:405–9.
11. Gutierrez-Padilla JF, Mendoza-Garcia M, Plascencia-Perez S, Renoirte-Lopez K, Garcia-Garcia G, et al. (2010) Screening for CKD and Cardiovascular Disease Risk Factors Using Mobile Clinics in Jalisco, Mexico. Am J Kidney Dis 55 3: 474–484.
12. Garcia-Garcia G, Renoirte-Lopez K, Marquez-Magaña I (2010) Disparities in renal care in Jalisco, Mexico. Semin Nephrol 30:3–7.
13. Méndez-Durán A, Méndez-Bueno FJ, Tapia-Yáñez T, Montes AM, Aguilar-Sánchez L (2010) Epidemiología de la insuficiencia renal crónica en México. Diálisis y Trasplante 31 1: 7–11.
14. INEGI Statistic and Geography National Institute (2010) Available: www.censo2010.org.mx. Accessed 2012 June 16.
15. Garcia-Diaz R, Sosa-Rub S (2011) Analysis of the distributional impact of out-of-pocket health payments: evidence from a public health insurance program for the poor in Mexico. J Health Econ 30: 707–718.
16. Frenk J (2006) Bridging the divide: global lessons from evidence-based health policy in Mexico. Lancet 368: 954–61.
17. Homedes N, Ugaldez A (2009) Twenty-Five Years of Convoluted Health Reforms in Mexico. PLOS Med 6 8: e1000124
18. Lakin J (2010) The end of insurance? Mexico's Seguro Popular, 2001–2007. J Health Politics, Policy and Law 35 3:313–352.
19. Eibenschutz C, Támez S, Camacho I (2008) Inequality and erroneous social policy produce inequity in Mexico. Rev Salud Pública 10:119–132.
20. Laurell AC, Herrera-Ronquillo J (2010) La segunda reforma de salud: Aseguramiento y compra-venta de servicios. Salud Colectiva 6 2:137–148.
21. Laurell AC (2011) Los seguros de salud mexicanos: cobertura universal incierta. Ciência & Saúde Coletiva 16 6: 2796–2806.
22. Támez S, Eibenschutz C (2008) Popular Health Insurance: key piece of inequity in health in Mexico. Rev Salud Pública 10: 133–145.

23. Urbina M (2008) Sistema de protección social en salud. Seguro popular en salud. Evaluación y consistencia de resultados. México,DF: Coneval. Available: http://www.coneval.gob.mx/contenido/cmsconeval/rw/resource/coneval/eval_mon/1742.pdf. Accessed 2012 June 16.

24. Frenk J, González-Pier E, Gómez-Dantés O, Lezana MA, Knaul FM (2006) Comprehensive reform to improve health system performance in Mexico. Lancet 368: 1524–34.

25. Gakidou E, Lozano R, Gonzalez-Pier, Abbott-Klafter J, Barofsky JT, et al. (2006) Assessing the effect of the 2001–2006 Mexican health reform: an interim report card. 368: 1920–35.

26. González-Pier E, Gutiérrez-Delgado C, Stevens G, Barraza-Lloréns M, Porras-Condey R, et al. (2006) Priority setting for health interventions in Mexico's System of Social Protection in Health. Lancet 368: 1608–18.

27. Knaul FM, Arreola-Ornelas H, Méndez-Carniado O, Bryson-Cahn C, Barofsky J, et al. (2006) Evidence is good for your health system: policy reform to remedy catastrophic and impoverishing health spending in Mexico. Lancet 368:1828–41.

28. Lozano R, Soliz P, Gakidou E, Abbott-Klafter J, Feehan DM, et al. (2006) Benchmarking of performance of Mexican states with effective coverage. Lancet 368: 1729–1741.

29. Editorial (2012) A crucial juncture for health in Mexico. Lancet 380: 76.

30. Laurell AC (2007) Health system reform in Mexico: a critical review. Intl J Health Services 37 3:515–535.

31. Lustig N (2007) Politicas publicas y salud en Mexico. Revista Nexos 358. Available: Http://historic.nexos.com.mx/vers_imp.php?id_article=1494&id_rubrique= 651. Accessed: 20/04/2012

32. Támez Gonsales S, Valle Arcos RI (2005) Desigualdad social reforma neoliberal en salud. Rev Mex Social 67:321–356.

33. Sosa-Rubí SG, Salinas-Rodríguez A, Galárraga O (2011) Impacto del Seguro Popular en el gasto catastrófico y de bolsillo en el México rural y urbano, 2005–2008. Salud Pública De México 53(Supp 4), 425–435.

34. Victora CG, Peters DH (2009) Seguro Popular in Mexico: is premature evaluation healthy? Lancet 373:1404–1405.

35. Malterud K (2001)Qualitative Research: standards, challenges, and guidelines. Lancet 358: 483–488.

36. Wacquant L (2003) Ethnografeast: a progress report on the practice and promise of ethnography. Ethnography 4:5–14.

37. Cueto-Manzano A, Rojas-Campos E (2007) Status of renal replacement therapy and peritoneal dialysis in Mexico. Perit Dial Int 27 2:142–148.

38. Garcia-Garcia G, Briseno-Renteria G, Luquin-Arellano VH, Gao Z, Gill J, et al. (2007) Survival among patients with kidney failure in Jalisco, Mexico. J Am Soc Nephrol 18: 1922–1927.

39. López-Cervantes M, Rojas-Russell ME, Tirado-Gómez LL, Durán-Arenas L, Pacheco-Domínguez RL, et al. (2010) Enfermedad renal crónica y su atención mediante tratamiento sustitutivo en México. México: Universidad Nacional Autónoma de México.

40. Garcia-Garcia G, Monteon-Ramos FJ, Garcia-Bejarano H, Garcia-Bejarano H, Gomez-Navarro B, et al. (2005) Renal replacement therapy among disadvantaged populations in Mexico: a report from the Jalisco Dialysis and Transplant Registry. Kidney Int (Suppl 97): S58–S61.

41. Consejo Estatal de Poplación Jalisco (2011) Diez Problemas de la Población de Jalisco: una perspectiva sociodemongráfica. Mexico: Gobierno de Jalisco and COEPO.

42. Latour B. (1987) Science in Action: how to follow scientists and engineers through society. Cambridge: Harvard University Press.

43. Corbin J, Strauss A (1991) Nursing Model for Chronic Illness Management Based upon the Trajectory framework. Scholarly Inq Nurs Practice 5: 155–174.

44. Becker H, Geer B, Hughes EC, Strauss A (1961) Boys in White: Student Culture in Medical School. Chicago: University of Chicago Press.

45. Goffman E (1961) Asylums. New York: Doubleday.

46. Bello AK, Nwankwo E, Nahas ME (2005)Prevention of chronic kidney disease: A global challenge. Kid Intl 68 98:S11–S17.

47. Nugent RA, Fathima SF, Feigl AB, Chyung D (2001) The Burden of Chronic Kidney Disease on Developing Nations: A 21st Century Challenge in Global Health. Nephron Clin Pract 118:c269–c277.

48. Whitehead M, Dahlgren G, Evans T (2001) Equity and health sector reforms: can low-income countries escape the medical poverty trap? Lancet 358: 833–6.

16

Measuring and Estimating GFR and Treatment Effect in ADPKD Patients: Results and Implications of a Longitudinal Cohort Study

Piero Ruggenenti[1,2⑨], Flavio Gaspari[1⑨], Antonio Cannata[1], Fabiola Carrara[1], Claudia Cella[1], Silvia Ferrari[1], Nadia Stucchi[1], Silvia Prandini[1], Bogdan Ene-Iordache[1], Olimpia Diadei[1], Norberto Perico[1], Patrizia Ondei[2], Antonio Pisani[3], Erasmo Buongiorno[4], Piergiorgio Messa[5], Mauro Dugo[6], Giuseppe Remuzzi[1,2]*, for the GFR-ADPKD Study Group

1 Clinical Research Center for Rare Diseases Aldo & Cele Daccò, Mario Negri Institute for Pharmacological Research, Bergamo, Italy, 2 Unit of Nephrology, Azienda Ospedaliera Ospedali Riuniti di Bergamo, Bergamo, Italy, 3 Azienda Ospedaliera Universitaria Federico II, Napoli, Italy, 4 Presidio Ospedaliero V. Fazzi, Lecce, Italy, 5 Fondazione IRCCS Ca' Granda Ospedale Maggiore Policlinico, Milano, Italy, 6 Azienda ULSS 9 – Ospedale S. Maria di Ca' Foncello, Treviso, Italy

Abstract

Trials failed to demonstrate protective effects of investigational treatments on glomerular filtration rate (GFR) reduction in Autosomal Dominant Polycystic Kidney Disease (ADPKD). To assess whether above findings were explained by unreliable GFR estimates, in this academic study we compared GFR values centrally measured by iohexol plasma clearance with corresponding values estimated by Chronic Kidney Disease Epidemiology Collaboration (CKD-Epi) and abbreviated Modification of Diet in Renal Disease (aMDRD) formulas in ADPKD patients retrieved from four clinical trials run by a Clinical Research Center and five Nephrology Units in Italy. Measured baseline GFRs and one-year GFR changes averaged 78.6 ± 26.7 and 8.4 ± 10.3 mL/min/1.73 m^2 in 111 and 71 ADPKD patients, respectively. CKD-Epi significantly overestimated and aMDRD underestimated baseline GFRs. Less than half estimates deviated by $<10\%$ from measured values. One-year estimated GFR changes did not detect measured changes. Both formulas underestimated GFR changes by 50%. Less than 9% of estimates deviated $<10\%$ from measured changes. Extent of deviations even exceeded that of measured one-year GFR changes. In ADPKD, prediction formulas unreliably estimate actual GFR values and fail to detect their changes over time. Direct kidney function measurements by appropriate techniques are needed to adequately evaluate treatment effects in clinics and research.

Editor: Jean-Claude Dussaule, INSERM, France

Funding: The authors have no support or funding to report.

Competing Interests: The authors have declared that no competing interests exist.

* E-mail: giuseppe.remuzzi@marionegri.it

⑨ These authors contributed equally to this work.

Introduction

Seven to ten percent of patients requiring chronic renal replacement therapy because of end-stage renal disease (ESRD) are affected by Autosomal Dominant Polycystic Kidney Disease (ADPKD) [1–3]. Renal function loss in ADPKD is largely related to the development and growth of cysts and concomitant disruption of normal renal tissue [4]. Thus, experimental and clinical studies tested drugs that specifically target factors - such as cyclic AMP and mammalian Target of Rapamycin (mTOR) related pathways [5,6] - that appear to be involved in the dysregulation of epithelial cell growth, secretion, and matrix deposition that is characteristic of the disease [7–11]. The enthusiasm on this line of research, however, was stifled by the results of recent trials showing no appreciable protective effect of sirolimus or everolimus therapy against progressive glomerular filtration rate (GFR) decline in two large cohorts of ADPKD patients [12,13]. In both trials the GFR was estimated (eGFR) by using prediction formulas - the "Chronic Kidney Disease Epidemiology Collaboration" (CKD-Epi) and the

"abbreviated Modification of Diet in Renal Disease" (aMDRD) equations – that are based on serum creatinine level, taken as an endogenous marker of glomerular filtration [Levey A, et al. (2000) J Am Soc Nephrol 11: 155A, Abstract] [14]. These formulas, however, has been repeatedly challenged and there is increasing evidence that their use might generate misleading information in particular in subjects with normal or near normal kidney function [15–19] [Porrini E et al. (2010) American Society of Nephrology, Renal Week 2010, Denver, CO, November 16–21, Abstract F-PO1244]. Thus, direct measurements of the GFR by gold-standard techniques based on the use of exogenous markers of glomerular filtration such as inulin, iohexol or radio-labeled tracers [20–24] would be needed to adequately assess a treatment effect on GFR decline in this population. To test this hypothesis we took advantage from a cohort of ADPKD patients prospectively monitored by serial GFR measurements and estimations in the setting of controlled clinical trials coordinated by the Mario Negri Institute for Pharmacological Research in Italy. In this population we evaluated the relationships between GFR values centrally measured (mGFR) at inclusion and at one-year follow-up and the concomitant GFR estimates obtained by prediction formulas (eGFR). To this purpose the GFR was measured by using the iohexol plasma clearance technique [21], a procedure previously validated by comparative analyses with inulin renal clearance showing that iohexol is a reliable marker of glomerular filtration in normal subjects as well as in patients with different degree of renal insufficiency [21]. Compared to renal inulin clearance this procedure does not require urine collection or continuous infusion of the filtration marker, and compared to ^{51}Cr-EDTA and ^{99m}Tc-DTPA plasma clearance techniques [25,26], it allows avoiding the use of radiolabeled tracers. Both advantages facilitate kidney function monitoring in everyday clinical practice and in research [21,27–29]. Thus, the availability of direct GFR measurements allowed to test the reliability of prediction formulas in patients with ADPKD and to assess whether and to which extent their use can affect the statistical power of a clinical trial aimed to detect the protective effect of a given intervention on progressive renal function loss in this population.

Methods

This was a fully academic, internally funded study with no sponsor or company involvement in study design and data recording, analysis, interpretation and reporting. All considered trials conformed to the Declaration of Helsinki guidelines and were approved by the "Comitato di Bioetica della Azienda Ospedaliera Ospedali Riuniti di Bergamo". In addition, for the ALADIN Study Ethics Committees of Lecce, Milan, Naples, and Treviso approved the trial. All included patients provided written consent to trial participation. Data were handled in respect of patient anonymity and confidentiality.

Study population

We used measured and estimated GFR data obtained from homogeneous cohorts of adult ADPKD subjects with baseline eGFR >30 mL/min/1.73 m^2 (by aMDRD equation) who had been included in four studies designed, conducted, and monitored by the Investigators of the Clinical Research Center for Rare Diseases *"Aldo e Cele Daccò"* of the Mario Negri Institute (Bergamo, Italy). The "Safety and Efficacy of Long-acting Somatostatin Treatment in Autosomal Dominant Polycystic Kidney Disease" study [30] and the "Sirolimus Treatment in Patients with Autosomal Dominant Polycystic Kidney Disease" I (SIRENA I, EUDRACT N°: 2006-003427-37) [31] and II (SIRENA II, EUDRACT N°: 2007-005047-21) studies were run in cooperation with the Nephrology Unit in Bergamo, whereas the "Effects of Long-acting Somatostatin on Disease Progression in Patients with Autosomal Dominant Polycystic Kidney Disease and Moderate to Severe Renal Insufficiency Therapy" (ALADIN, EUDRACT N°: 2005-005552-41) study involved also four Units in Lecce, Milan, Naples, and Treviso, all in Italy. The first two studies evaluated the short-term effects of six-month therapy with Sandostatin-LAR® Depot (Novartis Farma S.p.A., Origgio, Varese, Italy) or Rapamune® (Wyeth-Lederle S.p.A., Aprilia, Latina, Italy) on kidney volumes and function in the setting of a randomized, cross-over design. The other two studies evaluated the long-term effect of three-year treatment with the two agents on kidney volumes and mGFR decline in the setting of a randomized, parallel-group design. Baseline data were obtained from all studies (Somatostatin study: 10, SIRENA I: 21, SIRENA II: 4, ALADIN: 76), whereas one-year data were available only from the ALADIN study.

All studies excluded ADPKD patients with evidence of concomitant systemic, renal parenchymal (proteinuria ≥1 gr/24 hours) or

urinary tract disease, diabetes, cancer, psychiatric disorders, as well as pregnant or lactating women or fertile women without effective contraception. Considered variables were recorded according to similar timetables in case record forms and databases which had a similar frame. Thus, the homogeneity in patient characteristics, study design and organization, monitored variables, and data handling procedures allowed the merging of data in a common meta-database and all considered outcomes could be analyzed with a minimized risk of reasonably predictable biases.

GFR measurement and estimation

GFR was centrally determined at the laboratory of the Clinical Research Center at patient inclusion and one year apart by using the iohexol plasma clearance technique. GFR was determined by the plasma clearance of iohexol. Briefly, on the morning of renal function evaluation, 5 ml of iohexol solution (Omnipaque 300, GE Healthcare, Milan, Italy) was injected intravenously over 2 minutes. Blood samples were then taken at 120, 180, 240, 300, 360, 420, and 480 min for patients with expected mGFR≤40 mL/min, and at 120, 150, 180, 210, and 240 min for those with expected mGFR>40 mL/min. Blood iohexol plasma levels were measured by high-performance-liquid chromatography. The clearance of iohexol was calculated according to a one-compartment model (CL$_1$) by the formula: CL$_1$ = Dose/AUC, where AUC is the area under the plasma concentration-time curve. According to Bröchner-Mortensen [32], plasma clearances were then corrected by using the formula CL = (0.990778×CL$_1$)−(0.001218×CL$_1^2$). GFR values were then normalized to 1.73 m^2 of body surface area (BSA).

The procedure has remarkable precision over a wide range of kidney function [33] as documented by the low mean intra-individual coefficient of variation (5.59%) and good reproducibility index (6.28%) observed in repeated measurements in subjects with near-terminal kidney failure, normal GFR or even hyperfiltration.

The morning of each iohexol clearance study, serum creatinine concentration was measured with the modified rate Jaffé method using an automatic device (Beckman Synchron LX20 Pro, Beckman Coulter S.p.A., Cassina De' Pecchi, Italy) and demographic and anthropometric data considered in CKD-Epi and aMDRD equations [Levey A, et al. (2000) J Am Soc Nephrol 11: 155A, Abstract] [14] were recorded. For CKD-Epi estimates, measured serum creatinine values were standardized to the isotope-dilution-mass-spectrometry method by the equation provided by Beckman-Coulter. GFR values estimated by both models were normalized.

Statistical analysis

Data were expressed as mean ± standard deviation (SD) or median. The relationships between measured and estimated GFR values at baseline, as well as between one-year changes in measured and estimated GFRs, were studied by regression analyses considering Pearson correlation coefficient and Lin concordance correlation coefficient as an index to evaluate the degree to which pairs of observations fall on the 45° line through the origin [34]. Additional sensitivity analyses were performed by using the Deming regression. Analyses were performed in the study group as a whole and in two subgroups with baseline mGFR≥ or <70 mL/min/1.73 m^2 considered separately.

Bias, mean percent error (MPE) and mean percent absolute error (MAPE) were determined as previously described [35]. Scatter was defined as the median absolute difference between measured and estimated GFR. Taking into account that the reproducibility of the iohexol plasma clearance is 6.28% [33], the eGFR values lying within the ±10% error range were a priori considered as virtually identical to mGFR values. The trend of the errors was represented by Bland-Altman analysis: the differences between estimated and measured GFRs (or estimated and measured one-year GFR differences) were plotted versus the mean of estimated and measured GFRs (or estimated and measured one-year GFR differences). Data were compared by paired or unpaired t-test, Mann-Whitney test, chi-square test or one way analysis of variance (ANOVA), as appropriate. The statistical significance level was defined as p<0.05. All analyses were performed by MedCalc (11.3.3 version) or MS Excel.

Results

Patient characteristics

Baseline data were available from 111 patients. They were relatively young and predominantly male subjects (Table 1). Thirty-three patients were overweight and 13 obese (according to a body mass index between 25 and 30 kg/m^2 or exceeding 30 kg/m^2, respectively). Serum creatinine exceeded the upper limit of the normal range (1.30 mg/dL) in 39 cases. The GFR was less than the lower limit of the normal range (80–120 mL/min/1.73 m^2) in 62 cases. Only six patients were hyperfiltering (mGFR>120 mL/min/1.73 m^2). No patient was on concomitant treatment with drugs known to interfere with creatinine tubular handling.

Relationships between measured and estimated GFR at baseline

The GFRs estimated by CKD-Epi and aMDRD formulas were significantly correlated (p<0.001) with measured GFRs (Figure 1,

Left and Right Panel, respectively). The "r" correlation (0.908 vs. 0.891) and Lin concordance (0.899 vs. 0.872) coefficient were slightly higher with CKD-Epi than aMDRD estimates. Similar results were obtained by using the Deming regression model. Analyses indicated a proportional difference (slope statistically different from 1) and a constant negative difference (intercept significantly different from 0) for the CKD-Epi and aMDRD formulas respectively. CKD-Epi significantly overestimated and aMDRD underestimated mGFR values, respectively (Table 2). Mean percent errors vs. actual values showed similar trends, whereas mean absolute percent errors were similar with the two estimates (Table 2). Overall, less than half of the estimates deviated by <10% from actual values. The accuracy was poor for both estimates, although the percentage of acceptable estimates was slightly higher with CKD-Epi than aMDRD. With both formulas, scatter and mean absolute differences between measured and estimated GFR changes ranged between 7 and 11 mL/min/1.73 m^2. On the basis of the results of Bland-Altman analyses, the performance of the two equations was similarly poor at any degree of renal function, with a trend to greater errors for higher levels of mGFR (Figure 2). The differences between the upper and lower limits of agreement were 48.3 mL/min/1.73 m^2 and 50.1 mL/min/1.73 m^2 for the CKD-Epi and the aMDRD formula, respectively. However, the mean bias was negligible since it reflects the mean of over- and underestimation of individual mGFR values. The absolute differences between measured and estimated GFR values significantly increased (CKD-Epi: p<0.01,

Table 1. Patients characteristics at inclusion.

	Whole study group	Patients with baseline and one-year data	Patients with baseline data only
n	111	71	40
Age (yr)	38.20±7.87	37.15±7.98	40.06±7.40
Male sex – no. (%)	62(55.86)	34(47.89)	28(70.00)
Height (cm)	171.12±9.50	170.01±9.85	173.08±8.62
Weight (Kg)	73.28±14.65	72.49±14.58	74.68±14.86
Body Mass Index (kg/m^2)†	24.91±3.86	24.96±3.91	24.81±3.83
Body Surface Area (m^2)\$	1.85±0.21	1.83±0.21	1.88±0.21
Systolic Blood Pressure (mmHg)	130.21±15.50	127.74±15.49	136.06±14.08^
Diastolic Blood Pressure (mmHg)	84.91±11.22	84.07±12.22	86.89±8.25
Serum creatinine (mg/dL)ǀ	1.21±0.46	1.12±0.45	1.37±0.46^*
Uric Acid (mg/dL)	5.41±1.61	5.18±1.63	5.83±1.50^
GOT/AST (U/L)	19.99±6.36	19.61±7.24	20.69±4.33
GPT/ALT (U/L)	20.09±11.07	19.48±12.39	21.21±8.17
Proteinuria (g/24 h)	0.25±0.52	0.28±0.62	0.16±0.13
Albuminuria (µg/min)	52.86±65.02	61.89±79.63	40.81±35.36
GFR (mL/min/1.73 m^2)	78.56±26.70	83.13±27.52	70.45±23.38^
Antihypertensive therapy - no. (%)	73 (65.77)	44 (61.97)	29 (72.50)
ACEi – no. (%)	55 (49.55)	33 (46.48)	23 (57.50)
CCB – no. (%)	12 (10.81)	8 (11.27)	4 (10.00)
ARBs – no. (%)	23 (20.72)	16 (22.54)	7 (17.50)
Antihypertensive drugs - no.	2 (1–3)	2 (1–3)	1 (1–2)

Data are mean±SD.
†The body mass index is the weight in kilograms divided by the square of the height in meters.
\$The body surface area is calculated with the Dubois&Dubois formula.
ǀTo convert values for serum creatinine to micromoles per liter, multiply by 88.4.
*p<0.05 vs. whole study group;
^p<0.05 vs. patients with baseline and one-year data.

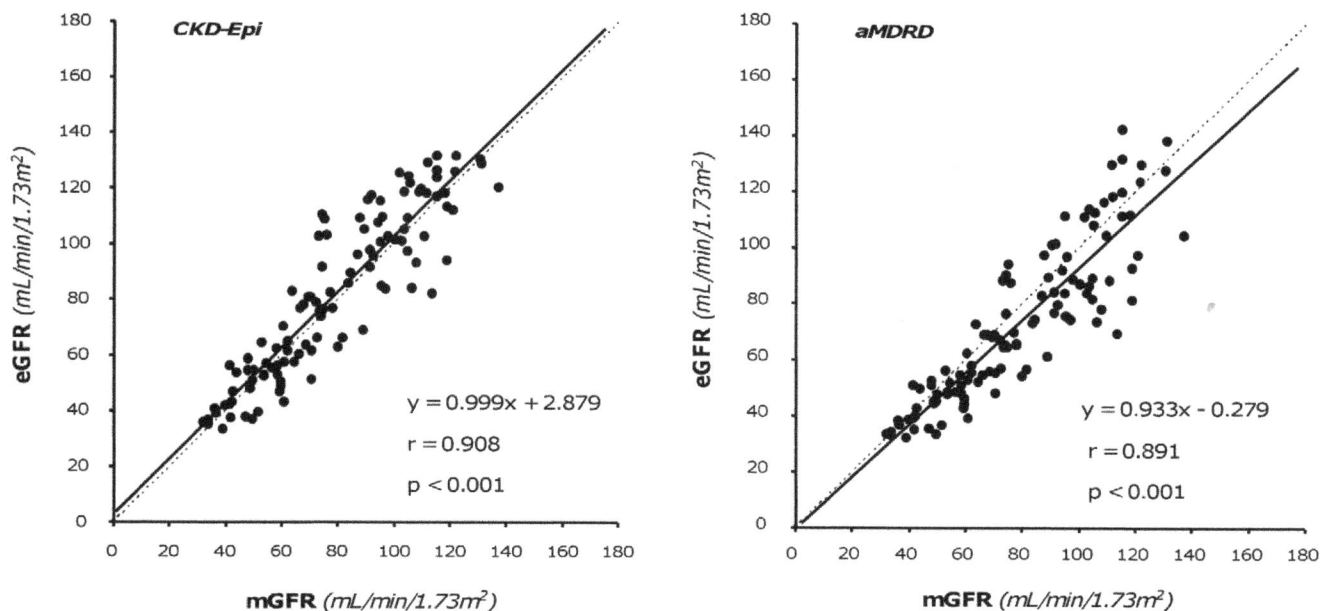

Figure 1. Correlation between estimated and measured by iohexol plasma clearance GFR. Values estimated by CKD-Epi and aMDRD formulas are shown in the left and right panel respectively. Dot lines are identity lines; continuous lines are regression lines.

Table 2. Performance of CKD-Epi and aMDRD equations in predicting GFR at inclusion in 111 ADPKD patients as a whole and ranked according to mGFR<70 (n = 45) and ≥70 (n = 66) mL/min/1.73 m².

		Overall	mGFR<70	mGFR≥70
CKD-Epi	**Estimated GFR**	81.37±29.39^	52.85±12.58	100.82±20.18^
	Bias	2.81±12.32	0.85±7.99	4.15±14.46
	Mean % Error	3.84±15.74	2.15±14.91	4.98±16.30
	Mean Absolute % Error	12.50±10.24	11.94±9.01	12.88±11.06
	Scatter	7.01	4.69	9.88
	Mean Absolute Differences	9.58±8.20	6.26±4.96	11.84±9.18
	Estimates within 10%	51.35	51.11	51.52
	Pearson Coefficient	0.908	0.775	0.715
	Lin Coefficient	0.899	0.760	0.692
aMDRD	**Estimated GFR**	73.01±27.95*	47.82±10.39*	90.18±22.59°
	Bias	−5.55±12.79	−4.17±7.08	−6.49±15.51
	Mean % Error	−6.93±14.69	−7.23±13.01	−6.72±15.82
	Mean Absolute % Error	13.32±9.23	11.76±9.01	14.38±9.29
	Scatter	8.92	4.60	11.24
	Mean Absolute Differences	10.76±8.82	6.34±5.18	13.77±9.53
	Estimates within 10%	41.44	51.11	34.85
	Pearson Coefficient	0.891	0.770	0.729
	Lin Coefficient	0.872	0.712	0.672

Iohexol plasma clearance: overall: 78.56±26.70 mL/min/1.73 m²; GFR<70: 51.99±10.49 mL/min/1.73 m²; GFR≥70: 96.67±17.63 mL/min/1.73 m².
Data are mean±SD or median.
Estimated GFR, Bias, Scatter and Mean Absolute Differences are in mL/min/1.73 m².
*p<0.001;
°p<0.01;
^p<0.05 vs. iohexol plasma clearance.

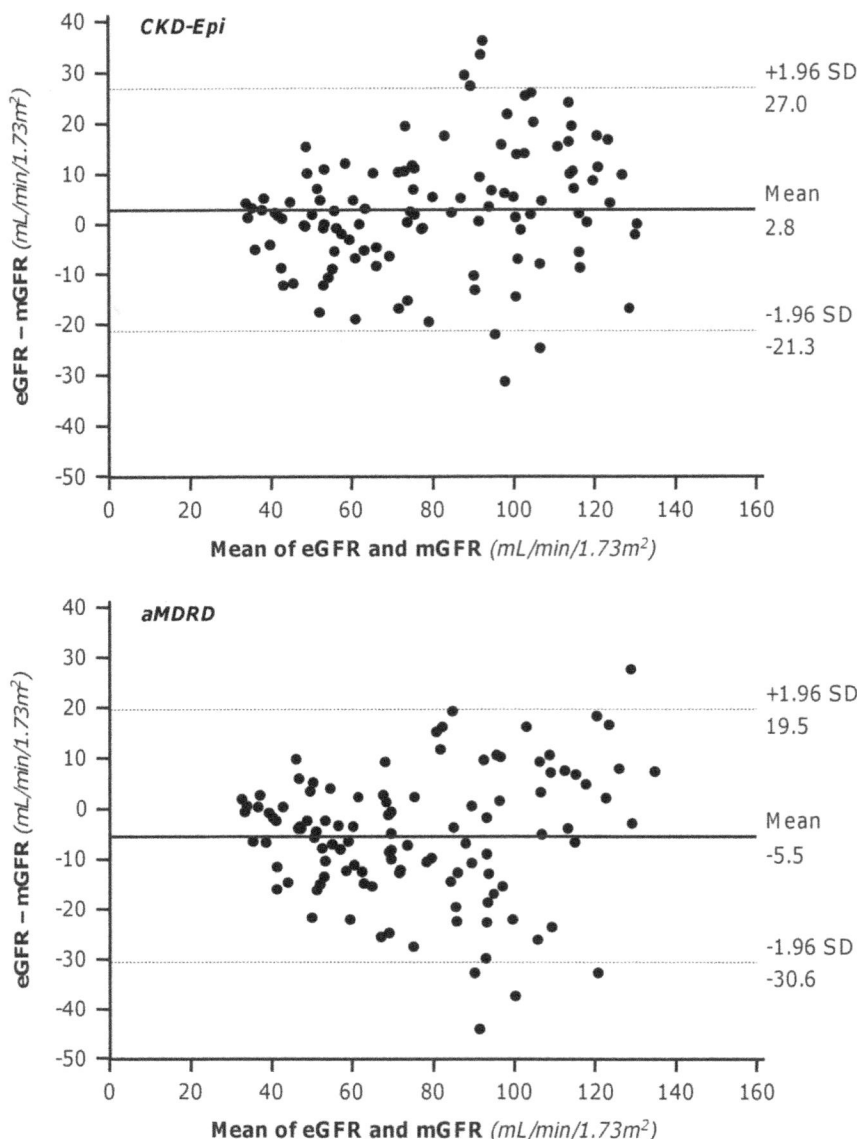

Figure 2. Agreement between measured and estimated GFR values. Bland-Altman plot of the difference between GFR estimated (eGFR) by the CKD-Epi (Upper panel) and by aMDRD (Lower panel) formulas and measured GFR (mGFR) vs. the mean of the two determinations. Straight line and dashed lines indicate mean difference and 95% limits of agreement, respectively.

$r = 0.248$; aMDRD: $p<0.001$, $r = 0.462$) for increasing levels of baseline mGFR (Figure 3). Analyses considering separately subjects with mGFR at inclusion $<$ or ≥ 70 mL/min/1.73 m^2 (Figure 4) showed that the accuracy of both prediction formulas was poor in either group (Table 2).

Relationships between measured and estimated GFR changes at one year vs. baseline

Measured and estimated one-year GFR data were available in 71 of the 111 included patients. Demography, clinical and laboratory characteristics at inclusion of patients with or without one-year outcome data were similar, with the exception of mGFR and serum creatinine levels (Table 1). Consistently with data in the whole study group, baseline mGFR values were significantly overestimated and underestimated by CKD-Epi and aMDRD formulas, respectively. At one year the difference between

estimated and measured GFRs was still significant only when CKD-Epi estimates were considered (Table 3).

Overall, at one-year, mGFR decreased by 8.4 mL/min/1.73 m^2 vs. baseline, a reduction that CKD-Epi and aMDRD significantly underestimated by 59% and 53%, respectively (Table 3). Bias, mean percent errors and mean absolute percent errors of estimated vs. measured one-year GFR changes were similar with the two equations (Table S1). Only 8.57% and 5.71% of the CKD-Epi and aMDRD estimates deviated by less than 10% from actual values, respectively. The accuracy was poor for both estimates, although the percentage of acceptable estimates was slightly higher with the CKD-Epi than with the aMDRD formula. With both formulas, scatter and mean absolute differences between measured and estimated GFR changes approximated 10 mL/min/1.73 m^2 (Table S1), a value that exceeded the 8.4 mL/min/1.73 m^2 GFR change actually measured at one year (Table 3). No significant

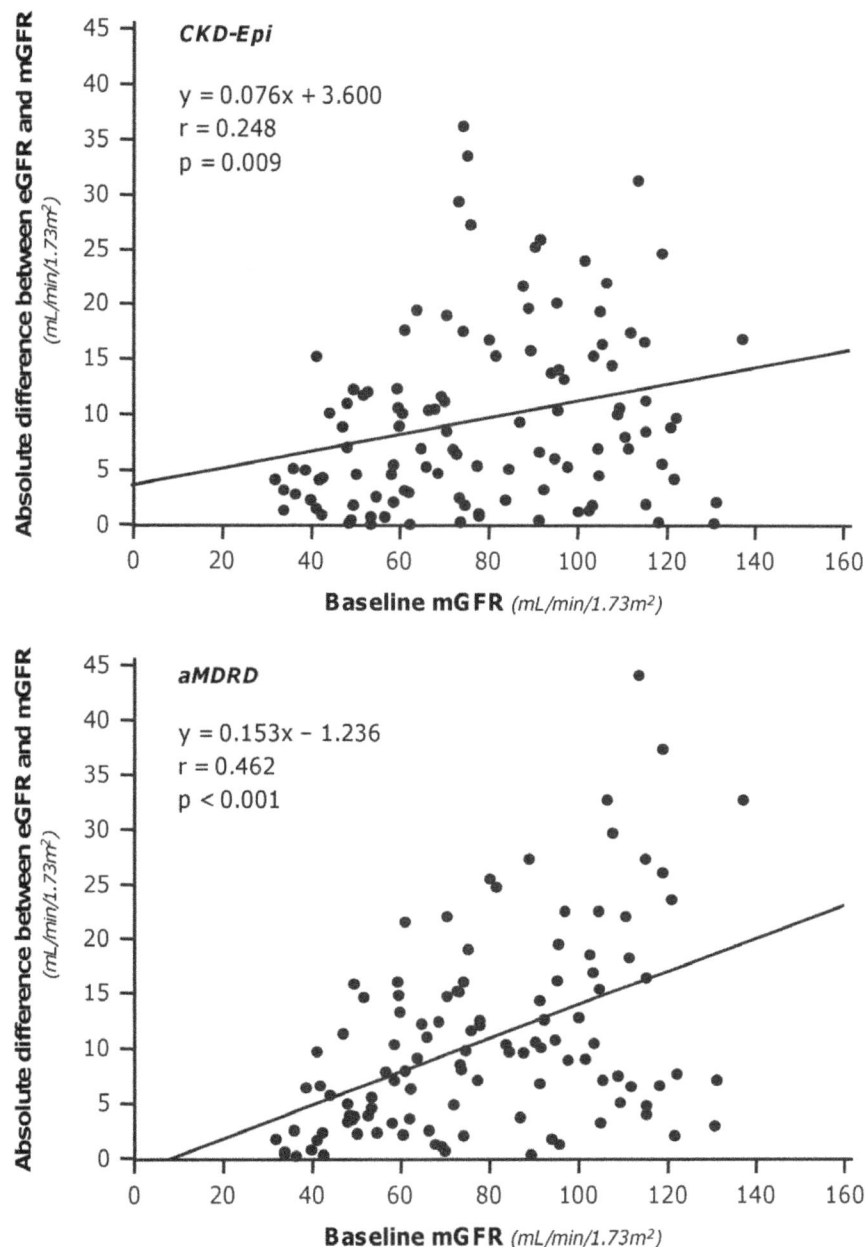

Figure 3. Absolute differences between measured and estimated GFR values vs baseline measured GFR. The absolute differences significantly increase for both CKD-Epi (Upper panel) and aMDRD (Lower panel) formulas for increasing values of GFR. Continuous lines are regression lines.

correlation was found between mGFR changes and changes estimated either by the CKD-Epi and the aMDRD formula (Figure 5). At Bland-Altman analyses, the performance of the two equations was similarly poor at any level of renal function changes (Figure 6). The differences between the upper and lower limits of agreement were 48.3 mL/min/1.73 m² and 49.8 mL/min/1.73 m² for the CKD-Epi and the aMDRD formula, respectively. The absolute differences between measured and estimated GFR changes significantly increased (CKD-Epi: p = 0.020 r = 0.275; aMDRD: p = 0.004, r = 0.335) for increasing levels of baseline mGFR (Figure 7). Actually, the analysis of the subgroups of subjects with mGFR at inclusion < or ≥70 mL/min/1.73 m² showed that the accuracy in assessing GFR change by both CKD-Epi and

aMDRD formulas was poorer for mGFR higher than 70 mL/min/1.73 m² (Table 3). Nevertheless, as shown in Figure 8, even in subjects with mGFR<70 mL/min/1.73 m² the extent of GFR changes predicted by both formulas was fully independent of actually measured changes. Consistently, in this subgroup of subjects estimates of one-year GFR changes based on CKD-Epi and aMDRD equations deviated with large percent errors from actual changes measured by iohexol plasma clearance (Table S1).

Discussion

The key findings of our present analysis in a relatively large cohort of adult ADPKD patients who had their GFR values

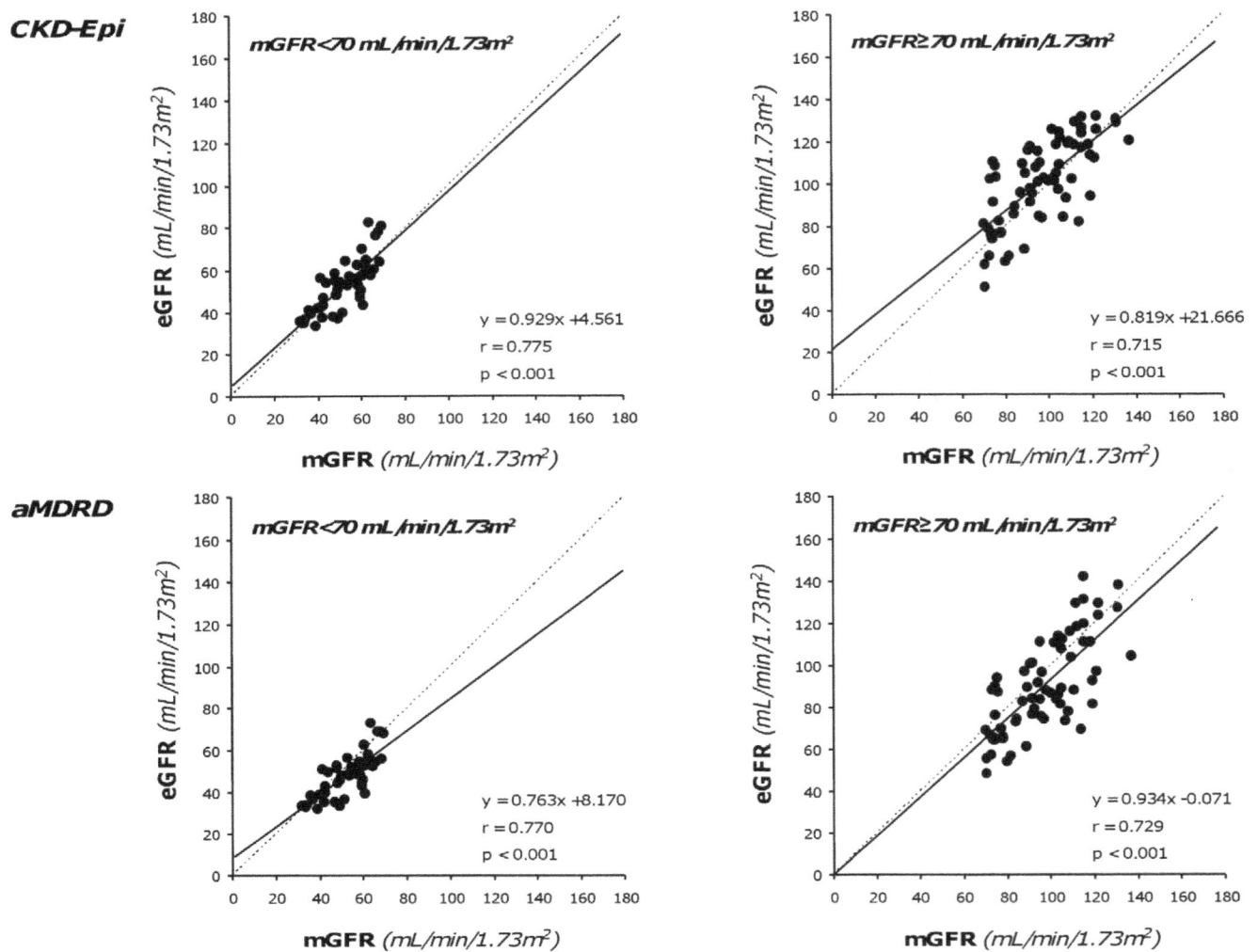

Figure 4. Relationship between GFR values ranked according to renal function. Correlation between GFR measured by iohexol plasma clearance and GFR estimated by the CKD-Epi (Upper panels) and aMDRD (Lower panels) formulas in patients with baseline GFR< or $\geq$70 mL/min/ 1.73 m^2 considered separately (Left and Right panels, respectively). Dot lines are identity lines; continuous lines are regression lines.

centrally measured by a gold standard procedure such as the iohexol plasma clearance technique [21] and at the same time estimated by the CKD-Epi and aMDRD prediction formulas, can be summarized in the following 3 points:

i.   GFR values estimated by the two formulas significantly correlated with measured GFRs. Data, however, were biased by a significant overestimation with the CKD-Epi and underestimation with the aMDRD formula. Moreover, there was a wide and unpredictable deviation of estimated data from measured values, with less than 50 percent of GFR values being predicted with an adequate accuracy by the two equations.

ii. One-year GFR changes estimated by both prediction formulas failed to correlate to any appreciable extent with measured changes. Moreover, data were biased by a systematic underestimation of measured GFR changes that averaged 50 percent with both formulas. Again, there was a wide and unpredictable deviation of estimated from measured GFR changes, with less than nine percent of GFR changes being reliably predicted by the two equations. Of

note, deviations of estimated data even exceeded the actually measured GFR changes.

iii. Because of imprecise estimation of actual GFR values and unreliable prediction of GFR changes over time, both CKD-Epi and aMDRD equations fail to provide useful information in the setting of clinical trials aimed to test the effect of experimental treatments on progressive renal function loss in patients with ADPKD.

In a previous prospective analysis of ADPKD patients with baseline GFR>70 mL/min/1.73 m^2, GFR slopes calculated on the basis of serial GFR measurements by iothalamate clearance better correlated with a series of baseline predictors of disease progression than GFR slopes calculated by using aMDRD and Cockcroft-Gault GFR estimates [36]. The above findings can be explained by the bias in calculating GFR slopes using creatinine-based prediction equations. Actually, other Authors have suggested that in early stages of CKD the variability in serum creatinine levels might reflect creatinine production related to muscle mass or protein intake more than glomerular filtration [36].

Table 3. Measured and estimated one-year GFR changes vs. baseline in 71 ADPKD patients as a whole and ranked according to mGFR<70 (n = 25) and ≥70 (n = 46) mL/min/1.73 m².

		Overall	mGFR<70	mGFR≥70
Iohexol	Baseline GFR	83.13±27.52	52.64±10.28	99.69±18.03
	One-Year GFR	74.70±27.83	45.52±9.77	90.56±20.58
	GFR Change	−8.43±10.31	−7.13±7.51	−9.13±11.57
CKD-Epi	Baseline GFR	86.84±29.56^	54.10±12.05	104.63±18.31^
	One-Year GFR	81.84±32.41*	47.00±14.40	100.78±21.96*
	GFR Change	−4.99±8.96^	−7.10±6.29	−3.85±10.00°
aMDRD	Baseline GFR	77.94±28.54°	48.74±9.70^	93.81±22.04^
	One-Year GFR	73.41±29.97	42.74±11.68	90.08±22.75
	GFR Change	−4.53±9.73^	−6.00±5.46	−3.72±11.39^

Data are in mL/min/1.73 m²; mean±SD.
*p<0.001;
°p<0.01;
^p<0.05 vs. iohexol plasma clearance.

Our present data confirm that prediction formulas, including the CKD-Epi equation - not considered in previous studies - are far from accurate in estimating GFR and are fully unreliable in estimating GFR changes in subjects with ADPKD, and provide formal evidence that this limitation is independent of kidney function and applies also to individuals with more severe renal insufficiency. This is in harmony with cross-sectional data by Orskov and colleagues [37] showing that the performance of prediction formulas, including CKD-Epi and aMDRD in estimating renal function, was poor across a wide range of GFRs from CKD stage 1 to 5. Here we extend these data by providing the fully novel evidence that the CKD-Epi and aMDRD formulas do not allow any useful information to predict GFR changes over time, a limitation that, again, applies also to subjects with lower GFRs to start with. These findings are in line with previous observations in other population, such as in kidney transplant recipients, showing that predictive performance of GFR equations, including aMDRD and Cockcroft-Gault formulas, in detecting renal function changes over time was remarkably inferior to that of GFR measurements with iohexol plasma clearance [35]. On the other hand, the wide variability of GFR estimates we observed in our ADPKD patients might be explained by changes in tubular creatinine handling that could be specific to the disease. Creatinine accumulating into non-communicating cysts, in particular in those originating from proximal tubuli, cannot be excreted into urine [1] and might back-diffuse into the circulation. We speculate that this would induce serum creatinine changes that are independent of glomerular filtration and that might bias any GFR estimation based on serum creatinine levels.

As demonstrated in our present analyses, both underestimation and dispersion of data synergistically converge to decrease the power of statistical analyses aimed to demonstrate a treatment effect on GFR. In this perspective, failure to detect any, even marginal, correlation between measured and estimated GFR changes over one year follow-up, definitely challenged the reliability of any clinical trial using CKD-Epi and aMDRD equations to test the effects of experimental treatments in ADPKD [12,13]. Similar considerations apply to the several prediction formulas developed over the last 40 years for GFR estimation that are flawed (even to a larger extent) by the same limitations described for the above equations.

In another perspective, an encouraging implication of the above findings is that the results of studies based on the use of prediction formulas cannot be taken to definitely discard the idea that mTOR inhibitors may be suitable for the treatment of ADPKD [6].

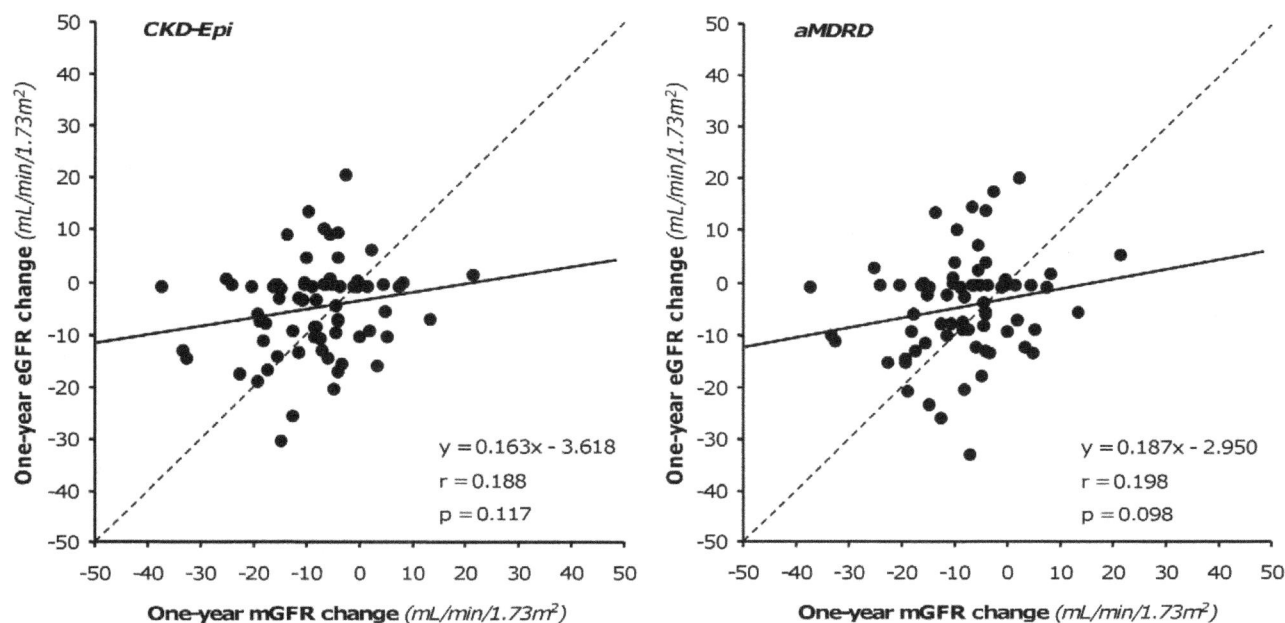

Figure 5. Relationship between measured and estimated 1-year GFR changes. Correlation between measured 1-year GFR changes vs. baseline and corresponding changes estimated by CKD-Epi (Left panel) and aMDRD (Right panel) formulas. Dot lines are identity lines; continuous lines are regression lines.

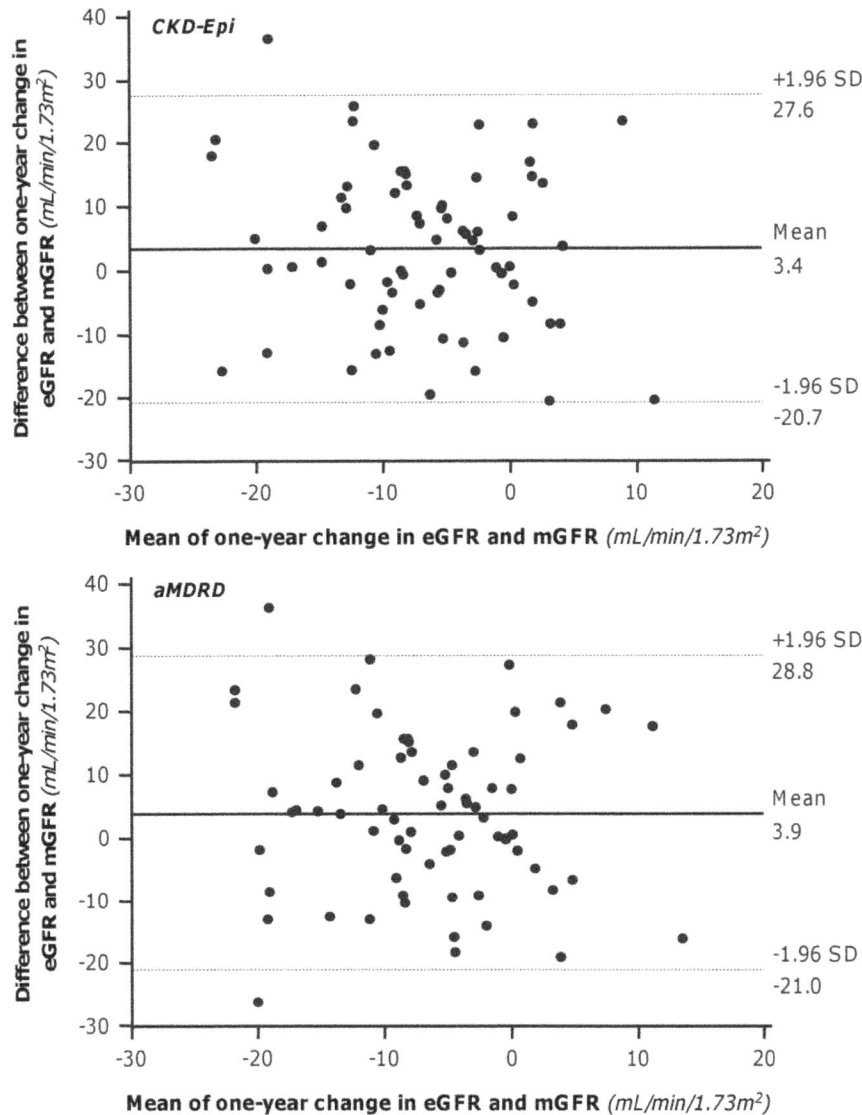

Figure 6. Bland-Altman plots of measured and estimated 1-year changes. Graphs show the agreement between estimated by CKD-Epi (Upper panel) or by aMDRD (Lower panel) formulas and corresponding measured 1-year GFR changes vs. baseline. Straight line and dashed lines indicate mean difference and 95% limits of agreement, respectively.

Limitations and Strengths

The major limitation of our study was the *post-hoc* nature of an observational analysis of subjects included in trials originally designed for other purposes. Moreover, since longitudinal data were available only for a subgroup, GFR changes over time could be analyzed in a relatively small number of patients. Finally, the availability of only two sequential GFR measurements per patient did not allow comparative analyses between slopes of measured and estimated GFRs. Thus, our present findings can be considered as hypothesis generating and merit confirmation in ad hoc studies formally comparing GFR changes over time directly measured by gold standard procedures and indirectly estimated by using prediction formulas. A major strength was that all patients were monitored according to predefined and standardized guidelines and by using a standard procedure for GFR measurement largely applied to monitor renoprotective effects of given treatments on renal function in patients with CKD participating to clinical trials

[38–42]. Iohexol plasma clearance also showed a good agreement with inulin renal clearance (the gold standard for renal function assessment) in subjects with different degree of renal function [21,28,29]. Consistently, GFR decline measured in our study patients was quite similar to that previously reported after the fourth decade of age in ADPKD patients prospectively monitored by serial GFR measurements by using the iothalamate plasma clearance technique [43].

Moreover, finding that no patients was on concomitant treatments known to affect creatinine tubular handling, avoided the confounding effect of GFR-independent changes in serum creatinine levels that might have further reduced the reliability of prediction formulas that use serum creatinine as an endogenous marker of glomerular filtration. Our present data also had a large external validity since selection criteria allowed identifying a study population which is representative of the average population of ADPKD patients who refer to a Nephrology Unit in every day

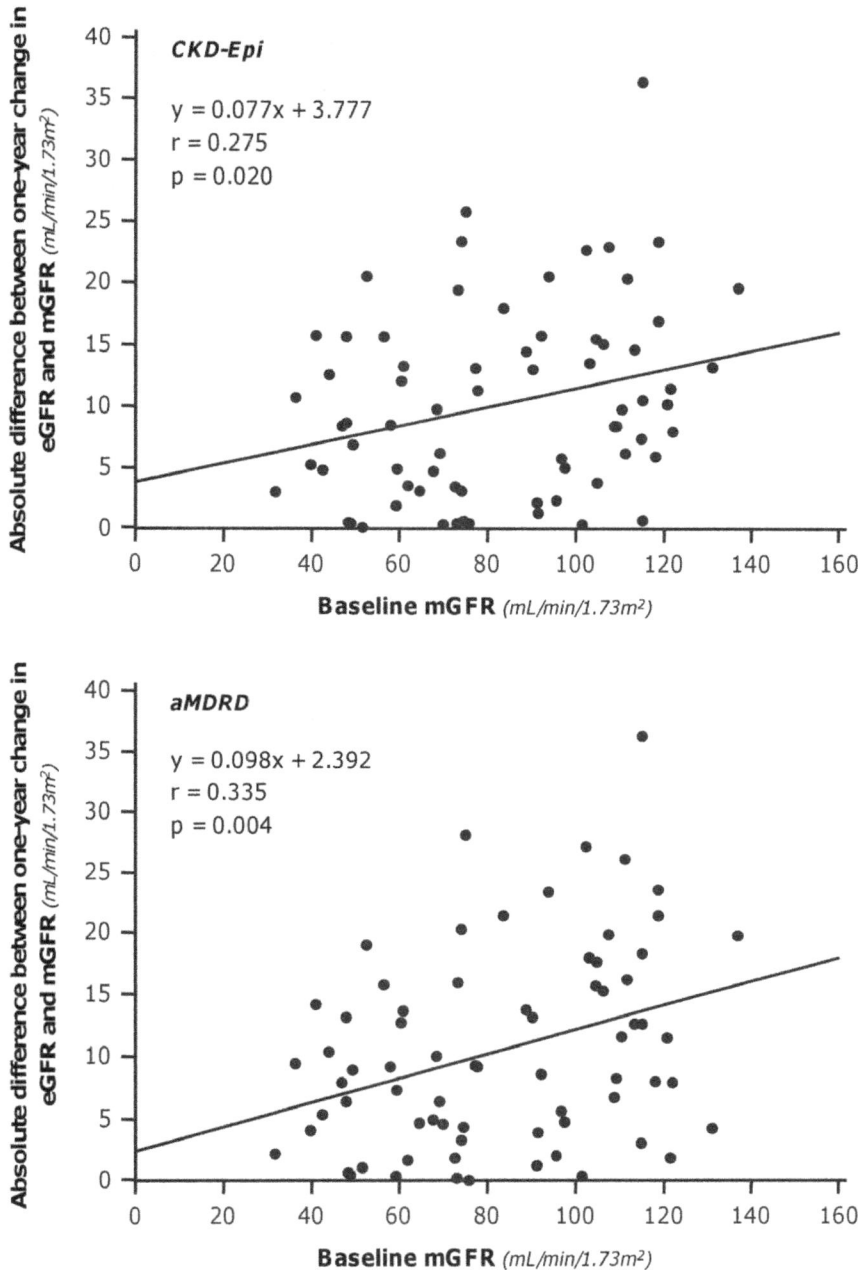

Figure 7. Absolute differences between measured and estimated 1-year GFR changes vs baseline measured GFR. The absolute differences between 1-year GFR changes for both CKD-Epi (Upper panel) and aMDRD (Lower panel) formulas significantly increase for increasing values of GFR. Continuous lines are regression lines.

clinical practice. Moreover, GFR estimates were based on serum creatinine levels measured in laboratories of different centers by using validated local procedures, which faithfully reflects how prediction formulas are routinely used in real life.

Conclusions

In our present series of patients with ADPKD, independent of their kidney function, prediction formulas, including those that have been most recently implemented to improve the performance in GFR estimation [14] unreliably estimated actual GFR values and failed to detect their changes over time. Study findings suggest that these surrogate outcome variables are not appropriate to assess progression of ADPKD and response to treatment in research and clinics. Long-term, adequately powered clinical trials with direct measurement of kidney function by appropriate techniques may help better evaluating the efficacy of therapeutic strategies in this clinical setting, as well as in other chronic kidney diseases.

Supporting Information

Table S1 Performance of CKD-Epi and aMDRD equations in predicting one-year GFR changes vs. baseline in 71 ADPKD

CKD-Epi

aMDRD

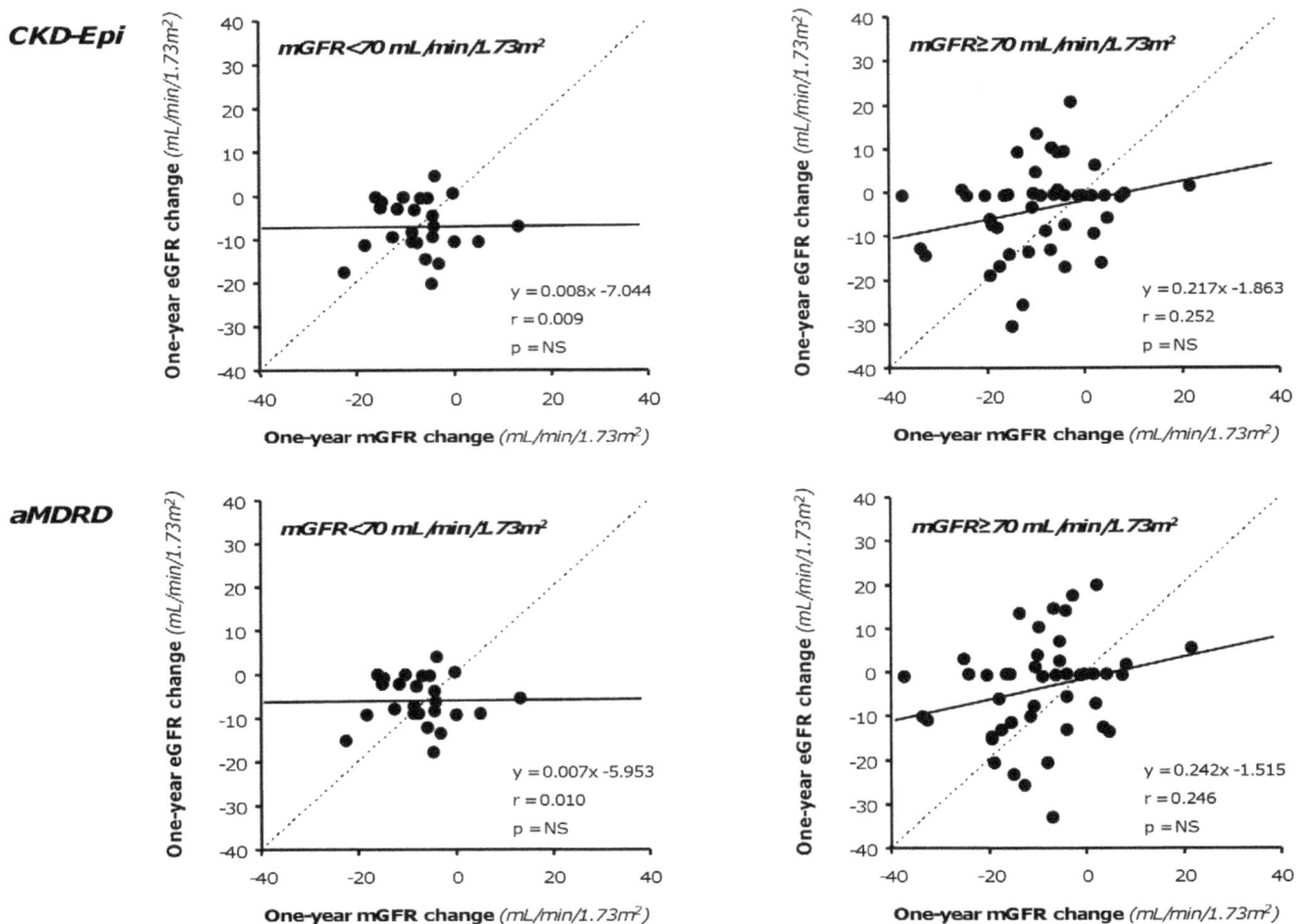

Figure 8. Relationship between 1-year GFR changes ranked according to renal function. Correlation between measured 1-year GFR changes vs. baseline and corresponding changes estimated by CKD-Epi (Upper panels) and aMDRD (Lower panels) formulas in patients with baseline GFR< or ≥70 mL/min/1.73 m² considered separately (Left and Right panels, respectively). Dot lines are identity lines; continuous lines are regression lines.

patients as a whole and ranked according to mGFR<70 (n = 25) and ≥70 (n = 46) mL/min/1.73 m².

Acknowledgments

The authors are indebted to the staff of the Nephrology Units of Involved Centers and to Rodolfo Flores Bravo, Andrea Panozo, Felipe Rodriguez de Leon, Patricia Espindola; Luca Barcella, Stefano Rota, Veruska Lecchi, Sunira Karki, Sujiata Rai, Sergio Brescianini, Paola Carrara, Svitlana Yakymchuck, of the Clinical Research Center for Rare Diseases "Aldo & Cele Daccò" of the Mario Negri Institute, for their assistance in patient care and monitoring; to Annalisa Perna for supervising the statistical analyses, Nadia Rubis and Giulia Gherardi for monitoring data handling and to Manuela Passera for assistance in the preparation of the manuscript. Novartis Farma S.p.A., (Origgio, Varese, Italy) and Wyeth-Lederle S.p.A. (Aprilia, Latina, Italy) supplied the study drugs Sandostatin-LAR® Depot and Rapamune®, respectively

GFR-ADPKD Study Organization

Principal investigator — G. Remuzzi (Bergamo); Study coordinator — P. Ruggenenti (Bergamo); Coordinating center — Mario Negri Institute for Pharmacological Research, Clinical Research Center for Rare Diseases Aldo e Cele Daccò, Villa Camozzi, Ranica (Bergamo); Participating centers — *Bergamo (Unit of Nephrology and Clinical Research Center)*: G. Remuzzi, P. Ruggenenti, N. Perico, P. Ondei, S. Rota, S. Prandini, M. Trillini, A. Panozo, R. Flores Bravo, F. Rodriguez De Leon, B. Bikbov, M. Sghirlanzoni, V. Lecchi, S. Yakymchuck, P. Carrara, R. Sujata,, S. Pavia, E. Vergani, E. Carozzi, A. Ferraris, S. Brescianini, E. Camoni; C. Valentino, G. Natali, P. Brambilla; *Napoli (Unit of Nephrology)* B. Visciano, R. Rossano, R. Casolaro, G. Pisani, P. Avolio, M. Imbriaco; *Lecce (Unit of Nephrology)*: A. De Pascalis, A. Mauro, M Murrone; *Milano (Unit of Nephrology)*: R. Cerutti, S. Verdesca, L. Forzenigo; *Treviso (Unit of Nephrology)* A. Mauro, R. Stefanato, C. Tuono, F. Grava, L.Cancian; Monitoring and Drug Distribution (Mario Negri Institute) — N. Rubis, G. Gherardi, O. Diadei, K. Pagani, V. Bendinelli, M. Sabatella, A. Villa (Ranica); Carriers (Mario Negri Institute) — S. Gelmi (Ranica); Database and Data Validation (Mario Negri Institute) — B. Ene-Iordache, S. Carminati (Ranica); Data Analysis (Mario Negri Institute) — A. Perna (Ranica); Laboratory Measurements (Mario Negri Institute) — F. Gaspari, F. Carrara, S. Ferrari, N. Stucchi, A. Cannata, C. Cella (Ranica); Regulatory Affairs (Mario Negri Institute) — P. Boccardo (Ranica).

Author Contributions

Conceived and designed the experiments: PR FG GR NP. Performed the experiments: FG AC FC CC SF NS. Analyzed the data: CC FC BEI. Contributed reagents/materials/analysis tools: FG AC FC CC SF NS. Wrote the paper: PR FG GR NP. Contributed to data analyses and interpretation: PR FG GR NP. Wrote the initial draft of the manuscript: PR FG GR NP. Coordinated the activities of the Laboratory of the Clinical Research Center where all the GFR measurements were centralized: FG.

Performed all the laboratory analyses: AC FC CC SF NS. Contributed to the statistical analyses: CC FC. Coordinated the activities of the Day Hospital of the Clinical Research Center where the clearance studies were performed: SP. Monitored all the activities of the clinical trials: OD.

Generated the data bases and contributed to data handling: BE-I. Contributed to patient identification, monitoring and care: NP PO AP EB PM MD.

References

1. Torres VE, Harris PC, Pirson Y (2007) Autosomal dominant polycystic kidney disease. Lancet 369: 1287–1301.
2. Dalgaard OZ (1957) Bilateral polycystic disease of the kidneys; a follow-up of two hundred and eighty-four patients and their families. Acta Med Scand Suppl 328: 1–255.
3. Stengel B, Billon S, Van Dijk PC, Jager KJ, Dekker FW, et al. (2003) Trends in the incidence of renal replacement therapy for end-stage renal disease in Europe, 1990–1999. Nephrol Dial Transplant 18: 1824–1833.
4. King BF, Reed JE, Bergstralh EJ, Sheedy PF, 2nd, Torres VE (2000) Quantification and longitudinal trends of kidney, renal cyst, and renal parenchyma volumes in autosomal dominant polycystic kidney disease. J Am Soc Nephrol 11: 1505–1511.
5. Gabow PA (1993) Autosomal dominant polycystic kidney disease. N Engl J Med 329: 332–342.
6. Perico N, Remuzzi G (2010) Do mTOR inhibitors still have a future in ADPKD? Nat Rev Nephrol 6: 696–698.
7. Torres VE, Harris PC (2007) Polycystic kidney disease: Genes, proteins, animal models, disease mechanisms and therapeutic opportunities. J Intern Med 261: 17–31.
8. Tao Y, Kim J, Schrier RW, Edelstein CL (2005) Rapamycin markedly slows disease progression in a rat model of polycystic kidney disease. J Am Soc Nephrol 16: 46–51.
9. Wu M, Arcaro A, Varga A, Wogetseder A, Le Hir M, et al. (2009) Pulse mTOR inhibitor treatment effectively controls cyst growth but leads to severe parenchymal and glomerular hypertrophy in rat polycystic kidney disease. Am J Physiol Renal Physiol 297: F1597–F1605.
10. Shillingford JM, Murcia NS, Larson CH, Low SH, Hedgepeth R, et al. (2006) The mTOR pathway is regulated by polycystin-1, and its inhibition reverses renal cystogenesis in polycystic kidney disease. Proc Natl Acad Sci U S A 103: 5466–5471.
11. Qian Q, Du H, King BF, Kumar S, Dean PG, et al. (2008) Sirolimus reduces polycystic liver volume in ADPKD patients. J Am Soc Nephrol 19: 631–638.
12. Serra AL, Poster D, Kistler AD, Krauer F, Raina S, et al. (2010) Sirolimus and kidney growth in autosomal dominant polycystic kidney disease. N Engl J Med 363: 820–829.
13. Walz G, Budde K, Mannaa M, Nurnberger J, Wanner C, et al. (2010) Everolimus in patients with autosomal dominant polycystic kidney disease. N Engl J Med 363: 830–840.
14. Levey AS, Stevens LA, Schmid CH, Zhang YL, Castro AF, 3rd, et al. (2009) A new equation to estimate glomerular filtration rate. Ann Intern Med 150: 604–612.
15. Rule AD, Larson TS, Bergstralh EJ, Slezak JM, Jacobsen SJ, et al. (2004) Using serum creatinine to estimate glomerular filtration rate: accuracy in good health and in chronic kidney disease. Ann Intern Med 141: 929–937.
16. Poggio ED, Wang X, Greene T, Van Lente F, Hall PM (2005) Performance of the modification of diet in renal disease and Cockcroft-Gault equations in the estimation of GFR in health and in chronic kidney disease. J Am Soc Nephrol 16: 459–466.
17. Ruggenenti P, Perna A, Remuzzi G (2005) Preventing Microalbuminuria in Type 2 Diabetes. N Engl J Med 352: 834.
18. Fontsere N, Salinas I, Bonal J, Bayes B, Riba J, et al. (2006) Are prediction equations for glomerular filtration rate useful for the long-term monitoring of type 2 diabetic patients? Nephrol Dial Transplant 21: 2152–2158.
19. Chudleigh RA, Dunseath G, Evans W, Harvey JN, Evans P, et al. (2007) How reliable is estimation of glomerular filtration rate at diagnosis of type 2 diabetes? Diabetes Care 30: 300–305.
20. Heath DA, Knapp MS, Walker WH (1968) Comparison between inulin and 51Cr-labelled edetic acid for the measurement of glomerular filtration-rate. Lancet 2: 1110–1112.
21. Gaspari F, Perico N, Ruggenenti P, Mosconi L, Amuchastegui CS, et al. (1995) Plasma clearance of nonradioactive iohexol as a measure of glomerular filtration rate. J Am Soc Nephrol 6: 257–263.
22. Price M (1972) Comparison of creatinine clearance to inulin clearance in the determination of glomerular filtration rate. J Urol 107: 339–340.
23. Brochner-Mortensen J, Giese J, Rossing N (1969) Renal inulin clearance versus total plasma clearance of 51Cr-EDTA. Scand J Clin Lab Invest 23: 301–305.
24. Rehling M, Moller ML, Thamdrup B, Lund JO, Trap-Jensen J (1984) Simultaneous measurement of renal clearance and plasma clearance of 99mTc-labelled diethylenetriaminepenta-acetate, 51Cr-labelled ethylenediami-netetra-acetate and inulin in man. Clin Sci (Lond) 66: 613–619.
25. Brandstrom E, Grzegorczyk A, Jacobsson L, Friberg P, Lindahl A, et al. (1998) GFR measurement with iohexol and 51Cr-EDTA. A comparison of the two favoured GFR markers in Europe. Nephrol Dial Transplant 13: 1176–1182.
26. Effersoe H, Rosenkilde P, Groth S, Jensen LI, Golman K (1990) Measurement of renal function with iohexol. A comparison of iohexol, 99mTc-DTPA, and 51Cr-EDTA clearance. Invest Radiol 25: 778–782.
27. Brown SC, O'Reilly PH (1991) Iohexol clearance for the determination of glomerular filtration rate in clinical practice: evidence for a new gold standard. J Urol 146: 675–679.
28. Erley CM, Bader BD, Berger ED, Vochazer A, Jorzik JJ, et al. (2001) Plasma clearance of iodine contrast media as a measure of glomerular filtration rate in critically ill patients. Crit Care Med 29: 1544–1550.
29. Berg UB, Back R, Celsi G, Halling SE, Homberg I, et al. (2011) Comparison of plasma clearance of iohexol and urinary clearance of inulin for measurement of GFR in children. Am J Kidney Dis 57: 55–61.
30. Ruggenenti P, Remuzzi A, Ondei P, Fasolini G, Antiga L, et al. (2005) Safety and efficacy of long-acting somatostatin treatment in autosomal-dominant polycystic kidney disease. Kidney Int 68: 206–216.
31. Perico N, Antiga L, Caroli A, Ruggenenti P, Fasolini G, et al. (2010) Sirolimus therapy to halt the progression of ADPKD. J Am Soc Nephrol 21: 1031–1040.
32. Brochner-Mortensen J (1972) A simple method for the determination of glomerular filtration rate. Scand J Clin Lab Invest 30: 271–274.
33. Gaspari F, Perico N, Matalone M, Signorini O, Azzollini N, et al. (1998) Precision of plasma clearance of iohexol for estimation of GFR in patients with renal disease. J Am Soc Nephrol 9: 310–313.
34. Lin LI (1989) A concordance correlation coefficient to evaluate reproducibility. Biometrics 45: 255–268.
35. Gaspari F, Ferrari S, Stucchi N, Centemeri E, Carrara F, et al. (2004) Performance of different prediction equations for estimating renal function in kidney transplantation. Am J Transplant 4: 1826–1835.
36. Rule AD, Torres VE, Chapman AB, Grantham JJ, Guay-Woodford LM, et al. (2006) Comparison of methods for determining renal function decline in early autosomal dominant polycystic kidney disease: the consortium of radiologic imaging studies of polycystic kidney disease cohort. J Am Soc Nephrol 17: 854–862.
37. Orskov B, Borresen ML, Feldt-Rasmussen B, Ostergaard O, Laursen I, et al. (2010) Estimating glomerular filtration rate using the new CKD-EPI equation and other equations in patients with autosomal dominant polycystic kidney disease. Am J Nephrol 31: 53–57.
38. (1997) Randomised placebo-controlled trial of effect of ramipril on decline in glomerular filtration rate and risk of terminal renal failure in proteinuric, non-diabetic nephropathy. The GISEN Group (Gruppo Italiano di Studi Epidemiologici in Nefrologia). Lancet 349: 1857–1863.
39. Barnett AH, Bain SC, Bouter P, Karlberg B, Madsbad S, et al. (2004) Angiotensin-receptor blockade versus converting-enzyme inhibition in type 2 diabetes and nephropathy. N Engl J Med 351: 1952–1961.
40. Kuypers DR, Neumayer HH, Fritsche L, Budde K, Rodicio JL, et al. (2004) Calcium channel blockade and preservation of renal graft function in cyclosporine-treated recipients: a prospective randomized placebo-controlled 2-year study. Transplantation 78: 1204–1211.
41. Schwartz GJ, Furth S, Cole SR, Warady B, Munoz A (2006) Glomerular filtration rate via plasma iohexol disappearance: pilot study for chronic kidney disease in children. Kidney Int 69: 2070–2077.
42. Schutzer KM, Svensson MK, Zetterstrand S, Eriksson UG, Wahlander K (2010) Reversible elevations of serum creatinine levels but no effect on glomerular filtration during treatment with the direct thrombin inhibitor AZD0837. Eur J Clin Pharmacol 66: 903–910.
43. Grantham JJ, Chapman AB, Torres VE (2006) Volume progression in Autosomal Dominant Polycystic Kidney Disease: The major factor determining clinical outcomes. Clin J Am Soc Nephrol 1: 148–157.

17

-374 T/A RAGE Polymorphism is Associated with Chronic Kidney Disease Progression in Subjects Affected by Nephrocardiovascular Disease

Ivano Baragetti[1]*, Giuseppe Danilo Norata[2,3,4]*, Cristina Sarcina[1], Andrea Baragetti[2,3], Francesco Rastelli[1], Laura Buzzi[1], Liliana Grigore[3,5], Katia Garlaschelli[3], Claudio Pozzi[1], Alberico Luigi Catapano[2,5]

1 Nephrology and Dialysis Unit, Bassini Hospital, Cinisello Balsamo, Milan, Italy, 2 Department of Pharmacological and Biomolecular Sciences, Università degli Studi di Milano, Milan, Italy, 3 Center for the Study of Atherosclerosis, Italian Society for the Study of Atherosclerosis (SISA) Lombardia Chapter, Bassini Hospital, Cinisello Balsamo, Milan, Italy, 4 The Blizard Institute, Barts and The London School of Medicine and Dentistry, Queen's Mary University, London, United Kingdom, 5 Multimedica IRCCS, Milano, Italy

Abstract

Background: Chronic kidney disease (CKD) patients present elevated advanced glycation end products (AGEs) blood levels. AGEs promote inflammation through binding to their receptor (RAGE), located on the membrane of mesangial cells, endothelial cells and macrophages. Several genetic polymorphisms influence RAGE transcription, expression and activity, including the substitution of a thymine with an adenine (T/A) in the position -374 of the gene promoter of RAGE. Our study investigates the role of -374 T/A RAGE polymorphism in CKD progression in subjects affected by nephrocardiovascular disease.

Methods: 174 patients (119 males (68.4%) mean age 67.2 ± 0.88 years; 55 females (31.6%): mean age 65.4 ± 1.50 years) affected by mild to moderate nephrocardiovascular CKD were studied. Each subject was prospectively followed for 84 months, every 6–9 months. The primary endpoint of the study was a rise of serum creatinine concentrations above 50% of basal values or end stage renal disease.

Results: Carriers of the A/A and T/A genotype presented higher plasma levels of interleukin 6 (A/A 29.5 ± 15.83; T/A 30.0 ± 7.89, vs T/T 12.3 ± 5.04 $p=0.01$ for both) and Macrophages chemoattractant protein 1 (A/A 347.1 ± 39.87; T/A 411.8 ± 48.41, vs T/T 293.5 ± 36.20, $p=0.04$ for both) than T/T subjects. Carriers of the A allele presented a faster CKD progression than wild type patients (Log-Rank test: Chi square $=6.84$, $p=0,03$). Cox regression showed that -374 T/A RAGE polymorphism ($p=0.037$), albuminuria ($p=0.01$) and LDL cholesterol ($p=0.038$) were directly associated with CKD progression. HDL cholesterol ($p=0.022$) and BMI ($p=0.04$) were inversely related to it. No relationship was found between circulating RAGE and renal function decline.

Conclusions: -374 T/A RAGE polymorphism could be associated with CKD progression and inflammation. Further studies should confirm this finding and address whether inhibiting RAGE downstream signalling would be beneficial for CKD progression.

Editor: Shree Ram Singh, National Cancer Institute, United States of America

Funding: The authors have no support or funding to report.

Competing Interests: The authors have declared that no competing interests exist.

* E-mail: ivano.baragetti@icp.mi.it (IB); danilo.norata@unimi.it (GDN)

Introduction

Oxidative stress (OS) is one of the main causes associated with chronic kidney disease progression (CKD). Beyond aging, diabetes and hypertension, several mechanisms contribute the production of reactive oxygen species (H_2O_2, OH^-, $O^{\cdot}$) in CKD, including vitamin C deficiency due to malnutrition [1], impairment of antioxidant mechanisms [2,3], inflammation [4] and increased levels of advanced glycation end products (AGEs), as a consequence of their impaired renal clearance [5]. The interaction between AGEs and their receptor (RAGE) located on monocytes [6], T- lymphocytes [7] and endothelial cells [8,9], enhances NF-kB-mediated [10] cellular production of cytokines, including interleukin-1 (IL-1), interleukin 6 (IL-6), Tumor Necrosis Factor α (TNF-α) and cell adhesion molecules. These events induce OS and reduce endothelial nitric oxide synthetase activity, thus resulting in endothelial dysfunction, a hallmark of cardiovascular complications, especially in diabetic patients [11].

RAGE is present either as a transmembrane receptor or as soluble protein (sRAGE). The latter acts as a decoy for circulating AGEs thus limiting the interaction between AGEs and membrane RAGE [12]. The gene is located on chromosome 6 (6p21.32

region). The transcription of the RAGE towards the soluble form rather than the membrane anchored form depends on two different types of post-transcriptional splicing of the messenger RNA respectively, which in turn generate two types of t-RNA [13]. It is known that higher sRAGE levels exert a protective role, in fact they are related to a lower risk of microvascular complication in type 2 diabetic patients [14]. There are several polymorphisms which could influence the transcription, the alternative splicing of the m-RNA, thus influencing the ratio between membrane and soluble RAGE, or the receptor affinity for AGEs [15,16].

A relatively frequent polymorphism consisting in a substitution of thymine with adenine (T/A) in -374 position of the gene promoter, leading in a 3 fold increase of transcriptional activity (17), was associated with protection toward the development of cardiovascular disease (T/A or A/A individuals) in both diabetic and non-diabetic individuals [17,18], although not all studies are consistent with these findings [19,20]. Also the association between the -374 T/A RAGE polymorphism and diabetic nephropathy is unclear. Whereas in some studies a protective role of -374 A genotype in diabetic nephropathy was showed [17], this finding was not confirmed by others [21]. Indeed two studies observed the prevalence of the A allele in patients affected by diabetic nephropathy [22,23].

Therefore we prospectively investigated the role of this single-nucleotide polymorphism (SNP) in the decline of renal function in patients with mild to moderate kidney dysfunction.

Materials and Methods

Ethics Statement

This trial has been conducted according to the principles of the Declaration of Helsinki. The trial was a substudy of CHECK Trial. It was approved by the Ethics Committee of the University of Study of Milan (Ethics committee UNIMI, approved on 06-02-2001, protocol n Pr.0003). Each patient signed an informed consent before participating to the trial.

Patients and Study Design

174 patients have been studied (119 males (68.4%): mean age 67.2 ± 0.88 years; 55 females (31.6%): mean age 65.4 ± 1.50 years). All subjects were outpatients chronically followed in Nephrology Division of Bassini Hospital (Cinisello Balsamo-Italy). Patients affected by mild to moderate chronic kidney dysfunction (mean GFR of 65 ± 5.65 ml/min) were enrolled. The enrolment lasted 1 month (from 1st January 2005 to 1st February 2005). Subjects were divided into three groups, on the basis of their -374 T/A RAGE genotype (wild type, heterozygous for the A allele, homozygous for the A allele). Patients groups were matched for all anthropometric, clinical and biohumoral parameters. Patients affected by any inflammatory or infective pathologies, congenital or hereditary kidney diseases, glomerulonephritis, malignant neoplasia, cardio-vascular events in the 6 months before (acute myocardial infarction, stroke, transient brain ischemic attacks, acute coronary syndrome, carotid thromboarterectomy, percutaneous coronary angioplasty, arterial angioplasty at the inferior limbs, coronary by-pass, arterial by-pass at the inferior limbs), major surgery in the previous 6 months, acute heart failure in the 6 months before, chronic heart failure NYHA III and IV, have been excluded from the trial. At the enrolment medical history (comprehensive of a drug history) was investigated and examined, including arterial pressure measurement (systolic, diastolic and mean blood pressure; the mean values of three measurements performed every 15

minutes were registered), weight and height (for BMI calculation) and waist circumference measurement.

Basal blood and urine samples were taken for the following laboratory tests: urea, creatinine, electrolytes, calcium, phosphorus, PTH, uric acid, glycated haemoglobin, blood glucose, haemoglobin, bicarbonates, iron assessment, albumin, lipid profile, PCR, interleukin 6, interleukin 8, macrophage chemoattractant protein 1, leptin, adiponectin, circulating RAGEs, albuminuria, urinary sodium and urinary urea and a genotyping for the -374 T/A RAGE polymorphism.

GFR was assessed both as calculated creatinine clearance (using the 24 hours urine collection) and as estimated GFR, using the Levey's formula [24].

Each subject was prospectively followed for 84 months and visited every 6–9 months, even blood samples were taken for the routine clinical biohumoral analyses (comprehensive serum creatinine). 24 hour urine was collected and sent to our central laboratory together with blood samples every visit.

The endpoint of the study was a rise of serum creatinine plasma concentrations above 50% of the basal values or severe renal dysfunction requiring dialysis treatment in the short period.

Patients who neeeded dialysis urgently went to our observation as late referrals, having not respected the follow-up schedule.

Laboratory Methods

Blood and urine samples were collected after over-night fasted. After centrifugation at 3.000 rpm for 12 minutes, samples were stored at $-80°C$.

In sera determinations of cardiometabolic markers (total cholesterol, HDL, triglycerides, and glycemia) as well as hepatic enzymes (ALT, AST, γGT, CPK), creatinine and uric acid levels were executed with colorimetric method using Cobas Mira Plus analyzer (Horiba®, ABX, France) [25].

LDL cholesterol fraction was calculated using Friedewald formula as described.

Fresh samples of blood were used for determination of: glycated haemoglobin (HPLC, %), urea (enzymatic method, mg/dL), hemoglobin (g/dL), leukocytes count (10^3 uL), emogas-analysis for electrolytes detection, plasmatic albumin (electrophoresis, g/dL), inorganic phosphorus (molybdate test, mg/dL), parathyroid hormone (ECLIA, pg/mL), iron (ferrozine assay, ug/dL), ferritin (ECLIA, ng/mL), transferrin and C-reactive protein (immunoturbidimetric, mg/dL). IL-6, IL-8 and MCP-1 levels were assessed with BIO-PLEX™ assay (Bio-Rad, Hercules, CA, USA). Plasma adiponectin levels (all the isoforms) were measured using a commercial available ELISA kit (Assaypro, Winfield, MO, USA) whereas leptin levels in plasma samples were assessed through RIA method (Leptin Tin Human Millipore®, St. Charles, Missouri, USA) as described [26,27].

Genotyping

Genomic DNA was extracted using the Flexigene DNA kit (Qiagen, Milan, Italy) [28]. Genotyping for the -374 T/A RAGE polymorphism was performed on 1 μL (10 to 200 ng of DNA), using a TaqMan allelic discrimination test. The primers used were the following: FW 5'--3', REV 5'--3' and the probes were FAM--BQ1 and Texas Red- BQ2.

Peripheral Blood Mononuclear Cells and Macrophages mRNA Analysis

-374 T/A RAGE polymorphism was assessed with real time PCR. Briefly blood diluted 1:3 in PBS (15 ml) was layered onto 4 ml of Ficoll Hipaque (Amersham) and centrifuged at 1500 rpm for 35 min. Peripheral blood mononuclear cells were removed from the interface and washed twice (10 min 1500 rpm) in PBS before being counted. Total RNA was extracted and underwent reverse transcription as described [29,30]. Three μL of cDNA were amplified by real-time quantitative PCR with 1X Syber green universal PCR mastermix (BioRad). The specificity of the Syber green fluorescence was tested by plotting fluorescence as a function of temperature to generate a melting curve of the amplicon. The primers used are described elsewhere [31,32]. The melting peaks of the amplicons were as expected (not shown). Each sample was analyzed in duplicate using the IQ-Cycler (BioRad). The PCR amplification was related to a standard curve ranging from 10^{-11} M to 10^{-14} M.

sRAGE Levels Determination

sRAGE levels were determined via ELISA assay using Quantikine® Human RAGE kit (R&D System, Minneapolis, USA) as described [33]. Briefly, pre-coated microplates with monoclonal antibody specifics for RAGE's extracellular domain were used. Firstly, 100 μL of Assay Diluent, 50 μL of sample (plasma stored at −20°C) and 50 μL of RAGE standard solutions (5000 pg/mL–2500 pg/mL–1250 pg/mL–625 pg/mL–312 pg/mL–156 pg/mL–78 pg/mL) were added. After two hours of incubation period at 25°C, the content of each well was aspired and four wash cycles with Wash Buffer solution were made. Then, the RAGE conjugate was added to react with the antibody and the microplate was exposed to two hours of incubation at 25°C. After another cycle of washes, Substrate Solution was added and the colour developed proportionally to the amount of RAGE bound in the initial step. Finally, Stop Solution (H_2SO_4 2 N) was added to stop the reaction and via spectrometer lecture was made at 450 nm. Results were expressed as pg/mL.

Left Ventricular Mass was Evaluated with Echocardiography

Echocardiograms were performed at rest with patients supine in the left lateral side, using standard parasternal and apical views. The overall monodimensional left ventricular measurements and the bidimensional (apical four and two chamber) views have been obtained according to the recommendations of the American Society of Echocardiography. All tracings have been done and read by a single observer blinded to the clinical characteristics of the patients under observation. LV mass has been derived using the formula described by Devereux and colleagues [34]:

LV Mass (grams) = 0.80×1.04 [(VSTd+LVIDd+PWTd)^3−(L-VIDd)^3]+0.6, where VSTd is ventricular septal thickness at end diastole, LVIDd is LV internal dimension at end diastole, and PWTd is LV posterior wall thickness at end diastole. Left ventricular mass has been corrected for height$^{2.7}$ (LVMI), and expressed in units of grams/meter (g/m$^{2.7}$). The presence of left ventricular hypertrophy (LVH) has been defined for LVMI>51 g/m$^{2.7}$ in either gender.

Carotid Intima-media Thickness

Intima plus media thickness (IMT) of both carotid arteries has been evaluated by high resolution US scan, Biosound 2000 SA (Minneapolis, In, USA) with a 8-MHz transducer as described [35]. Carotid artery has been scanned at the internal, at the bifurcation and at the common carotid artery (CCA). At each longitudinal projection the far-wall IMT, as defined by Wendelhag [36], was measured in five standardized points, in the first centimetre proximal to the bulb dilation. Carotid plaque has been defined as IMT>1.3 mm. IMT has been measured on CCA

outside the plaque, if any was present. Each patient's IMT has been calculated taking the averages of ten measurements, 5 in the left and 5 in the right carotid artery.

Endothelial Functionality Assessment – Flow-Mediated Dilatation

Endothelial function was evaluated non-invasively by B-mode ultrasonography (SA 6000C-MT, Medison, South Korea) as described elsewhere [31]. Briefly, each subject was requested to lie at rest for 10 min in a temperature-controlled room (21°C±1), and the first scan of brachial artery in the left arm was taken.

This was followed by inflation of a standard pneumatic tourniquet placed around the upper arm at a pressure of 200 mmHg. After cuff removal, electrocardiography was monitored continuously during the study and measurements were taken at the end diastole.

Vessel images were taken at rest and during reactive hyperemia: FMD was calculated 90–210 sec after the deflation of a pneumatic tourniquet. NMD was calculated as the percentage in variation between the basal diameter and the maximum diameter after sublingual administration or glyceryl trinitrate 0.3 mg.

Statistical Analysis

Statistical analysis was performed using the statistical package STATA/SE 9.2 for Windows XP. Results of the continuous variables were expressed as Mean ± Standard Error.

The three groups of patients (T/T, T/A and A/A -374 RAGE genotypes) were compared each other in terms of anthropometric, clinical, instrumental and biohumoral parameters using a one-way ANOVA. The post Hoc analysis was performed using the Bonferroni's Test. The distribution of sexes, diabetes, medications, smoke habitude among the three groups was assessed with a Chi square. The significance was assumed for p values <0.05.

The survival analysis was performed using the Kaplan Mayer method. The rate of survival was compared between the three groups of patients using the Log-Rank test. The significance was assumed for p values <0.05.

Finally two separate Cox multivariate models were generated including in the analysis the -374 T/A RAGE genotype, sRAGE and all the principal variables of nephrological interest as covariates and the rising of serum creatinine concentrations or dialysis as the outcome variable. The Enter method was used. The significance was assumed for p values <0.05.

Results

The anthropometric and biohumoral characteristics of patients enrolled in the trial are shown in table 1. The -374 T/A RAGE distribution was in Hardy-Weinberg equilibrium with 31.6% of patients having the T/T genotype, 50.0% the T/A genotype and 18.4% the A/A genotype.

No significant differences among the genotypes were observed according to age, sex, gender, mean arterial pressure, presence of diabetes, BMI, waist circumference, smoking habits and previous cardiovascular events (table 1).

The same was true for kidney and metabolic function; indeed electrolytes assessments, calcium-phosphorus metabolism, glyco-metabolic control, nutritional parameters, uric acid, hemoglobin, iron assessment, bicarbonates serum concentrations, total cholesterol, HDL and LDL cholesterol, triglycerides, PCR, interleukin 8, adiponectin and leptin plasma concentrations were similar among the genotypes (Table 1). Carries of the A allele showed significantly higher plasma levels of interleukin 6 (T/T: 12.3±5.04, T/A: 30.0±7.89, A/A: 29.5±15.83, respectively; p<0.01: T/A and A/

Table 1. Baseline characteristics of the population according to genotype.

	RAGE T/T	RAGE T/A	RAGE A/A	Chi square	p
Sex (n° M/F)	35/20	62/25	22/10	0.90	0.63
Diabetes (n°- %)	40 (72.7)	60 (69.0)	22 (68.8)	0.26	0.87
Smoke (n°- %)	9 (16.4)	18 (20.7)	7 (21.9)	0.53	0.76
Past cardiovascular events (n°-%)	8 (14.5)	23 (26.4)	8 (25)	2.89	0.23
				F test	p
Age (years)	64,9±1,22	67,3±1,19	67.5±1.91	1.0	0,37
BMI (Kg/m^2)	29,2±0,77	29,2±0.65	29.4±1.03	0.01	0.98
Waist circumference (cm)	103.5±1,96	102.6±1,63	105.1±2.63	0.87	0.41
Mean arterial pressure (mmHg)	107.5±2.57	102.1±1.30	101.1±1.89	2.98	0.054
PTH (pg/mL)	98.7±21.27	72.5±11.13	77.3±11.68	0.85	0,42
Hemoglobin (g/dL)	13.3±0.23	13.1±0.22	13.3±0.30	0.23	0.79
Glycated Hemoglobin (%)	6.7±0.20	6.9±0.77	6.9±0.21	0.75	0.47
Uric acid (mg/dL)	6.1±0.20	6.7±0.54	6.4±0.27	0.34	0.71
Urea (mg/dL)	57.2±4.47	66.1±4.84	58.8±5.86	0.95	0.38
Creatinine (mg/dL)	1.48±0.14	1.6±0.12	1.4±0.12	0.47	0.62
eGFR (mL/min)	67.7±5.43	57.2±3.62	65.0±7.30	1.41	0.24
Calculated GFR (mL/min)	70.3±9.42	59.2±4.91	58.1±12.29	0.73	0.48
Na (mmol/L)	134.6±0.76	133.9±0.06	134.4±0.09	0.29	0.74
K (mmol/L)	4.3±0.10	4.3±0.07	4.2±0.11	0.56	0.56
Ca x P product (mg/dL)	29.5±1.30	30.3±1.18	28.1±1.69	0.57	0.56
Serum Bicarbonates (mmol/L)	26.6±0.61	25.9±0.36	27.3±0.61	1.77	0.17
Serum Iron (μg/dL)	55.7±5.62	59.7±3.59	47.9±7.13	1.26	0.28
Transerrin (mg/dL)	244±10.02	255.6±6.26	264.2±14.2	0.89	0.41
Ferritin (ng/mL)	175±26.06	161.3±21.61	116.6±20.65	1.03	0.36
Albumin (g/dL)	4.3±0.04	4.2±0.04	4.2±0.10	1.49	0.22
Total cholesterol (mg/dL)	19.9±6.25	203.7±5.22	207.8±7.36	0.59	0.55
HDL cholesterol (mg/dL)	52±2.40	48.4±1.37	50.8±2.57	1.04	0.35
LDL cholesterol (mg/dL)	117.2±5.59	122.9±4.67	126.4±7.32	0.53	0.58
Triglycerides (mg/dL)	40.5±4.26	38.1±3.33	38.0±5.59	0.11	0.89
24 h urinary sodium (mmol/24 h)	164.7±11.63	162.6±8.10	182.2±19.25	0.63	0.53
24 h urinary urea (g/24 h)	2.0±0.98	2.1±1.02	2.4±0.37	1.01	0.36
CRP (mg/dL)	0.33±0.067	0.30±0.055	0.44±0.165	0.59	0.55
Albuminuria (mg urinary albumin/ mmol urinary creatinine	43.7±13.83	73.1±16.37	24.3±9.78	2.22	0.11
LVM (g/h$^{2.7}$)	50.6±2.45	53.2±1.89	57.2±3.78	1.29	0.27
Carotid Intima-Media Thickness (mm)	0.78±0.029	0.79±0.025	0.76±0.031	0.12	0.88
Flow mediated brachial artery dilation (%)	13.6±1.08	11.2±0.84	15.3±3.07	2.11	0.12
Adiponectin (μg/mL)	18.2±1.46	19.5±1.32	18.2±2.17	0.27	0.76
Leptin (ng/mL)	19.9±3.82	20.0±2.18	19.0±4.14	0.02	0.97
Serum RAGE (pg/mL)	1633.8±137.22	1950.7±108.7	1626.8±121.1	2.42	0.09
Interleukin 6 (pg/mL)	12.3±5.04	30.0±7.89	29.5±15.83	1.13	0.01
Interleukin 8 (mg/dL)	70.1±24.98	47.5±10.44	56.1±19.77	0.46	0.63
Macrophages chemoactrant protein 1 (pg/mL)	293.5±36.20	411.8±48.41	347.1±39.87	1.63	0.04

The anthropometric parameters, the prevalence of past cardiovascular events (myocardial infarction, acute coronary syndrome, stroke, transient ischemic attacs, by-passes at the inferior limbs, angioplasty, aorto-coronary by-passes) and biohumoral parameters are compared between patients carrying the −374 T/T,T/A and A/A genotypes of RAGE. Significance have been taken for p values <0.05, using a single way ANOVA: the post-hoc analysis showed a statistically significant difference between T/T and T/A subjects vs A/A subjects in terms of Interleukin 6 and Macrophages chemoattractant protein 1. No differences have been seen in terms of renal function, albuminuria, intermediate cardiovascular organ damage, inflammatory parameters or nutritional parameters between the three groups of subjects.

A vs T/T) and macrophages chemoattractant protein 1 (T/T: 293.5±36.20, T/A: 411.8±48.41, A/A: 347.1±39.87, respectively; p = 0.04: T/A and A/A vs T/T) compared to T/T subjects while plasma levels of sRAGE were only slightly increased (T/T: 1633.8±137.22 pg/mL, T/A: 1950.7±108.7 and A/A: 1626.8±121.1 pg/mL, p = 0,09).

The presence of the -374 T/A SNP was not associated with subclinical cardiovascular disease, in fact carotid intima-media thickness, flow mediated brachial artery vasodilation and left ventricular mass were not statistically different among the RAGE genotypes. Finally the distribution of anti-hypertensive, anti-diabetic or lipid-lowering therapies was similar among the three groups (table 2).

During the follow-up period we observed 40 events comprehensive of the serum creatinine increase of more than 50% of the basal values and need of dialysis (22%).

Survival analysis showed a faster decline of renal function in carriers of the A allele compared to TT subjects (Log-Rank test: Chi square = 6.34, p = 0,018) (fig. 1).

Differences in renal survival were also maintained when the three genotypes were analyzed independently; with a significant difference in terms of survival between T/T subjects and T/A and A/A subjects (Log-Rank test: Chi square = 6.84, p = 0,03) (fig. 2).

Overall T/T subjects presented a mean percentage of endpoint achievement of 89±0.04% at 67 months, those belonging to T/A group showed a mean percentage of endpoint achievement 70±0.04% at 75 months and patients carrying the A/A genotype 75±0.07% at 74 months.

Furthermore multivariate analysis was then performed to identify among albuminuria, LDL-cholesterol, HDL-cholesterol, -374 T/A RAGE, BMI, GFR, mean arterial pressure, haemoglobin levels and calcium-phosphorus product, the main predictors of renal function decline (Table 3). As expected, albuminuria resulted the main predictor [Wald test 6.550 and a mean Hazard ratio of 1.015 (increased risk of reaching the end point of 1.5% for each mg/l in more of albuminuria) (IC 95%: 1.003–1.025), p = 0.01] followed by the-374 RAGE polymorphism [Wald test of 4.330 and a mean Hazard ratio of 2.724 (increased risk of reaching the end point of 2.724 fold higher for subjects carrying the A allele than

those carrying T/T genotype) (IC 95%: 1.060–6.998), p = 0.037], LDL cholesterol [Wald test of 4.310 and an Hazard ratio of 1.009 (increased risk of reaching the end point of 0.9% per each mg/dl increase of LDL cholesterol) (IC 95%:.1.000–1.017, p = 0.038)], HDL cholesterol [Wald test of 5.253 and an Hazard Ratio of 0.958 (decreased risk of reaching the end point of 5% per each mg/dl in more of HDL cholesterol) (IC 95%: 0.941–0.995, p = 0.022)] and BMI [Wald test of 4.215 and an Hazard ratio of 0.933 (decreased risk of reaching the end point of 0.7% per each Kg/m² in more of BMI) (IC 95%: 0.873–0.997, p = 0.040)].

In the second multivariate model including albuminuria, LDL-cholesterol, HDL-cholesterol, sRAGE, BMI, GFR, mean arterial pressure, haemoglobin levels and calcium-phosphorus product, only albuminura [Wald test 6.5 and a mean Hazard ratio of 1.016 (increased risk of reaching the end point of 1.6% for each mg/l in more of albuminuria) (IC 95%: 1.004–1.029), p = 0.01] followed by HDL cholesterol [Wald test of 5.26 and a mean Hazard ratio of 0.97 (reduced risk of reaching the end point of 3% per each mg/dl in more of HDL cholesterol) (IC 95%: 0.94–0.99), p = 0.031] predictors of CKD progression (Table 4).

Discussion

Our results show that CKD patients with the −374 RAGE A allele have a poor CKD prognosis compared to carriers of the TT genotype. Although the role of −374 T/A RAGE in CKD progression has not been extensively investigated, some cross-sectional studies showed an association of the A allele with CKD in diabetic subjects [22,23], in contrast with the protective role exerted by this allele toward cardiovascular disease [21]. To the best of our knowledge, our trial is the first which prospectively shows a direct relationship between −374 T/A RAGE polymorphism and the decline of kidney function in patients with cardiovascular renal disease. Of note, a recent meta-analysis showed that other SNPs known to affect RAGE transcription are not associated with the prevalence of diabetic nephropathy [37] further supporting the relevance of our finding.

This finding suggests that the presence of the T allele is protective toward the decline of kidney function compared to a

Table 2. Prevalence of medications according to genotypes.

Medication yes/no (n°- % of all patients studied)	RAGE T/T (n° = 55)	RAGE T/A (n° = 87)	RAGE A/A (n° = 32)	Chi square	p
ASA/Ticlopidine	22/33(40.0)	37/50 (42.5)	18/14(56.3)	2.37	0.30
Allopurinol	12/43(21.8)	14/73(16.1)	4/28(12.5)	1.39	0.49
Statins or fibrates	20/35(36.4)	28/59 (32.2)	16/16(50.0)	3.2	0.20
β blockers or αβ Blockers	10/45(18.2)	20/67 (23.0)	6/26(18.8)	0.56	0.75
Clonidine	0/55 (0)	3/84 (3.4)	1/31(3.1)	1.90	0.38
α antagonists	2/53 (3.6)	11/76(12.6)	2/30(6.3)	3.75	0.15
Calcium channel blockers (DDP and NDDP)	10/45(18.2)	26/61(29.9)	10/22(31.3)	2.84	0.24
Diuretics	18/37(32.7)	32/55 (36.8)	13/19 (40.6)	0.57	0.75
ARBs	21/34(38.2)	26/61 (29.9)	10/22 (31.3)	1.09	0.57
ACE inhibitors	28/27(50.9)	36/51 (41.4)	17/15 (53.1)	1.91	0.38
Oral antidiabetics	27/28 (49)	33/54 (37.9)	15/17 (46.9)	1.93	0.37
Insulin	7/48 (12.7)	19/68 (21.8)	2/30(6.3)	4.88	0.09

Medications: no differences have been found between patients carrying −374 T/T, T/A and A/A genotypes in terms of antihypertensive or antidiabetic therapy. A Pearson Chi square test was used, keeping a significant difference for p values <0.05.

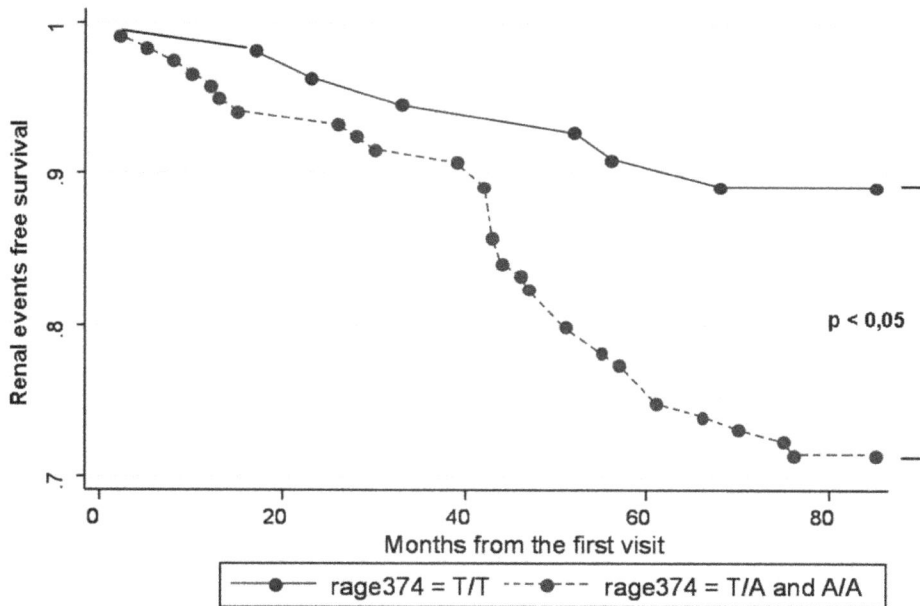

Figure 1. Renal survival of patients carrying –374 T/T and the A allele. The figure shows that the subjects carrying the A allele present a faster decline of renal function than wild type patients. The main endpoint of the analysis was an increase of serum creatinine over 50% or the beginning of chronic dialysis. The figure shows a total of 40 events: 6 in T/T subjects, 34 in subjects carrying the A allele.

potential protective effect of the A allele in cardiovascular disorders showed in previous studies [21]. The molecular mechanisms behind this effect need further investigations. The presence of the -374 A allele is associated with increased RAGE transcription [16]; however, while the increase in RAGE plasma levels observed in carriers of the A allele was not statistically significant we cannot exclude that specific isoforms of RAGE are differently affected. Indeed, the transcription of the RAGE

towards the soluble form rather than the membrane form depends on a different post-transcriptional splicing of the messenger RNA (38). It is known that higher sRAGE levels exert a protective role, in fact they are related to a lower risk of microvascular complication in type 2 diabetic patients [14]. However sRAGE levels are contributed both by the original spliced isoforms but also by the cleaved membrane receptor [38], with potentially different roles. Of note, in vitro experiments have shown that AGEs-RAGE

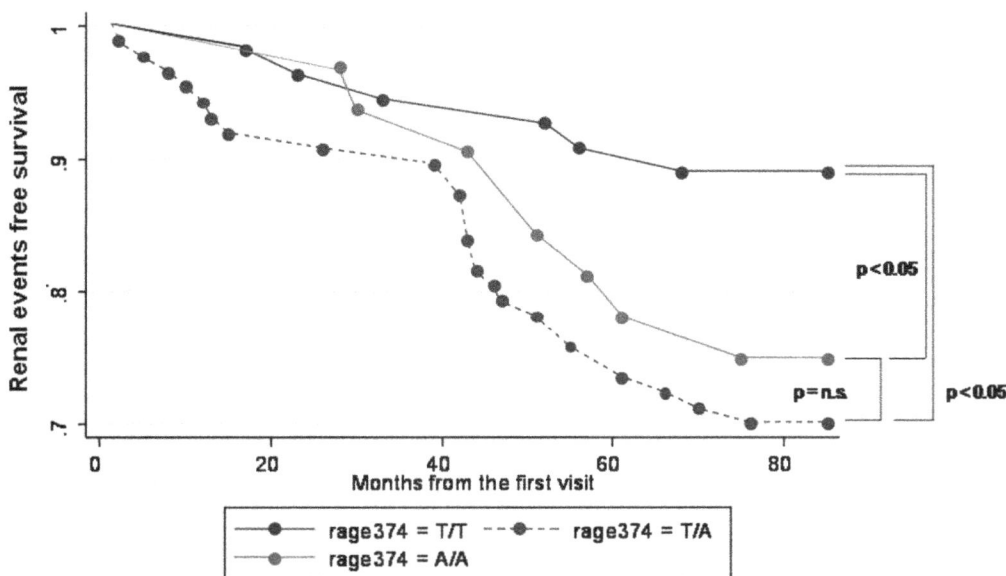

Figure 2. Renal survival of wild-type, heterozygous and homozygous patients for the A allele. The figure shows that T/A and A/A subjects present a faster decline of renal function than T/T patients. The main end point of the analysis was an increase of serum creatinine over 50% or the beginning of chronic dialysis. Figure shows a total of 40 events: 6 in T/T subjects, 26 in T/A subjects and 8 in A/A subjects.

Table 3. Cox regression for the decline of renal function including -374 T/A RAGE.

Covariates	Beta	Beta Standard Error	wald	p	Hazard Ratio	CI Hazard ratio
Haemoglobin (g/dL)	−0.156	0.114	1.854	0.172	0.855	0.584–1.070
GFR (mL/min)	−0.005	0.007	0.477	0.490	0.995	0.982–1.009
Albuminuria (mg/L)	0.015	0.006	6.550	0.01	1.015	1.003–1.025
Mean arterial pressure (mmHg)	0.21	0.015	2.011	0.153	1.021	0.992–1.051
-374 A RAGE	1.002	0.481	4.330	0.037	2.724	1.060–6.998
Ca x P product (mg/dL)	0.059	0.032	3.285	0.070	1.060	0.995–1.130
HDL Cholesterol (mg/dL)	−0.033	0.014	5.253	0.022	0.958	0.941–0.995
LDL Cholesterol (mg/dL)	0.008	0.004	4.310	0.038	1.009	1.000–1.017
BMI (Kg/m^2)	−0.059	0.034	4.215	0.040	0.933	0.873–0.997

Cox regression. Table shows that −374 A RAGE genotype, together with albuminuria, LDL cholesterol, HDL cholesterol and BMI are significantly associated with the decline of renal function. −374 A allele for RAGE, albuminuria and LDL cholesterol are predictor of CKD progression, while HDL cholesterol and BMI are inversely associated with renal function decline.

interaction is involved in the progression of renal damage by inducing mesangial fibrosis, glomerular sclerosis and the expression of vascular endothelial grow factor (VEGF) and MCP1 by mesangial cells [39,40], which in turn could support monocyte mesangial infiltration in early phase of diabetic nephropathy [41]. AGEs-RAGE interaction stimulates mesangial cells production of insulin grow factor-1 and 2, platelet derived grow factor (PDGF) and transforming grow factor–β (TGF-β), which further promote mesangial production of type IV collagen, laminin and fibronectin [39–41]. Moreover AGEs-RAGE interaction also increases TGF-β expression by podocytes and proximal tubular cells, leading to glomerulosclerosis and tubule-interstitial fibrosis [42]. Furthermore in vivo experiments in rats showed that infusion of AGE-albumin induced glomerular hypertrophy, overexpression of type IV collagen, laminin B1 and TGF-β [42,43,44]. AGEs-RAGE interaction and also other metabolic factors such as HDL also increases TGF-β expression by podocytes and proximal tubular cells, leading to glomerulosclerosis and tubule-interstitial fibrosis [45,46]. All these aspects clearly point to an involvement of the AGEs-RAGE in CKD progression. AGEs promote inflammation [47] by binding RAGE on the surface of macrophages, lymphocytes, endothelial cells and mesangial cells; the observation

that in our cohort carriers of the A allele present increased levels of MCP-1 and IL-6 could support the concept of an higher inflammatory mediated kidney function decline in A carriers.

Cox analysis showed that also albuminuria and LDL cholesterol were independent predictors of CKD progression in agreement with the CKD protective effects of therapies aimed at improving proteinuria such as RAS inhibitors or lipid profile [48] such as HMGCoA reductase inhibitors [49].

The Cox analysis also showed an inverse relationship between BMI and CKD progression. Although this finding could seem somehow confounding, given that BMI, an obesity marker as waist circumference, is a risk factor for the development and the progression of chronic renal dysfunction [50], our data support the hypothesis that BMI could inversely reflect patient's lean mass and malnutrition, which is highly prevalent among CKD patients at risk of progression [51].

We have to acknowledge some limitations of our study: firstly, we enrolled patients who already presented some degree of renal dysfunction which could result in minor differences among the genotypes. However, the long follow-up (84 months) allowed to appreciate prospectively the association of the A allele to kidney function decline compared to that of TT.

Table 4. Cox regression for the decline of renal function including the levels of the soluble form of RAGE.

Covariates	Beta	Beta Standard Error	wald	p	Hazard Ratio	CI Hazard ratio
Hemoglobin (g/dL)	−0.145	0.112	1.850	0.176	0.841	0.656–1.080
GFR (mL/min)	−0.001	0.004	0.423	0.948	1.004	0.987–1.013
Albuminuria (mg/L)	0.013	0.005	6.500	0.010	1.016	1.004–1.029
Mean arterial pressure (mmHg)	0.20	0.012	2.014	0.080	1.019	0.998–1.042
Tertiles sRAGE (pg/mL)	−0.003	0.005	0.530	0.590	1.001	0.991–1.005
Ca x P product (mg/dL)	0.061	0.038	3.310	0.185	1.045	0.978–1.116
HDL Cholesterol (mg/dL)	−0.034	0.014	5.260	0.031	0.969	0.942–0.997
LDL Cholesterol (mg/dL)	0.075	0.048	2.102	0.105	1.007	0.998–1.016
BMI (Kg/m^2)	−0.118	0.015	2.015	0.099	0.938	0.861–1.012

Cox regression. Table 3b shows that replacing sRAGE rather than −374 A RAGE genotype in the same model showed in table 3a, only albuminuria, and HDL cholesterol are significantly associated with the decline of renal function.

Secondly, we investigated a relatively limited number of CKD patients, however the frequencies of the -374T/A genotypes are similar to those reported in larger cohorts [18,20], thus suggesting that our findings could set the stage for further confirmation in larger CKD cohorts. We cannot exclude that studying prospectively a cohort of subjects, all with a normal renal function and a longer follow-up could result in additional predictors.

In conclusion, our data support the role of AGEs-RAGE system in the progression of chronic renal dysfunction and suggest a potential target to further improve the management of CKD progression toward dialysis given that the conventional strategies are not sufficiently effective. Future studies addressing markers of

inflammation and of angiogenesis are needed to clarify the pathophysiological mechanisms of AGEs-RAGE system activation and the association between the chronic inflammatory status and the consecutive kidney remodelling in relation to the RAGE status.

Author Contributions

Conceived and designed the experiments: IB GDN LB LG CP ALC. Performed the experiments: CS AB FR KG. Analyzed the data: AB IB. Contributed reagents/materials/analysis tools: GDN AB KG. Wrote the paper: IB GDN AB ALC.

References

1. Locatelli F, Canaud B, Eckardt KU, Stenvinkel P, Wanner C, et al. (2003) Oxidative stress in end-stage renal disease: an emerging threat to patient outcome. Nephrol Dial Transplant 18: 1272–1280.
2. Mimic-Oka J, Simic T, Ekmescic V, Dragicevic P (1995) Erythrocyte glutathione peroxidase and superoxide dismutase activities in different stages of chronic renal failure. Clin Nephrol 44: 44–48.
3. Vaziri ND, Dicus M, Ho ND, Boroujerdi-Rad L, Sindhu RK (2003) Oxidative stress and dysregulation of superoxide dismutase and NADPH oxidase in renal insufficiency. Kidney Int 63: 179–185.
4. Cachofeiro V, Goicochea M, de Vinuesa SG, Oubina P, Lahera V, et al. (2008) Oxidative stress and inflammation, a link between chronic kidney disease and cardiovascular disease. Kidney Int Suppl: S4–9.
5. Bohlender JM, Franke S, Stein G, Wolf G (2005) Advanced glycation end products and the kidney. Am J Physiol Renal Physiol 289: F645–659.
6. Kirstein M, Aston C, Hintz R, Vlassara H (1992) Receptor-specific induction of insulin-like growth factor I in human monocytes by advanced glycosylation end product-modified proteins. J Clin Invest 90: 439–446.
7. Imani F, Horii Y, Suthanthiran M, Skolnik EY, Makita Z, et al. (1993) Advanced glycosylation endproduct-specific receptors on human and rat T-lymphocytes mediate synthesis of interferon gamma: role in tissue remodeling. J Exp Med 178: 2165–2172.
8. Rashid G, Benchetrit S, Fishman D, Bernheim J (2004) Effect of advanced glycation end-products on gene expression and synthesis of TNF-alpha and endothelial nitric oxide synthase by endothelial cells. Kidney Int 66: 1099–1106.
9. Bucala R, Tracey KJ, Cerami A (1991) Advanced glycosylation products quench nitric oxide and mediate defective endothelium-dependent vasodilatation in experimental diabetes. J Clin Invest 87: 432–438.
10. Yamagishi S, Nakamura K, Matsui T, Noda Y, Imaizumi T (2008) Receptor for advanced glycation end products (RAGE): a novel therapeutic target for diabetic vascular complication. Curr Pharm Des 14: 487–495.
11. Widlansky ME, Gokce N, Keaney JF Jr, Vita JA (2003) The clinical implications of endothelial dysfunction. J Am Coll Cardiol 42: 1149–1160.
12. Falcone C, Emanuele E, D'Angelo A, Buzzi MP, Belvito C, et al. (2005) Plasma levels of soluble receptor for advanced glycation end products and coronary artery disease in nondiabetic men. Arterioscler Thromb Vasc Biol 25: 1032–1037.
13. Ramasamy R, Yan SF, Schmidt AM (2009) RAGE: therapeutic target and biomarker of the inflammatory response–the evidence mounts. J Leukoc Biol 86: 505–512.
14. Grossin N, Wautier MP, Meas T, Guillausseau PJ, Massin P, et al. (2008) Severity of diabetic microvascular complications is associated with a low soluble RAGE level. Diabetes Metab 34: 392–395.
15. Yan SF, Ramasamy R, Schmidt AM (2010) The RAGE axis: a fundamental mechanism signaling danger to the vulnerable vasculature. Circ Res 106: 842–853.
16. Hudson BI, Stickland MH, Futers TS, Grant PJ (2001) Effects of novel polymorphisms in the RAGE gene on transcriptional regulation and their association with diabetic retinopathy. Diabetes 50: 1505–1511.
17. Pettersson-Fernholm K, Forsblom C, Hudson BI, Perola M, Grant PJ, et al. (2003) The functional -374 T/A RAGE gene polymorphism is associated with proteinuria and cardiovascular disease in type 1 diabetic patients. Diabetes 52: 891–894.
18. Falcone C, Geroldi D, Buzzi MP, Emanuele E, Yilmaz Y, et al. (2008) The -374T/A RAGE polymorphism protects against future cardiac events in nondiabetic patients with coronary artery disease. Arch Med Res 39: 320–325.
19. Kucukhuseyin O, Aydogan HY, Isbir CS, Isbir T (2009) Associations of -374T/A polymorphism of receptor for advanced glycation end products (RAGE) gene in Turkish diabetic and non-diabetic patients with coronary artery disease. In Vivo 23: 949–954.
20. Kirbis J, Milutinovic A, Steblovnik K, Teran N, Terzic R, et al. (2004) The -429 T/C and -374 T/A gene polymorphisms of the receptor of advanced glycation end products gene (RAGE) are not risk factors for coronary artery disease in Slovene population with type 2 diabetes. Coll Antropol 28: 611–616.
21. dos Santos KG, Canani LH, Gross JL, Tschiedel B, Pires Souto KE, et al. (2005) The -374A allele of the receptor for advanced glycation end products gene is

associated with a decreased risk of ischemic heart disease in African-Brazilians with type 2 diabetes. Mol Genet Metab 85: 149–156.
22. Lindholm E, Bakhtadze E, Sjogren M, Cilio CM, Agardh E, et al. (2006) The -374 T/A polymorphism in the gene encoding RAGE is associated with diabetic nephropathy and retinopathy in type 1 diabetic patients. Diabetologia 49: 2745–2755.
23. Abdel-Azeez HA, El-Okely AM (2009) Association of the receptor for advanced glycation end products (RAGE) -374 T/A gene polymorphism and circulating soluble RAGE with nephropathy in type 1 diabetic patients. Egypt J Immunol 16: 95–106.
24. Goolsby MJ (2002) National Kidney Foundation Guidelines for chronic kidney disease: evaluation, classification, and stratification. J Am Acad Nurse Pract 14: 238–242.
25. Norata GD, Baragetti I, Raselli S, Stucchi A, Garlaschelli K, et al. (2010) Plasma adiponectin levels in chronic kidney disease patients: relation with molecular inflammatory profile and metabolic status. Nutr Metab Cardiovasc Dis 20: 56–63.
26. Norata GD, Garlaschelli K, Grigore L, Raselli S, Tramontana S, et al. (2010) Effects of PCSK9 variants on common carotid artery intima media thickness and relation to ApoE alleles. Atherosclerosis 208: 177–182.
27. Norata GD, Raselli S, Grigore L, Garlaschelli K, Dozio E, et al. (2007) Leptin:adiponectin ratio is an independent predictor of intima media thickness of the common carotid artery. Stroke 38: 2844–2846.
28. Predazzi IM, Norata GD, Vecchione L, Garlaschelli K, Amati F, et al. (2012) Association between OLR1 K167N SNP and Intima Media Thickness of the Common Carotid Artery in the General Population. PLoS One 7: e31086.
29. Norata GD, Garlaschelli K, Ongari M, Raselli S, Grigore L, et al. (2006) Effects of fractalkine receptor variants on common carotid artery intima-media thickness. Stroke 37: 1558–1561.
30. Ammirati E, Cianflone D, Banfi M, Vecchio V, Palini A, et al. (2010) Circulating CD4+CD25hiCD127lo Regulatory T-Cell Levels Do Not Reflect the Extent or Severity of Carotid and Coronary Atherosclerosis. Arterioscler Thromb Vasc Biol 30: 1832–1841.
31. Norata GD, Grigore L, Raselli S, Redaelli L, Hamsten A, et al. (2007) Postprandial endothelial dysfunction in hypertriglyceridemic subjects: molecular mechanisms and gene expression studies. Atherosclerosis 193: 321–327.
32. Norata GD, Raselli S, Grigore L, Garlaschelli K, Vianello D, et al. (2009) Small dense LDL and VLDL predict common carotid artery IMT and elicit an inflammatory response in peripheral blood mononuclear and endothelial cells. Atherosclerosis 206: 556–562.
33. Norata GD, Garlaschelli K, Grigore L, Tibolla G, Raselli S, et al. (2009) Circulating soluble receptor for advanced glycation end products is inversely associated with body mass index and waist/hip ratio in the general population. Nutr Metab Cardiovasc Dis 19: 129–134.
34. Devereux RB, Alonso DR, Lutas EM, Gottlieb GJ, Campo E, et al. (1986) Echocardiographic assessment of left ventricular hypertrophy: comparison to necropsy findings. Am J Cardiol 57: 450–458.
35. Ammirati E, Cianflone D, Vecchio V, Banfi M, Vermi AC, et al. (2012) Effector Memory T cells Are Associated With Atherosclerosis in Humans and Animal Models. J Am Heart Assoc 1: 27–41.
36. Wendelhag I, Wiklund O, Wikstrand J (1993) Atherosclerotic changes in the femoral and carotid arteries in familial hypercholesterolemia. Ultrasonographic assessment of intima-media thickness and plaque occurrence. Arterioscler Thromb 13: 1404–1411.
37. Kang P, Tian C, Jia C (2012) Association of RAGE gene polymorphisms with type 2 diabetes mellitus, diabetic retinopathy and diabetic nephropathy. Gene 500: 1–9.
38. Kalea AZ, Schmidt AM, Hudson BI (2011) Alternative splicing of RAGE: roles in biology and disease. Front Biosci 16: 2756–2770.
39. Wendt TM, Tanji N, Guo J, Kislinger TR, Qu W, et al. (2003) RAGE drives the development of glomerulosclerosis and implicates podocyte activation in the pathogenesis of diabetic nephropathy. Am J Pathol 162: 1123–1137.
40. Ehlermann P, Eggers K, Bierhaus A, Most P, Weichenhan D, et al. (2006) Increased proinflammatory endothelial response to S100A8/A9 after preactivation through advanced glycation end products. Cardiovasc Diabetol 5: 6.

41. Yamagishi S, Fukami K, Ueda S, Okuda S (2007) Molecular mechanisms of diabetic nephropathy and its therapeutic intervention. Curr Drug Targets 8: 952–959.

42. Fukami K, Ueda S, Yamagishi S, Kato S, Inagaki Y, et al. (2004) AGEs activate mesangial TGF-beta-Smad signaling via an angiotensin II type I receptor interaction. Kidney Int 66: 2137–2147.

43. Yamagishi S, Inagaki Y, Okamoto T, Amano S, Koga K, et al. (2003) Advanced glycation end products inhibit de novo protein synthesis and induce TGF-beta overexpression in proximal tubular cells. Kidney Int 63: 464–473.

44. Ziyadeh FN, Hoffman BB, Han DC, Iglesias-De La Cruz MC, Hong SW, et al. (2000) Long-term prevention of renal insufficiency, excess matrix gene expression, and glomerular mesangial matrix expansion by treatment with monoclonal antitransforming growth factor-beta antibody in db/db diabetic mice. Proc Natl Acad Sci U S A 97: 8015–8020.

45. Vlassara H, Striker LJ, Teichberg S, Fuh H, Li YM, et al. (1994) Advanced glycation end products induce glomerular sclerosis and albuminuria in normal rats. Proc Natl Acad Sci U S A 91: 11704–11708.

46. Norata GD, Callegari E, Marchesi M, Chiesa G, Eriksson P, et al. (2005) High-density lipoproteins induce transforming growth factor-beta2 expression in endothelial cells. Circulation 111: 2805–2811.

47. Yang CW, Vlassara H, Peten EP, He CJ, Striker GE, et al. (1994) Advanced glycation end products up-regulate gene expression found in diabetic glomerular disease. Proc Natl Acad Sci U S A 91: 9436–9440.

48. Bianchi S, Bigazzi R, Campese VM (2010) Intensive versus conventional therapy to slow the progression of idiopathic glomerular diseases. Am J Kidney Dis 55: 671–681.

49. Baigent C, Landray MJ, Reith C, Emberson J, Wheeler DC, et al. (2011) The effects of lowering LDL cholesterol with simvastatin plus ezetimibe in patients with chronic kidney disease (Study of Heart and Renal Protection): a randomised placebo-controlled trial. Lancet 377: 2181–2192.

50. Burton JO, Gray LJ, Webb DR, Davies MJ, Khunti K, et al. (2012) Association of anthropometric obesity measures with chronic kidney disease risk in a non-diabetic patient population. Nephrol Dial Transplant 27: 1860–1866.

51. Reaich D, Price SR, England BK, Mitch WE (1995) Mechanisms causing muscle loss in chronic renal failure. Am J Kidney Dis 26: 242–247.

18

Maintenance of Hypertensive Hemodynamics does not Depend on ROS in Established Experimental Chronic Kidney Disease

Diana A. Papazova[1], Arianne van Koppen[1], Maarten P. Koeners[1], Ronald L. Bleys[2], Marianne C. Verhaar[1], Jaap A. Joles[1]

1 Department of Nephrology & Hypertension, University Medical Center Utrecht, Utrecht, The Netherlands, **2** Department of Anatomy, University Medical Center Utrecht, Utrecht, The Netherlands

Abstract

While the presence of oxidative stress in chronic kidney disease (CKD) is well established, its relation to hypertensive renal hemodynamics remains unclear. We hypothesized that once CKD is established blood pressure and renal vascular resistance (RVR) no longer depend on reactive oxygen species. CKD was induced by bilateral ablation of 2/3 of each kidney. Compared to age-matched, sham-operated controls all ablated rats showed proteinuria, decreased glomerular filtration rate (GFR), more renal damage, higher mean arterial pressure (MAP), RVR and excretion of oxidative stress markers and hydrogen peroxide, while excretion of stable nitric oxide (NO) metabolites tended to decrease. We compared MAP, RVR, GFR and fractional excretion of sodium under baseline and during acute Tempol, PEG-catalase or vehicle infusion in rats with established CKD vs. controls. Tempol caused marked reduction in MAP in controls (96 ± 5 vs.79 ± 4 mmHg, $P<0.05$) but not in CKD (130 ± 5 vs. 127 ± 6 mmHg). PEG-catalase reduced MAP in both groups (controls: 102 ± 2 vs. 94 ± 4 mmHg, $P<0.05$; CKD: 118 ± 4 vs. 110 ± 4 mmHg, $P<0.05$), but did not normalize MAP in CKD rats. Tempol and PEG-catalase slightly decreased RVR in both groups. Fractional excretion of sodium was increased by both Tempol and PEG-catalase in both groups. PEG-catalase decreased TBARS excretion in both groups. In sum, although oxidative stress markers were increased, MAP and RVR did not depend more on oxidative stress in CKD than in controls. Therefore reactive oxygen species appear not to be important direct determinants of hypertensive renal hemodynamics in this model of established CKD.

Editor: Michael Bader, Max-Delbrück Center for Molecular Medicine (MDC), Germany

Funding: MCV is supported by the Netherlands organization for Scientific Research (NWO) Vidi grant 016.096.359. The funders had no role in study design, data collection and analysis, decision to publish, or preparation of the manuscript.

Competing Interests: The authors have declared that no competing interests exist. The corresponding author Jaap A. Joles, DVM, PhD serves as a member of PLOS ONE Editorial board. This does not alter the authors' adherence to all the PLOS ONE policies on sharing data and materials.

* E-mail: J.A.Joles@umcutrecht.nl

Introduction

Chronic kidney disease (CKD) is associated with hypertension. Patients with mild to moderate renal insufficiency have increased levels of oxidative stress [1–5] i.e. unfavourable redox balance in which pro-oxidants gain the upper hand over anti-oxidants. This results in a net increase in reactive oxygen species (ROS), leading to cellular and tissue damage. Experimentally increasing ROS (superoxide anion and hydrogen peroxide) in the renal medulla induces hypertension [6,7].

Several studies support the hypothesis that antioxidants may play an important role in the pathogenesis of chronic renal failure and that antioxidant intervention can slow the progression of renal insufficiency in different experimental models of renal disease [8]. On the other hand, with the notable exception of a single study in hemodialysis patients [9], clinical studies showed no beneficial effects of antioxidants in the CKD population [8,10,11].

Tempol (4-hydroxy-2,2,6,6-tetramethyl-piperidine-1-oxyl) is a stable low-molecular-weight (172.25 g/mol) cell-permeable super-oxide dismutase (SOD) mimetic that has been used to reduce oxidative injury in cell and animal models. Chronic Tempol administration has been shown to ameliorate oxidative stress and

lower arterial pressure in various rat models of hypertension: spontaneously hypertensive rats (SHR) [12], Dahl salt-sensitive rats [13], mineralocorticoid-induced hypertension [14], lead-induced hypertension [15], and erythropoietin-induced hypertension in uremic rats [16]. Acute Tempol administration decreases mean arterial pressure (MAP) and renal vascular resistance (RVR) in SHR [17,18] and in two-kidney one-clip hypertension [19]. Although in the remnant kidney model, chronic Tempol administration decreases oxidative stress, it has only been shown to prevent or reduce increase of blood pressure for 10–14 days after nephrectomy [20,21].

Catalase, an H_2O_2 detoxifying enzyme, has been shown to prevent hypertension induced by the infusion of H_2O_2 in the renal medulla [7]. Polyethylene glycol (PEG)-catalase was preferred to catalase, since the conjugation of catalase with PEG enhances cell association and increases cellular enzyme activity [22]. PEG-catalase prevents the markedly increased vascular and urinary H_2O_2 levels and rise in blood pressure in hypertension induced by adenosine receptor blockade [23]. In angiotensin-induced hypertension, although blood pressure was markedly decreased during the first days of PEG-catalase administration, this effect waned after only three days [24].

While the presence of oxidative stress as a feature of CKD is well established, its relation to hypertension and related hemodynamics in CKD has not been systematically addressed. In the current study we hypothesized that ROS are not important determinants of hypertensive renal hemodynamics in long-term, established experimental CKD. To this end we developed a novel bilateral renal ablation model that was staged by the level of proteinuria. In order to differentiate hypertensive effects of superoxide and H_2O_2, we studied acute effects of the SOD mimetic Tempol or PEG-catalase on blood pressure (BP) and renal hemodynamics in rats with established CKD and age-matched sham-operated control rats. Furthermore, we investigated the effect of both these interventions on oxidative stress in CKD and control rats.

Materials and Methods

Ethics statement

The study protocol was approved by the Utrecht University Committee on Animal Experiments, and conformed to Dutch Law on Laboratory Animal Experiments (DEC number 2010.II.05.097 and DEC number 2012.II.03.053).

Animals

Male inbred Lewis rats (Lew/CRl), 180–200 g, were purchased from Charles River, Germany and housed in a climate-controlled facility with a 12:12-hour light: dark cycle under standard conditions.

In order to develop established CKD in this strain, the rats were subjected to partial ablation of both kidneys. Via laparotomy under isoflurane anaesthesia (5% induction, 1.5–2% maintenance), branches of both renal arteries were coagulated, resulting in loss of approximately 2/3 of total renal mass in a one-step procedure. Age-matched control rats were sham-operated (CON). All rats received an intramuscular injection of analgesia straight after and one day after surgery (Buprenorphine, 0.05 mg/kg). 24-h urine samples were collected weekly for determination of protein excretion, with the rats in individual metabolic cages while fasting, as described [25]. Blood samples were collected from the tail vein for determination of plasma urea and creatinine. CKD was initially accelerated with N(omega)-nitro-L-arginine (L-NNA), a NO-synthase inhibitor (50 mg/L) in drinking water [11] and the standard powdered chow (CRM-FG; Special Diet Services Ltd., Witham, Essex, UK) was supplemented with 6% NaCl until proteinuria exceeded 200 mg/day after a median of 8 weeks (range: 6–9 weeks). Subsequently L-NNA was withdrawn causing proteinuria to initially fall and subsequently increase slowly as

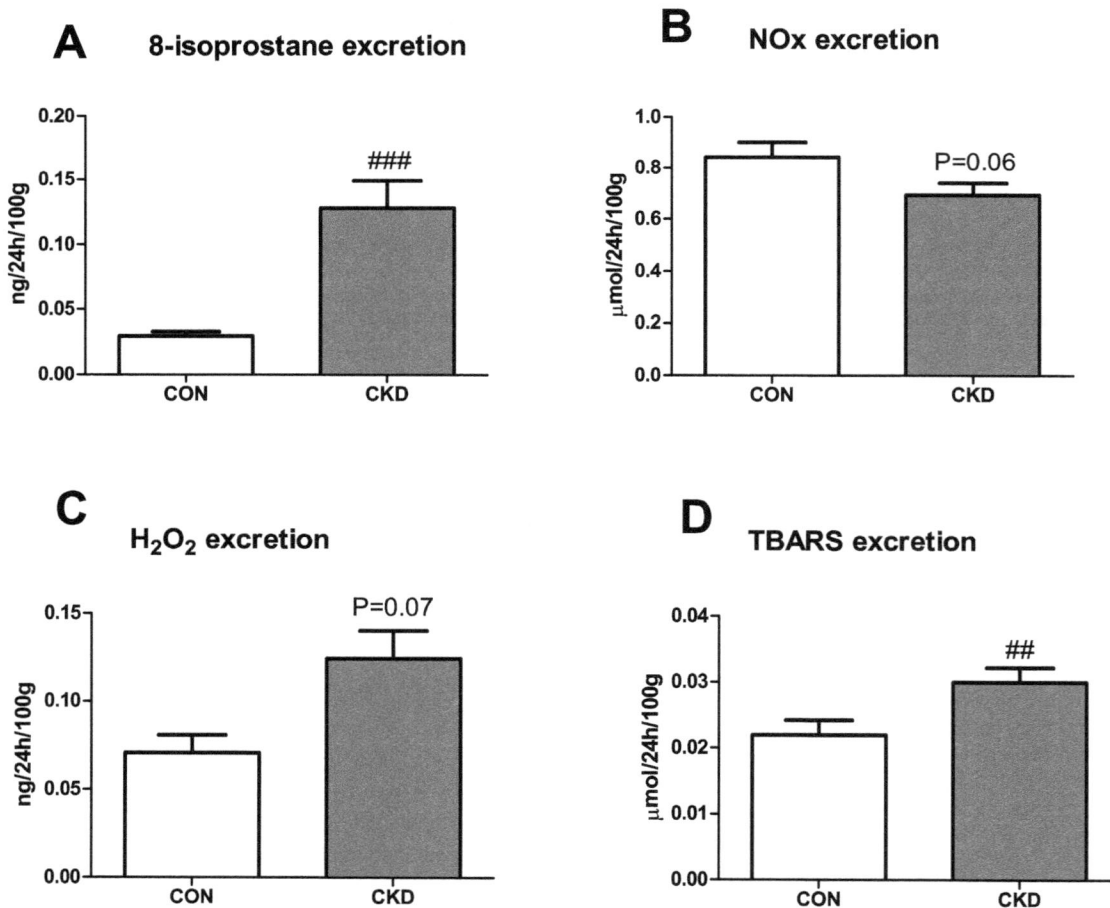

Figure 1. 24 h excretions of 8-isoprostanes (panel A), NO metabolites (NOx, panel B), hydrogen peroxide (panel C) and lipid peroxides (TBARS, panel D) in CKD vs. CON rats. Mean ± SEM. ###P<0.001, ##P<0.01 vs. CON.

described by Quiroz et al. [26] (data not shown). Terminal experiments were planned within a week when proteinuria exceeded 100 mg/day. This time point was reached after a median of 35 weeks (range: 22–56 weeks). This approach ensured that staging of CKD was similar in all rats. Previously we have shown that proteinuria predicts target organ injury in hypertensive rats [27]. Timing of terminal experiments in sham-operated controls was determined by their age-matched CKD litter mates.

One week prior to termination 24 h urinary excretion of markers of oxidative stress (thiobarbituric acid reactive substances (TBARS), 8-isoprostane (EIA kit, Cayman Chemical, Michigan, USA) and hydrogen peroxide (Amplex Red Hydrogen Peroxide/Peroxidase Assay Kit (Molecular probes, OR, USA)) were measured. Urinary excretion of stable NO metabolites $NO_2 + NO_3$ (NOx) were determined by fluorometric quantification of nitrite content [28]. Rats underwent a terminal measurement under anaesthesia as described. L-NNA, Tempol, PEG-catalase, BSA and Buprenorphine were purchased from Sigma-Aldrich. Isoflurane was purchased from Abbott.

Terminal experiment protocol

On the day of the experiment the trachea was intubated with a 16-G catheter (Venisystems, Abbocath-T, Abbott, Ireland) under isoflurane anesthesia (5% induction, 1.5–2% maintenance). The femoral artery was cannulated in order to obtain direct measurement of MAP and a Transonic flow probe was placed on the left renal artery to measure renal blood flow (RBF) [17,29], allowing calculation of renal vascular resistance (RVR: MAP/RBF). Urine was collected allowing measurement of kidney function (glomerular filtration rate, GFR: inulin clearance). During surgery, animals received an intravenous infusion of a 150 mmol/L NaCl solution containing 6% bovine serum albumin (BSA) at a rate of 100 µl/kg/min. Following surgery, the infusion was switched to a 150 mmol/L NaCl solution with 1% BSA, containing inulin for measurement of GFR, which was maintained at the same infusion rate throughout the experiment. Following a 60 min equilibration period, after which both signals were stable, baseline data were collected for 15 min. Thereafter, to investigate renal vascular reactivity we continuously infused the SOD mimetic Tempol (180 µmol/kg/h, CKD n = 6, CON n = 4), PEG-catalase (2000 units/kg/h, CKD n = 8, CON n = 5) or vehicle (NaCl, 0.9% 6 ml/kg/h, CKD n = 4, CON n = 4) after baseline measurements. Following a 45 min equilibration period, after which both signals were stable, intervention data were collected for 15 min. This dose for Tempol was chosen because it has already been shown by others that 72–90 µmol/kg is an effective dose and acute response was very rapid to intravenous Tempol in anaesthetized rat with spontaneous hypertension [30]. A dose of 174 µmol/kg caused a decrease in MAP with more than 30 mmHg and when given in an effective dose (72–90 µmol/kg), Tempol reduced the blood

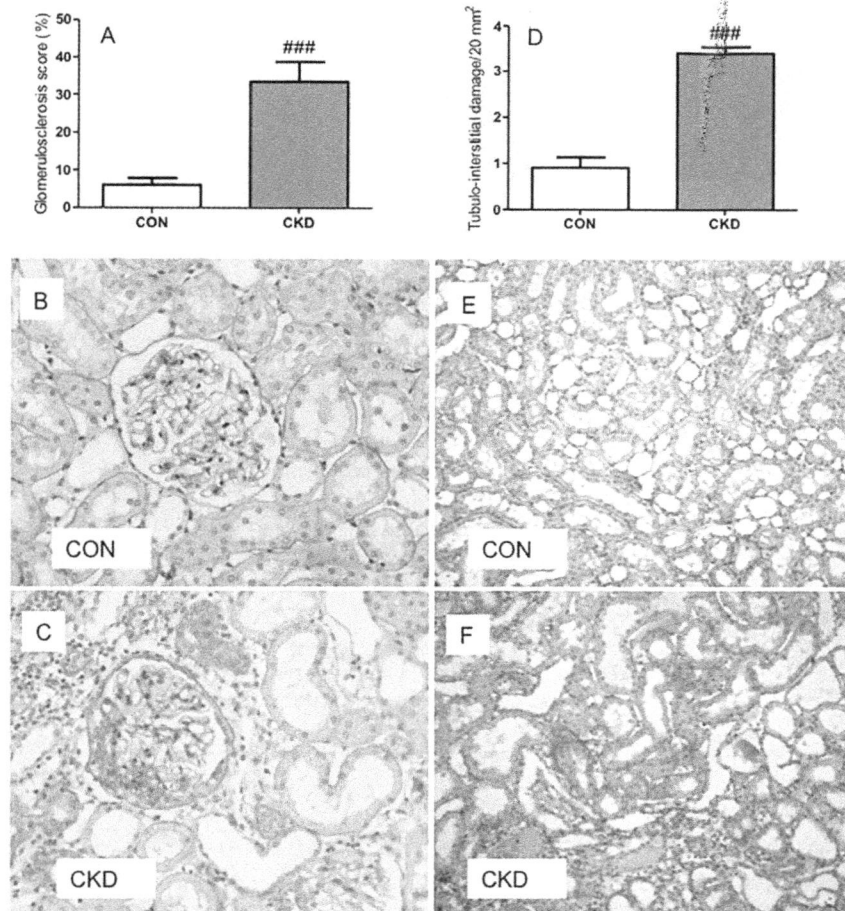

Figure 2. Bilateral ablation (C and F) induced more glomerulosclerosis (panel A) and tubulo-interstitial damage (panel D) in CKD rats compared to controls (B and E) on PAS-stained sections. Means ± SEM. Unpaired t-test: ###P<0.001 vs. CON.

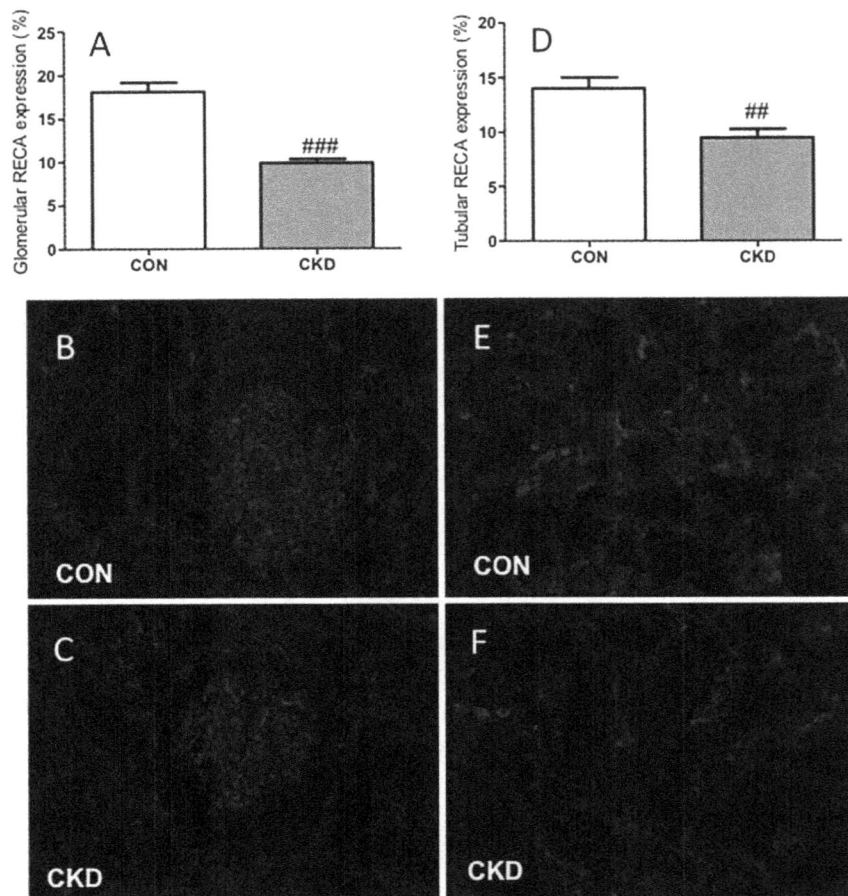

Figure 3. Less (RECA)$^+$ pixels (green) were found in CKD rats compared to CON rats in both glomeruli (panel A) and tubular fields (panel D). Immunohistochemical labeling is shown in CON rats (panels B and E) and in CKD rats (panels C and F). Means ± SEM. Unpaired t-test: ###P<0.001; ##P<0.01 vs. CON.

Table 1. Characterisation of CKD vs. control (CON) rats: organ weights, clinical signs and renal injury.

	CON	CKD
N	13	18
Body weight (BW) g	560±14	540±11
Total renal weight (mg/100 g BW)	664±13	591±10 ###
Heart weight (mg/100 g BW)	244±5	280±14 #
Total wet lung weight (mg/100 g BW)	309±6	337±6 ##
Diuresis (ml/24 h/100 g)	3.15±0.3	5.45±0.68 #
Proteinuria (mg/24 h)	16±4	152±9###
Hematocrit (%)	45.2±0.3	42.6±0.5 ###
Plasma urea (mmol/L)	6.76±0.18	10.47±0.38 ###
Plasma creatinine (μmol/L)	34±4	50±6 #
Plasma Na (mmol/L)	146.6±1.5	145.7±1.3
Plasma K (mmol/L)	4.25±0.12	4.22±0.07

Mean ± SEM, t-test: # P<0.05, ##P<0.01, ###P<0.001 vs. CON.

pressure in all hypertensive models with evidence of oxidative stress [31]. Moreover, Tempol administration ameliorated 8-isoprostane excretion in several hypertensive models [32,33]. Fractional excretions of sodium and potassium (FE Na and FE K) were calculated using standard formulae.

Oxidative stress protocol

To investigate the effect of antioxidants on oxidative stress in our CKD model, we administered Tempol (180 μmol/kg), PEG-

Table 2. Gene expression of renin, AT1, ACE1 and VEGF-A in CON and CKD rats. Data are presented as log fold change relative to CON.

	CON	CKD
renin	0.0±0.37	−1.6±0.35 #
AT1	0.0±0.15	−0.7± 0.24
ACE1	0.0±0.17	−0.1±0.59
VEGF-A	0.0±0.10	−1.4±0.46 #

Means ± SEM. Unpaired T-test. #P<0.05 vs. CON.

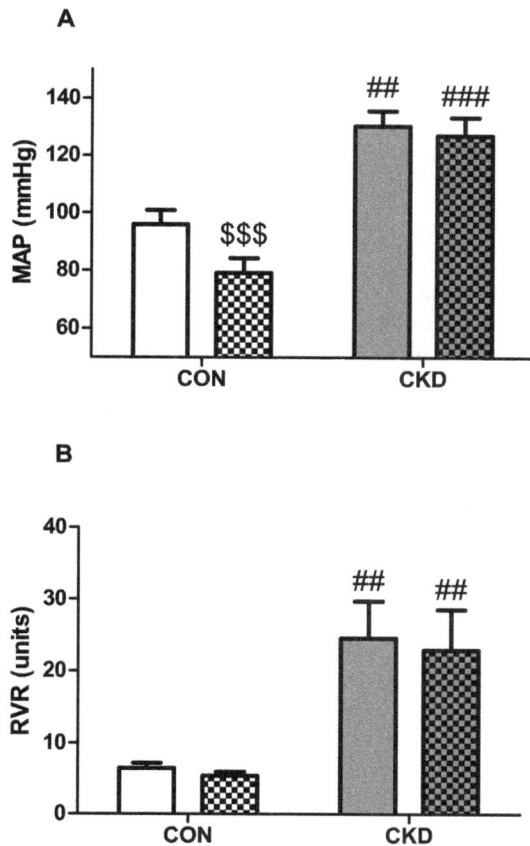

Figure 4. Mean arterial pressure (MAP) (panel A) and renal vascular resistance (RVR) (panel B) prior to baseline (plain bars) and during Tempol (bars with squares) in CON (n = 4, white bars) and CKD (n = 6, grey bars) rats. Mean ± SEM. Two-way RM ANOVA (P CKD vs. CON = 0.001, P Tempol vs. baseline < 0.001, P Interaction = 0,002 for panel A; P CKD vs. CON = 0.030, P Tempol vs. baseline = NS, P Interaction = NS for panel B), ## P<0.01, ### P< 0.001 vs. CON. $$$ P<0.001 vs. baseline (paired observations).

Figure 5. Mean arterial pressure (MAP) (panel A) and renal vascular resistance (RVR) (panel B) prior to baseline (plain bars) and during PEG-catalase (striped bars) in CON (n = 5, white bars) and CKD (n = 8, grey bars) rats. Mean ± SEM. Two-way RM ANOVA (P CKD vs. CON = 0.017, P PEG-catalase vs. baseline <0.001, P Interaction = NS for panel A; P CKD vs. CON = 0.001, P PEG-catalase vs. baseline <0.001, P Interaction = NS for panel B). ## P<0.01, ### P<0.001 vs. CON. && P<0.01, &&& P<0.001 vs. baseline (paired observations).

catalase (2000 IU/kg) or vehicle (0.9 % NaCl) iv (tail vein) in a separate cohort of CKD rats. Administration of antioxidant or vehicle was time-matched (between 17:30 and 18:30 h) and followed by collection of urine in metabolic cages overnight. We compared TBARS excretion between age-matched CKD (n = 6) and CON (n = 6) rats, treated in a repeated-design experiment with Tempol, PEG-catalase or vehicle in random sequence.

Renal morphology

Directly after performing the terminal experiment protocol, rats were sacrificed and tissues were collected and fixed in 4% paraformaldehyde for embedding in paraffin or were snap frozen. Glomerulosclerosis (GS) and tubulo-interstitial injury (TI) were scored on PAS-stained paraffin-embedded slides [34]. Furthermore, endothelial cells in the glomeruli and tubuli were stained with rat endothelial cell antigen (RECA). (RECA)$^+$ pixels were counted in glomeruli and tubular fields using ImageJ Software (Rasband, W.S., ImageJ, U.S. National Institutes of Health, Bethesda, MD) [35]. In order to evaluate whether Tempol and PEG-catalase caused changes in thesympathetic nervous system, we performed immunohistochemistry using an antibody against marker for sympathetic nerves: tyrosine hydroxylase (TH) [36].

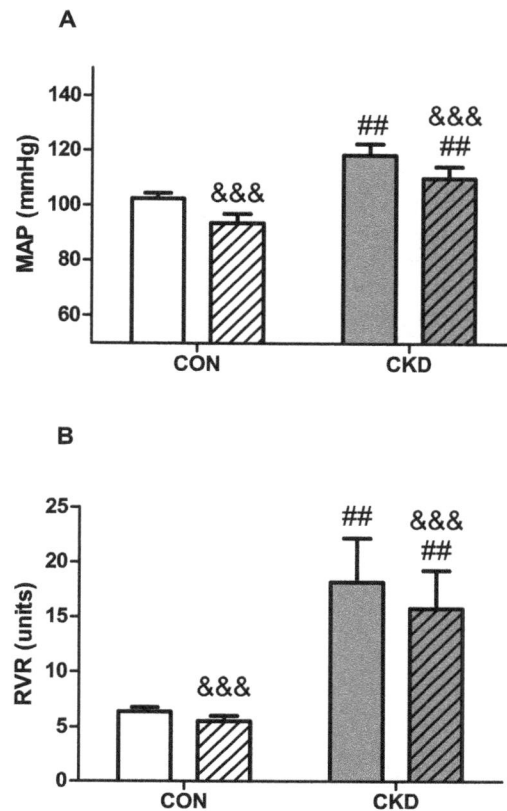

Snap frozen kidney slices were incubated overnight with anti-TH antibody (P40101-0, Pel-Freez Biologicals, 1:500).

Gene expression

To determine whether Tempol and PEG-catalase affected renin-angiotensin system (RAS), gene expression of angiotensin II receptor type 1 (AT1), angiotensin converting enzyme 1 (ACE1) and renin in renal tissue was assessed by qPCR as described [35]. Using the same method we assessed the renal expression of vascular endothelial growth factor (VEGF-A), which is responsible for angiogenesis and endothelial cell proliferation [37]. The following TaqMan Gene Expression Assays (Applied Biosystems) were used : (AT1: Rn01435427_m1), (ACE1:Rn00561094_m1), (renin: Rn00561847_m1), (VEGF-A: Rn00582935_m1), (beta-actin: Rn00667869_m1) and (beta-2-microglobulin: Rn00560865_m1). Cycle time (Ct) values for all genes were normalized for mean Ct-values of beta-actin and beta-2-micro-glubulin which we previously determined to be the two most stable housekeeping genes for renal tissue for all groups.

Statistics

Values are expressed as mean ± SEM. Data were compared with unpaired T-test, one way analysis of variance (ANOVA) and

A

B

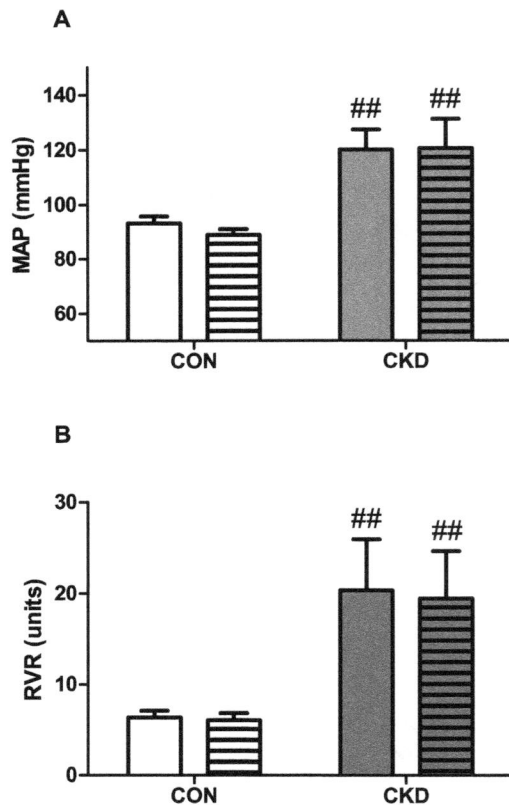

Figure 6. Mean arterial pressure (MAP) (panel A) and renal vascular resistance (RVR) (panel B) prior to baseline (plain bars) and during infusion of vehicle (bars with horizontal lines) in CON (n = 4, white bars) and CKD (n = 4, grey bars) rats. Mean ± SEM. Two-way RM ANOVA (P CKD vs. CON = 0.020, P vehicle vs. baseline = NS, P Interaction = NS for panel A; P CKD vs. CON = 0.040, P vehicle vs. baseline = NS, P Interaction = NS for panel B). ## P<0.01 vs. CON.

two-way ANOVA for repeated measurements when appropriate. Tukey test was used as a post-hoc test (P<0.05).

Results

Ablation of 2/3 of each kidney leads to established CKD

In the CKD group, 3 of the initial 21 animals died during follow-up which resulted in n = 18 of CKD animals, an 85% survival rate. Mortality was either spontaneous (1 rat) or caused by intestinal ischemia in the first week after bilateral ablation possibly due to manipulating the intestines during surgery (2 rats). Survival rate of all sham-operated CON rats was 100%. CKD rats showed slightly lower body weight vs. CON rats (Table 1). All organ weights were corrected for body weight. Renal mass was lower (P<0.01) and heart and wet lungs heavier in CKD rats (P<0.05 and P<0.01 respectively). CKD rats showed increased diuresis (P<0.01) and proteinuria (P<0.001). All CKD rats had mild anemia (P<0.001), higher plasma urea (P<0.001) and creatinine (P<0.05). Markers of oxidative stress were increased in CKD: TBARS and 8-isoprostane excretion were significantly higher (P<0.01 and P<0.001 respectively), whereas H_2O_2 excretion tended to increase (P = 0.07) vs. CON rats (Fig. 1). NOx excretion tended to decrease in CKD vs. CON (P = 0.06). In CKD rats, the expression of renin and VEGF-A were lower in comparison to

CON rats. No differences in expression of AT1 and ACE1 were found (Table 2). CKD rats showed marked glomerulosclerosis and tubulo-interstitial injury (both P<0.001) (Fig. 2). Counts of RECA-positive pixels indicated lower numbers of endothelial cells in the glomeruli and the tubular fields of CKD rats vs. CON rats (Fig. 3). Visual impression showed no difference in tyrosine hydroxylase expression (Supplemental Figure S1).

Tempol decreased MAP in CON but not in CKD and did not affect RVR

CKD increased MAP (P = 0.001) and Tempol decreased MAP (P<0.001, Fig. 4A). However, the effect of Tempol was different in CKD than in CON, resulting in strong interaction (P<0.01), and when individual groups were compared with the post-hoc test, we found that infusion of Tempol significantly decreased MAP in CON (P<0.001) but had no effect on MAP in CKD. All CKD rats had higher RVR vs. CON rats (P<0.01) and Tempol had no significant effect on RVR (Fig. 4B).

PEG-catalase decreased MAP and RVR in CON and CKD

PEG-catalase significantly reduced MAP (P<0.001) in both CON and CKD, and in the post-hoc analysis, PEG-catalase-induced reductions in MAP were all significant (Fig. 5A). For RVR, the same pattern was observed: PEG-catalase decreased RVR in both CON and CKD (P<0.001), and in the post-hoc analysis all PEG-catalase-induced reductions in RVR were significant (Fig. 5B).

Vehicle

Infusion of vehicle (0.9 % NaCl) did not affect either MAP (Fig. 6A) or RVR (Fig 6B).

Tempol and PEG-catalase reduced GFR in CON and increased FE Na in CKD

CKD rats had lower GFR vs. CON rats (P<0.001, Table 3). Tempol had different effects on GFR in CKD and CON, resulting in interaction (P<0.05), and when groups were compared with the post-hoc test, Tempol markedly reduced GFR in CON (P<0.001), but not in CKD. Similarly, PEG-catalase had different effects on GFR in CKD and CON (P<0.05), and reduced GFR in CON (P<0.001), but not in CKD. This pattern for GFR was also observed during vehicle infusion.

CKD rats had higher FE Na (P<0.01) and FE K (P<0.001) than CON rats (Table 3). During Tempol infusion FE Na tended to decrease in CON (NS), but was markedly increased in CKD (P<0.01), both compared to their own baseline. This pattern resulted in a significant interaction for FE Na (P<0.05). During PEG-catalase effects on FE Na were similar to those observed for Tempol: no change in CON but a marked increase in CKD (P< 0.001), resulting in significant interaction (P<0.01). FE K was not affected by either Tempol or PEG-catalase, and neither FE Na nor FE K were affected by vehicle infusion.

Comparison of changes induced by Tempol, PEG-catalase and vehicle

Figure 7 depicts the changes in MAP and RVR after acute administration of Tempol, PEG-catalase or vehicle in CON and CKD rats. For change in MAP an overall effect of all three interventions was observed (P<0.001) as well as interaction (P< 0.01, Fig. 7A). Tempol infusion decreased MAP by nearly 15 mmHg in CON rats (P<0.001) but MAP remained unchanged in CKD rats when compared with the change caused by vehicle infusion in the same condition. However, when comparing change

Table 3. Glomerular filtration rate (GFR) and fractional electrolyte excretion prior to (baseline) and after intervention (Tempol, PEG-catalase, vehicle).

	CON		CKD		P-value		
	baseline	Tempol	baseline	Tempol	CKD-cat	Tempol	Interaction
N	4		6				
GFR (µl/min/100g)	672±65	485±60 $$	302±18 ###	262±21 ##	<0.001	=0.003	=0.029
FE Na (%)	0.28±0.12	0.23±0.13	1.02±0.26	1.91±0.54 # $$	=0.042	=0.066	=0.043
FE K (%)	26.09±1.94	25.11±0.73	64.22±4.61 ###	62.43±3.90 ###	<0.001	=0.665	=0.898
	baseline	PEG-catalase	baseline	PEG-catalase	CKD	PEG-catalase	Interaction
N	5		8				
GFR (µl/min/100g)	784±105	510±112 &&&	354±40 ###	273±24 ##	<0.001	<0.001	=0.021
FE Na (%)	0.15±0.04	0.12±0.04	0.47±0.08	0.79±0.14 ### &&&	=0.005	=0.026	=0.009
FE K (%)	30.47±3.53	28.67±3.56	63.42±5.41 ###	60.96±4.98 ###	<0.001	=0.501	=0.915
	baseline	vehicle	baseline	vehicle	CKD	vehicle	Interaction
N	4		4				
GFR (µl/min/100g)	741±102.13	523±107 §	303±32 ##	240±28 #	=0.013	=0.007	=0.066
FE Na (%)	0.17±0.04	0.16±0.05	1.27±0.60	1.60±0.92	=0.145	=0.364	=0.342
FE K (%)	30.67±0.79	26.77±1.94	73.50 ±8.58 ##	73.45±7.64 ##	=0.001	=0.273	=0.284

Mean ± SEM, ANOVA RM, Tukey post-hoc test for comparison between groups ### P<0.001, ## P<0.01, #P<0.05 vs. CON; $$P<0.01 Tempol vs. baseline; &&& P<0.001 PEG-catalase vs. baseline; § P<0.05 vehicle vs. baseline.

in MAP caused by PEG-catalase administration, the opposite was observed: MAP decreased slightly in CON rats but was significantly lower in CKD rats (P<0.05) when compared to change caused by vehicle infusion in the same condition. Changes in RVR were not significantly different (Fig. 7B). One-hour acute infusion of Tempol or PEG-catalase in terminal setting did not cause any changes in the renal expression of RAS and VEGF-A genes or in tyrosine hydroxylase staining in comparison to vehicle infusion in both CON and CKD (Supplemental Table S1 and Supplemental Figure S1).

Comparison of TBARS excretion induced by Tempol, PEG-catalase or vehicle

Intravenous administration of Tempol did not affect excretion of TBARS in CON and CKD groups compared to vehicle, whereas PEG-catalase decreased TBARS excretion in CKD group (P<0.05) and showed a trend to decrease in CON group compared to vehicle (P = 0.09) (Fig. 8).

Discussion

The main novel finding of this study is that in established CKD, MAP and RVR do not depend on ROS. This was demonstrated by the failure to alter MAP in CKD rats by acute scavenging of superoxide with Tempol. Reducing H_2O_2 with PEG-catalase did not normalize MAP in CKD rats. Furthermore, in CKD rats, Tempol had no effect on TBARS excretion while PEG-catalase reduced it.

Parameters of oxidative stress are increased and antioxidant enzyme activities are decreased in patients with various degrees of CKD [38–40]. Important endogenous antioxidant enzymes are SOD(s) that convert superoxide to H_2O_2, which is in turn disposed of by two other enzymes, catalase and glutathione peroxidase. In experimental CKD a marked down-regulation of hepatic and renal cytoplasmic and mitochondrial SOD was found as well as

down-regulation of renal catalase and glutathione peroxidase protein abundance and catalase activity [41,42].

Effect of Tempol and PEG-catalase on MAP

In CKD rat models chronic Tempol administration only ameliorated hypertension for 10–14 days after nephrectomy [20,21]. Our data suggests that in long-term experimental CKD, once hypertension is established, other mechanisms contribute to its maintenance. Because Tempol caused a marked decrease in MAP in CON but not in CKD rats, maintenance of hypertension in our model of CKD appears not to depend on superoxide. Although Tempol infusion reduces superoxide levels, it results in accumulation of H_2O_2 that might serve as an important hypertensive factor [7] and has been reported to induce renal vasoconstriction [43,44]. The lack of antihypertensive effects of Tempol might be explained by the need of a fully functional system of other (non-SOD) antioxidant enzymes to drive the H_2O_2 generated from superoxide dismutation to CO_2 and H_2O. In contrast to Tempol, we found that acute administration of PEG-catalase did decrease MAP in CKD. However, MAP was not normalized to control levels in response to PEG-catalase, suggesting that H_2O_2 is not solely responsible for hypertension in established CKD. Increased production of ROS can reduce the availability of vasodilators such as nitric oxide (NO), which can lead to functional NO deficiency and thus contribute to maintenance of hypertension. Indeed, CKD rats in the present study showed a tendency to lower levels of urinary NOx excretion vs. CON rats. However, VEGF-A gene expression and endothelial cell staining, although both clearly reduced in CKD rats, were not affected acutely by Tempol and PEG-catalase. Other factors than oxidative stress that can affect the blood pressure are RAS and the sympathetic nervous system. We found no changes in either gene expression of AT1, ACE1 or renin (Supplemental Table S1) or in detection of sympathetic nerves between treatment groups (Supplemental Figure S1). Thus, at least these levels of expression,

A

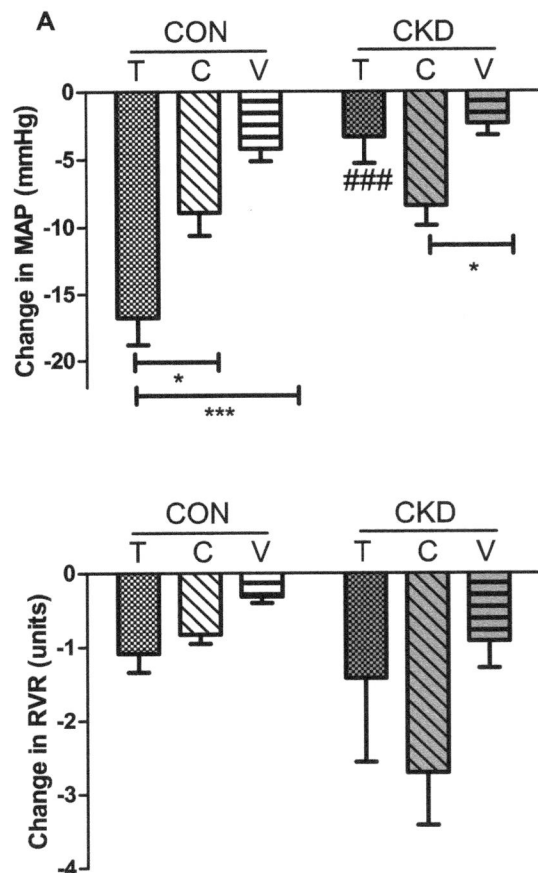

Figure 7. Changes in MAP (panel A) and RVR (panel B) in CON (white bars) and CKD rats (grey bars) during infusion of Tempol (T, bars with squares), PEG-catalase (C, bars with stripes) and vehicle (V, bars with horizontal lines). Mean ± SEM. P CKD vs. CON = 0.0011, P Interventions = 0.0028, P Interaction = 0.0014, for panel A; P CKD vs. CON = NS, P Interventions = NS, P Interaction = NS for panel B). Tukey post-hoc test for comparison between groups: ### P<0.01 vs. CON. Between groups: *P<0.05. **P<0.01 ***P< 0.001.

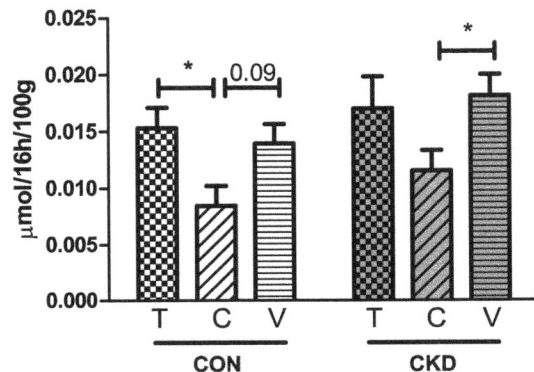

Figure 8. 16h TBARS excretion in CON rats (white bars) and CKD rats (grey bars) after intravenous administration of Tempol (T, bars with squares), PEG-catalase (C, bars with stripes) or vehicle (V, bars with horizontal lines). Mean ± SEM. P CON vs. CKD = NS; P Interventions = 0.003; P Interaction = NS. Tukey post hoc test for comparison between groups: *P<0.05.

mesenteric arteries from CKD rats incubated with Tempol and PEG-catalase showed a significant increase rather than decrease in myogenic constriction suggesting that superoxide and H_2O_2 may be involved in pathological loss of the myogenic response [47].

Effect of Tempol and PEG-catalase on TBARS excretion

Tempol showed no effect on urinary TBARS excretion in neither CON nor CKD rats suggesting that it failed to reduce oxidative stress in both groups. Similar to the effect on MAP in the acute experiment, PEG-catalase reduced TBARS excretion in both CON and CKD. This once again suggests that oxidative stress is not the main force driving maintenance of hypertension in this established model of CKD.

Effect of Tempol and PEG-catalase on FE Na

A striking finding in this study is that FE Na in CKD rats was increased by both Tempol and PEG-catalase in comparison to CON rats suggesting that excessive ROS modulate natriuresis. In agreement with our observation, it has been demonstrated that ROS decreases sodium excretion [48]. It has been shown that ROS have multiple anti-natriuretic tubular actions [49]. Our data suggests, as indicated by the increase of FE Na, that Tempol and PEG-catalase decreased tubular reabsorption. The observation that both Tempol and PEG-catalase had no effects on MAP and RBF suggests that, in this model of CKD, they acted mainly via tubular mechanisms and thus can only affect BP indirectly and hence slowly. We observed a time-dependent reduction of GFR in all groups. However, relative to baseline, the reduction in the vehicle control group was smaller than the one observed in the Tempol and PEG-catalase control groups. Moreover, no significant difference was observed between the baseline and vehicle measurements in the CKD groups.

In conclusion, in the current study we show that in established CKD MAP and RVR did not depend more on ROS than in CON. Our findings suggest that antioxidant therapy in experimental CKD, although it can prevent the increase in BP in early stages, might not be effective in reducing BP once CKD is established.

these known regulators of blood pressure and renal perfusion were not acutely affected by Tempol and PEG-catalase.

Effect of Tempol and PEG-catalase on RVR

Tempol and PEG-catalase had limited effects on RVR in CKD suggesting that renal resistance vessels are not sensitive to renal vasoconstrictor effects of ROS in this model. We found no other reports on renal hemodynamics during acute treatment with either Tempol or PEG-catalase in rats with established CKD. Because we chose for a systemic intravenous rather than renal intra-arterial administration of Tempol and PEG-catalase we cannot evaluate their direct effects on the kidney. One might hypothesize that ROS-mediated vasoconstriction in the extrarenal circulation contributes to hypertension in established, long-term CKD. Although increased myogenic tone preceded structural vascular changes and hypertension in rats with CKD induced by renal mass reduction [45], ultimately, loss of myogenic response of the mesenteric arteries was observed [46]. Moreover, segments of the

Supporting Information

Figure S1 Immunohistochemical labeling of renal tissue for tyrosine hydroxylase (TH) in CON rats (first row) and CKD rats (second row) to detect sympathetic nerves (green, white arrows).

Table S1 Gene expression of renin, AT1, ACE1 and VEGF-A in CON and CKD rats (first cohort), after intravenous infusion of with Tempol, PEG-catalase or vehicle in terminal setting. Data are presented as log fold change relative to the calibrator (vehicle treated animals in CON and CKD groups). Means ± SEM.

Acknowledgments

We thank Paula Martens, Adele Dijk, Krista den Ouden, Jan Willem de Groot and Petra de Bree for their expert laboratory assistance.

Author Contributions

Conceived and designed the experiments: DAP AvK MCV JAJ. Performed the experiments: DAP. Analyzed the data: DAP AvK MPK RLB MCV JAJ. Contributed reagents/materials/analysis tools: MPK, RLB. Wrote the paper: DAP JAJ MCV.

References

1. Galle J (2001) Oxidative stress in chronic renal failure. Nephrol Dial Transplant 16: 2135-2137.
2. Himmelfarb J (2004) Linking oxidative stress and inflammation in kidney disease: which is the chicken and which is the egg? Semin Dial 17: 449–454.
3. Oberg BP, McMenamin E, Lucas FL, McMonagle E, Morrow J, et al. (2004) Increased prevalence of oxidant stress and inflammation in patients with moderate to severe chronic kidney disease. Kidney Int 65: 1009–1016.
4. Tepel M (2003) Oxidative stress: does it play a role in the genesis of essential hypertension and hypertension of uraemia? Nephrol Dial Transplant 18: 1439–1442.
5. Vaziri ND (2004) Roles of oxidative stress and antioxidant therapy in chronic kidney disease and hypertension. Curr Opin Nephrol Hypertens 13: 93–99.
6. Makino A, Skelton MM, Zou AP, Roman RJ, Cowley AW, Jr. (2002) Increased renal medullary oxidative stress produces hypertension. Hypertension 39: 667–672.
7. Makino A, Skelton MM, Zou AP, Cowley AW, Jr. (2003) Increased renal medullary H2O2 leads to hypertension. Hypertension 42: 25–30.
8. Chen J, He J, Ogden LG, Batuman V, Whelton PK (2002) Relationship of serum antioxidant vitamins to serum creatinine in the US population. Am J Kidney Dis 39: 460–468.
9. Boaz M, Smetana S, Weinstein T, Matas Z, Gafter U, et al. (2000) Secondary prevention with antioxidants of cardiovascular disease in endstage renal disease (SPACE): randomised placebo-controlled trial. Lancet 356: 1213–1218.
10. Kamgar M, Zaldivar F, Vaziri ND, Pahl MV (2009) Antioxidant therapy does not ameliorate oxidative stress and inflammation in patients with end-stage renal disease. J Natl Med Assoc 101: 336–344.
11. Mann JF, Lonn EM, Yi Q, Gerstein HC, Hoogwerf BJ, Pogue J, et al. (2004) Effects of vitamin E on cardiovascular outcomes in people with mild-to-moderate renal insufficiency: results of the HOPE study. Kidney Int 65: 1375–1380.
12. Schnackenberg CG, Wilcox CS (1999) Two-week administration of tempol attenuates both hypertension and renal excretion of 8-Iso prostaglandin f2alpha. Hypertension 33: 424–428.
13. Nishiyama A, Yoshizumi M, Hitomi H, Kagami S, Kondo S, et al. (2004) The SOD mimetic tempol ameliorates glomerular injury and reduces mitogen-activated protein kinase activity in Dahl salt-sensitive rats. J Am Soc Nephrol 15: 306–315.
14. Beswick RA, Zhang H, Marable D, Catravas JD, Hill WD, et al. (2001) Long-term antioxidant administration attenuates mineralocorticoid hypertension and renal inflammatory response. Hypertension 37: 781–786.
15. Vaziri ND, Ding Y, Ni Z (2001) Compensatory up-regulation of nitric-oxide synthase isoforms in lead-induced hypertension; reversal by a superoxide dismutase-mimetic drug. J Pharmacol Exp Ther 298: 679–685.
16. Rancourt ME, Rodrigue ME, Agharazii M, Lariviere R, Lebel M (2010) Role of oxidative stress in erythropoietin-induced hypertension in uremic rats. Am J Physiol 23: 314–320.
17. Koeners MP, Braam B, Joles JA (2011) Perinatal inhibition of NF-kappaB has long-term antihypertensive effects in spontaneously hypertensive rats. J Hypertens 29: 1160–1166.
18. Schnackenberg CG, Welch WJ, Wilcox CS (1998) Normalization of blood pressure and renal vascular resistance in SHR with a membrane-permeable superoxide dismutase mimetic: role of nitric oxide. Hypertension 32: 59–64.
19. Guron GS, Grimberg ES, Basu S, Herlitz H (2006) Acute effects of the superoxide dismutase mimetic tempol on split kidney function in two-kidney one-clip hypertensive rats. J Hypertens 24: 387–394.
20. Hasdan G, Benchetrit S, Rashid G, Green J, Bernheim J, et al. (2002) Endothelial dysfunction and hypertension in 5/6 nephrectomized rats are mediated by vascular superoxide. Kidney Int 61: 586–590.
21. Quiroz Y, Ferrebuz A, Vaziri ND, Rodriguez-Iturbe B (2009) Effect of chronic antioxidant therapy with superoxide dismutase-mimetic drug, tempol, on progression of renal disease in rats with renal mass reduction. Nephron Exp Nephrol 112: e31–e42.
22. Hughes JM, Bund SJ (2004) Influence of experimental reduction of media/lumen ratio on arterial myogenic properties of spontaneously hypertensive and Wistar-Kyoto rats. Clin Sci (Lond) 106: 163–171.
23. Sousa T, Pinho D, Morato M, Marques-Lopes J, Fernandes E, et al. (2008) Role of superoxide and hydrogen peroxide in hypertension induced by an antagonist of adenosine receptors. Eur J Pharmacol 588: 267–276.
24. Sousa T, Oliveira S, Afonso J, Morato M, Patinha D, et al. (2012) Role of H(2)O(2) in hypertension, renin-angiotensin system activation and renal medullary disfunction caused by angiotensin II. Br J Pharmacol 166: 2386–2401.
25. Bongartz LG, Braam B, Verhaar MC, Cramer MJ, Goldschmeding R, et al. (2010) Transient nitric oxide reduction induces permanent cardiac systolic dysfunction and worsens kidney damage in rats with chronic kidney disease. Am J Physiol Regul Integr Comp Physiol 298: R815–R823.
26. Quiroz Y, Pons H, Gordon KL, Rincon J, Chavez M, et al. (2001) Mycophenolate mofetil prevents salt-sensitive hypertension resulting from nitric oxide synthesis inhibition. Am J Physiol Renal Physiol 281: F38–F47.
27. Blezer EL, Schurink M, Nicolay K, Bar PR, Jansen GH, et al. (1998) Proteinuria precedes cerebral edema in stroke-prone rats: a magnetic resonance imaging study. Stroke 29: 167–174.
28. Attia DM, Ni ZN, Boer P, Attia MA, Goldschmeding R (2002) Proteinuria is preceded by decreased nitric oxide synthesis and prevented by a NO donor in cholesterol-fed rats. Kidney Int 61: 1776–1787.
29. Racasan S, Joles JA, Boer P, Koomans HA, Braam B (2003) NO dependency of RBF and autoregulation in the spontaneously hypertensive rat. Am J Physiol Renal Physiol 285: F105–F112.
30. Patel K, Chen Y, Dennehy K, Blau J, Connors S, et al. (2006) Acute antihypertensive action of nitroxides in the spontaneously hypertensive rat. Am J Physiol Regul Integr Comp Physiol 290: R37–R43.
31. Wilcox CS, Pearlman A (2008) Chemistry and antihypertensive effects of tempol and other nitroxides. Pharmacol Rev 60: 418–469.
32. Knight SF, Yuan J, Roy S, Imig JD (2010) Simvastatin and tempol protect against endothelial dysfunction and renal injury in a model of obesity and hypertension. Am J Physiol Renal Physiol 298: F86–F94.
33. Moreno JM, Rodriguez G, I, Wangensteen R, Osuna A, Bueno P, et al. (2005) Cardiac and renal antioxidant enzymes and effects of tempol in hyperthyroid rats. Am J Physiol Endocrinol Metab 289: E776–E783.
34. Koeners MP, Braam B, van der Giezen DM, Goldschmeding R, Joles JA (2008) A perinatal nitric oxide donor increases renal vascular resistance and ameliorates hypertension and glomerular injury in adult fawn-hooded hypertensive rats. Am J Physiol Regul Integr Comp Physiol 294: R1847–R1855.
35. van Koppen A., Joles JA, Bongartz LG, van den Brandt J., Reichardt HM, et al. (2012) Healthy bone marrow cells reduce progression of kidney failure better than CKD bone marrow cells in rats with established chronic kidney disease. Cell Transplant 21: 2299–2312.
36. Mulder J, Hokfelt T, Knuepfer MM, Kopp UC (2013) Renal sensory and sympathetic nerves reinnervate the kidney in a similar time-dependent fashion after renal denervation in rats. Am J Physiol Regul Integr Comp Physiol 304: R675–R682.
37. Tanaka T, Nangaku M (2013) Angiogenesis and hypoxia in the kidney. Nat Rev Nephrol 9: 211–222.
38. Hasselwander O, Young IS (1998) Oxidative stress in chronic renal failure. Free Radic Res 29: 1–11.
39. Martin-Mateo MC, Sanchez-Portugal M, Iglesias S, de PA, Bustamante J (1999) Oxidative stress in chronic renal failure. Ren Fail 21: 155–167.
40. Mimic-Oka J, Simic T, Djukanovic L, Reljic Z, Davicevic Z (1999) Alteration in plasma antioxidant capacity in various degrees of chronic renal failure. Clin Nephrol 51: 233–241.
41. Sindhu RK, Ehdaie A, Farmand F, Dhaliwal KK, Nguyen T, et al. (2005) Expression of catalase and glutathione peroxidase in renal insufficiency. Biochim Biophys Acta 1743: 86–92.
42. Vaziri ND, Rodriguez-Iturbe B (2006) Mechanisms of disease: oxidative stress and inflammation in the pathogenesis of hypertension. Nat Clin Pract Nephrol 2: 582–593.
43. Erdei N, Bagi Z, Edes I, Kaley G, Koller A (2007) H2O2 increases production of constrictor prostaglandins in smooth muscle leading to enhanced arteriolar tone in Type 2 diabetic mice. Am J Physiol Heart Circ Physiol 292: H649–H656.
44. Gao YJ, Lee RM (2005) Hydrogen peroxide is an endothelium-dependent contracting factor in rat renal artery. Br J Pharmacol 146: 1061–1068.

45. Savage T, McMahon AC, Mullen AM, Nott CA, Dodd SM, et al. (1998) Increased myogenic tone precedes structural changes in mild experimental uraemia in the absence of hypertension in rats. Clin Sci (Lond) 95: 681–686.

46. Vettoretti S, Ochodnicky P, Buikema H, Henning RH, Kluppel CA, et al. (2006) Altered myogenic constriction and endothelium-derived hyperpolarizing factor-mediated relaxation in small mesenteric arteries of hypertensive subtotally nephrectomized rats. J Hypertens 24: 2215–2223.

47. Vavrinec P, van Dokkum RP, Goris M, Buikema H, Henning RH (2011) Losartan protects mesenteric arteries from ROS-associated decrease in myogenic constriction following 5/6 nephrectomy. J Renin Angiotensin Aldosterone Syst 12: 184–194.

48. Zou AP, Li N, Cowley AW, Jr. (2001) Production and actions of superoxide in the renal medulla. Hypertension 37: 547–553.

49. Garvin JL, Ortiz PA (2003) The role of reactive oxygen species in the regulation of tubular function. Acta Physiol Scand 179: 225–232.

19

Urine MicroRNA as Potential Biomarkers of Autosomal Dominant Polycystic Kidney Disease Progression: Description of miRNA Profiles at Baseline

Iddo Z. Ben-Dov[1¤]*, Ying-Cai Tan[2,3], Pavel Morozov[1], Patricia D. Wilson[4], Hanna Rennert[2,3], Jon D. Blumenfeld[5], Thomas Tuschl[1]

1 Laboratory of RNA Molecular Biology, Howard Hughes Medical Institute, The Rockefeller University, New York, New York, United States of America, 2 Molecular Pathology Laboratory, New York Presbyterian Hospital, Cornell University, New York, New York, United States of America, 3 Pathology and Laboratory Medicine, Weill Medical College, Cornell University, New York, New York, United States of America, 4 Centre for Nephrology, University College London Medical School, London, United Kingdom, 5 Rogosin Institute, Weill Medical College of Cornell University, New York, New York, United States of America

Abstract

Background: Autosomal dominant polycystic kidney disease (ADPKD) is clinically heterogenic. Biomarkers are needed to predict prognosis and guide management. We aimed to profile microRNA (miRNA) in ADPKD to gain molecular insight and evaluate biomarker potential.

Methods: Small-RNA libraries were generated from urine specimens of ADPKD patients (N = 20) and patients with chronic kidney disease of other etiologies (CKD, N = 20). In this report, we describe the miRNA profiles and baseline characteristics. For reference, we also examined the miRNA transcriptome in primary cultures of ADPKD cyst epithelia (N = 10), normal adult tubule (N = 8) and fetal tubule (N = 7) epithelia.

Results: In primary cultures of ADPKD kidney cells, miRNA cistrons mir-143(2) (9.2-fold), let-7i(1) (2.3-fold) and mir-3619(1) (12.1-fold) were significantly elevated compared to normal tubule epithelia, whereas mir-1(4) members (19.7-fold), mir-133b(2) (21.1-fold) and mir-205(1) (3.0-fold) were downregulated (P<0.01). Expression of the dysregulated miRNA in fetal tubule epithelia resembled ADPKD better than normal adult cells, except let-7i, which was lower in fetal cells. In patient biofluid specimens, mir-143(2) members were 2.9-fold higher in urine cells from ADPKD compared to other CKD patients, while expression levels of mir-133b(2) (4.9-fold) and mir-1(4) (4.4-fold) were lower in ADPKD. We also noted increased abundance mir-223(1) (5.6-fold), mir-199a(3) (1.4-fold) and mir-199b(1) (1.8-fold) (P<0.01) in ADPKD urine cells. In ADPKD urine microvesicles, miR-1(2) (7.2-fold) and miR-133a(2) (11.8-fold) were less abundant compared to other CKD patients (P< 0.01).

Conclusions: We found that in ADPKD urine specimens, miRNA previously implicated as kidney tumor suppressors (miR-1 and miR-133), as well as miRNA of presumed inflammatory and fibroblast cell origin (miR-223/miR-199), are dysregulated when compared to other CKD patients. Concordant with findings in the primary tubule epithelial cell model, this suggests roles for dysregulated miRNA in ADPKD pathogenesis and potential use as biomarkers. We intend to assess prognostic potential of miRNA in a followup analysis.

Editor: David Long, UCL Institute of Child Health, United Kingdom

Funding: IZB was supported by Grant Award Number UL1RR024143 from the National Center for Research Resources, a component of the National Institutes of Health (NIH) and NIH Roadmap for Medical Research. IZB was also supported in part by a fellowship from the American Physicians Fellowship for Medicine in Israel. The work described in this manuscript was also supported in part by grant number UH2TR000933 awarded by the NIH Common Fund, through the Office of Strategic Coordination/Office of the NIH Director. The funders had no role in study design, data collection and analysis, decision to publish, or preparation of the manuscript.

Competing Interests: The authors have declared that no competing interests exist.

* E-mail: iddo@hadassah.org.il

¤ Current address: Nephrology and Hypertension Services, Hadassah - Hebrew University Medical Center, Jerusalem, Israel.

Introduction

Autosomal dominant polycystic kidney disease (ADPKD) is characterized by unpredictable progression rate and incidence of complications. Research of potential therapeutics is hampered by lack of short-term surrogate markers of therapeutic effects. Reduction in glomerular filtration rate is a late occurrence in the course of the disease that manifests only after >60% of normal renal parenchyma has sustained permanent damage.

The diagnostic criteria for ADPKD are based on renal ultrasonography and a positive family history [1]. Ideally, biomarkers of disease progression should reflect short-term changes in rate of cyst development, akin to blood pressure, cholesterol and glycated hemoglobin measurements to predict long-term benefits of respective medications. Accordingly, biomarkers could be used to support early detection, assess progression risk, monitor disease progression, identify factors involved in the disease pathogenesis, and inform on the success of therapeutic interventions [2]. Currently, biomarkers for ADPKD are lacking. Although there is an inverse association of GFR with total kidney volume, significant inter-subject variation in this relationship [3] limits its role as a biomarker for the individual patient. Recently, NMR spectroscopy of urine small molecules reliably discriminated ADPKD patients with moderately advanced disease from ADPKD patients with end-stage renal disease, patients with chronic kidney disease of other etiologies, and healthy siblings. The prognostic potential of these profiles was not studied [4].

MicroRNAs (miRNA) are small regulatory non-coding RNAs expressed in plants and animals. miRNA primary transcripts (pri-miRNA) are transcribed by RNA polymerase II from independent promoters, or processed from intronic regions, and are thus governed by regulatory mechanisms common to protein-coding genes. Accordingly, abundance of miRNAs, like protein coding mRNAs, is tuned both by cell-specific and cell non-specific regulation. Some miRNA are ubiquitous, while others are strictly limited to a cell type or lineage. Of approximately 600 known human miRNAs [5], most of which are detectable by deep-sequencing in a given cell type, only the highest expressed miRNAs are able to exert regulation on their target mRNA transcripts [6]. Developmental, physiologic and disease processes can alter miRNA levels. In addition to human cells, miRNAs are also found in body fluids. miRNA are released from cells, and are protected from extracellular nuclease activity by the miRNA ribonucleoprotein complex [7] or enclosing membrane vesicle [8]. Indeed, urine [9] has been used as source of protein biomarkers in polycystic kidney disease. Several features favor a role for miRNAs in biomarker discovery. Specifically, they can be assayed using high throughput platforms, are relatively simple to analyze compared to protein or mRNA profiling, and have been occasionally found to outperform mRNA-based biomarker discovery in cancer diagnosis [10,11].

Our broad aim in this study is to examine miRNAs in ADPKD in an attempt to translate methodological advantages of miRNA profiling to the need for biomarkers in assessment of disease progression in ADPKD. miRNAs were profiled from nanogram amounts of input total RNA in clinical biofluid specimens from ADPKD patients and other chronic kidney disease (CKD) patients using deep sequencing of multiplexed small-RNA cDNA libraries. In the current report, we describe the urine miRNA profiles in relation to study group. In addition, since cystic proliferation of tubular epithelial cells is pivotal in ADPKD, we profiled miRNA in primary cultures of cyst-derived epithelial cells from ADPKD explants and normal kidneys as a cell culture model for the disease. We intend to evaluate prediction of kidney outcome by baseline miRNA abundance in a followup study.

Subjects and Methods

Ethics Statement

This study was approved by the Institutional Review Boards of the Rockefeller University Hospital and the Weill Medical College of Cornell University. Clinical data and specimens were collected after obtaining participants' written informed consent.

Cell culture samples

Primary tubule epithelial cell cultures were derived from microdissected renal tubules and explanted kidney tissues from adults without parenchymal kidney disease prepared for transplant donation but deemed unsuitable due to renal vascular structural abnormalities (N = 8) or early stage ADPKD (N = 6, National

Disease Research Interchange, Philadelphia); from surgical nephrectomy of end stage kidneys from patients with ADPKD (N = 4, PKD Foundation, Kansas) or from normal fetal kidneys after elective pregnancy termination (N = 7, Anatomic Gift Foundation, Philadelphia). Primary epithelial cells were grown to confluence in cell-type-specific supplemented media according to published techniques (**Figure S1**) [12–14]. Details of harvesting and expression markers in specimens used in this study were previously described [15]. RNA from immortalized tubular cells [16] and podocytes [17] were obtained for additional perspective.

Urine specimens

We collected urine specimens from 20 patients with ADPKD and 20 patients with CKD of other etiologies, matched for age, sex, ethnicity/race and CKD stage (**Table 1**). Patients with active immune disorders affecting the kidneys were excluded. This component of the study is registered at *ClinicalTrials.gov* (identifier: NCT01114594). ADPKD patients enrolled in this study were also registered into an ongoing data repository (*ClinicalTrials.gov* identifier: NCT00792155). Total RNA was extracted from 50 ml urine sediment cells and from the ensuing cell-free, ultrafiltration-retained supernatant, a ~250-fold concentrate of urine particles and macromolecules >100 kDa, thus including vesicle-enclosed RNA (VS2042, Vivaproducts Inc., Littleton MA) (see **Figure S2**). Small-RNA cDNA libraries were constructed and sequenced with modifications for small amounts of input RNA. Details of head-to-head comparison between precipitation-purified and silica column-purified RNA are shown in **Figure S3** [18].

Sequencing and annotation of small-RNA cDNA libraries

Extracted total RNA was subjected to barcoded adapter ligation, and the reverse-transcribed small-RNA libraries were deep sequenced on Illumina Genome Analyzer II, as previously described [19]. The resulting sequence files were trimmed and split into the separate samples according to the barcode sequences. Extracted reads were assigned annotations by aligning to the genome and small-RNA databases. For miRNA annotation we used contemporary in-house definitions [5].

We display miRNA according to our recently published definitions [5]. Briefly, reads from multi-copy miRNA are summed into single entries. For example, miR-24-1 and miR-24-2 are represented by miR-24-1(2); the number in parenthesis symbolizes the number of members. Alternatively, reads from miRNA that share pri-miRNA cistronic transcription units are collapsed into miRNA cistron (precursor) clusters. For example, cluster-mir-23a(3) represents miR-23a, miR-24-2 and miR-27a. Lastly, miRNA with extensive sequence similarity are collapsed into sequence families. For example, miR-23a and miR-23b are members of seqfam-miR-23a(2). For analysis of differential expression we employ the cistron cluster arrangement, as cistron cluster members are co-transcribed and their levels are thus highly correlated [20]. However, when analyzing extracellular RNA (urine exosomes), secretion into the biofluid and stability in the biofluid affect miRNA levels, eliminating correlation between cistron cluster members [19].

Statistical analysis

PASW 17.0 Statistics (www.spss.com) and the edgeR package for RNA sequencing on R platform [21,22] were used for statistical analyses. Patient characteristics were compared between ADPKD and other-CKD groups using standard *t*-tests. Individual patient/sample miRNA data are displayed in supplementary tables as counts derived from deep sequencing reads. In addition, counts are aggregated according to miRNA sequence families and

Table 1. Clinical characteristics of study patients and biochemical features of study specimens*.

Type of specimen	N	Gender	Age, years	eGFR, ml/min/1.73 m²	CKD stage
		M/F	mean±SD [range]	mean±SD [range]	1/2/3/4
Primary cultures	ADPKD:10	n/a	n/a	n/a	n/a
	Normal: 8	n/a	n/a	n/a	n/a
	Fetal: 7	n/a	n/a	n/a	n/a
Urine specimens	ADPKD: 20	10/10	48±13 [25–70]	57±32 [20–130]	5/3/8/4
	CKD:20	10/10	50±12 [29–69]	57±26 [20–102]	5/3/8/4

*, Abbreviations: eGFR, estimated glomerular filtration rate; CKD, chronic kidney disease; ADPKD, autosomal dominant polycystic kidney disease; n/a, not assessed or not applicable.

precursor cluster cistrons and presented in the respective supplementary tables (see above). Analyses of differential expression between ADPKD and non-ADPKD groups of samples were conducted under the assumption that gene (miRNA) counts in RNA deep sequencing data follow negative binomial distribution. The R/Bioconductor statistical package edgeR was developed with the negative binomial distribution assumption at its core. In generalized linear negative binomial models fitted with edgeR, the dependent variables are the genewise miRNA counts (expressed as counts per million miRNA counts, CPM) while the independent variable we included were disease group (e.g. ADPKD vs. other CKD urine cell pellets) and patient sex (when relevant). Fold-change values in miRNA abundance between the two groups of samples are calculated as the ratio of mean CPM in ADPKD to the mean CPM in the non-ADPKD group, and transformed to log base 2. P-values for coefficients in the model are computed by genewise likelihood ratio tests (or quasi-likelihood F-tests). Dispersion, which reflects biological variation, is estimated using the Cox-Reid method, and is inherent in the modeling procedure. Thus, within group variability impacts the statistical inference. Nominal P-values<0.05 are considered significant, provided that false detection rate (FDR) computed with the Benjamini-Hochberg method is less than 0.2.

Results

We profiled miRNA in various specimens obtained from ADPKD and non-ADPKD patients. Clinical and biochemical characteristics of the study patients and samples are summarized in **Tables 1 and 2**, and further described in **Table S1 in File S1**.

Figure 1 provides an outline perspective of the abundant miRNA across the study samples, aggregated by gender and specimen type, and presented as a heatmap. In the following sections, findings are depicted according to the type of specimen: primary cultures of human kidney cyst-lining or normal tubular epithelia as *ex vivo* disease model; urine sediment cells; and microvesicles retained following urine centrifugation and ultrafiltration.

MicroRNA content in primary cultures of renal tubule epithelia

Small-RNA categories were obtained from primary tubule epithelial cell cultures grown from microdissected renal tubules of adults (i) without parenchymal kidney disease (N = 8), (ii) with early stage (pre-dialysis) ADPKD (N=6), (iii) end-stage ADPKD kidneys (N=4), and from normal fetal kidneys (N=7) (**Table S1 in File S1**). Based on the addition of defined amounts of synthetic calibrator oligoribonucleotides [23], the miRNA content in input total RNA was 5.8 fmol/µg (interquartile range (IQR) 3.5–7.9 fmol/µg), with no significant differences between study groups.

miRNA profiles diverged in accordance with sample groups (**Figure S4**). Sequence reads derived from let-7i(1) (2.3-fold), mir-143(2) (9.1-fold) and mir-3619(1) (11.8-fold) were upregulated, and mir-1(4) (20-fold), mir-133b(2) (20.8-fold) and mir-205(1) (3.1-fold) cistron members were downregulated in primary cultures of cyst

Table 2. Clinical characteristics of study patients and biochemical features of study specimens*.

Type of specimen	Group	Total RNA	Total small RNA	Total miRNA	miRNA, fmol/µg	Urine miRNA
		ng/ml urine	read counts/10⁶	read counts/10⁵	of total RNA	fmol/l
Primary cultures	ADPKD	n/a	1.0, 0.6–1.3	4.7, 2.7–7.7	4.2, 2.8–6.7	n/a
	Normal	n/a	0.9, 0.9–1.1	5.1, 4.0–6.4	5.0, 3.2–9.5	n/a
	Fetal	n/a	1.3, 1.2–1.3	5.6, 4.3–6.2	6.9, 6.0–7.9	n/a
Urine cells	ADPKD	2.9, 1.4–11	3.5, 2.2–4.9	8.4, 4.4–16	8.1, 4.2–14	30, 8.2–83
	CKD	2.9, 1.4–7.8	3.5, 2.3–4.3	5.0, 2.7–13	7.4, 4.5–19	18, 5.6–163
Urine UF retentates	ADPKD	0.3, 0.2–0.7**	0.48, 0.28–1.2	0.17, 0.12–0.26	6.4, 3.7–9.6†	1.8, 1.0–3.7
	CKD	0.6, 0.3–0.8	0.55, 0.24–1.2	0.17, 0.07–0.35	2.8, 2.2–4.0	1.8, 0.9–4.0

*, Abbreviations: CKD, chronic kidney disease; ADPKD, autosomal dominant polycystic kidney disease; UF, ultrafiltration; n/a, not assessed or not applicable.
**, P-value = 0.056 (Mann-Whitney U test).
†, P-value = 0.02 (Mann-Whitney U test).

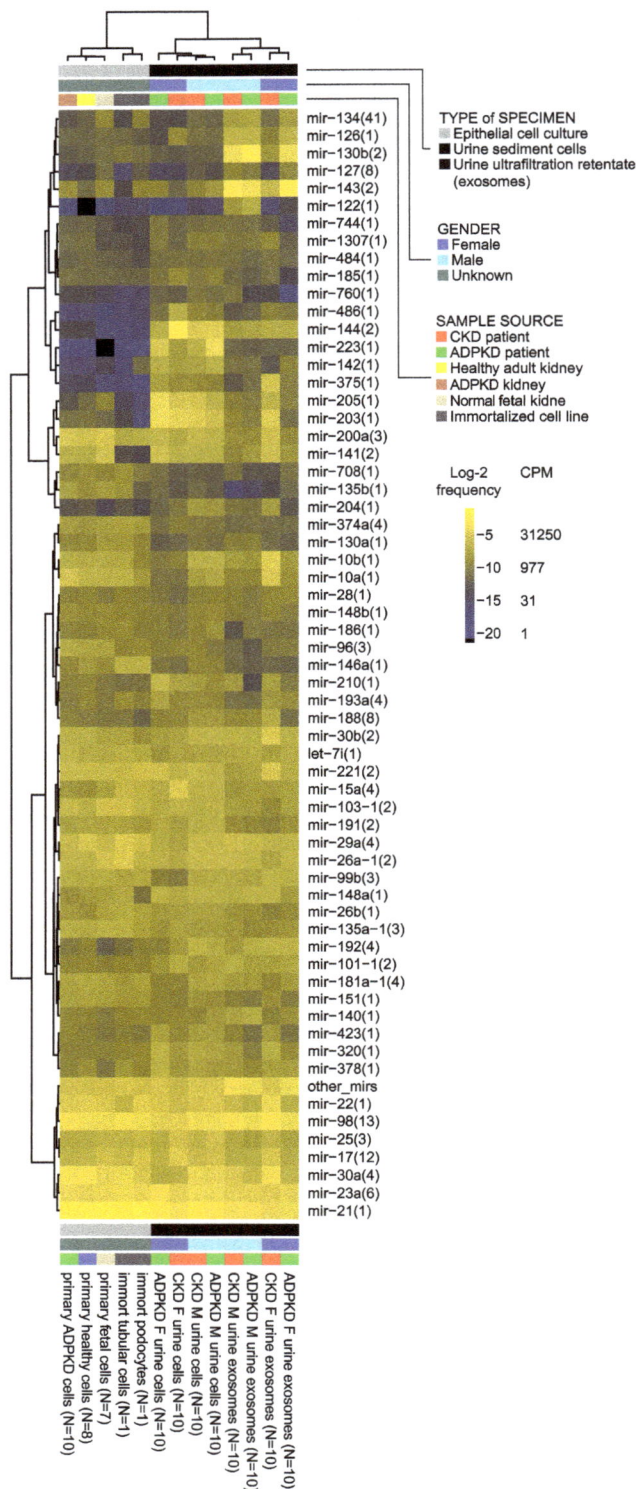

Figure 1. Hierarchically clustered study samples grouped by type and clinical characteristics. including additional non-study specimens for reference (columns) and miRNA cistrons (rows). High relative read frequency (log$_2$-transformed) is indicated by bright yellow shades; low frequencies in dark blue. Corresponding numerical data is presented in the supplementary tables. Abbreviations: ADPKD, autosomal dominant polycystic kidney disease; CKD, chronic kidney disease; immort, immortalized; CPM, counts per million; F, female; M, male.

epithelial cells compared to normal kidney-derived cells (P-values<0.01, FDR<0.2) (**Table 3**) (see **Tables S2, S3, S4, S5 in File S1** for complete count data and miRNA cluster and sequence family definitions). Resembling ADPKD-derived cells, fetal cells had similarly lower levels of mir-1(4) and mir-133b(2) members and higher levels of mir-143(2) and mir-3619(1) members compared to normal adult tubular epithelial cells (P-values<0.05, FDR<0.2) (**Table 3**).

Segmental origin of the cultured cells, determined in all specimens except end-stage ADPKD kidneys, e.g. proximal straight tubule (PST), thick ascending limb (TAL) and collecting duct (CT) had no impact upon miRNA profiles. However, cells originating in cysts of end-stage ADPKD kidneys had higher content of mir-21(1) (1.6-fold), mir-30a(4) (1.5-fold) and mir-101(2) (3.2-fold) and lower content of mir-143(2) (10-fold), compared to PST, TAL or CT-derived cells (P-values<0.01, FDR<0.2). For perspective, we provide miRNA profiles of immortalized kidney epithelial cell lines of tubular and podocyte origin (**Figure 1** and see **Tables S6, S7, S8 in File S1** for details and differential expression). None of the top 15 miRNA precursor clusters or top 40 miRNA sequence families were differentially expressed in immortalized compared to primary cells (**Table S8 in File S1**), suggesting that miRNA expression and regulatory function in immortalized cell lines may recapitulate their respective properties in primary cultures of kidney epithelial cells. Presence of SV40-miR-S1 and downregulation of miR-141/miR-200c in immortalized cells were the most striking differences in miRNA profiles compared to primary cells (**Table S7 in File S1**).

MicroRNA content in urine of ADPKD and other CKD patients

We collected urine specimens from 20 patients with ADPKD and 20 patients with chronic kidney disease (CKD) of other etiologies, matched for age, sex, ethnicity/race and CKD stage (**Table 1**). Yields of total RNA extracted from urine sediment cells and from cell-free, ultrafiltration-retained supernatant specimens (containing microvesicles) and small-RNA annotation categories are summarized in **Table 2 and Table S1 in File S1**. In *sediment cell* RNA, total RNA yield (2.9 ng per ml of urine), small-RNA annotation categories and calculated total miRNA content (7.4–8.1 fmol per μg total RNA) did not differ by disease group or gender. In *cell-free ultrafiltration-retained material* total RNA yields were 2-fold lower, but miRNA content per μg total RNA were 2.3-fold higher in ADPKD compared to non-ADPKD CKD specimens, and thus molar miRNA concentrations were overall similar; 68–104 fM (**Table 2**, and see also **Table S1 in File S1**).

Abundance of specific miRNA in urine cells and cell-free ultrafiltration-retained specimens is depicted in **Tables S9, S10, S11, S12, S23, S14 in File S1**. Compared with CKD of other etiologies, in urine cells from ADPKD mir-143(2) cluster members were upregulated, whereas mir-1(4) and related mir-133b(2) were downregulated. Moreover, there was an increased relative abundance of mir-223(1), mir-199a(3) and mir-199b(1) in ADPKD (**Table 4**). In cell-free urine ultrafiltration-retained specimens, relative abundance of mir-1(4) cistron members was lower in ADPKD compared to other CKD patients (**Table 5**).

MicroRNA sequence variants in primary cultures of normal, cyst-lining and fetal cells

We found 138 unique miRNA sequence variants across primary culture specimens relative to the reference genome, according to published criteria (**Table S15 in File S1**) [5]. Sequence variants are predominantly due to RNA editing but may represent genetic

Table 3. miRNA cistron clusters differentially expressed between ADPKD-derived and normal kidney-derived primary tubular epithelial cultures[*].

	CPM (log$_{10}$)	ADPKD (N = 10) vs. normal adult (N = 8)			fetal (N = 7) vs. normal adult (N = 8)		
		FC (log$_2$)	P-value	FDR	FC (log$_2$)	P-value	FDR
cluster-hsa-let-7i(1)	4.1	1.2	3.7E-04	2.6E-02	−0.1	7.6E-01	8.9E-01
cluster-hsa-mir-143(2)	3.5	3.2	3.6E-03	1.5E-01	2.3	2.8E-02	1.2E-01
cluster-hsa-mir-205(1)	2.9	−1.6	9.1E-05	8.9E-03	1.9	5.0E-05	9.8E-04
cluster-hsa-mir-1-1(4)	2.8	−4.3	4.5E-04	2.6E-02	−5.8	2.0E-04	3.1E-03
cluster-hsa-mir-133b(2)	1.2	−4.4	2.9E-05	8.6E-03	−4.5	7.6E-05	1.4E-03
cluster-hsa-mir-3619(1)	0.8	3.6	8.1E-05	8.9E-03	2.0	3.6E-02	1.4E-01

[*], Cutoff for presentation in this table is p-value<0.05 and FDR<0.2 in the ADPKD vs. normal comparison.

variation. Non-parametric analysis revealed that the relative abundance of 9 sequence variants (related to 8 unique miRNAs) was altered in primary ADPKD cells compared to normal cells (at $\alpha = 0.1$, **Figure 2A**). A composite score derived from the relative expression of these sequence variants (the score was defined as the number of variants with expression above median minus number of variants with expression below median) strongly discriminated ADPKD from normal renal cells (**Figure 2B**; area under the ROC curve 0.975, P = 0.001). Intriguingly, relative expression of sequence variants in urine sediment cell RNA (**Table S16 in File S1**) followed similar trends for 6 of the 8 miRNA above, and a similarly derived score discriminated ADPKD from other CKD patients' urine cells (**Figure 2C**; area under the ROC curve 0.713, P = 0.037).

Table 4. miRNA cistron clusters differentially expressed between ADPKD (N = 20) and other CKD (N = 20) patient urine sediment cells[*].

	log$_{10}$CPM	log$_2$FC	P-value	FDR
cluster-hsa-mir-223(1)	4.6	2.5	1.3E-06	1.7E-04
cluster-hsa-mir-142(1)	3.9	1.3	3.8E-03	5.8E-02
cluster-hsa-mir-143(2)	3.4	1.6	1.6E-04	6.9E-03
cluster-hsa-mir-133b(2)	3.3	−2.3	3.2E-03	5.2E-02
cluster-hsa-mir-652(1)	3.1	0.9	6.3E-03	9.1E-02
cluster-hsa-mir-338(1)	2.6	1.9	2.7E-05	2.2E-03
cluster-hsa-mir-450a-1(4)	2.5	1.2	4.4E-04	1.1E-02
cluster-hsa-mir-199a-1(3)	2.5	1.4	1.2E-03	2.5E-02
cluster-hsa-mir-199b(1)	2.4	1.8	7.8E-05	4.8E-03
cluster-hsa-mir-582(1)	2.4	1.6	2.7E-04	8.3E-03
cluster-hsa-mir-3613(1)	2.1	1.0	1.0E-02	1.4E-01
cluster-hsa-mir-1-1(4)	2.0	−2.1	3.6E-04	9.8E-03
cluster-hsa-mir-618(1)	1.8	1.5	2.7E-03	4.8E-02
cluster-hsa-mir-2115(1)	1.6	1.4	2.3E-04	7.9E-03
cluster-hsa-mir-873(2)	1.5	1.2	1.7E-03	3.2E-02
cluster-hsa-mir-2355(1)	1.5	1.9	1.4E-06	1.7E-04
cluster-hsa-mir-551a(1)	1.2	1.8	1.7E-04	6.9E-03
cluster-hsa-mir-139(1)	1.1	−1.4	1.1E-03	2.4E-02
cluster-hsa-mir-370(1)	0.8	−1.9	1.5E-02	2.0E-01

[*], Cutoff for presentation in this table is p-value<0.05 and FDR<0.2.

Mining of small-RNA reads to discover novel microRNA

Examination of sequence reads (21 to 23 nt length) that mapped to the human genome but had no matching small-RNA annotation in primary culture libraries (normal-, ADPKD- and fetal-derived cells) revealed that no single sequence exceeded a level corresponding to 0.02% of total miRNA (i.e., 200 reads per million miRNA reads). A miRNA of this level typically ranks ~250 in abundance (namely, be outcompeted in terms of argonaute occupancy and potential for target repression by ~250 higher-ranked miRNA). Thus, the existence of a previously unidentified yet biologically important kidney tubule epithelial miRNA is effectively ruled-out [6].

Discussion

In this study, we obtained expression profiles of miRNA in ADPKD patient-derived primary cell cultures and urine RNA. Sequence profiles were generated by sequencing of multiplexed small-RNA cDNA libraries constructed in-house from as low as 5 ng total RNA per sample. This technical achievement has not been reported with currently available commercial kits [24,25]. Advantages of multiplexing include shorter processing time, less labor-intensive, lower sequencing costs (we estimate 25 USD per sample for reagents and sequencing at 5 Mio reads/sample plus 75 USD per sample for labor), minimization of batch effects and thus improving the prospects for clinical research utility [23].

We studied primary cultures of epithelial cells lining ADPKD cysts as a basic model of the disease [12,14,26]. Similar cell systems were also reported to harbor phenotypic differences

Table 5. Mature miRNA differentially expressed between ADPKD (N = 20) and other CKD (N = 20) patient urine exosomal preparations[*].

	log$_{10}$CPM	log$_2$FC	P-value	FDR
hsa-miR-133a(2)	4.3	−4.0	5.0E-04	3.9E-02
hsa-miR-1(2)	4.1	−3.1	6.8E-04	3.9E-02
hsa-miR-671	4.0	1.9	6.3E-03	2.4E-01
hsa-miR-378	4.0	−1.6	1.4E-02	3.9E-01
hsa-miR-221	3.8	1.1	3.5E-02	7.9E-01
hsa-miR-98	2.7	−3.4	4.7E-02	8.7E-01

[*], Cutoff for presentation in this table is p-value<0.05.

A

miR	pre-miR pos	change	Genomic coords	pre-miR region	Pos in region	CY1	CY2	CY3	CY4	CY5	CY6	CY7	CY8	CY9	CY10	CY13	CY14	CY15	CY16	CY17	CY18	CY19	CY20	Mann-Whitney P-value
						ADPKD primary cultures										Normal primary cultures								
hsa-mir-21	10	G→c	chr17:57918633:+	5p	10	25%	33%	30%	30%	18%	36%	29%	24%	15%	0%	40%	45%	62%	23%	38%	30%	33%	29%	0.026
hsa-mir-196a-2†	64	C→t	chr12:54385599:+	miR-196a-2*	18	96%	0%	0%	0%	100%	0%	0%	69%	0%	ND	75%	62%	ND	100%	82%	96%	94%	89%	0.050
hsa-mir-30b	33	G→a	chr8:135812812:-	loop	1	ND	0%	0%	0%	ND	0%	0%	0%	0%	0%	44%	58%	0%	0%	48%	63%	0%	0%	0.038
hsa-mir-200b	44	C→a	chr1:1102537:+	loop	12	ND	ND	ND	100%	ND	100%	100%	100%	ND	ND	ND	100%	ND	ND	0%	ND	ND	97%	0.078
hsa-mir-22	71	T→a	chr17:1617207:-	3p	1	30%	14%	14%	13%	13%	9%	11%	14%	19%	0%	5%	11%	6%	10%	9%	12%	10%	10%	0.026
hsa-mir-27a	73	C→t	chr19:13947260:-	3p	1	0%	0%	5%	0%	0%	3%	0%	0%	0%	0%	8%	4%	17%	0%	25%	18%	0%	16%	0.008
hsa-mir-27a	73	C→a	chr19:13947260:-	3p	1	19%	0%	24%	15%	0%	31%	0%	0%	9%	0%	15%	10%	40%	11%	6%	54%	10%	53%	0.073
hsa-mir-25	71	C→a	chr7:99691193:-	3p	1	0%	0%	0%	68%	0%	80%	0%	0%	77%	ND	0%	0%	0%	0%	0%	0%	0%	0%	0.083
hsa-mir-324	68	G→t	chr17:7126626:-	3p	1	76%	0%	0%	0%	0%	0%	0%	0%	0%	0%	67%	94%	0%	82%	0%	0%	0%	78%	0.056

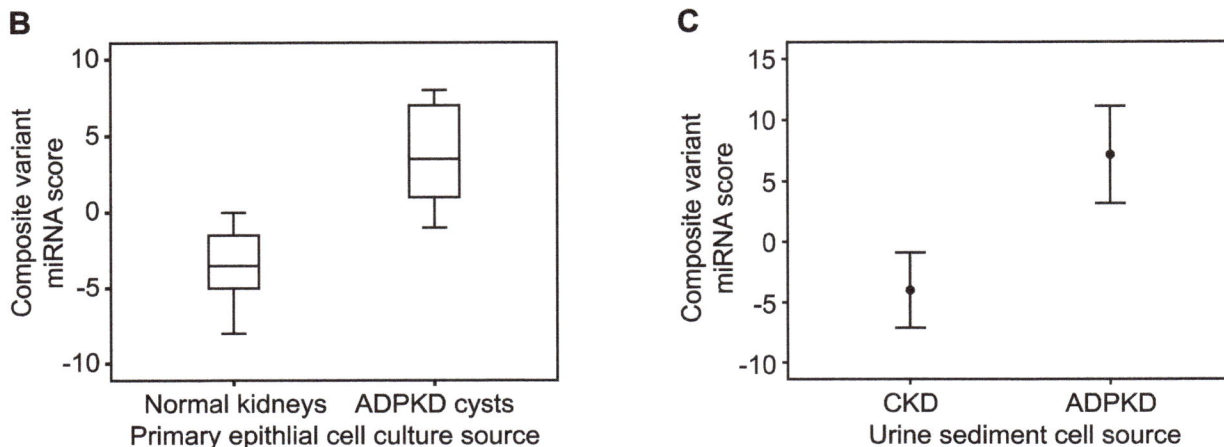

†, rs11614913:C->C/T

Figure 2. miRNA sequence variants that were found to be differentially expressed between ADPKD and non-ADPKD specimens. (A) miRNA sequence variants that were found to be differentially expressed between ADPKD cyst-derived primary cultures and normal adult kidney derived cultures (see complete list in Table S15 in File S1). **(B)** Box plot showing a composite score derived from the information in (A). The median frequency of each miRNA variant across the samples was used to generate the score; 1 point was added (or reduced) for each miRNA variant with frequency above (or below) the median frequency. **(C)** Bar plot showing a composite score derived in a manner similar to (B) from patient' urine sediment cell sequence data (contributing miRNA variants are depicted in Table S16 in File S1).

compared to normal cells, such as higher rates of proliferation, secretion and cell-matrix adhesion, decreased cell migration and abnormal polarization of specific membrane proteins such as EGFR [27–29]. Examination of miRNA profiles generated from these cells showed modest differences between ADPKD and normal renal epithelial cells. These differences were to an extent reminiscent of changes seen between normal fetal and adult cells. In line with the previously reported failure to switch-off fetal proteins [30], this finding may point to transcriptional alterations that contribute to the pathogenesis of cyst formation.

Compared to normal cells, ADPKD and fetal cells had lower levels of mir-1(4) and mir-133b(2) and higher levels of mir-143(2) and mir-3619(1) members. mir-143(2) members (predominantly miR-145) are highly abundant throughout the urinary tract, particularly in the lower segments. In contrast, mir-1(4) and mir-133b(2) are not abundantly expressed in kidneys (see below). Nonetheless, mir-1(4) and mir-133b(2) were reportedly downregulated in renal cell carcinoma (RCC) specimens and cell lines, and transfection experiments suggested that these clusters of miRNAs may be tumor suppressive in the kidney [31]. While epidemiological data do not demonstrate that patients with ADPKD bear an increased risk for RCC [32], a recent surgical specimen-based study showed 5% prevalence of RCC in ADPKD [33]. It is thus intriguing that in cultures of both fetal tubule cells and in cells obtained from ADPKD cysts, levels of mir-1(4) and mir-133b(2) cluster members were consistently lower (~25–60-fold) than in normal kidney cells, in which they constituted ~0.19% of all

miRNA (ranking 41 of 350 detectable miRNA clusters). It should be noted that mir-1(4) and mir-133b(2) have crucial roles in muscle development. Transcription of mir-1(4) clusters is regulated by prototypical myocyte differentiation factors [34] and mir-1(4) members inhibit cardiomyocyte growth and proliferation [35]. In our miRNA expression database, respective abundance of mir-1(4) and mir-133b(2) was 27.2% and 0.18% in fetal heart; 19.4% and 0.14% in adult heart; and 54.1% and 2.3% in adult skeletal muscle (Williams Z and Tuschl T, unpublished). In light of these abundance data, the functional importance of mir-1(4) and mir-133b(2) members in kidney cells, in which their level of expression is ~100-fold lower than myocytes, remains to be clarified.

We hypothesized that transcriptome-wide urine miRNA profiles would differ between ADPKD and other chronic kidney diseases, and that alterations discovered in the primary culture model may be recapitulated in the patient specimens. Indeed, abundance of specific miRNA in cellular and extracellular (exosome) specimens differed in ADPKD and non-ADPKD patients. Increased levels of mir-143(2) (urine cells) and decrease in mir-1(4) and mir-133b(2) members (urine cells and extracellular RNA) were found in ADPKD patients, extending the findings from primary cultures to clinical specimens. mir-499(1), albeit rare in kidney cells, was also significantly lower in ADPKD cell-free urine RNA compared to non-ADPKD specimens. miR-499 is encoded within an intron of the sarcomeric myosin gene, Myh7b [36], providing an additional link between ADPKD and suppression of muscle-enriched miRNA.

We observed higher levels of the lymphocyte/monocyte associated miR-223 and fibroblast-enriched miR-199a and miR-199b in ADPKD urine specimens. Monocyte infiltration [37–39] and myofibroblast transition [40] have been implicated in the pathogenesis of ADPKD. Moreover, increased levels of urine monocyte chemoattractant protein-1 (MCP1), possibly secreted by cyst epithelium, has been shown to precede increases in serum creatinine in ADPKD [41] is a potential biomarker [42]. This implies that participation of these cell types in the pathogenic process can be detected and monitored by examining spot urine samples.

In addition to analyzing differential expression (also possible with RT-PCR and hybridization-based profiling methods), we made use of information uniquely attainable by RNA sequencing. In primary culture profiles, we searched for yet undiscovered human miRNA. However, since miRNA action depends on stoichiometric interaction with their mRNA targets, exceedingly rare miRNA, even if processed and handled as prototypical miRNA, are unlikely to convey detectable post-transcriptional regulation. A study employing large-scale miRNA decoy and sensing libraries combined with RNA sequencing showed that only the most abundant miRNAs in a cell mediate target suppression and that ~60% of detected miRNAs had no discernible activity [6]. The authors proposed that miRNAs expressed at levels below 1,000 reads per million (RPM, namely 0.1% of all miRNA) do not mediate substantial regulation on natural targets. Accordingly, our finding that no un-annotated sequence in the cultured cell libraries surpassed 200 RPM practically rules-out the existence of unidentified miRNA likely to mediate target suppression in kidney tubule epithelium. Conversely, similar considerations *support* a functional role for mir-1(4) and mir-133b(2) members in normal kidney epithelial cells, in which they are present at ~1,900 RPM (0.19%), see above.

Genome-encoded and post-transcriptional alterations in miRNA sequence have bearings on miRNA stability and target repression [43], and may contribute to the biomarker potential of miRNA profiling. We mined our small-RNA libraries for variation in miRNA sequence and found evidence for previously reported miRNA SNPs and both reported and unreported RNA modifications. A subgroup of these modifications was associated with disease etiology in both primary cultures and urine sediment cells. These findings represent another unique advantage of RNA sequencing in the process of biomarker discovery.

Conclusion

We profiled miRNA in ADPKD and non-ADPKD-derived kidney epithelial cells and in two sets of ADPKD and non-ADPKD patient urine specimens. We propose a role for repression of mir-1(4) and mir-133b(2) members in the pathogenesis of ADPKD, and for their potential use as biomarkers for monitoring disease progression and response to evolving treatments. However, prospective, longitudinal studies of these miRNA members are required to establish their role as biomarkers of ADPKD. Indeed, we intend to examine prediction of ADPKD progression in a followup longitudinal study of the study participants reported herein. We also suggest that enrichment of monocyte- and fibroblast-specific miRNA in urine from ADPKD patients' urine supports their role in disease progression. Finally, we have demonstrated the feasibility of multiplexed small-RNA cDNA library preparation and sequencing from nanogram-scale input total RNA, and its utility in generating research hypotheses and in the process of biomarker discovery.

Supporting Information

Figure S1 Phase contrast images of confluent normal renal tubule and ADPKD cystic epithelial cell monolayers. (**A**) primary fetal, (**B**) primary adult, (**C**) primary early ADPKD and (**D**) primary end-stage ADPKD.

Figure S2 Electron micrographs of a representative urine ultrafiltration retentate specimen showing vesicular structures of different sizes; uranyl-acetate ('negative') stain.

Figure S3 Parallel miRNA profiling from selected split urine ultrafiltration retentate samples. (exosome preparations). (**A**) Experimental design – urine specimens were homogenized with TRIzol LS (Life Technologies – Invitrogen), RNA was extracted with chloroform, and the aqueous phase split and subjected to either isopropanol precipitation or miRNeasy silica column purification (Qiagen). For precipitation, glycogen (15 µg) was added prior to isopropanol, and precipitation carried out overnight at $-20°C$. (**B**) Differentially extracted miRNA (silica column vs. isopropanol precipitation) as determined with edgeR [22] by adjusting for specimen (blocking factor). Seven miRNA were differentially extracted at P-value<0.05; however, false detection rate (FDR) was >0.2 in all cases. Six of seven miRNA were enriched in column purifications compared to precipitation. Average GC content of enriched miRNA was 51% (range 36 to 68%), and average minimum free energy of optimal secondary structure -2.0 kcal/mol (range -3.5 to 0 kcal/mol). As opposed to Kim YK et al [18], we did not observe depletion of miR-141 or other miRNA with low GC content and stable secondary structure. We suggest that prolonged incubation in the presence of glycogen as co-precipitant may account for relatively more efficient recovery of these miRNA by isopropanol precipitation in our study [18].

Figure S4 miRNA profiles in primary cultures of renal tubule epithelia. (**a**) Hierarchically clustered samples (columns) and miRNA cistrons (rows). High relative read frequency (log2-transformed) is indicated by bright yellow shades; low frequencies in dark blue. Selected miRNA cistrons are color-shaded to denote dysregulation in ADPKD-descended cultures. (**b**) MA plot generated showing miRNA cistron differential expression between normal adult kidney and ADPKD cyst-derived epithelial cultures (R/Bioconductor; 'edgeR' package). (**c**) Multidimensional scaling (MDS) plot of primary culture samples according to miRNA cistron expression profiles (R/Bioconductor; 'limma' package).

File S1 Contains. **Table S1. Small RNA annotation categories across types of study samples, given as percentage of all post-filtering reads. Table S2. Tusch$_1$ lab miRNA group definitions. Table S3. Merged mature miRNA profiles of primary kidney cell cultures. Table S4. miRNA precursor (cistron) cluster profiles of primary kidney cell cultures. Table S5. miRNA sequence family profiles of primary kidney cell cultures. Table S6. Merged mature miRNA profiles of pooled primary and immortalized kidney cell cultures. Table S7. miRN$_A$ precursor (cistron) profiles of pooled primary and immortalized kidney cell cultures. Table S8. miRN$_A$ sequence family profiles of pooled primary and immortalized kidney cell cultures. Table S9. Merged mature miRNA profiles of patients' urine sediment cells. Table**

S10. iRNA precursor (cistron) cluster profiles of patients' urine sediment cells. Table S11. miRNA sequence family profiles of patients' urine sediment cells. Table S12. merged mature miRNA profiles of patients' urine exosome preparations. Table S13. miRNA precursor (cistron) cluster profiles of patients' urine exosome preparations. Table S14. miRNA sequence family profiles of patients' urine exosome preparations. Table S15. miRNA sequence variants in profiles generated from primary kidney cell cultures. Table S16. miRNA sequence variants in profiles generated from patients' urine sediment cells.

Author Contributions

Conceived and designed the experiments: IZB HR JDB TT. Performed the experiments: IZB YCT. Analyzed the data: IZB PM. Contributed reagents/materials/analysis tools: PDW PM. Wrote the paper: IZB. Revised the manuscript: PDW HR JDB TT.

References

1. Pei Y, Obaji J, Dupuis A, Paterson AD, Magistroni R, et al. (2009) Unified criteria for ultrasonographic diagnosis of ADPKD. J Am Soc Nephrol 20: 205–212.
2. Myrvang H (2011) Polycystic kidney disease: Urinary fingerprints unique to patients with ADPKD. Nat Rev Nephrol 7: 244.
3. Grantham JJ, Torres VE, Chapman AB, Guay-Woodford LM, Bae KT, et al. (2006) Volume progression in polycystic kidney disease. The New England journal of medicine 354: 2122–2130.
4. Gronwald W, Klein MS, Zeltner R, Schulze BD, Reinhold SW, et al. (2011) Detection of autosomal dominant polycystic kidney disease by NMR spectroscopic fingerprinting of urine. Kidney Int 79: 1244–1253.
5. Farazi TA, Horlings HM, Ten Hoeve JJ, Mihailovic A, Halfwerk H, et al. (2011) MicroRNA sequence and expression analysis in breast tumors by deep sequencing. Cancer research 71: 4443–4453.
6. Mullokandov G, Baccarini A, Ruzo A, Jayaprakash AD, Tung N, et al. (2012) High-throughput assessment of microRNA activity and function using microRNA sensor and decoy libraries. Nat Meth 9: 840–846.
7. Arroyo JD, Chevillet JR, Kroh EM, Ruf IK, Pritchard CC, et al. (2011) Argonaute2 complexes carry a population of circulating microRNAs independent of vesicles in human plasma. Proceedings of the National Academy of Sciences of the United States of America 108: 5003–5008.
8. Fleissner F, Goerzig Y, Haverich A, Thum T (2012) Microvesicles as novel biomarkers and therapeutic targets in transplantation medicine. American journal of transplantation : official journal of the American Society of Transplantation and the American Society of Transplant Surgeons 12: 289–297.
9. Kistler AD, Mischak H, Poster D, Dakna M, Wuthrich RP, et al. (2009) Identification of a unique urinary biomarker profile in patients with autosomal dominant polycystic kidney disease. Kidney international 76: 89–96.
10. Lu J, Getz G, Miska EA, Alvarez-Saavedra E, Lamb J, et al. (2005) MicroRNA expression profiles classify human cancers. Nature 435: 834–838.
11. Rosenfeld N, Aharonov R, Meiri E, Rosenwald S, Spector Y, et al. (2008) MicroRNAs accurately identify cancer tissue origin. Nature biotechnology 26: 462–469.
12. Wilson PD (1991) Monolayer cultures of microdissected renal tubule epithelial segments. J Tiss Culture Methods 13: 137–142.
13. Wilson PD, Dillingham MA, Breckon R, Anderson RJ (1985) Defined human renal tubular epithelia in culture: growth, characterization, and hormonal response. The American journal of physiology 248: F436–443.
14. Wilson PD, Schrier RW, Breckon RD, Gabow PA (1986) A new method for studying human polycystic kidney disease epithelia in culture. Kidney Int 30: 371–378.
15. Wilson PD, Devuyst O, Li X, Gatti L, Falkenstein D, et al. (2000) Apical plasma membrane mispolarization of NaK-ATPase in polycystic kidney disease epithelia is associated with aberrant expression of the beta2 isoform. Am J Pathol 156: 253–268.
16. Rohatgi R, Battini L, Kim P, Israeli S, Wilson PD, et al. (2008) Mechanoregulation of intracellular Ca2+ in human autosomal recessive polycystic kidney disease cyst-lining renal epithelial cells. Am J Physiol Renal Physiol 294: F890–899.
17. Saleem MA, O'Hare MJ, Reiser J, Coward RJ, Inward CD, et al. (2002) A conditionally immortalized human podocyte cell line demonstrating nephrin and podocin expression. Journal of the American Society of Nephrology : JASN 13: 630–638.
18. Kim YK, Yeo J, Kim B, Ha M, Kim VN (2012) Short structured RNAs with low GC content are selectively lost during extraction from a small number of cells. Molecular cell 46: 893–895.
19. Williams Z, Ben-Dov IZ, Elias R, Mihailovic A, Brown M, et al. (2013) Comprehensive profiling of circulating microRNA via small RNA sequencing of cDNA libraries reveals biomarker potential and limitations. Proceedings of the National Academy of Sciences of the United States of America 110: 4255–4260.
20. Landgraf P, Rusu M, Sheridan R, Sewer A, Iovino N, et al. (2007) A mammalian microRNA expression atlas based on small RNA library sequencing. Cell 129: 1401–1414.
21. Robinson MD, McCarthy DJ, Smyth GK (2010) edgeR: a Bioconductor package for differential expression analysis of digital gene expression data. Bioinformatics 26: 139–140.
22. McCarthy DJ, Chen Y, Smyth GK (2012) Differential expression analysis of multifactor RNA-Seq experiments with respect to biological variation. Nucleic Acids Res 40: 4288–4297.
23. Hafner M, Renwick N, Brown M, Mihailovic A, Holoch D, et al. (2011) RNA-ligase-dependent biases in miRNA representation in deep-sequenced small RNA cDNA libraries. RNA 17: 1697–1712.
24. Muthukumar T, Dadhania D, Ding R, Snopkowski C, Naqvi R, et al. (2005) Messenger RNA for FOXP3 in the Urine of Renal-Allograft Recipients. The New England journal of medicine 353: 2342–2351.
25. Hanke M, Kausch I, Dahmen G, Jocham D, Warnecke JM (2007) Detailed Technical Analysis of Urine RNA-Based Tumor Diagnostics Reveals ETS2/Urokinase Plasminogen Activator to Be a Novel Marker for Bladder Cancer. Clin Chem 53: 2070–2077.
26. Wilson PD (2009) In vitro methods in Renal Research. In: E. D. . Avner, W. . Harmon and P. . Niaudet, editors. Pediatric Nephrology. Lippincott Williams & Wilkins.
27. Wilson PD (2004) Polycystic kidney disease: new understanding in the pathogenesis. The international journal of biochemistry & cell biology 36: 1868–1873.
28. Wilson PD (2001) Polycystin: new aspects of structure, function, and regulation. J Am Soc Nephrol 12: 834–845.
29. Wilson PD (2004) Polycystic kidney disease. The New England journal of medicine 350: 151–164.
30. Burrow CR, Devuyst O, Li X, Gatti L, Wilson PD (1999) Expression of the beta2-subunit and apical localization of Na+-K+-ATPase in metanephric kidney. The American journal of physiology 277: F391–403.
31. Kawakami K, Enokida H, Chiyomaru T, Tatarano S, Yoshino H, et al. (2012) The functional significance of miR-1 and miR-133a in renal cell carcinoma. Eur J Cancer 48: 827–836.
32. Orskov B, Sorensen VR, Feldt-Rasmussen B, Strandgaard S (2012) Changes in causes of death and risk of cancer in Danish patients with autosomal dominant polycystic kidney disease and end-stage renal disease. Nephrol Dial Transplant 27: 1607–1613.
33. Jilg CA, Drendel V, Bacher J, Pisarski P, Neeff H, et al. (2013) Autosomal Dominant Polycystic Kidney Disease: Prevalence of Renal Neoplasias in Surgical Kidney Specimens. Nephron Clin Pract 123: 13–21.
34. Zhao Y, Samal E, Srivastava D (2005) Serum response factor regulates a muscle-specific microRNA that targets Hand2 during cardiogenesis. Nature 436: 214–220.
35. Meder B, Katus HA, Rottbauer W (2008) Right into the heart of microRNA-133a. Genes & development 22: 3227–3231.
36. van Rooij E, Quiat D, Johnson BA, Sutherland LB, Qi X, et al. (2009) A family of microRNAs encoded by myosin genes governs myosin expression and muscle performance. Developmental cell 17: 662–673.
37. Karihaloo A, Koraishy F, Huen SC, Lee Y, Merrick D, et al. (2011) Macrophages promote cyst growth in polycystic kidney disease. J Am Soc Nephrol 22: 1809–1814.
38. Swanson MS, Dreyfuss G (1988) Classification and purification of proteins of heterogeneous nuclear ribonucleoprotein particles by RNA-binding specificities. Mol Cell Biol 8: 2237–2241.
39. Ta MH, Harris DC, Rangan GK (2013) Role of interstitial inflammation in the pathogenesis of polycystic kidney disease. Nephrology (Carlton) 18: 317–330.
40. Schieren G, Rumberger B, Klein M, Kreutz C, Wilpert J, et al. (2006) Gene profiling of polycystic kidneys. Nephrol Dial Transplant 21: 1816–1824.
41. Zheng D, Wolfe M, Cowley BD Jr, Wallace DP, Yamaguchi T, et al. (2003) Urinary excretion of monocyte chemoattractant protein-1 in autosomal dominant polycystic kidney disease. J Am Soc Nephrol 14: 2588–2595.
42. Meijer E, Boertien WE, Nauta FL, Bakker SJ, van Oeveren W, et al. (2010) Association of urinary biomarkers with disease severity in patients with autosomal dominant polycystic kidney disease: a cross-sectional analysis. Am J Kidney Dis 56: 883–895.
43. Slaby O, Bienertova-Vasku J, Svoboda M, Vyzula R (2012) Genetic polymorphisms and microRNAs: new direction in molecular epidemiology of solid cancer. Journal of cellular and molecular medicine 16: 8–21.

20

Serum CXCL16 as a Novel Marker of Renal Injury in Type 2 Diabetes Mellitus

Leping Zhao[1]ⓨ, Fan Wu[2]ⓨ, Leigang Jin[3], Tingting Lu[3], Lihui Yang[1], Xuebo Pan[3], Chuanfeng Shao[1], Xiaokun Li[3], Zhuofeng Lin[2,3]*

1 The affiliated Yueqing Hospital of Wenzhou Medical University, Wenzhou Zhejiang, China, **2** Engineering Research Center of Bioreactor and Pharmaceutical Development, Ministry of Education, Jilin Agricultural University, Changchun, Jilin, China, **3** School of Pharmacy, Wenzhou Medical University, Chashan College Park, Wenzhou Zhejiang, China

Abstract

Background: Soluble C-X-C chemokine ligand 16 (CXCL16), a scavenger receptor for oxidized low density lipoprotein, has been shown to promote atherogenic effects *in vivo* and to predict long-term mortality in acute coronary syndrome. The aim of this study was to explore the association of circulating CXCL16 levels with diabetic subjects with and without renal disease.

Methodology/Principal Findings: One hundred twenty Chinese subjects, which included patients with type 2 diabetes mellitus (T2DM), diabetic nephropathy (DN), and CKD, as well as healthy controls, were enrolled in this study. Serum CXCL16 levels were examined by immunoassay and other clinical biochemical parameters were tested based on standard methods. Our results indicated that, HDL and LDL cholesterol levels are significantly different in DN but not in T2D patients in comparison with healthy subjects. On the other hand, Serum CXCL16 levels were significantly increased in DN subjects compared with age and gender matched healthy and T2DM subjects (p<0.05 respectively). However, no significant changes in serum CXCL16 levels were found between T2DM and healthy subjects. Furthermore, serum CXCL16 concentration negatively correlated with estimated glomerular filtrate rate, creatinine clearance rate and blood albumin, and positively with 24 h proteinuria, blood urea nitrogen (BUN), creatinine, and uric acid after adjusting for age, gender and BMI in subjects with DN. Multiple stepwise regression analyses indicated that serum CXCL16 levels were independently associated with serum 24 h proteinuria, and BUN (p<0.05 respectively).

Conclusion: Serum CXCL16 may be an indicator of renal injury in subjects with T2DM. Understanding the exact mechanism of elevated CXCL16 in subjects with DN requires further study.

Editor: Utpal Sen, University of Louisville, United States of America

Funding: This work was supported by grants from "Scientific Technological Projects of Wenzhou", H20100026 (Z. Lin), H2009 (X. Pan), and Natural Science Project of Zhejiang Province, Y2110339 (Z. Lin) and LY12H07002 (L.Zhao). The funders had no role in study design, data collection and analysis, decision to publish, or preparation of the manuscript.

Competing Interests: The authors have declared that no competing interests exist.

* E-mail: zhuofenglin@wzmc.edu.cn

ⓨ These authors contributed equally to this work.

Introduction

C-X-C chemokine ligand 16 (CXCL16), a member of the scavenger receptors, appears to be the primary receptor for oxidized low-density lipoprotein (oxLDL) based on atherogenesis studies[1–5]. It has been shown to promote atherogenic effects *in vivo* through the endocytosis of oxLDL and activation of proinflammatory cascades following ligand binding[1,4,6]. For instance, CXCL16 was found to be associated with long-term mortality after adjustment for other risk factors in patients with acute coronary syndrome[7]. Additionally, CXCL16 levels were increased significantly with severity of renal injury caused by hypercholesterolemia and oxLDL generation after unilateral ureteral obstruction[8,9]. Furthermore, CXCL16 was found to be expressed in podocytes and to act as a scavenger receptor for oxLDL in the pathology of glomerular kidney diseases, notably membranous nephropathy[10]. Recent, our study indicated that

serum CXCL16 levels were significantly increased in CKD and gout subjects and were independently associated with a change of renal function[11,12]. Taken together, these findings implicate that CXCL16 plays an important role in the pathogenesis of renal disease.

Diabetic nephropathy (DN) is a progressive kidney disease and a well-known complication of long-standing diabetes[13]. DN is the most frequent reason for dialysis in many Western countries. Early diagnosis may enable development of specific drugs and early initiation of therapy, thereby postponing or even preventing the need for renal replacement therapy. Our previous work showed that serum CXCL16 levels in DN were significantly higher than those of CKD patients without diabetes[12]. However, whether CXCL16 levels can be attributed to the onset and development of DN from the early stages of diabetes is still unclear. To explore the physiological and pathological characteristics of CXCL16 in

Table 1 Anthropometric parameters and biochemical index among subjects with T2DM, DN, CKD and healthy.

Variables	Controls (n = 30)	T2DM (n = 30)	DN (n = 30)	CKD (n = 30)	p for trend
Age (years)	47.56±1.60	49.81±2.06	48.65±1.71	49.13±1.89	NS
Gender, male (%)	63%	75%	65%	60.9%	NS
BMI (kg/m²)	22.58±0.66	24.07±0.79	22.76±0.500	22.78±0.70	NS
Hypertension					
Systolic pressure (mmHg)	116.0±2.86	120.0±8.94	149.1±3.5^c	117.7±3.15†††	<0.001
Diastolic pressure (mmHg)	74.86±1.85	83.07±2.56^a	88.55±3.39^c	78.82±2.16†	0.002
The presence of hypertension (%)	0	30%	60%	0	-
Lipid profiles					
Total Cholesterol (mmol/L)	4.82±0.17	5.26±0.30	5.12±0.30	5.83±0.63	NS
HDL-cholesterol (mmol/L)	1.31±0.06	1.24±0.07	1.06±0.09^a	1.16±0.09	0.032
LDL-cholesterol (mmol/L)	2.64±0.11	2.47±0.24	2.86±0.27^a	3.68±0.46	0.017
Triglyceride (mmol/L)	1.34±0.15	1.85±0.50	2.17±0.28^a	1.93±0.34	NS
Glucose metabolism					
Fasting glucose (mmol/L)	4.99±0.11	9.49±0.51^c	6.10±0.37^c	4.66±0.13	<0.001
2h glucose (mmol/L)	6.20±0.30	18.39±0.94^c	11.29±1.49^c	6.64±0.53	<0.001
Fasting insulin (IU/L)	6.75±0.90	12.36±2.73^c	15.28±3.62^c	8.28±2.82	<0.001
Laboratory values					
BUN (mmol/L)	5.16±0.38	5.05±0.32	14.38±2.13^c	6.97±0.93††	<0.001
Creatinine (mg/dL)	62.91±3.798	62.16±3.199	382.4±64.70^c	154.0±34.25††	<0.001
Uric acid (μmol/L)	298.7±13.24	288.7±14.35	432.1±41.95^b	386.0±23.78	<0.001
CCR (mL/min)	91.49±4.23	98.05±4.48	36.35±7.65^c	45.76±6.83††	<0.001
eGFR	102.0±3.08	108.8±3.97	31.95±7.87^c	57.30±6.32††	0.012
24 h proteinuria (mg/24 h)	52.3±5.71	61.8±12.56	902.7±300.5^c	723.3±216.5†	0.045
24 h proteinuria positive (%)	0	0	27(90%)	23(76%)	-
Albumin (g/L)	41.31±2.08	40.83±0.60	29.96±1.48^c	25.34±1.78†	<0.001
hs-CRP (mg/L)	480.0±130.1	8892±1231^c	1280.4±188.6^c	789.7±139.5	<0.001

NS: not significant. Results are expressed as frequencies, mean±SD, or median (interquartile range) as appropriate. ^{a}, p<0.05 vs. Healthy; ^{b}, p<0.01 vs. Healthy; ^{c}, p<0.001 vs. Healthy; †, p<0.05 vs. DN; ††, p<0.05 vs. DN; †††, p<0.05 vs. DN.

subjects with diabetes and DN, we measured the serum CXCL16 levels in 120 Chinese subjects and analyzed its association with a cluster of metabolic parameters. Our data demonstrate that serum CXCL16 levels are significantly increased in subjects with DN, but not diabetes, and they are independently associated with renal function in DN.

Materials and Methods

Subjects

A total of 120 Chinese subjects including those with type 2 diabetic mellitus (T2DM, n = 30), diabetic nephropathy (DN, n = 30), chronic kidney disease (CKD, n = 30) and their respective age and sex-matched controls (n = 30) were recruited from the 2nd affiliated Hospital of Wenzhou Medical University. T2DM was diagnosed according to American Diabetic Association criteria (2007), and DN was classified according to either the presence of microalbuminuria (30 to 300 mg albumin/24 hours or an albumin to creatinine ratio [ACR] of 3.4 to 34.0 mg/mmol [30 to 300 mg/g]) or macroalbuminuria (>300 mg albumin/24 hours or ACR >34 mg/mmol [300 mg/g]). DN was also classified on the basis of renal biopsy. Patients with a sustained reduction (≥3 months) in estimated glomerular filtration rate (eGFR) of ≤60 ml min^{-1} 1.73 m^{-2} based on the simplified Modification of Diet in

Renal Disease formula were recruited as CKD subjects in the present study. The eGFR values were determined based on our previous report[14]. CKD patients with other complications such as coronary heart disease, diabetes and other relevant diseases would be excluded in the present study. All subjects in the T2DM, DN and CKD groups did not receive any treatment before recruitment. Subjects with following conditions were excluded from this study: biliary obstructive diseases, acute or chronic viral hepatitis, cirrhosis, known hyperthyroidism or hypothyroidism, presence of cancer, current treatment with systemic corticosteroids, and pregnancy. We also included 30 healthy subjects who underwent a routine health examination at the 2nd Affiliated Hospital of Wenzhou Medical College, had no history of medical disease, and were not taking regular medication. All healthy subjects were selected based on the results of a physician's questionnaire and laboratory tests. All studies were approved by the Ethics Committee of Wenzhou Medical College, and all patients provided written informed consent.

Clinical Data and Laboratory test

All subjects were assessed after overnight fasting for at least 10 hours. Data on demographic characteristics, medical history, current medications, and blood samples were collected from all subjects at the time of enrollment. Blood samples were immedi-

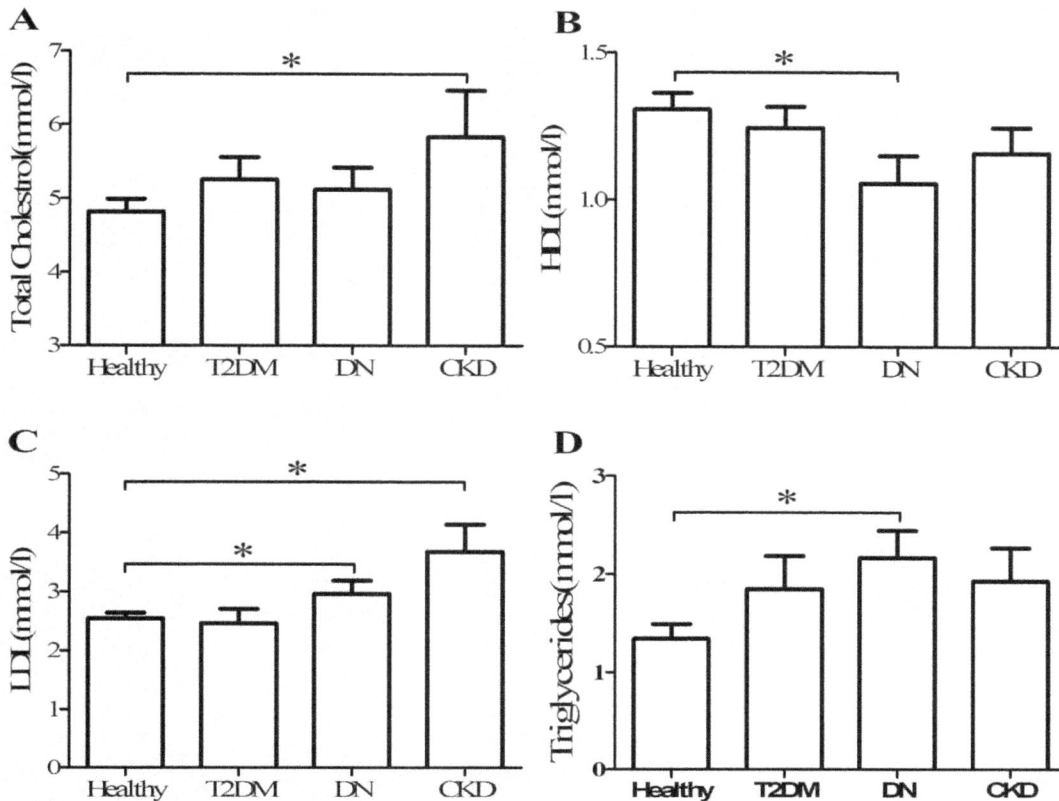

Figure 1. Serum concentration of total cholesterol(A), HDL (B), LDL (C), and triglycerides (D) among T2DM, DN, CKD, and healthy subjects. *, p<0.05.

ately centrifuged, separated into aliquots, and stored at $-80°C$ for future batched assays. Serum creatinine, phosphate, and albumin were measured with standard commercial assays. Serum CXCL16 (R&D, Minneapolis, MN, USA) and CRP (Antibody and Immunoassay Services, HK)concentrations were measured in duplicate with commercially available enzyme-linked immunosorbent assays according to the manufacturers' instructions in the Core Laboratory of School of Pharmacy, Wenzhou Medical College. All other clinical biochemistry tests were processed in the Clinical Examination Laboratory of the 2nd Affiliated Hospital of Wenzhou Medial College after a single thaw.

Statistical analysis

All analyses were performed with Statistical Package for Social Sciences version 13.0 (SPSS, Chicago, IL), and the statistical analysis was done similarly as described by Lin Z. et al[15]. Normally distributed data were expressed as mean ± SD. Data that were not normally distributed, as determined using the Kolmogorox-Smirnov test, were logarithmically transformed before analysis and expressed as the median with interquartile range. Student's unpaired t-test was used for comparison between the two groups. Pearson's correlations were used for comparisons between groups when appropriate, and multiple testing was corrected using Bonferroni correction. The variables which correlated significantly with serum CXCL16 (after Bonferroni correction for multiple testing) were selected to enter into stepwise logistic regression. In all statistical tests, P-values <0.05 were considered significant.

Results

Characteristics of Study Subjects

Characteristics of T2DM patients (n = 30), DN patients (n = 30), CKD patients (n = 30), and age- and gender-matched healthy subjects (n = 30) are described in Table 1. Compared to the subjects with T2DM, DN patients had higher systolic pressure, fasting insulin, BUN, creatinine, uric acid, phosphate, and 24 h proteinuria compared with T2DM and healthy subjects. They also had lower fasting glucose, 2-h glucose, creatinine clearance rate (CCR), eGFR, blood albumin, and high sensitive C-reactive protein (hs-CRP) levels. Compared to the subjects with DN, CKD disease control subjects had higher total cholesterol, LDL, HDL, CCR, and eGFR levels, and they had lower systolic pressure, diastolic pressure, fasting glucose, 2-h glucose, fasting insulin, BUN, and creatinine levels (Table 1, all p<0.05).

In lipid profiles, plasma concentrations of total cholesterol were similar in T2DM, DN and CKD patients, and higher than in controls(Figure 1A); whereas HDL cholesterol levels were clearly lower only in DN and CKD than that in healthy but not in T2DM(Figure 1B). LDL cholesterol levels were also higher in DN and CKD than that in T2DM and healthy (Figure 1C). Eventually, triglyceride levels were uniformly higher in T2DM, DN and CKD than that in healthy (Figure 1D). These data suggested that HDL and LDL cholesterol levels are significantly different in DN but not in T2DM patients in comparison with healthy subjects.

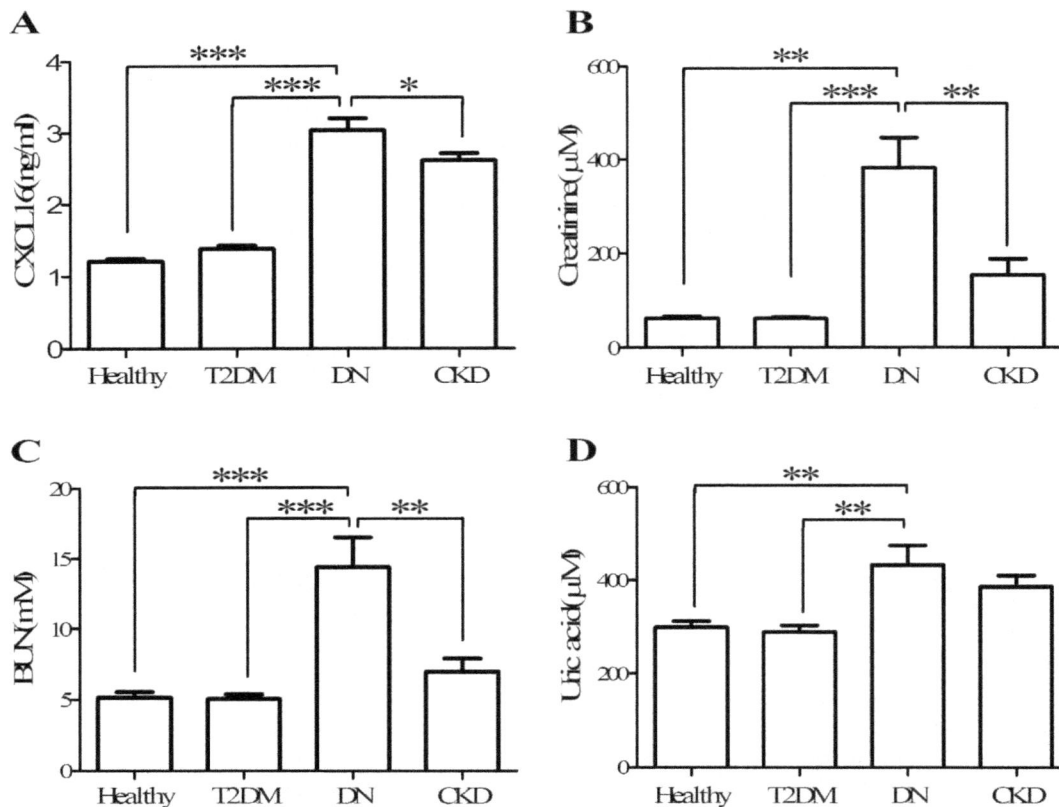

Figure 2. Serum concentration of CXCL16 (A), creatinine (B), BUN (C), and uric acid (D) among T2DM, DN, CKD, and healthy subjects. *, $p < 0.05$; **, $p < 0.01$; ***, $p < 0.001$.

Serum CXCL16 levels are increased in patients with diabetic nephropathy, but not in T2DM

Consistent with our previous reports [11,12], our data show that fasting serum CXCL16 levels were significantly increased in subjects with CKD (2.65 ± 0.11 ng/ml) compared with healthy subjects (1.30 ± 0.05 ng/ml, $p < 0.05$). Serum CXCL16 levels in subjects with DN (3.04 ± 0.16 ng/ml) were also significantly increased compared with T2DM subjects and healthy controls ($p < 0.05$, Figure 2A). No significant changes in serum CXCL16 levels were observed between T2DM and healthy subjects (1.31 ± 0.03 vs. 1.23 ± 0.04 ng/ml). Additionally, circulating CXCL16 levels were significantly higher in subjects with DN than in age- and gender-matched CKD subjects ($p < 0.05$, Figure 2A), and this is consistent with our previous study [12].

Serum CXCL16 levels were strongly associated with renal function in subjects with DN

Creatinine, BUN, and uric acid are conventional biomarkers reflecting the decline of renal function in CKD patients [16,17]. As shown in Figure 2B, 2C, and 2D, serum CXCL16 levels paralleled trends of creatinine, BUN, and uric acid levels among T2DM, DN, and healthy subjects, suggesting that circulating CXCL16 levels may be related to the change of renal function in these patients. To further explore the relationship between CXCL16 and renal function in subjects with DN, correlation analyses were performed. As shown in Table 2 and Figure 3, circulating CXCL16 levels were negatively correlated with endogenous creatinine clearance rate (CCR), eGFR and blood albumin, and

they positively correlated with creatinine, BUN, uric acid and 24 h proteinuria in DN subjects after adjustment for age, gender and BMI ($p < 0.05$ respectively).

Table 2 Correlation of serum CXCL16 levels with anthropometric parameters, biochemical indexes and other relevant factors in subjects with DN (n = 30).

	Serum CXCL16		Serum CXCL16*	
	r	p	r	p
Age	0.217	NS	-	-
Gender	−0.204	NS	-	-
BMI	0.251	0.042	-	-
Systolic stress	0.362	0.013	0.285	NS
CCR	−0.438	0.002	−0.402	0.013
eGFR	−0.454	0.006	−0.406	0.015
CRP	0.494	0.004	0.298	NS
Blood albumin	−0.409	0.007	−0.331	0.036
24 h proteinuria	0.532	<0.001	0.476	<0.001
BUN	0.497	0.004	0.484	0.008
Creatinine	0.512	0.003	0.445	0.015
Uric acid	0.357	0.011	0.293	0.042

*Adjusted for age, gender, and BMI. NS: not significant.

A

B

C

D

E

F

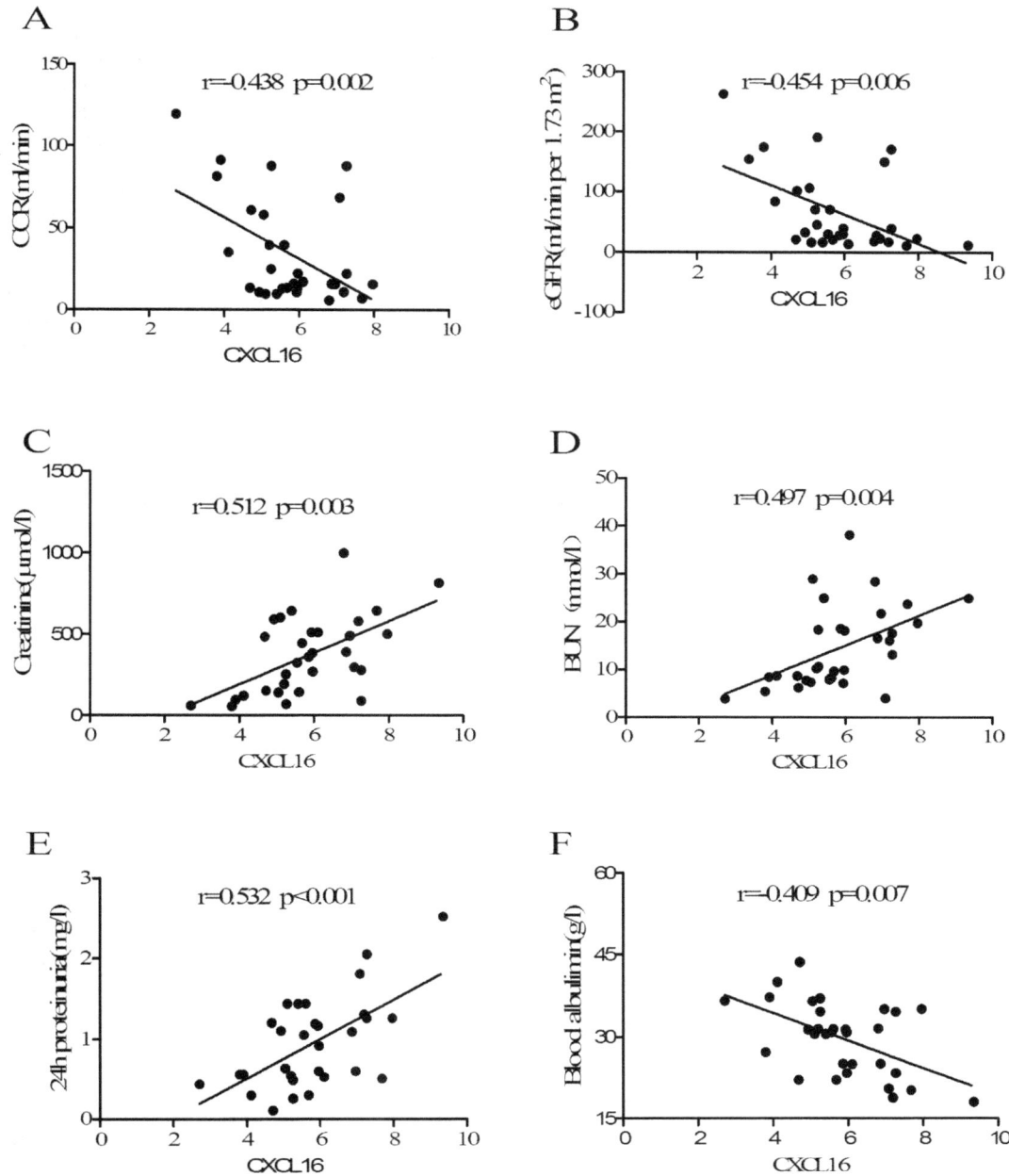

Figure 3. Correlation of serum CXCL16 levels with CCR (A), eGFR (B), creatinine (C), BUN (D), 24 h proteinuria (E), and blood albumin (F) in subjects with DN.

Serum CXCL16 levels were independently associated with albumin, BUN and uric acid in subjects with DN

To determine whether serum CXCL16 was independently associated with anthropometric parameters and other relevant factors, multiple stepwise regression analysis involving all the parameters with significant correlations to serum CXCL16 was performed. Our results revealed that serum CXCL16 was independently associated with 24 h proteinuria and BUN after adjustment for age, gender and BMI in all subjects in the present study (P≤0.004, respectively, Table 3). Thus, all other parameters including CCR, eGFR, blood albumin, uric acid and creatinine were all excluded during regression analysis.

Discussion

Our primary aim in this study was to characterize the clinical manifestation of CXCL16 in conjunction with pathophysiologic measures in diabetes and DN and to explore the relationship between CXCL16 and renal injury in diabetes patients. Our results suggest that CXCL16 is involved in the pathogenesis of renal dysfunction in diabetes patients as supported by two novel findings. First, serum CXCL16 levels were significantly increased in diabetes patients with renal disease when compared with healthy subjects. Furthermore, no significant changes in serum CXCL16 levels were found between healthy and T2DM subjects. Second, HDL and LDL cholesterol levels were significantly

Table 3 Multiple stepwise regression analysis showing variables independently associated with serum CXCL16 level.

Independent variables	Standardized β	B(95% CI)	t	P
24 h proteinuria	0.588	0.802(0.403 to 1.201)	4.138	<0.001
BUN	0.369	0.047(0.003 to 0.092)	0.311	0.004

different only in subjects with DN and not in T2DM patients without renal injury in comparison with heatlhy subjects. Taken together, these data suggest that CXCL16 may be a novel biomarker involved in the onset and deterioration of renal injury in diabetic patients, and the increased serum CXCL16 levels may be related to the abnormality of cholesterol metabolism in DN subjects.

CXCL16, a chemokine that is mainly expressed on dendritic cells and macrophages, plays an important role in the recruitment of T cells and NK cells[18–21]. While much is known from animal-based studies, little is known about CXCL16 in human subjects, particularly in patients with diabetes mellitus. Previous studies have indicated that serum CXCL16 levels are significantly higher in active SLE patients with renal disease than in active SLE patients without renal disease[22]. Furthermore, our previous studies showed that serum CXCL16 levels are significantly increased in subjects with CKD and gout, and these levels are significantly associated with renal function[11,12]. In the present study, we point to a new pathological manifestation of CXCL16 in the context of diabetic nephropathy. Our data showed that there were no significant changes in serum CXCL16 levels between healthy and T2DM subjects (Figure 1A). However, serum CXCL16 concentrations were significantly increased in DN subjects compared with T2DM and healthy subjects (Figure 1A). These results are consistent with our previous report on CKD subjects with T2DM [12]. This suggests that the elevation of CXCL16 in DN patients may be involved in the pathological progression of kidney disease in T2DM subjects.

Diabetes mellitus (DM) is one of the most prevalent diseases and is associated with increased incidence of structural and functional derangements in the kidneys, eventually leading to end-stage renal disease. Diabetic nephropathy is an important complication in diabetes patients. eGFR, CCR, creatinine, and BUN are conventional biomarkers reflecting changes in renal function in CKD and DN patients [16,17,23,24]. As shown in Table 1, several biomarkers of renal function including creatinine, BUN, uric acid, 24 h proteinuria, eGFR, and CCR in DN patients were significantly increased compared with T2DM subjects without renal disease. We also found that serum CXCL16 concentrations followed changes in a similar manner to creatinine, BUN, and uric acid among the subjects with T2DM, DN and CKD (Figure 1B, C, and D). On the other hand, elevated serum CXC16 levels in subjects with renal damage were already confirmed by our and other studies reports[9–12,25]. In the present study, our data indicated that, elevated serum CXCL16 levels were observed in both DN and CKD patients, even though both of them have different pathogenesis. Take together, these data implied that increased CXCL16 levels in relevant subjects are related to renal damage.

Our previous study indicated that serum CXCL16 levels are significantly increased in subjects with CKD and gout and are independently associated with the change of renal function in these subjects[11,12]. In the present study, our data indicated that serum CXCL16 levels were strongly associated with eGFR, CCR, creatinine, BUN, and uric acid in DN patients (Table 2, Figure 3), suggesting that elevated CXCL16 levels are closely related to glomerular injury and declining renal function in DN patients. Meanwhile, multiple logistic regression analysis also showed that serum CXCL16 was independently associated with changes in 24 h proteinuria and BUN. Taken together, these results indicate that serum CXCL16 levels are elevated in renal damage patient independently from diabetes. However, the mechanism responsible for the elevation of CXCL16 concentration and its role in the pathophysiology of DN is not fully understood. We speculate that the elevation of CXCL16 expression in subjects with DN may be related to the abnormalites of cholesterol metabolism especially in LDL and HDL. This is supported by the facts that elevation of CXCL16 following with higher levels of oxLDL were found in streptozotocin-induced diabetic mice[26], increased glomerular CXCL16 expression was also accompanied by high levels of oxidized low-density lipoprotein in subjects with glomerular kidney diseases in human[10].

Previous studies indicated that, CXCL16 plays a major role in the uptake of oxidized LDL by podocytes but not by mesangial and tubular renal cells[25]. Furthermore, abnormalities of podocyte structure and function, particularly with regard to LDL metabolism, play a major role in the onset of albuminuria both in diabetic and non diabetic nephropathy[25]. In the present study, we found that the abnormalities of LDL and HDL cholesterol levels were occurred only when overt kidney damage is present, irrespective of glycemic abnormalities in diabetes patients(Table 1 and Figure 2B,C). Take together, these results implied that the LDL-podocyte dysfunction-oxLDL-CXCL16 axis plays an important role in the onset and development of DN. Furthermore, the novel finding of abnormalities of cholesterol metabolism only in diabetic patients with kidney damage may be potentially useful to understand why diabetic nephropathy does occur only in a cohort of diabetic patients.

In summary, this study provides clinical evidence revealing that serum concentrations of CXCL16 are increased in subjects with DN and are independently associated with the loss of renal function. These data imply that CXCL16 may be a novel marker that predicts renal injury in T2DM subjects. There are several limitations in this study. The first one is that the sample size of this study cohort is relatively small. Furthermore, the cross-sectional nature of this study does not allow us to address the causal relationship between CXCL16 and the pathogenesis of DN in patients. Further prospective studies with larger sample sizes are needed to determine whether CXCL16 can be used as a potential biomarker for diagnosing and evaluating the onset and development of DN among DM subjects.

Author Contributions

Conceived and designed the experiments: LZ ZL. Performed the experiments: LZ FW TL LJ LY XP CS. Analyzed the data: LZ FW LJ. Contributed reagents/materials/analysis tools: LJ LY XP. Wrote the paper: LZ FW XL ZL.

References

1. Agostini C, Cabrelle A, Calabrese F, Bortoli M, Scquizzato E, et al. (2005) Role for CXCR6 and its ligand CXCL16 in the pathogenesis of T-cell alveolitis in sarcoidosis. American journal of respiratory and critical care medicine 172: 1290–1298.

2. Aslanian AM, Charo IF (2006) Targeted disruption of the scavenger receptor and chemokine CXCL16 accelerates atherosclerosis. Circulation 114: 583–590.

3. Moore KJ, Freeman MW (2006) Scavenger receptors in atherosclerosis: beyond lipid uptake. Arteriosclerosis, thrombosis, and vascular biology 26: 1702–1711.

4. Sheikine Y, Sirsjo A (2008) CXCL16/SR-PSOX–a friend or a foe in atherosclerosis? Atherosclerosis 197: 487–495.

5. Wuttge DM, Zhou X, Sheikine Y, Wagsater D, Stemme V, et al. (2004) CXCL16/SR-PSOX is an interferon-gamma-regulated chemokine and scavenger receptor expressed in atherosclerotic lesions. Arteriosclerosis, thrombosis, and vascular biology 24: 750–755.

6. Barlic J, Zhu W, Murphy PM (2009) Atherogenic lipids induce high-density lipoprotein uptake and cholesterol efflux in human macrophages by up-regulating transmembrane chemokine CXCL16 without engaging CXCL16-dependent cell adhesion. Journal of immunology 182: 7928–7936.

7. Jansson AM, Aukrust P, Ueland T, Smith C, Omland T, et al. (2009) Soluble CXCL16 predicts long-term mortality in acute coronary syndromes. Circulation 119: 3181–3188.

8. Okamura DM, Lopez-Guisa JM, Koelsch K, Collins S, Eddy AA (2007) Atherogenic scavenger receptor modulation in the tubulointerstitium in response to chronic renal injury. American journal of physiology Renal physiology 293: F575–585.

9. Schramme A, Abdel-Bakky MS, Gutwein P, Obermuller N, Baer PC, et al. (2008) Characterization of CXCL16 and ADAM10 in the normal and transplanted kidney. Kidney international 74: 328–338.

10. Gutwein P, Abdel-Bakky MS, Schramme A, Doberstein K, Kampfer-Kolb N, et al. (2009) CXCL16 is expressed in podocytes and acts as a scavenger receptor for oxidized low-density lipoprotein. The American journal of pathology 174: 2061–2072.

11. Gong Q, Wu F, Pan X, Yu J, Li Y, et al. (2012) Soluble C-X-C chemokine ligand 16 levels are increased in gout patients. Clinical biochemistry 45: 1368–1373.

12. Lin Z, Gong Q, Zhou Z, Zhang W, Liao S, et al. (2011) Increased plasma CXCL16 levels in patients with chronic kidney diseases. European journal of clinical investigation 41: 836–845.

13. Berkman J, Rifkin H (1973) Unilateral nodular diabetic glomerulosclerosis (Kimmelstiel-Wilson): report of a case. Metabolism: clinical and experimental 22: 715–722.

14. Lin Z, Zhou Z, Liu Y, Gong Q, Yan X, et al. (2011) Circulating FGF21 levels are progressively increased from the early to end stages of chronic kidney diseases and are associated with renal function in Chinese. PloS one 6: e18398.

15. Lin Z, Wu Z, Yin X, Liu Y, Yan X, et al. (2010) Serum levels of FGF-21 are increased in coronary heart disease patients and are independently associated with adverse lipid profile. PloS one 5: e15534.

16. Coresh J, Selvin E, Stevens LA, Manzi J, Kusek JW, et al. (2007) Prevalence of chronic kidney disease in the United States. JAMA: the journal of the American Medical Association 298: 2038–2047.

17. Fliser D, Kollerits B, Neyer U, Ankerst DP, Lhotta K, et al. (2007) Fibroblast growth factor 23 (FGF23) predicts progression of chronic kidney disease: the Mild to Moderate Kidney Disease (MMKD) Study. Journal of the American Society of Nephrology: JASN 18: 2600–2608.

18. Chandrasekar B, Bysani S, Mummidi S (2004) CXCL16 signals via Gi, phosphatidylinositol 3-kinase, Akt, I kappa B kinase, and nuclear factor-kappa B and induces cell-cell adhesion and aortic smooth muscle cell proliferation. The Journal of biological chemistry 279: 3188–3196.

19. Gough PJ, Garton KJ, Wille PT, Rychlewski M, Dempsey PJ, et al. (2004) A disintegrin and metalloproteinase 10-mediated cleavage and shedding regulates the cell surface expression of CXC chemokine ligand 16. Journal of immunology 172: 3678–3685.

20. Shimaoka T, Nakayama T, Fukumoto N, Kume N, Takahashi S, et al. (2004) Cell surface-anchored SR-PSOX/CXC chemokine ligand 16 mediates firm adhesion of CXC chemokine receptor 6-expressing cells. Journal of leukocyte biology 75: 267–274.

21. Shimaoka T, Nakayama T, Kume N, Takahashi S, Yamaguchi J, et al. (2003) Cutting edge: SR-PSOX/CXC chemokine ligand 16 mediates bacterial phagocytosis by APCs through its chemokine domain. Journal of immunology 171: 1647–1651.

22. Wu T, Xie C, Wang HW, Zhou XJ, Schwartz N, et al. (2007) Elevated urinary VCAM-1, P-selectin, soluble TNF receptor-1, and CXC chemokine ligand 16 in multiple murine lupus strains and human lupus nephritis. Journal of immunology 179: 7166–7175.

23. Kouroumichakis I, Papanas N, Zarogoulidis P, Liakopoulos V, Maltezos E, et al. (2012) Fibrates: therapeutic potential for diabetic nephropathy? European journal of internal medicine 23: 309–316.

24. Mathiesen ER, Ringholm L, Feldt-Rasmussen B, Clausen P, Damm P (2012) Obstetric nephrology: pregnancy in women with diabetic nephropathy–the role of antihypertensive treatment. Clinical journal of the American Society of Nephrology: CJASN 7: 2081–2088.

25. Awad AS, Rouse M, Liu L, Vergis AL, Rosin DL, et al. (2008) Activation of adenosine 2A receptors preserves structure and function of podocytes. Journal of the American Society of Nephrology: JASN 19: 59–68.

26. Gutwein P, Abdel-Bakky MS, Doberstein K, Schramme A, Beckmann J, et al. (2009) CXCL16 and oxLDL are induced in the onset of diabetic nephropathy. Journal of cellular and molecular medicine 13: 3809–3825.

21

A Retrospective Case-Control Analysis of the Outpatient Expenditures for Western Medicine and Dental Treatment Modalities in CKD Patients in Taiwan

Ren-Yeong Huang[1], Yuh-Feng Lin[2,3,4], Sen-Yeong Kao[5], Yi-Shing Shieh[6], Jin-Shuen Chen[2]*

1 Department of Periodontology, School of Dentistry, Tri-Service General Hospital, National Defense Medical Center, Taipei, Taiwan, 2 Division of Nephrology, Department of Internal Medicine, Tri-Service General Hospital, National Defense Medical Center, Taipei, Taiwan, 3 Division of Nephrology, Department of Medicine, Shuang Ho Hospital, New Taipei City, Taiwan, 4 Graduate Institute of Clinical Medicine, Taipei Medical University, Taipei, Taiwan, 5 School of Public Health, National Defense Medical Center, Taipei, Taiwan, 6 Department of Oral Diagnosis, School of Dentistry, Tri-Service General Hospital, National Defense Medical Center, Taipei, Taiwan

Abstract

Background: To determine if expenditures for dentistry (DENT) correlate with severity of chronic kidney disease (CKD).

Methods: A total of 10,457 subjects were enrolled from January 2008 to December 2010, divided into three groups: healthy control (HC) group (n = 1,438), high risk (HR) group (n = 3,392), and CKD group (n = 5,627). Five stages were further categorized for the CKD group. OPD utilization and expenditures for western medicine (WM), DENT, and TCM (traditional Chinese medicine) were analyzed retrospectively (2000–2008) using Taiwan's National Health Insurance Research Database. Three major areas were analyzed among groups CKD, HR and HC in this study: 1) demographic data and medical history; 2) utilization (visits/person/year) and expenditures (9-year cumulative expenditure, expenditure/person/year) for OPD services in WM, DENT, and TCM; and 3) utilization and expenditures for dental OPD services, particularly in dental filling, root canal and periodontal therapy.

Results: OPD utilization and expenditures of WM increased significantly for the CKD group compared with the HR and HC groups, and increased steadily along with the severity of CKD stages. However, overall DENT and TCM utilization and expenditures did not increase for the CKD group. In comparison among different CKD stages, the average expenditures and utilization for DENT including restorative filling and periodontal therapy, but not root canal therapy, showed significant decreases according to severity of CKD stage, indicating less DENT OPD utilization with progression of CKD.

Conclusions: Patients with advanced CKD used DENT OPD service less frequently. However, the connection between CKD and DENT service utilization requires further study.

Editor: Giuseppe Remuzzi, Mario Negri Institute for Pharmacological Research and Azienda Ospedaliera Ospedali Riuniti di Bergamo, Italy

Funding: This study is based in part on data from the NHIRD provided by the Bureau of NHI, Department of Health, and managed by National Health Research Institutes in Taiwan and supported by the National Science Council of Taiwan under grant DOH97-HP-1101, DOH-98-1110, DOH99-HP-1106, DOH100-HP-1102, DOH101-HP-1103, and DOH102-HP-1103. The funders had no role in study design, data collection and analysis, decision to publish, or preparation of the manuscript.

Competing Interests: The authors have declared that no competing interests exist.

* E-mail: dgschen@ndmctsgh.edu.tw

Introduction

Chronic kidney disease (CKD) affects an increasing number of people around the world, and the prevalence of CKD appears to have increased over the past decade [1]. Evidence from the United States Renal Data System 2011 suggests that from the year 2000, Taiwan has had the highest incidence and prevalence of end-stage renal disease (ESRD) among all of the countries examined, with approximately 400 per million of the population affected [2], and ESRD is one of the leading causes of death in Taiwan [3]. In response, the government of Taiwan has launched a project of multidisciplinary care for CKD patients since 2004. It has been demonstrated that CKD is linked to many morbidities, creating a heavy burden on the medical insurance system [4]. Expenditures for CKD create significant economic burdens on patients as well

and have become a major challenge for medical care systems [5]. Nevertheless, in light of the health-related expenditures, CKD treatment has been shown to be cost effective as it slows disease progression and prevents the development of comorbidities [5,6].

CKD, a complex comorbid condition with multiple manifestations, is closely linked with cardiovascular disease, hypertension, anemia, diabetes, malnutrition, dyslipidemia, bone and mineral disorders, all of which increase the chances of morbidity, mortality, and healthcare costs [2,7,8]. In recent years, numerous studies have demonstrated higher rates of oral pathology in CKD patients with one or more oral symptoms; thus, a variety of changes occur in the oral cavity are strongly correlated with CKD itself or with CKD therapy [9,10,11]. In addition, poor oral health status is closely associated with markers of malnutrition, inflammation and increased risk of death for patients undergoing

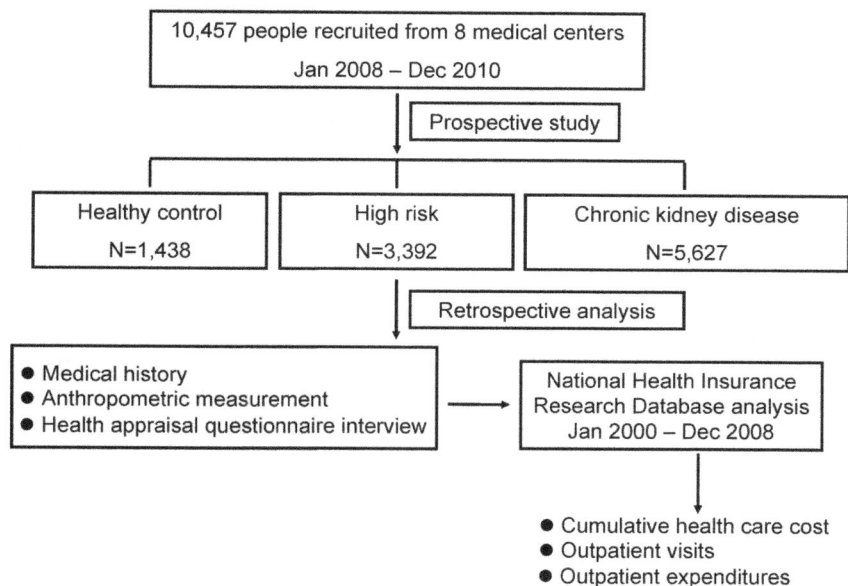

Figure 1. Flow chart of the selection process of the study participants.

hemodialysis [12,13]. Although the exact causality between diseases is intricate [11,14], studies have demonstrated that poor oral health conditions and its severe consequences are closely associated with the incidence or progression of CKD [15,16,17]. Accordingly, it is widely accepted that CKD can have a critical impact on oral health; likewise, poor oral health has been linked to CKD [11].

Treatment of CKD through multidisciplinary approaches may improve patient outcomes and be cost-effective [6,18,19,20]. On the basis of these findings, it should be emphasized that monitoring and maintaining the oral health status of CKD patients, as well as in patients who are considered for renal dialysis or as transplant candidates is essential. This would justify an increased attention to and better awareness of dental care in CKD patients. Furthermore, it might be possible to achieve better clinical and economic outcomes for CKD patients if patients are comprehensively evaluated and referred to the relevant specialty early, including dental services. However, to date, there is no retrospective epidemiologic study from a general population performed by analyzing a nationwide hospital-based database to investigate the relationship between the utilization and expenditures of dental services and CKD progression.

Recent publications focusing on medical care expenditures in CKD have concentrated mainly on Western Medicine (WM), including hospitalization [21,22], pharmacy services [23,24] and individual co-morbidity costs [4,25,26,27,28,29]. Despite the emerging studies that have investigated possible associations between oral health and CKD [11], the correlation between Dentistry (DENT) and Traditional Chinese Medicine (TCM) outpatient (OPD) utilization and expenditures and the progression of kidney disease in the CKD population is largely unknown.

To the best of our knowledge, there are no large, hospital-based studies which outline the relationship between DENT and TCM utilization and expenditures for CKD patients. The objective of this study was designed to use a nationwide case control cohort to investigate DENT OPD utilization and associated expenditures in patients at various stages of CKD.

Methods

Study design and populations

A case-control study was conducted over 3 years. Three study groups, including healthy control (HC), high risk (HR) and chronic kidney disease (CKD), were collected throughout the period January 1, 2008, to December 31, 2010. A total of 10,457 Taiwan people all covered by the National Health Insurance Program (NHIP) from 8 medical centers located in different regions of Taiwan were the subjects of this study. Participants recruited for this study were randomly selected from the participating medical centers. The design for this study is a cluster randomized without age- or gender-match. This kind of design is vulnerable to lack of comparability; however, this design makes it easy to increase sample size and calculate expenditure more accurately. A detailed medical history, anthropometric measurements, laboratory analyses, and a health appraisal questionnaire eliciting demographic, socioeconomic and behavioral risk factors were conducted through face-to-face interviews with each participant by well-trained investigators at the initial visit. Written informed consent was obtained from all study participants. At the end of the three-year study, all participants' claims data were analyzed, and their OPD utilization and expenditure, particularly in WM, DENT, and TCM, were analyzed retrospectively from the National Health Insurance Research Database (NHIRD). A flow chart summarizing the selection process of the study participants is given in Figure 1. This study protocol involving human subjects was reviewed and approved by the Institutional Review Board of Tri-Service General Hospital, National Defense Medical Center and other participating medical centers.

Definition of participants

All eligible participants were categorized into 3 mutually exclusive categories: "HC", "HR", and "CKD," based on estimated glomerular filtration rate (eGFR) and medical history. The level of eGFR was calculated using the Modification of Diet in Renal Disease study equation [30].

Individuals in the HC group, eGFR ≥ 60 (mL/min/1.73 m^2) without renal abnormalities or family history of renal diseases, were recruited from health examination in the communities or participating hospital-affiliated health evaluation units.

Patients in the HR group were eGFR ≥ 60 (mL/min/1.73 m^2) and had to meet one of the following criteria: (1) diagnosed diabetes mellitus (DM), hypertension, cardiovascular disease; (2) family member diagnosed with CKD or receiving dialysis treatment.

The CKD stages were defined according to clinical practice guidelines developed under the Kidney Disease: Improving Global Outcomes (KDIGO) classification system established by the National Kidney Foundation [31], with further classification of stage 3 disease into stage3a (eGFR <60 and ≥ 45 mL/min/1.73 m^2) and stage3b (eGFR <45 and ≥ 30 mL/min/1.73 m^2) [32].

Basic data collection

A face-to-face interview was conducted to obtain participants' information regarding socioeconomic status (gender, age, residence district, occupation, household income, marital status and education level) and oral health behavior (alcohol consumption, betel nut chewing and cigarette smoking habits). The geographic locations of residency were grouped into three categories of northern, central, and southern Taiwan.

Anthropometric evaluation included measurements of wrist circumference, body weight and height to calculate body mass index (BMI). According to the Bureau of Health Promotion, Department of Health, Taiwan, BMI less than 18.5 was defined as underweight, 18.5–24 as normal, between 24 and 27 as overweight, and higher than 27 as obese [33].

Retrospective analysis of past 9 years OPD utilization and expenditure of WM, DENT and TCM

Data source and validation. This hospital-based study recruited individuals from the NHIRD provided by the Bureau of National Health Insurance (BNHI), and released by National Health Research Institutes (NHRI), Miaoli, Taiwan (http://www.nhri.org.tw/nhird/). Taiwan initiated the National Health Insurance (NHI) program in March 1995 to offer affordable medical care for all residents. In addition, Taiwan has the highest incidence and prevalence of end-stage renal disease globally [2]. In response, the government of Taiwan launched a project of multidisciplinary care for CKD patients in 2004. This service is available throughout Taiwan and is covered by the NHI program. Furthermore, dental care is widely available and covered by the NHI program in Taiwan.

A distinctive characteristic of the NHIRD is its comprehensive coverage of 99% of the population, for whom the NHI program has provided universal medical coverage, comprehensive benefits, and unrestricted access to any medical institution of the patient's choice [34]. Moreover, regular justifications and claims of the medical charts are performed by the BNHI of Taiwan to ensure the fidelity of the coding system in the database. The dataset after merging from Taiwan's NHIRD was transcribed for further statistical analysis. Thus, NHIRD provides a good statistical representation for analyzing epidemiological profiles of the entire population of Taiwan. Several high-quality international peer-reviewed studies have been published based on the NHIRD data, supporting its validity for medical research [35,36,37,38,39].

Analysis of WM, DENT, and TCM utilization and expenditure. The OPD prescription and therapeutic coding system for WM (01–15, 22, 23, 81, 82, 83, 84) DENT (40–49), and TCM (60–69) of each participant were retrieved and transcribed

from the NHIRD. Utilization and expenditures for WM, DENT and TCM, including cumulative medical care expenditures, annual OPD visits, and OPD expenditure per person from January 2000 to December 2008 were further analyzed.

Analysis of DENT expenditure and utilization. OPD expenditures and utilization of DENT were defined according to diagnostic code and NHI therapeutic procedure codes. The coding system by the NHI in Taiwan is performed according to the International Classification of Diseases, Ninth Revision, Clinical Modification (ICD-9-CM). Diagnostic and therapeutic procedure codes were used to define expenditure and utilization of the three most common DENT procedures: restorative therapy (ICD-9-CM code: 5210–5219; therapeutic code: 89001–89012), root canal therapy (ICD-9-CM code: 5220–5229; therapeutic code: 90001–90020), and periodontal therapy (ICD-9-CM code: 5230–5239; therapeutic code: 91001–91014). These patients' first ambulatory care visits for DENT treatment between January 1, 2000, and December 31, 2008, were assigned as the index date use of medical care.

Statistical analyses

All statistical analyses were carried out using the SAS 9.13 system (SAS system for windows, version 8.2. SAS Institute Inc. Cary. NC) and SPSS 18.0 software package (SPSS Inc., Chicago, Illinois). Mean expenditures and frequency of medical care visits where appropriate were used to describe the characteristics of the study groups. Statistical differences in categorical variables and in continuous variables between the three groups were determined using the chi-square test and one-way analysis of variance (ANOVA), respectively. Differences between each group/stage were assessed by Scheffe post hoc tests. Level of statistical significance was set at $P<0.05$.

Results

Demographic differences among subjects

Among the 10,457 eligible participants, clinical diagnosis was made and three mutually exclusive patient groups were categorized. Data were collected for 1,438 patients in the HC group, 3,392 patients in the HR group, and 5,627 patients in the CKD group. The number of subjects for each CKD stage (stage 1 to stage 5) was 917 (stage 1), 1108 (stage 2), 763 (stage 3a), 780 (stage 3b), 1036 (stage 4), and 1023 (stage 5). Of all the eligible individuals, significant differences existed in demographic characteristics and socioeconomic status among groups (all $p<0.001$) (Table 1). The majority of the patients in the CKD group were older, with a mean age 61.04 ± 15.21 years compared with 57.59 ± 14.30 yrs and 46.62 ± 15.15 yrs in the HR and HC groups, respectively. Of the analyzed socioeconomic variables, patients in the CKD group were more likely to be unemployed (56.7%), have a household income $\leq 40,000$ NT$ (71.8%), and lower education achievement<college level (84.3%) when compared with other groups (Table 1).

Family history, anthropometric measurements and oral health habits of participants

Among the eligible individuals, significant differences existed in family history among groups, with a higher prevalence of diabetes mellitus, heart diseases, and cerebrovascular diseases (CVDs) observed in CKD and HR patients than in HC patients (all $p<0.001$) (Table 2).

The anthropometric evaluations of body mass index (BMI) and waist circumference showed significant differences among groups ($p<0.001$) (Table 2). Only a minority of eligible individuals were

Table 1. Demographic characteristics and socioeconomic status of eligible subjects.

Variables	HC (n = 1,438)		HR (n = 3,392)		CKD (n = 5,627)		P^a
	n	%	n	%	n	%	
Gender							<0.001
Male	477	33.2	1,554	45.8	3,247	57.7	
Female	961	66.8	1,838	54.2	2,380	42.3	
Age (years)							<0.001
mean ±SD	46.62±15.15	57.59±14.30	61.04±15.21	<0.001			
<45	680	47.3	616	18.2	796	14.1	
45–64	551	38.3	1,589	46.8	2,285	40.6	
65–74	138	9.6	794	23.4	1,386	24.6	
>75	69	4.8	393	11.6	1,160	20.6	
Living district (area of Taiwan)							<0.001
Northern	619	43.0	1,206	35.6	2,419	43.0	
Central	413	28.7	1,127	33.2	1,373	24.4	
Southern	406	28.3	1,059	31.2	1,835	32.6	
Marital status							<0.001
Married (%)	1,017	70.7	2,754	81.2	4,496	79.9	
Single (%)	334	23.2	326	9.6	546	9.7	
Other (%)	88	6.1	312	9.2	585	10.4	
Occupation							<0.001
None	362	25.2	1,638	48.3	3,191	56.7	
Government	104	7.2	149	4.4	242	4.3	
Agriculture	11	0.8	64	1.9	135	2.4	
Business	135	9.4	319	9.4	445	7.9	
Labor	121	8.4	282	8.3	405	7.2	
Others	705	49	940	27.7	1,210	21.5	
Household income (NT$)							<0.001
None (%)	224	15.6	1,238	36.5	2,481	44.1	
<40,000 (%)	387	26.9	987	29.1	1,559	27.7	
4–90,000 (%)	520	36.2	814	24.0	1,092	19.4	
>90,000 (%)	306	21.3	353	10.4	495	8.8	
Education level							<0.001
<Junior high (%)	267	18.6	1,442	42.5	2,864	50.9	
Senior high (%)	598	41.6	1,323	39.0	1,879	33.4	
>College (%)	572	39.8	628	18.5	883	15.7	

Unless otherwise indicated, values are number (percentage). The eligible subjects were recruited patient from 2008 to 2010. N = 10,457.
Abbreviations: CKD, chronic kidney disease; HC, healthy control; HR, high risk; NT$, new Taiwan dollars.
[a]Chi-square test. P<0.05 was considered statistically significant.

considered obese, with a BMI>27 (28.1%) and waist circumference >91 cm (31.2%) (Table 2).

Subjects' oral health habits, including alcohol and betel nut use, and cigarette smoking, all considered to have negative effects on oral health, were summarized (Table 2). The most frequent habits among all participants were cigarette smoking (19.7%), alcohol use (13.6%), and betel nut use (3.7%). Participants in the CKD and HR groups were more likely to have these oral habits than were those in the HC group (all p<0.001) (Table 2).

OPD utilization and expenditure in WM, DENT and TCM

Figure 2 shows the cumulative OPD expenditures per person in WM, DENT and TCM from 2000 to 2008. In general, patients with CKD had greater overall expenditures in WM than for DENT and TCM. Interestingly, the cumulative expenditures for WM for the CKD group exhibited remarkable annual increase when compared with the HR and HC groups, whereas this tendency was not observed for DENT (Figure 2B) and TCM (Figure 2C) expenditures.

The annual number of OPD visits per person, and expenditures per person (NT$) for WM and DENT exhibited significant differences among the groups (Table 3). For WM, the CKD group had higher expenditures and OPD visits than the HC or HR groups; however, these trends were not observed for DENT (Table 3). These parameters steadily increased along with the severity of CKD stages (stage 1–5) in WM (p<0.01) (Table 3).

Table 2. Medical history, anthropometric measurements and oral habits of eligible patients.

Variables	HC (n = 1,438)		HR (n = 3,392)		CKD (n = 5,627)		P^b
	n	%	n	%	n	%	
Medical history							
Family history							
Diabetes mellitus	309	21.5	984	29.0	1,412	25.1	<0.001
Heart diseases	127	8.8	271	8.0	304	5.4	<0.001
CVDs	112	7.8	265	7.8	304	5.4	<0.001
Physical status							
BMI (Kg/m²)							<0.001
Underweight[a]	97	6.8	75	2.2	214	3.8	
Normal weight[a]	679	47.2	1,275	37.6	2,223	39.5	
Overweight[a]	292	20.3	1,041	30.7	1,626	28.9	
Obesity[a]	370	25.7	1,001	29.5	1,564	27.8	
Waist (cm)							<0.001
<70	293	20.4	268	7.9	394	7	
71–80	585	40.7	862	25.4	1,311	23.3	
81–90	293	20.4	1,262	37.2	1,930	34.3	
>91	266	18.5	1,001	29.5	1,992	35.4	
Oral habit							
Alcohol	121	8.4	461	13.6	838	14.9	<0.001
Betel nuts	19	1.3	122	3.6	248	4.4	<0.001
Cigarette	141	9.8	638	18.8	1,283	22.8	<0.001

The eligible subjects were recruited patient from 2008 to 2010. N = 10,457.
Abbreviations: BMI, body mass index; CKD, chronic kidney disease; CVDs, cerebrovascular diseases; HC, healthy control; HR, high risk.
[a]Underweight: BMI<18.5; Normal weight: BMI = 18.5–24; Overweight: BMI = 24–27; Obesity: BMI>27.
[b]Chi-square test. P<0.05 was considered statistically significant.

Interestingly, only the OPD visits for DENT services showed significant differences in different CKD stages (p = 0.034) although significant differences for DENT expenditures were not found (p = 0.166) (Table 3), suggesting that DENT expenditures did not increase as the patient's kidney disease became worse.

Utilization and expenditure of DENT therapeutic procedures

Annual OPD visits and expenditures per person for restorative and periodontal therapy exhibited significant differences among groups; however, for root canal therapy, only OPD visits presented considerable difference among all groups (p = 0.0063) (Table 4). At different CKD stages, the average expenditures and OPD visits for restorative filling and periodontal therapy (all p<0.0001), but not root canal therapy, showed significant decreases according to severity of CKD stages (Table 4), indicating less DENT utilization with progression of CKD.

Discussion

To the best of our knowledge, this is the first attempt to use a long-term, nationwide hospital-based cohort to investigate the relationship between DENT utilization and expenditures for CKD patients according to the progression of CKD stages. Our major findings were as follows: 1) group CKD demonstrated significant differences in terms of demographic data and socioeconomic performance when compared to groups HC and HR; 2) participants in group CKD had poor oral health habits compared

to group HC; 3) the medical care utilization and expenditures for WM services for patients with CKD were higher when compared to groups HC and HR, but DENT and TCM services showed no significant difference among the three groups; and 4) as for DENT services, the OPD visits and expenditures of the patients receiving restorative and periodontal therapy showed a significant decrease in group CKD, but not in groups HC and HR. Moreover, the OPD visits and expenditures for group CKD decreased significantly according to the progression of CKD. All these findings provide a new understanding of the relationship between CKD and DENT services, particularly in the treatment of restorative and periodontal therapy.

First, in our study we investigated socioeconomic and demographic data, finding that group CKD was more likely to be male, unemployed or earning a low income, and more than 50% likely to have less than a junior high diploma. A US study had similar findings, in that people with CKD and limited education or low income have more risk of disability because of socioeconomic disparities [40]. Moreover, patients in our CKD group were more likely to have bad oral habits than were other groups (Table 2). A cross-sectional study regarding the oral health status of adults in Taiwan found that demographic factors (i.e., gender, marital status, and income levels) are all significantly associated with general health [41]. Thus, our findings highlight the need for more attention to DENT needs for CKD patients.

As for oral health habits, we found that group CKD had the worst habits, including alcohol use, betel nut use and smoking. It has been shown that oral health-related factors (i.e., oral hygiene,

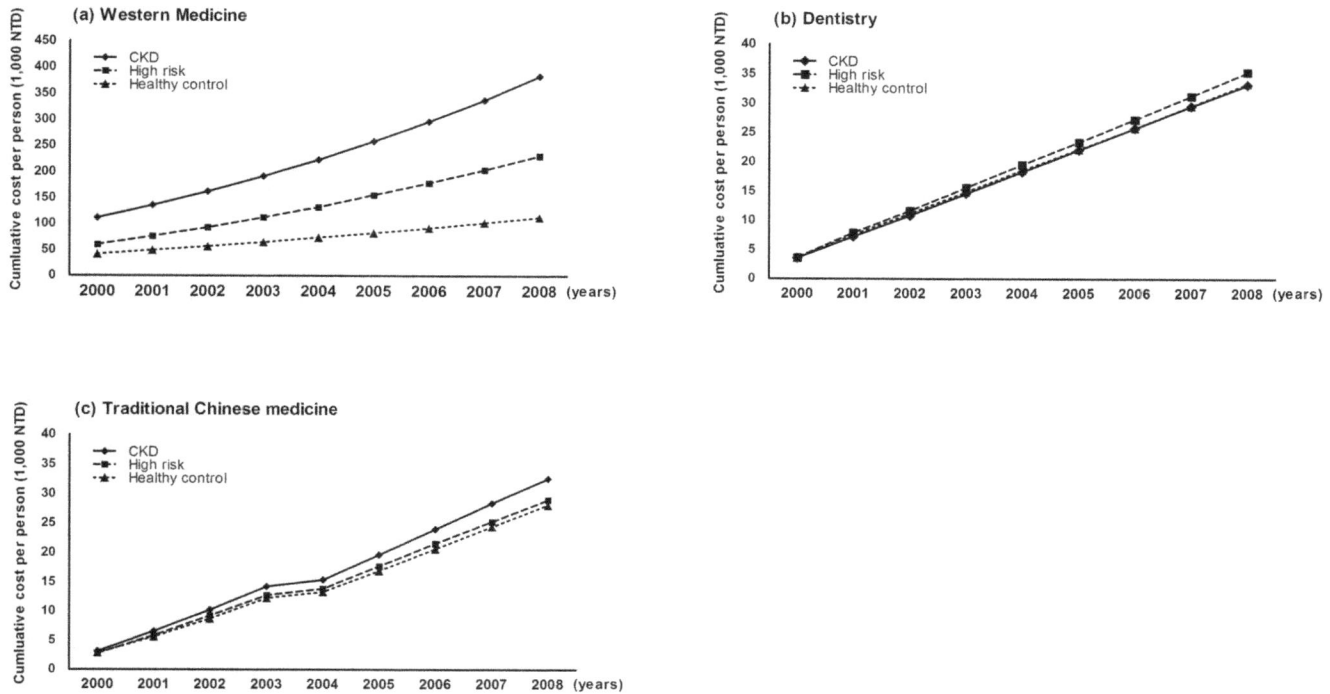

Figure 2. Cumulative OPD expenditures per person in WM, DENT, and TCM from 2000 to 2008. The eligible subjects were recruited from 2008 to 2010. N = 10,457. Abbreviations: CKD, chronic kidney disease; DENT, Dentistry; HC, healthy control; HR, high risk; OPD, outpatient; NT$, new Taiwan dollars; TCM, Traditional Chinese Medicine; WM, Western Medicine.

oral health status, dental care utilization, disease history, and lifestyle factors such as cigarette smoking, alcohol use, and betel nut chewing) are significantly associated with general and oral health [41]. A higher rate of concurrent usage of oral substances, particularly in the CKD group, indicates certain lifestyle patterns, which may confer a higher health risk [41]. However, previous studies demonstrated an inverse association between alcohol consumption and renal dysfunction [42,43] because beneficial oxidative activity on endothelial function has a protective property for kidneys [42,44]. Additionally, in Taiwan, CKD prevalence among betel-nut users is higher than in the non-users in all age groups [43]. The habit of betel-nut chewing may be associated with CKD, especially in males [43,45]. It has been reported that relative risk for oral cancer among those who chew betel-nut in the Taiwanese population is 58.4 (95% confidence interval 7.6 to 447.6) [46]. Generally, oral health status is significantly related to socio-economic status and strongly correlated with oral health behaviors and even general health. We strongly recommend

Table 3. The average annual number of OPD visits and expenditures per person in WM and DENT among eligible patients and different CKD stages from 2000 to 2008.

| Parameters | HC (n = 1,438) | HR (n = 3,392) | CKD (n = 5,627) | p^b | CKD | | | | | | |
					Stage 1	Stage 2	Stage 3a	Stage 3b	Stage 4	Stage 5	p^b
Western Medicine											
OPD visits (mean ± SD)	20.4±10.7	30.6±15.7	42.3±28.7	<0.01[c]	29.1±16.7	35.0±20.0	40.0±21.0	45.0±27.4	49.8±29.0	50.9±40.8	<0.01[e]
OPD expenditures[a] (NT$, mean)	12,986	26,427	42,213	<0.01[c]	244,703	340,972	404,935	452,443	505,490	532,729	<0.01[e]
Dentistry											
OPD visits (mean ± SD)	4.1±9.2	4.9±2.7	4.7±2.0	0.019[d]	4.3±2.3	4.7±2.2	4.4±1.7	4.8±1.8	5.5±2.4	4.4±1.5	0.034
OPD expenditures[a] (NT$, mean)	38,384	43,537	40,130	0.049	37,140	41,024	38,799	40,911	45,290	37,394	0.166

The eligible subjects were recruited patient from 2008 to 2010. N = 10,457.
Abbreviations: CKD, chronic kidney disease; DENT, Dentistry; HC, healthy control; HR, high risk NT$, new Taiwan dollars; OPD, outpatient; WM, Western Medicine.
[a]Expenditures were rounded to the nearest whole dollar.
[b]ANOVA. P<0.05 was considered statistically significant.
[c]Scheffe's test : CKD>HR>HC.
[d]Scheffe's test : HR>HC.
[e]Scheffe's test :Stage5>Stage4>Stage3b>Stage3a>Stage2>Stage1.

Table 4. The average annual number of OPD visits, and expenditures per person of different dental procedures among eligible patients and different CKD stages from 2000 to 2008.

Parameters	HC (n = 1,438)	HR (n = 3,392)	CKD (n = 5,627)	p^b	CKD Stage 1	Stage 2	Stage 3a	Stage 3b	Stage 4	Stage 5	p^b
Restorative therapy											
OPD visits (mean ± SD)	0.81±0.66	0.83±0.72	0.78±0.69	0.0027[c]	0.83±0.74	0.82±0.69	0.8±0.67	0.81±0.7	0.77±0.74	0.64±0.59	<0.0001[h]
OPD expenditures[a] (NT$, mean)	10,040	9,808	8,812	<0.0001[d]	9,786	9,457	9,025	8,962	8,462	7,174	<0.0001[h]
Root canal therapy											
OPD visits (mean ± SD)	0.38±0.34	0.43±0.42	0.42±0.39	0.0063[e]	0.43±0.36	0.43±0.42	0.41±0.35	0.45±0.41	0.43±0.42	0.41±0.34	0.436
OPD expenditures[a] (NT$, mean)	6,179	6,522	6,140	0.0705	6,217	6,256	6,023	6,626	5,970	5,803	0.3
Periodontal therapy											
OPD visits (mean ± SD)	0.76±0.68	0.87±0.86	0.78±0.76	<0.0001[f]	0.76±0.71	0.84±0.78	0.83±0.73	0.86±0.76	0.76±0.84	0.67±0.66	<0.0001[i]
OPD expenditures[a] (NT$, mean)	6,377	7,020	6,149	<0.0001[g]	6,153	6,640	6,488	6,697	5,835	5,262	<0.0001[i]

The eligible subjects were recruited patient from 2008 to 2010. N = 10,457.
Abbreviations: CKD, chronic kidney disease; DENT, Dentistry; HC, healthy control; HR, high risk NT$, new Taiwan dollars; OPD, outpatient; WM, Western Medicine.
[a]Expenditures were rounded to the nearest whole dollar.
[b]ANOVA. P<0.05 was considered statistically significant.
[c]Scheffe's test : HR>CKD.
[d]Scheffe's test : HC>HR>CKD.
[e]Scheffe's test : HR>CKD>HC.
[f]Scheffe's test : HR>CKD>HC.
[g]Scheffe's test : HR>HC>CKD.
[h]Scheffe's test : Stage1>Stage2>Stage3a>Stage3b>Stage4>Stage5.
[i]Scheffe's test : Stage3b>Stage2>Stage3a>Stage4>Stage5.

widespread public health care education targeting all three risky behaviors at the same time.

As for dental care, we found there was no difference in utilization and expenditure for dental care at different CKD stages, but the utilization of western medicine increased with the progression of CKD. Furthermore, the utilization and expenditure of periodontal therapy and restorative therapy both decreased with the progression of CKD stage (Table 4). But how can we explain this outcome? Recently, a survey was conducted from a representative database to examine self-reported dental status, dental care utilization, and dental insurance, by race/ethnicity [47], among community-dwelling older adults. The author found that Non-Hispanic White respondents reported better dental health, higher dental care utilization, and higher satisfaction with dental care compared to all other racial/ethnic groups. On the contrary, Chinese immigrants were more likely to report poor dental health, were less likely to report dental care utilization and dental insurance, and were less satisfied with their dental care compared to all other racial/ethnic groups [47]. Some factors including cost, physical disabilities, language barriers, dental fear and socio-psychological concerns may affect dental care service utilization by a specific population [41,47,48,49]. It has been shown that those with CKD had a 25% lower likelihood of having a dental visit [HR = 0.75, 95% CI (0.64–0.88)] than those without CKD after adjustment for confounders [50]. In addition, the uremic patients demonstrated more dental problems than healthy controls and seem to develop their problems before they progressed to dialysis [51]. Treatments for CKD and dental care are widely available and inexpensive in Taiwan. Take CKD care, for example. According to Lin et al [52], the medical expenditures per subject per year in years 1997, 1998 and 1999 were US$

129.7, 432.8 and 725.6 for CKD late stages, stages 3, 4 and 5. For dental care, from 1998 to 2005, the number of dentists at national level increased 30.5% from 8,020 to 10,465 and the population-dentist ratio decreased 22.0% (2,588 people per dentist in 1998 and 2,115 people per dentist in 2005). The percentage of insured population receiving dental service increased from 36.1% in 1998 to 40.8% in 2005. The dentist-to-population ratio (defined as the number of dentists per 10,000 people) was 5.0 in 2010 [53]. Thus, dental care for each participants is widely available and inexpensive in Taiwan.

It is essential to address the factors affecting the usage of dental care in CKD patients, as these may contribute to the progression of CKD stages. Greater attention to dental problems may be warranted during the progression of CKD to prevent deterioration of kidney function [51]. Furthermore, it is plausible that restorative and periodontal expenditure and utilization may provide contributory information on the deterioration of kidney function in patients with CKD [51]. Further studies to ascertain the nature of the association between oral health and CKD progression are needed.

This study has a few limitations that should be addressed. First, claims data were identified from the NHIRD under the principal payment code for DENT service and complete dental examination was not performed during face-to-face interview; however, to date, the decision criteria for subjects leading to dental treatment, including restorative or filling, endodontic and periodontal therapy is still judged by clinicians according to an imprecise coding system. Second, claims data may have minor inaccuracies even through these inaccuracies are rare. The accuracy of claims data of NHIRD is improved by a cross-checking system with full review by specialists. Thus, these inaccuracies would be unlikely to have significantly affected the results, considering the substantial sample size. Third, the study evaluated only the direct OPD expenditures, including WM, DENT and TCM expenditures. Information to determine the indirect economic burdens of CKD, such as work productivity loss and reduced quality of life, was not available. Furthermore, the current study may also suffer from detection bias. Indeed, it was not possible to capture the entire continuum of care of patients, as the NHIRD does not include information regarding the proportion of self-payment dental therapies such as denture fabrication, orthodontic treatment, dental implant placement and medical cosmetics treatment. Moreover, findings were based on a single integrated health system and may not be generalizable to larger populations because of hospital-based study design. A community- or population-based study will be needed to delineate the intricate relationship between CKD and oral health.

Since patients at advanced CKD stages in our study used DENT services less frequently, it would be very likely that individuals with more advanced CKD are older and less educated, and have lower income. Further multivariate regression analysis may have interesting findings regarding whether this association is dependent or not on some confounders such as demographics, socio-economic status and oral habits. In this study, from our collected data, we can offer some evidence regarding the factors on demographics, and socioeconomic status to support our conclusion. As for gender, our result showed a gender difference consistent with several previous studies in Taiwan [54,55,56]. It should be emphasized that 99% of Taiwan's population is covered by NHIP [34]. Thus, in terms of gender, there is no difference between the healthcare utilization for kidney disease [52,57]. As for age, there is no obvious finding that individuals with more advanced CKD are older. For the later stages, such as CKD Stage 4 and Stage 5, the majority of CKD patients in our study were age 45–64 (32.8% and 39.4%, respectively), greater than for other age groups, including age >75 (28.6% for CKD Stage 4 and 24.20% for CKD Stage 5) (data not shown). Therefore, "Age" may not correlate to healthcare utilization and expenditure. As for demographic characteristics, such as residential district, a similar distribution pattern was found in our investigated groups (Table 1). The residential district may not have a significant impact on healthcare utilization for recruited patients because of the universal coverage of NHIP in Taiwan [34]. As for socioeconomic status, such as household income, more subjects in CKD Stage 2 (24%) indicate low or no income than those in Stage 5 (22.10%) or Stage 1 (19.7%) (data not shown). Lower socioeconomic status is a risk factor for CKD and progression to end-stage renal disease; however, consistent with another study [58], GFR decline was

similar across income groups and patients with advanced CKD may not necessarily have lower income than those in other stages. For the "education level," CKD patients at Stage 4 and Stage 5 have a higher likelihood of lower educational achievement (<Junior high) (Table 1). However, subjects aged 45–64 (40.9%) had less education than those 65–74 (34.0%), and those >75 (21.8%) (data not shown). Thus, in fact, we found individuals with more advanced CKD may not necessarily be less educated or have less income. Consequently, the demographic and socioeconomic factors may have only a limited influence on the analysis procedure and result of this study. Nevertheless, we should be cautions about the interpretation of the results; the interacting effects of these covariates on the correlation between CKD stages and healthcare utilization and expenditure still require further investigation.

Despite these limitations, this study has several strengths, including the important advantage of relying on real-world population-based data, a relatively substantial sample size, face-to-face questionnaire interview for each participant, and the availability of laboratory results to ascertain CKD stage.

Conclusions

In conclusion, from the horizon of dental utilization and expenditures, this hospital-based research is the first to assess dental OPD utilization and expenditures in a population with CKD. Patients at advanced CKD stages used DENT services, including periodontal therapy and restorative filling, less frequently. However, a large and prospective study is warranted to clarify the connection between CKD stages and DENT utilization in CKD subjects.

Acknowledgments

The authors acknowledge Dr. Fu-Gong Lin, and Ms. Jing-Shu Huang (School of Public Health, National Defense Medical Center (N.D.M.C)) and Ms. Hui-Chih Liu (Graduate Institute of Life Sciences, N.D.M.C) for assistance with statistical analysis. The authors also appreciate Professor Mary Goodwin's help in manuscript editing.

Author Contributions

Conceived and designed the experiments: RYH YFL SYK YSS JSC. Performed the experiments: RYH JSC. Analyzed the data: RYH YFL SYK YSS JSC. Contributed reagents/materials/analysis tools: YFL SYK JSC. Wrote the paper: RYH JSC. Reviewed/critiqued statistical analysis: YFL YSS. Reviewed/critiqued the manuscript: YFL SYK YSS. Approved the final manuscript version: RYH YFL SYK YSS JSC.

References

1. Kerr M, Bray B, Medcalf J, O'Donoghue DJ, Matthews B (2012) Estimating the financial cost of chronic kidney disease to the NHS in England. Nephrol Dial Transplant 27 Suppl 3: iii73–iii80.
2. Liang CH, Yang CY, Lu KC, Chu P, Chen CH, et al. (2011) Factors affecting peritoneal dialysis selection in Taiwanese patients with chronic kidney disease. Int Nurs Rev 58: 463–469.
3. Chang JM, Hwang SJ, Tsukamoto Y, Chen HC (2012) Chronic kidney disease prevention–a challenge for Asian countries: report of the Third Asian Forum of Chronic Kidney Disease Initiatives. Clin Exp Nephrol 16: 187–194.
4. Frankenfield DL, Weinhandl ED, Powers CA, Howell BL, Herzog CA, et al. (2012) Utilization and costs of cardiovascular disease medications in dialysis patients in Medicare Part D. Am J Kidney Dis 59: 670–681.
5. Vekeman F, Yameogo ND, Lefebvre P, Bailey RA, McKenzie RS, et al. (2010) Healthcare costs associated with nephrology care in pre-dialysis chronic kidney disease patients. J Med Econ 13: 673–680.
6. Trivedi H (2010) Cost implications of caring for chronic kidney disease: are interventions cost-effective? Adv Chronic Kidney Dis 17: 265–270.
7. Yang M, Fox CH, Vassalotti J, Choi M (2011) Complications of progression of CKD. Adv Chronic Kidney Dis 18: 400–405.
8. Grima DT, Bernard LM, Dunn ES, McFarlane PA, Mendelssohn DC (2012) Cost-effectiveness analysis of therapies for chronic kidney disease patients on dialysis: a case for excluding dialysis costs. Pharmacoeconomics 30: 981–989.
9. Summers SA, Tilakaratne WM, Fortune F, Ashman N (2007) Renal disease and the mouth. Am J Med 120: 568–573.
10. Vesterinen M, Ruokonen H, Leivo T, Honkanen AM, Honkanen E, et al. (2007) Oral health and dental treatment of patients with renal disease. Quintessence Int 38: 211–219.
11. Akar H, Akar GC, Carrero JJ, Stenvinkel P, Lindholm B (2011) Systemic consequences of poor oral health in chronic kidney disease patients. Clin J Am Soc Nephrol 6: 218–226.
12. Chen LP, Chiang CK, Chan CP, Hung KY, Huang CS (2006) Does periodontitis reflect inflammation and malnutrition status in hemodialysis patients? Am J Kidney Dis 47: 815–822.
13. Chen LP, Chiang CK, Peng YS, Hsu SP, Lin CY, et al. (2011) Relationship between periodontal disease and mortality in patients treated with maintenance hemodialysis. Am J Kidney Dis 57: 276–282.
14. Proctor R, Kumar N, Stein A, Moles D, Porter S (2005) Oral and dental aspects of chronic renal failure. J Dent Res 84: 199–208.

15. Fisher MA, Taylor GW, Papapanou PN, Rahman M, Debanne SM (2008) Clinical and serologic markers of periodontal infection and chronic kidney disease. J Periodontol 79: 1670–1678.

16. Fisher MA, Taylor GW, Shelton BJ, Jamerson KA, Rahman M, et al. (2008) Periodontal disease and other nontraditional risk factors for CKD. Am J Kidney Dis 51: 45–52.

17. Grubbs V, Plantinga LC, Crews DC, Bibbins-Domingo K, Saran R, et al. (2011) Vulnerable populations and the association between periodontal and chronic kidney disease. Clin J Am Soc Nephrol 6: 711–717.

18. Foundation NK (2002) K/DOQI clinical practice guidelines for chronic kidney disease: evaluation, classification, and stratification. Am J Kidney Dis 39: S1–266.

19. Khan S, Amedia CA Jr. (2008) Economic burden of chronic kidney disease. J Eval Clin Pract 14: 422–434.

20. Luciano Ede P, Luconi PS, Sesso RC, Melaragno CS, Abreu PF, et al. (2012) [Prospective study of 2151 patients with chronic kidney disease under conservative treatment with multidisciplinary care in the Vale do Paraiba, SP]. J Bras Nefrol 34: 226–234.

21. Wiebe N, Klarenbach SW, Chui B, Ayyalasomayajula B, Hemmelgarn BR, et al. (2012) Adding specialized clinics for remote-dwellers with chronic kidney disease: a cost-utility analysis. Clin J Am Soc Nephrol 7: 24–34.

22. Bessette RW, Carter RL (2012) Predicting hospital cost in CKD patients through blood chemistry values. BMC Nephrol 12: 65.

23. Hassan Y, Al-Ramahi RJ, Aziz NA, Ghazali R (2009) Impact of a renal drug dosing service on dose adjustment in hospitalized patients with chronic kidney disease. Ann Pharmacother 43: 1598–1605.

24. Wish JB, Coyne DW (2007) Use of erythropoiesis-stimulating agents in patients with anemia of chronic kidney disease: overcoming the pharmacological and pharmacoeconomic limitations of existing therapies. Mayo Clin Proc 82: 1371–1380.

25. White CA, Jaffey J, Magner P (2007) Cost of applying the K/DOQI guidelines for bone metabolism and disease to a cohort of chronic hemodialysis patients. Kidney Int 71: 312–317.

26. Schiller B, Doss S, E DEC, Del Aguila MA, Nissenson AR (2008) Costs of managing anemia with erythropoiesis-stimulating agents during hemodialysis: a time and motion study. Hemodial Int 12: 441–449.

27. Higashiyama A, Okamura T, Watanabe M, Murakami Y, Otsuki H, et al. (2009) Effect of chronic kidney disease on individual and population medical expenditures in the Japanese population. Hypertens Res 32: 450–454.

28. Levin A, Chaudhry MR, Djurdjev O, Beaulieu M, Komenda P (2009) Diabetes, kidney disease and cardiovascular disease patients. Assessing care of complex patients using outpatient testing and visits: additional metrics by which to evaluate health care system functioning. Nephrol Dial Transplant 24: 2714–2720.

29. Wish J, Schulman K, Law A, Nassar G (2009) Healthcare expenditure and resource utilization in patients with anaemia and chronic kidney disease: a retrospective claims database analysis. Kidney Blood Press Res 32: 110–118.

30. Levey AS, Coresh J, Greene T, Stevens LA, Zhang YL, et al. (2006) Using standardized serum creatinine values in the modification of diet in renal disease study equation for estimating glomerular filtration rate. Ann Intern Med 145: 247–254.

31. Uhlig K, Berns JS, Kestenbaum B, Kumar R, Leonard MB, et al. (2010) KDOQI US commentary on the 2009 KDIGO Clinical Practice Guideline for the Diagnosis, Evaluation, and Treatment of CKD-Mineral and Bone Disorder (CKD-MBD). Am J Kidney Dis 55: 773–799.

32. Go AS, Chertow GM, Fan D, McCulloch CE, Hsu CY (2004) Chronic kidney disease and the risks of death, cardiovascular events, and hospitalization. N Engl J Med 351: 1296–1305.

33. Yeh CJ, Chang HY, Pan WH (2011) Time trend of obesity, the metabolic syndrome and related dietary pattern in Taiwan: from NAHSIT 1993–1996 to NAHSIT 2005–2008. Asia Pac J Clin Nutr 20: 292–300.

34. Wu JC, Liu L, Chen YC, Huang WC, Chen TJ, et al. (2011) Ossification of the posterior longitudinal ligament in the cervical spine: an 11-year comprehensive national epidemiology study. Neurosurg Focus 30: E5.

35. Yuh DY, Cheng GL, Chien WC, Chung CH, Lin FG, et al. (2013) Factors affecting treatment decisions and outcomes of root-resected molars: a nationwide study. J Periodontol 84: 1528–1535.

36. Kang JH, Lin HC (2012) Increased risk of multiple sclerosis after traumatic brain injury: a nationwide population-based study. Journal of Neurotrauma 29: 90–95.

37. Keller JJ, Chung SD, Lin HC (2012) A nationwide population-based study on the association between chronic periodontitis and erectile dysfunction. Journal of Clinical Periodontology 39: 507–512.

38. Kuo CF, Luo SF, Yu KH, Chou IJ, Tseng WY, et al. (2012) Cancer risk among patients with systemic sclerosis: a nationwide population study in Taiwan. Scand J Rheumatol 41: 44–49.

39. Wu MY, Hsu YH, Su CL, Lin YF, Lin HW (2012) Risk of herpes zoster in CKD: a matched-cohort study based on administrative data. Am J Kidney Dis 60: 548–552.

40. Plantinga LC, Johansen KL, Schillinger D, Powe NR (2012) Lower socioeconomic status and disability among US adults with chronic kidney disease, 1999–2008. Prev Chronic Dis 9: E12.

41. Wang TF, Chou C, Shu Y (2012) Assessing the effects of oral health-related variables on quality of life in Taiwanese adults. Qual Life Res 22: 811–825.

42. Schaeffner ES, Kurth T, de Jong PE, Glynn RJ, Buring JE, et al. (2005) Alcohol consumption and the risk of renal dysfunction in apparently healthy men. Arch Intern Med 165: 1048–1053.

43. Hsu YH, Liu WH, Chen W, Kuo YC, Hsiao CY, et al. (2011) Association of betel nut chewing with chronic kidney disease: a retrospective 7-year study in Taiwan. Nephrology (Carlton) 16: 751–757.

44. Presti RL, Carollo C, Caimi G (2007) Wine consumption and renal diseases: new perspectives. Nutrition 23: 598–602.

45. Chou CY, Cheng SY, Liu JH, Cheng WC, Kang IM, et al. (2009) Association between betel-nut chewing and chronic kidney disease in men. Public Health Nutr 12: 723–727.

46. Lu CT, Yen YY, Ho CS, Ko YC, Tsai CC, et al. (1996) A case-control study of oral cancer in Changhua County, Taiwan. J Oral Pathol Med 25: 245–248.

47. Shelley D, Russell S, Parikh NS, Fahs M (2011) Ethnic disparities in self-reported oral health status and access to care among older adults in NYC. J Urban Health 88: 651–662.

48. Yuen HK, Wolf BJ, Bandyopadhyay D, Magruder KM, Selassie AW, et al. (2010) Factors that limit access to dental care for adults with spinal cord injury. Spec Care Dentist 30: 151–156.

49. Rohn EJ, Sankar A, Hoelscher DC, Luborsky M, Parise MH (2006) How do social-psychological concerns impede the delivery of care to people with HIV? Issues for dental education. J Dent Educ 70: 1038–1042.

50. Grubbs V, Plantinga LC, Tuot DS, Powe NR (2012) Chronic kidney disease and use of dental services in a United States public healthcare system: a retrospective cohort study. BMC Nephrol 13: 16.

51. Thorman R, Neovius M, Hylander B (2009) Clinical findings in oral health during progression of chronic kidney disease to end-stage renal disease in a Swedish population. Scand J Urol Nephrol 43: 154–159.

52. Lin MY, Hwang SJ, Mau LW, Chen HC, Hwang SC, et al. (2010) Impact of late-stage CKD and aging on medical utilization in the elderly population: a closed-cohort study in Taiwan. Nephrol Dial Transplant 25: 3230–3235.

53. Huang CS, Cher TL, Lin CP, Wu KM (2013) Projection of the dental workforce from 2011 to 2020, based on the actual workload of 6762 dentists in 2010 in Taiwan. J Formos Med Assoc 112: 527–536.

54. Kuo HW, Tsai SS, Tiao MM, Yang CY (2007) Epidemiological features of CKD in Taiwan. Am J Kidney Dis 49: 46–55.

55. Chiang HH, Livneh H, Yen ML, Li TC, Tsai TY (2013) Prevalence and correlates of depression among chronic kidney disease patients in Taiwan. BMC Nephrol 14: 78.

56. Lin C, Hsu HT, Lin YS, Weng SF (2013) Increased risk of getting sudden sensorineural hearing loss in patients with chronic kidney disease: a population-based cohort study. Laryngoscope 123: 767–773.

57. Chang RE, Hsieh CJ, Myrtle RC (2011) The effect of outpatient dialysis global budget cap on healthcare utilization by end-stage renal disease patients. Soc Sci Med 73: 153–159.

58. Hidalgo G, Ng DK, Moxey-Mims M, Minnick ML, Blydt-Hansen T, et al. (2013) Association of Income Level With Kidney Disease Severity and Progression Among Children and Adolescents With CKD: A Report From the Chronic Kidney Disease in Children (CKiD) Study. Am J Kidney Dis 62: 1087–1094.

Permissions

The contributors of this book come from diverse backgrounds, making this book a truly international effort. This book will bring forth new frontiers with its revolutionizing research information and detailed analysis of the nascent developments around the world.

We would like to thank all the contributing authors for lending their expertise to make the book truly unique. They have played a crucial role in the development of this book. Without their invaluable contributions this book wouldn't have been possible. They have made vital efforts to compile up to date information on the varied aspects of this subject to make this book a valuable addition to the collection of many professionals and students.

This book was conceptualized with the vision of imparting up-to-date information and advanced data in this field. To ensure the same, a matchless editorial board was set up. Every individual on the board went through rigorous rounds of assessment to prove their worth. After which they invested a large part of their time researching and compiling the most relevant data for our readers.

The editorial board has been involved in producing this book since its inception. They have spent rigorous hours researching and exploring the diverse topics which have resulted in the successful publishing of this book. They have passed on their knowledge of decades through this book. To expedite this challenging task, the publisher supported the team at every step. A small team of assistant editors was also appointed to further simplify the editing procedure and attain best results for the readers.

Apart from the editorial board, the designing team has also invested a significant amount of their time in understanding the subject and creating the most relevant covers. They scrutinized every image to scout for the most suitable representation of the subject and create an appropriate cover for the book.

The publishing team has been an ardent support to the editorial, designing and production team. Their endless efforts to recruit the best for this project, has resulted in the accomplishment of this book. They are a veteran in the field of academics and their pool of knowledge is as vast as their experience in printing. Their expertise and guidance has proved useful at every step. Their uncompromising quality standards have made this book an exceptional effort. Their encouragement from time to time has been an inspiration for everyone.

The publisher and the editorial board hope that this book will prove to be a valuable piece of knowledge for researchers, students, practitioners and scholars across the globe.

List of Contributors

Ikechi G. Okpechi, Brian L. Rayner, Bongani M. Mayosi
Department of Medicine, Groote Schuur Hospital and University of Cape Town, Cape Town, South Africa

Lize van der Merwe
Department of Statistics, University of the Western Cape, Cape Town, South Africa

Adebowale Adeyemo
Centre for Research on Genomics and Global Health, National Human Genome Research Institute, Bethesda, Maryland, United States of America

Nicki Tiffin, Rajkumar Ramesar
Division of Human Genetics, Institute for Infectious Diseases and Molecular Medicine, University of Cape Town, Cape Town, South Africa

Simone Costa Alarcon Arias, Carla Perez Valente, Flavia Gomes Machado, Camilla Fanelli, Denise Maria Avancini Costa Malheiros, Roberto Zatz, Clarice Kazue Fujihara
Laboratory of Renal Pathophysiology (LIM-16), Renal Division, Department of Clinical Medicine, Faculty of Medicine, University of São Paulo, São Paulo, Brazil

Thales de Brito
Department of Pathology, Faculty of Medicine, University of São Paulo, São Paulo, Brazil

Clarice Silvia Taemi Origassa, Niels Olsen Saraiva Camara
Laboratory of Immunology, Nephrology Division, Faculty of Medicine, Federal University of São Paulo, São Paulo, Brazil

Rosana G. Bruetto, Ulysses S. Torres, Emmanuel A. Burdmann
Division of Nephrology, Hospital de Base, Sao Jose do Rio Preto Medical School (FAMERP), Sao Jose do Rio Preto, São Paulo, Brazil

Fernando B. Rodrigues
Department of Internal Medicine - Division of Emergency and Chest Pain Center, Hospital de Base, Sao Jose do Rio Preto Medical School (FAMERP), Sao Jose do Rio Preto, São Paulo, Brazil

Ana P. Otaviano
Division of Cardiology, Hospital de Base, Sao Jose do Rio Preto Medical School (FAMERP), Sao Jose do Rio Preto, São Paulo, Brazil

Dirce M. T. Zanetta
Public Health School, University of São Paulo, São Paulo, Brazil

Guoqiang Xie., Jing Xu., Chaoyang Ye., Dongping Chen, Chenggang Xu, Li Yang, Yiyi Ma, Xiaohong Hu, Lin Li, Lijun Sun, Xuezhi Zhao, Zhiguo Mao, Changlin Mei
Kidney Institute of CPLA, Division of Nephrology, Changzheng Hospital, Second Military Medical University, Shanghai, China

Maxim N. Petrov, Alexandr V. Tarasov, Olga A. Kost
Department of Chemistry, Lomonosov Moscow State University, Moscow, Russia

Valery Y. Shilo
Department of Nephrology, Moscow University for Medicine and Dentistry, Moscow, Russia

David E. Schwartz
Department of Anesthesiology, University of Illinois at Chicago, Chicago, Illinois, United States of America

Sergei M. Danilov
Department of Anesthesiology, University of Illinois at Chicago, Chicago, Illinois, United States of America
Institute for Personalized Respiratory Medicine, University of Illinois at Chicago, Chicago, Illinois, United States of America
National Cardiology Research Center, Moscow, Russia

Joe G. N. Garcia
Institute for Personalized Respiratory Medicine, University of Illinois at Chicago, Chicago, Illinois, United States of America

Yanlong Liu, Qi Gong, Xinxin Yan, Jian Xiao, Xiaojie Wang, Shaoqiang Lin
School of Pharmacy, Wenzhou Medical College, Zhejiang, China

Zhuofeng Lin
School of Pharmacy, Wenzhou Medical College, Zhejiang, China
School of Pharmacy, Jinan University, Guanghzou, China

Xiaokun Li
School of Pharmacy, Wenzhou Medical College, Zhejiang, China
The Key Lab of Pathobiology, National Ministry of Education, Jilin University, Changchun, China

Wenke Feng
School of Pharmacy, Wenzhou Medical College, Zhejiang, China
School of Medicine, University of Louisville, Louisville, Kentucky, United States of America

Zhihong Zhou
Division of Kidney, the 2nd Affiliated Hospital, Wenzhou Medical College, Zhejiang, China

Masashi Kitagawa, Tatsuyuki Inoue, Keiichi Takiue, Ayu Ogawa, Toshio Yamanari, Yoko Kikumoto, Haruhito Adam Uchida, Shinji Kitamura, Yohei Maeshima, Hirofumi Makino
Department of Medicine and Clinical Science, Okayama University Graduate School of Medicine, Dentistry and Pharmaceutical Sciences, Okayama, Japan

Hitoshi Sugiyama, Hiroshi Morinaga
Department of Medicine and Clinical Science, Okayama University Graduate School of Medicine, Dentistry and Pharmaceutical Sciences, Okayama, Japan
Department of Chronic Kidney Disease and Peritoneal Dialysis, Okayama University Graduate School of Medicine, Dentistry and Pharmaceutical Sciences, Okayama, Japan

Kazufumi Nakamura, Hiroshi Ito
Department of Cardiovascular Medicine, Okayama University Graduate School of Medicine, Dentistry and Pharmaceutical Sciences, Okayama, Japan

Wei-Tse Kao
Institute of Medicine, Chung Shan Medical University, Taichung, Taiwan

Jen-Pi Tsai
Institute of Medicine, Chung Shan Medical University, Taichung, Taiwan
Department of Nephrology, Buddhist Dalin Tzu Chi General Hospital, Chiayi, Taiwan

Shao-Chung Wang
Institute of Medicine, Chung Shan Medical University, Taichung, Taiwan
Department of Urology, Chung Shan Medical University Hospital, Taichung, Taiwan

Horng- Rong Chang
Institute of Medicine, Chung Shan Medical University, Taichung, Taiwan
Division of Nephrology, Department of Internal Medicine, Chung Shan Medical University Hospital, Taichung, Taiwan

Jia-Hung Liou
Institute of Medicine, Chung Shan Medical University, Taichung, Taiwan
Department of Pathology, Changhua Christian Hospital, Changhua, Taiwan
Department of Medical Technology, Jen-The Junior College of Medicine, Nursing and Management, Miaoli, Taiwan

Jong-Da Lian
Division of Nephrology, Department of Internal Medicine, Chung Shan Medical University Hospital, Taichung, Taiwan

Jia-fu Feng, Yu-wei Yang, Ping Zeng
Laboratory Medicine, Mianyang Central Hospital, Mianyang, Sichuan Province, China

Lin Zhang
Kidney Internal Medical Department, Mianyang Central Hospital, Mianyang, Sichuan Province, China

Ling Qiu, Xiu-zhi Guo, Yan Qin
Laboratory Medicine, Peking Union Medical College Hospital, Bejing, China

Xue-mei Li
Kidney Internal Medical Department, Peking Union Medical College Hospital, Bejing, China

Hong-chun Liu
Laboratory Medicine, The First Affiliated Hospital of Zhengzhou University, Zhengzhou, Henan Province, China

Xing-min Han, Yan-peng Li
Department of Nuclear Medicine, The First Affiliated Hospital of Zhengzhou University, Zhengzhou, Henan Province, China

Wei Xu, Shu-yan Sun, Li-qiang Wang
Laboratory Medicine, The First Bethune Hospital of Jilin University, Jilin, Jilin Province, China

Hui Quan, Li-jun Xia, Hong-zhang Hu
Laboratory Department, Nuclear Industrial 416 Hospital, Chengdu, Sichuan Province, China

Fang-cai Zhong
Laboratory Department, The First People's Hospital of Neijiang, Neijiang, Sichuan Province, China

Rong Duan
Kidney Internal Medical Department, The First People's Hospital of Neijiang, Neijiang, Sichuan Province, China

Zhichao Huang, Zhaohui Zhong, Lei Zhang, Ran Xu, Xiaokun Zhao
Department of Urology, Second Xiangya Hospital, Central South University, Changsha, Hunan, China

Fajun Fu
Department of Urology, Changsha Central Hospital, Changsha, Hunan, China
Vala Kolbrún Pálmadóttir, Hjalti Gudmundsson
Department of Internal Medicine, Landspitali University Hospital, Reykjavik, Iceland

Sverrir Hardarson
Department of Pathology, Landspitali University Hospital, Reykjavik, Iceland

Margrét B. Andrésdóttir, Margrét Árnadóttir
Division of Nephrology, Landspitali University Hospital, Reykjavik, Iceland

Thorvaldur Magnússon
Department of Internal Medicine, Akranes Hospital, Akranes, Iceland

Ying-Yong Zhao, Ya-Long Feng
Key Laboratory of Resource Biology and Biotechnology in Western ChinaMinistry of Education, the College of Life Sciences, Northwest University, Xi'an, Shaanxi, P.R. China

Xu Bai, Xiao-Jie Tan, Qibing Mei
Solution Center, Waters Technologies (Shanghai) Ltd., Shanghai, P.R. China

Rui-Chao Lin
Research and Inspection Center of Traditional Chinese Medicine and Ethnomedicine, National Institutes for Food and Drug Control, State Food and Drug Administration, Beijing, P.R. China

Bing Dai, Valentin David, Aline Martin, Jinsong Huang, Hua Li , L. Darryl Quarles
University of Tennessee Health Science Center, Medicine-Nephrology, Memphis, Tennessee, United States of America

Yan Jiao, Weikuan Gu
University of Tennessee Health Science Center, Orthopaedic Surgery, Memphis, Tennessee, United States of America

Gregory Papagregoriou, Kamil Erguler, Konstantinos Voskarides, Panayiota Koupepidou, Constantinos Deltas
Molecular Medicine Research Center and Laboratory of Molecular and Medical Genetics, Department of Biological Sciences, University of CyprusNicosia, Cyprus

Harsh Dweep, Norbert Gretz
Medical Research Center, University of Heidelberg, Mannheim, Germany

Yiannis Athanasiou
Department of Nephrology, Nicosia General Hospital, Nicosia, Cyprus

Alkis Pierides
Department of Nephrology, Hippocrateon Hospital, Nicosia, Cyprus

Kyriacos N. Felekkis
Department of Life and Health Sciences, University of Nicosia, Nicosia, Cyprus

Ciara Kierans, Cesar Padilla-Altamira
Department of Public Health and Policy, The University of Liverpool, Liverpool, United Kingdom

Guillermo Garcia-Garcia, Margarita Ibarra-Hernandez
Division of Nephrology, Hospital Civil de Guadalajara, University of Guadalajara Health Sciences Centre, Hospital 278, Jalisco, Mexico

Francisco J. Mercado
Depto Salud Pública, CUCS, Universidad Guadalajara, Guadalajara, Jalisco, Mexico

Flavio Gaspari, Antonio Cannata, Fabiola Carrara, Claudia Cella, Silvia Ferrari, Nadia Stucchi, Silvia Prandini, Bogdan Ene-Iordache, Olimpia Diadei, Norberto Perico
Clinical Research Center for Rare Diseases Aldo & Cele Daccò, Mario Negri Institute for Pharmacological Research, Bergamo, Italy

Piero Ruggenenti, Giuseppe Remuzzi
Clinical Research Center for Rare Diseases Aldo & Cele Daccò, Mario Negri Institute for Pharmacological Research, Bergamo, Italy
Unit of Nephrology, Azienda Ospedaliera Ospedali Riuniti di Bergamo, Bergamo, Italy

Patrizia Ondei
Unit of Nephrology, Azienda Ospedaliera Ospedali Riuniti di Bergamo, Bergamo, Italy

Antonio Pisani
Azienda Ospedaliera Universitaria Federico II, Napoli, Italy

Erasmo Buongiorno
Presidio Ospedaliero V. Fazzi, Lecce, Italy

Piergiorgio Messa
Fondazione IRCCS Ca' Granda Ospedale Maggiore Policlinico, Milano, Italy

Mauro Dugo
Azienda ULSS 9 – Ospedale S. Maria di Ca' Foncello, Treviso, Italy

Ivano Baragetti, Cristina Sarcina, Francesco Rastelli, Laura Buzzi, Claudio Pozzi
Nephrology and Dialysis Unit, Bassini Hospital, Cinisello Balsamo, Milan, Italy

Andrea Baragetti
Department of Pharmacological and Biomolecular Sciences, Università degli Studi di Milano, Milan, Italy
Center for the Study of Atherosclerosis, Italian Society for the Study of Atherosclerosis (SISA) Lombardia Chapter, Bassini Hospital, Cinisello Balsamo, Milan, Italy

Giuseppe Danilo Norata
Department of Pharmacological and Biomolecular Sciences, Università degli Studi di Milano, Milan, Italy
Center for the Study of Atherosclerosis, Italian Society for the Study of Atherosclerosis (SISA) Lombardia Chapter, Bassini Hospital, Cinisello Balsamo, Milan, Italy
The Blizard Institute, Barts and The London School of Medicine and Dentistry, Queen's Mary University, London, United Kingdom

Alberico Luigi Catapano
Department of Pharmacological and Biomolecular Sciences, Università degli Studi di Milano, Milan, Italy
Multimedica IRCCS, Milano, Italy

Katia Garlaschelli
Center for the Study of Atherosclerosis, Italian Society for the Study of Atherosclerosis (SISA) Lombardia Chapter, Bassini Hospital, Cinisello Balsamo, Milan, Italy

Liliana Grigore
Center for the Study of Atherosclerosis, Italian Society for the Study of Atherosclerosis (SISA) Lombardia Chapter, Bassini Hospital, Cinisello Balsamo, Milan, Italy
Multimedica IRCCS, Milano, Italy

Diana A. Papazova, Arianne van Koppen, Maarten P. Koeners, Marianne C. Verhaar, Jaap A. Joles
Department of Nephrology & Hypertension, University Medical Center Utrecht, Utrecht, The Netherlands

Ronald L. Bleys
Department of Anatomy, University Medical Center Utrecht, Utrecht, The Netherlands

Iddo Z. Ben-Dov, Pavel Morozov, Thomas Tuschl
Laboratory of RNA Molecular Biology, Howard Hughes Medical Institute, The Rockefeller University, New York, New York, United States of America

Ying-Cai Tan, HannaRennert
Molecular Pathology Laboratory, New York Presbyterian Hospital, Cornell University, New York, New York, United States of America
Pathology and Laboratory Medicine, Weill Medical College, Cornell University, New York, New York, United States of America

Patricia D. Wilson
Centre for Nephrology, University College London Medical School, London, United Kingdom

Jon D. Blumenfeld
Rogosin Institute, Weill Medical College of Cornell University, New York, New York, United States of America

Leping Zhao, Chuanfeng Shao, Lihui Yang
The affiliated Yueqing Hospital of Wenzhou Medical University, Wenzhou Zhejiang, China

Fan Wu
Engineering Research Center of Bioreactor and Pharmaceutical Development, Ministry of Education, Jilin Agricultural University, Changchun, Jilin, China

Zhuofeng Lin
Engineering Research Center of Bioreactor and Pharmaceutical Development, Ministry of Education, Jilin Agricultural University, Changchun, Jilin, China
School of Pharmacy, Wenzhou Medical University, Chashan College Park, Wenzhou Zhejiang, China

Leigang Jin, Tingting Lu, Xuebo Pan, Xiaokun Li
School of Pharmacy, Wenzhou Medical University, Chashan College Park, Wenzhou Zhejiang, China

Ren-Yeong Huang
Department of Periodontology, School of Dentistry, Tri-Service General Hospital, National Defense Medical Center, Taipei, Taiwan

Jin-Shuen Chen
Division of Nephrology, Department of Internal Medicine, Tri-Service General Hospital, National Defense Medical Center, Taipei, Taiwan

Yuh-Feng Lin
Division of Nephrology, Department of Internal Medicine, Tri-Service General Hospital, National Defense Medical Center, Taipei, Taiwan
Division of Nephrology, Department of Medicine, Shuang Ho Hospital, New Taipei City, Taiwan
Graduate Institute of Clinical Medicine, Taipei Medical University, Taipei, Taiwan

Sen-Yeong Kao
School of Public Health, National Defense Medical Center, Taipei, Taiwan

Yi-Shing Shieh
Department of Oral Diagnosis, School of Dentistry, Tri-Service General Hospital, National Defense Medical Center, Taipei, Taiwan

Index